# Nuclear Medicine

THE REQUISITES

SECOND EDITION

SERIES EDITOR **James H. Thrall,** MD

Professor of Radiology
Department of Radiology
Harvard Medical School;
Radiologist-in-Chief
Massachusetts General Hospital
Boston, Massachusetts

OTHER VOLUMES IN THE REQUISITES™ SERIES

Pediatric Radiology

Neuroradiology

Ultrasound

Musculoskeletal Imaging

Cardiac Radiology

Genitourinary Radiology

Thoracic Radiology

Mammography

Vascular and Interventional Radiology

Gastrointestinal Radiology

# Nuclear Medicine

## THE REQUISITES

### SECOND EDITION

**JAMES H. THRALL,** M.D.
Professor of Radiology
Department of Radiology
Harvard Medical School;
Radiologist-in-Chief
Massachusetts General Hospital
Boston, Massachusetts

**HARVEY A. ZIESSMAN,** M.D.
Professor of Radiology
Director, Division of Nuclear Medicine
Georgetown University Hospital
Washington, D.C.

*with 646 illustrations*

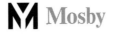 Mosby

*A Harcourt Health Sciences Company*

St. Louis   London   Philadelphia   Sydney   Toronto

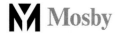

A Harcourt Health Sciences Company

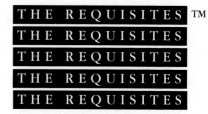

THE REQUISITES is a proprietary trademark
of Mosby, Inc.

Acquisitions Editor: Stephanie Donley
Project Manager: Patricia Tannian
Book Design Manager: Gail Morey Hudson

**SECOND EDITION**

**Copyright © 2001 by Mosby, Inc.**

Previous edition copyrighted 1995

Mosby, Inc.
*A Harcourt Health Sciences Company*
11830 Westline Industrial Drive
St. Louis, Missouri 63146

Printed in United States of America

**International Standard Book Number 0-323-00537-3**

00  01  02  03  04  GW/MV  9  8  7  6  5  4  3  2  1

# Preface

The second edition of *Nuclear Medicine: The Requisites* follows the philosophy and format of the first edition. As we noted in the preface to the previous edition, the specialty of nuclear medicine is "so dynamic that it is impossible to 'capture' the entire subject in a textbook." Since the pace of change has accelerated, this observation is more pertinent today than ever. Thus our book continues to have as its principal aims the efficient introduction of people to the field of nuclear medicine and a summary of the knowledge required for a concise review of the subject.

As before, the basic science chapters emphasize a clinical context for physics, instrumentation, and nuclear pharmacy. For this second edition we have added a new chapter dedicated to single-photon emission computed tomography (SPECT) and positron emission tomography (PET), reflecting the dramatic rise in importance of these tomographic methods in nuclear medicine. We have again illustrated and reinforced basic science concepts with practical examples from daily practice. We hope that using practical examples will help clarify scientific principles for the reader and help demystify some of the basic science aspects of nuclear medicine.

The enduring unifying theme in the clinically oriented chapters is the establishment of a logical progression from basic principles to clinical applications. We have continued to describe tracer mechanisms in detail, aiming to provide deductive tools for analyzing images rather than simply offer representative illustrations. Scintigraphic patterns represent the convolution of disease pathophysiology with tracer pharmacokinetics. Because no textbook or atlas can present every possible scintigraphic pattern, an understanding of the principles that underlie the creation of scintigraphic images permits diagnostic inference and the ability to tackle previously unencountered problems.

Two other features that we have expanded in this edition are the inclusion of image acquisition protocols for the major procedures and the reinforcement of important material in boxes and tables. We recognize that each nuclear medicine laboratory must develop its own protocols based on available equipment and other individual considerations. From this standpoint there is no single "correct" way to perform a nuclear medicine procedure. This is particularly true for SPECT and PET, in which observer preference varies widely among physicians and an infinite variety of parameters for difference acquisition sequences and processing algorithms is possible. The protocols included have been successfully used in our respective practices and can be considered points of departure for thinking about study acquisition and postprocessing.

As well as the new chapter on the basic science aspects of PET and SPECT, several important additions and revisions have been made to the clinical material. In the years since the first edition of *Nuclear Medicine: The Requisites* was published, nuclear cardiology has flourished and the dominant tracers are now those labeled with technetium-99m rather than thallium-201. The chapter on the cardiovascular system has been extensively rewritten to reflect this important change and to emphasize SPECT and PET applications.

The chapter on tumor imaging has been rewritten and updated to include many radiopharmaceuticals that have been approved for clinical use since the first edition, including radiolabeled monoclonal antibodies and peptides, notably Tc-99m CEA for colorectal cancer, Tc-99m ProstaScint for prostate cancer, and In-111 pentetreotide for neuroendocrine tumors. Special emphasis has been placed on the rapidly emerging role of F-18 FDG PET in tumor imaging. The section on lymphoscintigraphy for melanoma and breast cancer has been expanded because of the increasing importance of sentinel node biopsy and gamma probe detectors at surgery. This chapter alone has 20 new illustrations.

Major revisions have been made to most of the other chapters, and many new illustrations and tables have been included. All chapters have been updated with emphasis on new techniques and modern methodology. For example, Tc-99m MAG3 is now used routinely for renal studies in most laboratories. Emphasis is therefore placed on this radiopharmaceutical, although others are discussed as well. The chapter on infection and inflammation has a new section presenting Tc-99m HMPAO labeled white blood cells and comparing them with In-111 oxine labeled cells. This chapter has been significantly reorganized. Numerous new images illustrate clinical applications. The chapter on the hepatobiliary system has been updated to emphasize new techniques including optimal present-day cholescintigraphic methodology such as the pharmacological interventional use of morphine and cholecystokinin.

A novel feature of the first edition was the chapter "Pearls, Pitfalls, and Frequently Asked Questions." This chapter is designed to have a little fun while reemphasizing and highlighting some of the material presented in the text. Feedback from readers of the first edition was positive, and we hope you enjoy the chapter in this edition.

In keeping with the philosophy of the *Requisites in Radiology* series, we hope that residents will find our book useful in rapidly acquiring a working knowledge of nuclear medicine that will make their initial clinical experiences more meaningful and that they can continue to build on throughout their careers. We hope that radiologists and nuclear medicine specialists also find the book helpful as a quick reference and review.

**James H. Thrall**
**Harvey A. Ziessman**

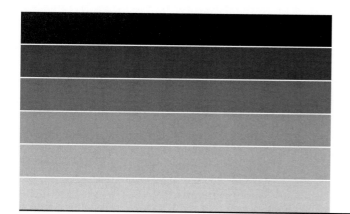

# Acknowledgments

We would like to acknowledge the help and support that we have received in preparing *Nuclear Medicine: The Requisites,* second edition, from colleagues at our respective institutions and across the country. New original illustrations and computer graphics were drawn by David M. Klemm in the Educational Media Department at Georgetown University Medical Center. Computer graphics and drawings were also done by Nancy Speroni, Director of the Radiology Photography Laboratory at the Massachusetts General Hospital.

Special appreciation goes to Patrice Rehm, M.D., for her critical review of chapters including, most importantly, those dealing with cardiology and oncology. Thanks go to Frank Atkins, Ph.D., and Ali Bonab, Ph.D., for reviewing the physics and instrumentation chapters. Ronald J. Callahan, Ph.D., Steven Dragotakes, and Allegra DiPietro helped in reviewing the chapter on nuclear pharmacy. We would also like to thank the many residents who have reviewed the chapters for us and made constructive recommendations and suggestions. Special thanks go to Suhny Abbarra, M.D., and Chris Grady, M.D.

Many colleagues contributed illustrations. Special thanks in the second edition go to John Hergenrother, Tsunehiro Yasuda, M.D., and Stephen Weise. Gloria Sprague did an excellent job of preparing chapters for the original manuscript.

We would like to thank our families for enduring the long hours of our additional absences from them to work on this book. We also acknowledge the fact that no one can work in isolation from colleagues, residents, fellows, and students. You are all also our friends and teachers and the enduring inspiration for this book.

**J.H.T.** and **H.A.Z.**

# Contents

# BASIC PRINCIPLES

# Basic Principles

---

Medical imaging is based on the interaction of energy with biological tissues. The kind of diagnostic information available in each modality is determined by the nature of these interactions. In conventional x-ray imaging the differential absorption of x-rays in air, water, fat, and bone allows the distinction of these tissues in the image. In ultrasonography the differing reflective properties of tissues are the basis for creating images. In magnetic resonance imaging the differences in hydrogen content and in the chemical and physical environments of hydrogen nuclei provide the basis for distinguishing tissues.

In nuclear medicine the body is imaged "from the inside out." Radiotracers, often in the form of complex radiopharmaceuticals, are administered internally. Diagnostic inference is gained by recording the distribution of the radioactive material in both time and space. Tracer pharmacokinetics and selective tissue uptake form the basis of diagnostic utility. To understand nuclear imaging procedures, one must understand a sequence of concepts, beginning with the physics of radioactivity, continuing through the process of detecting radiation and selecting appropriate radiopharmaceuticals, and ending with the uptake and distribution of those pharmaceuticals in health and disease.

## ATOMS AND THE STRUCTURE OF MATTER

Atoms are the building blocks of molecules and are the smallest structures that represent the physical and chemical properties of the elements. Each atom consists of a nucleus surrounded by orbiting electrons (Fig. 1-1). The nuclei are composed of protons and neutrons, collectively referred to as *nucleons*. *Proton*s are positively charged particles weighing approximately $1.67 \times 10^{-24}$ g. Their positive charge is equal in magnitude and opposite to the charge of an electron (Box 1-1). The element to which the atom belongs is determined by the number of protons in the nucleus. *Neutrons* are slightly heavier than protons and are electrically neutral, as the name implies.

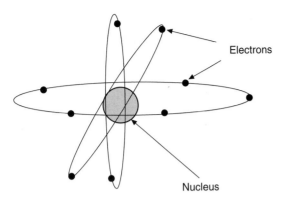

**Fig. 1-1** Bohr model of the atom. The nucleus contains protons and neutrons and has a radius of $10^{-14}$ m. The protons in the nucleus carry a positive charge. The orbital electrons carry a negative charge.

---

### Box 1-1   Summary of Physical Constants

| | |
|---|---|
| Speed of light in a vacuum (c) | $3.0 \times 10^8$ m/sec |
| Elementary charge (e) | $4.803 \times 10^{-10}$ esu |
| | $1.602 \times 10^{-19}$ coulomb |
| Rest mass of electron | $9.11 \times 10^{-28}$ g |
| Rest mass of proton | $1.67 \times 10^{-24}$ g |
| Planck's constant (h) | $6.63 \times 10^{-27}$ erg sec |
| Avogadro's number | $6.02 \times 10^{23} \dfrac{\text{molecules}}{\text{gram mole}}$ |
| 1 electron volt (eV) | $1.602 \times 10^{-12}$ erg |
| 1 calorie (cal) | $4.18 \times 10^7$ erg |
| 1 Angstrom (Å) | $10^{-10}$ m |
| Euler's number (e) (base of natural logarithms) | 2.718 |
| Atomic mass unit (U) | $1.66 \times 10^{-24}$ g (1/12 the mass of a carbon-12 atom) |

---

A shorthand notation has been developed to describe or define specific atoms. The notation is as follows:

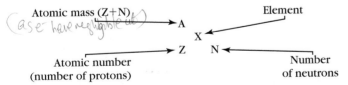

where X is the symbol for the element, Z is the number of protons, N is the number of neutrons, and A is the total number of neutrons and protons. Z is also referred to as the *atomic number* and A as the *mass number* or *atomic mass number.* A *nuclide* is an atom with a given number of neutrons and protons. A *radionuclide* is

simply an unstable nuclide or nuclear species that undergoes radioactive decay.

Several terms help define special relationships between different nuclides. The term *isotope* is used to denote nuclides with the same number of protons (Z), that is, the same element but different numbers of neutrons (N). For example, the element iodine has more than 20 isotopes. All except one (I-127) are radioisotopes or radionuclides, and several are of medical interest, including I-123, I-125, and I-131, which have the following notation:

$$\begin{array}{cccc} {}^{123}_{53}\text{I}_{70} & {}^{125}_{53}\text{I}_{72} & {}^{131}_{53}\text{I}_{78} & {}^{127}_{53}\text{I}_{74} \end{array}$$

Other special terms that are used are *isobar* to indicate the same A but different N and Z, *isotone* to indicate the same number of N but different Z and A, and *isomer* to indicate different *energy states* in nuclides with identical A, Z, and N. The most important isomers in nuclear medicine are technetium-99 and technetium-99m, in which the *m* denotes a *metastable* or prolonged intermediate state in the decay of molybdenum-99 to technetium-99.

---

### Bohr Model of the Atom

In the classic Bohr model of the atom, electrons are arranged in well-defined orbits around the nucleus (Figs. 1-1 and 1-2). The number of orbital electrons in each atom equals the atomic number, Z (the number of protons in the nucleus). The closest orbit, referred to as the K shell, is followed by the L, M, and N shells and so forth. The maximum number of electrons in the K shell is 2, in the L shell is 8, in the M shell is 18, and in the N shell is 32, except that no more than 8 electrons can be in the outermost shell of an atom. Fig. 1-2 is a simplified schematic of the Bohr model for potassium. The term *valence electron* is used to designate electrons in the outermost shell (Box 1-2). These electrons are important in defining the chemical properties of elements. For example, atoms with the outermost shell maximally filled are chemically unreactive. These are the inert gases helium, neon, argon, krypton, xenon, and radon.

Electrons have a negative charge equal to $1.6 \times 10^{-19}$ coulomb; as previously noted, protons have a positive charge of equal magnitude. Electrons are bound in their orbits by the electrical force between their negative charge and the positive charge of the nucleus. The highest binding energy is in the electrons in the shell closest to the nucleus (the K shell), with progressively lower binding energies in the more distant shells. Before an electron can be removed from its shell, the binding energy must be overcome. Interactions involving orbital electrons and ionizing electromagnetic radiation (x-rays

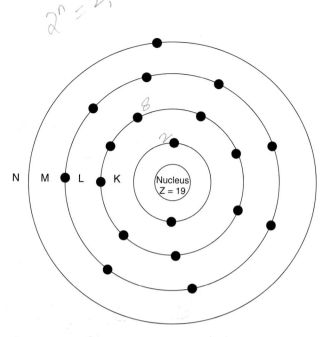

$2^n = 2_1$

8

ν

N  M  L  K  Nucleus
Z = 19

**Fig. 1-2**  Potassium atom. Potassium has an atomic number of 19, with 19 protons in the nucleus and 19 orbital electrons.

## Box 1-2  Terms Used to Describe Electrons

| TERM | COMMENT |
|---|---|
| Electron | Basic elementary particle |
| Orbital electron | Electron in one of the shells or orbits in an atom |
| Valence electron | Electron in the outermost shell of an atom; responsible for chemical characteristics and reactivity |
| Auger electron | Electron ejected from an atomic orbit by energy released during an electron transition |
| Photoelectron | Electron ejected from an atomic orbit as a consequence of an interaction with a photon (photoelectric interaction) and complete absorption of the photon's energy |
| Conversion electron | Electron ejected from an atomic orbit because of internal conversion phenomenon as energy is given off by an unstable nucleus (isomeric transition) |

Characteristic X ray
E. from electron transition
b/w shells

and gamma rays) are central to the way medical images are made and to the quality of the images.

It has long been recognized that the Bohr model of the atom is too simplistic to portray many atomic phenomena accurately. Nuclear physicists have developed sophisticated wave mechanical or quantum mechanical models in which probability density functions are used to describe spatial and temporal properties of electrons. However, the Bohr model can still be used to describe the basic interactions of interest in nuclear medicine.

## ELECTROMAGNETIC RADIATION

The term *electromagnetic radiation* or *electromagnetic waves* refers to energy in the form of oscillating electric and magnetic fields. Individual packets of electromagnetic radiation are referred to as *photons*. Photons with energy greater than 100 eV are classified as x-rays or gamma rays. Lower energy photons may be in the range of ultraviolet light, infrared, visible light, radar waves, or radio and television waves. The unit of energy used to describe these electromagnetic waves or radiations is the *electron volt*. (One electron volt is defined as the kinetic energy of an electron accelerated through a potential difference of 1 volt. One electron volt = $1.6 \times 10^{-19}$ joules or $1.6 \times 10^{-12}$ erg.)

### Mathematics of Electromagnetic Radiation

The relationship between the energy of x-rays and gamma rays (or other electromagnetic radiations) and their frequencies is given by the following equation:

$$E = h\nu$$

where $\nu$ is the frequency and $h$ is Planck's constant (Box 1-1).

Electromagnetic radiation travels with the speed of light ($c$). The relationship between frequency and wavelength is given by:

$$c = \nu\lambda$$

where $\lambda$ is the wavelength. Rearranging this equation to solve for v and substituting it into the previous equation yields:

$$E = \frac{hc}{\lambda}$$

Taking wavelength in angstroms (Å) and energy in keV and substituting the numerical value for $h$ and $c$, this becomes:

$$E\,(keV) = \frac{12.4}{\lambda\,(\text{Å})}$$

## RELATIONSHIP OF MASS AND ENERGY

In 1905, Albert Einstein published his famous equation $E = mc^2$, where $E$ is energy in ergs, $m$ is mass in

| Table 1-1 | Mass-energy equivalence for atomic particles | |
| --- | --- | --- |
| Particle | Mass (U) | Energy (MeV) |
| Electron | $5.486 \times 10^{-4}$ | 0.511 |
| Proton | 1.0073 | 938.20 |
| Neutron | 1.0087 | 939.5 |

grams, and $c$ is the velocity of light in a vacuum ($3 \times 10^{10}$ cm/sec). From this equation it is possible to calculate the energy equivalent of the various subatomic particles. By definition the unified or universal *atomic mass unit* (U) is equal to one twelfth the mass of a carbon-12 atom (Box 1-1). One U = $1.66 \times 10^{-24}$ g. Using this value for mass in Einstein's equation yields the following result:

$$E = (1.66 \times 10^{-24} \text{ g/U}) \times (3.0 \times 10^{10} \text{ cm/sec})^2$$
$$E = 1.5 \times 10^{-3} \text{ erg/U}$$
$$(1 \text{ erg} = 1 \text{ gcm}^2/\text{sec}^2)$$

Inserting the conversion factor between ergs and electron volts (Box 1-1) yields the relationship 1 U = 931.5 MeV. Table 1-1 provides the mass and energy relationships for the basic subatomic particles. The most important of these relationships in clinical nuclear medicine is the energy equivalence of the mass of an electron, which is 511 keV.

## Mass Deficit and Nuclear Binding Energy

The relationships between mass and energy are of fundamental importance in nuclear physics. By carefully determining the weight of atomic nuclei, physicists have shown that the theoretical sum of the component nucleons is always greater than the actual observed mass of the respective atomic nuclei. The difference is known as the *mass deficit*. The *nuclear binding energy* is defined as the energy equivalent of the mass deficit.

Energy equal to the difference in nuclear binding energy of the pretransformation and posttransformation nuclei is released in atomic fusion and atomic fission. The energy of hydrogen and atomic bombs comes from energy released when trillions of new atomic nuclei are formed. That is, the aggregate mass deficit of the posttransformation nuclei after a fusion or fission reaction is greater than that of the original nuclei.

The concept of mass deficit is also fundamental to the use of radionuclides in medical imaging. As a more stable atomic configuration is formed in the radioactive decay process, the mass deficit always increases. In many radionuclide decay schemes, part of the mass deficit is given off in the form of energetic electromagnetic radiation (photons) that can be detected and used to form medical images.

## RADIONUCLIDES AND THEIR RADIATIONS

Because of their physical properties, certain atoms are unstable and undergo radioactive decay. The daughter product in radioactive decay is always at a lower energy state than the parent. The energy difference or mass deficit between parent and daughter is equal to the total energy in the radiations given off. For each radionuclide, the type of radiation emitted, the energy of the radiation(s), and the half-life of the decay process are physical constants. These parameters are important in determining the suitability of a given radionuclide for medical use.

The types of radiation important in nuclear medicine are gamma rays, characteristic x-rays, negatrons (beta particles), positrons (beta particles), and alpha particles. (By definition the term *gamma ray* is used for photons originating in the nucleus and the term *x-ray* for photons originating outside the nucleus.)

Among the lighter atomic elements the number of protons and neutrons in the nucleus is roughly equal. As the atomic number, Z, increases, the ratio of neutrons to protons in stable nuclei increases. A plot of this ratio versus atomic number defines an empirical "line of stability" (Fig. 1-3). That is, the neutron/proton (N/P) ratio is greater than 1 for stable nuclei in the middle and upper atomic numbers. This observation is important in predicting the mode of radioactive decay of unstable nuclides. In general, the decay process tends to return the daughter nucleus closer to the line of stability. That is, if an unstable nucleus contains more neutrons than do stable isotopes of the same element, the mode of decay will reduce the N/P ratio, and vice versa for nuclei with fewer neutrons than predicted by the line of stability.

A system of schematic diagrams has been developed to illustrate radioactive decay. Positive emissions (alpha particles and positrons) and electron capture cause the daughter nucleus to have a lower atomic number. This is indicated by an arrow pointing down and to the left (Fig. 1-4). Following negative emissions (by beta particles [negatrons]), the daughter nucleus has a higher atomic number, which is indicated by an arrow pointing down and to the right (Fig. 1-5).

Complete decay schemes can be complex, with multiple pathways from parent to daughter. For practical purposes the decay schemes in this book are simplified to illustrate important general principles and specific aspects relevant to clinical nuclear medicine.

## Alpha Decay

Alpha particles are essentially helium nuclei with a +2 charge and an atomic mass number of 4. Alpha decay is common in the higher atomic number range of the periodic table of elements. For example, radium-226

(Ra-226) decays to radon-222 (Rn-222) by emitting an alpha particle (Fig. 1-4).

In the simplified scheme shown for Ra-226, three different alpha particles are shown (Fig. 1-4). One reaches the ground state of Rn-222 directly. The other two result in an excited state of Rn-222 with subsequent gamma ray emission to reach the ground state. (In the complete decay scheme for Ra-226 additional alpha particles are present, but they occur in low abundance.)

In all radioactive decay processes, mass and energy are conserved. The *transition energy* is the total energy released during the decay process. For alpha decay this energy is in the form of the kinetic energy of the alpha particle and energy released in the form of gamma radiation.

Alpha particles are undesirable in diagnostic applications because they result in high radiation to the patient. No currently used diagnostic radiopharmaceuticals include alpha-emitting radionuclides. On the other hand, a number of therapeutic agents have been designed to incorporate alpha particle emitters.

### Negatron Decay

The negatron decay process involves the conversion of a neutron into a proton, an electron, and a subatomic particle called an antineutrino. The electron is ejected from the atomic nucleus, thereby giving the decay

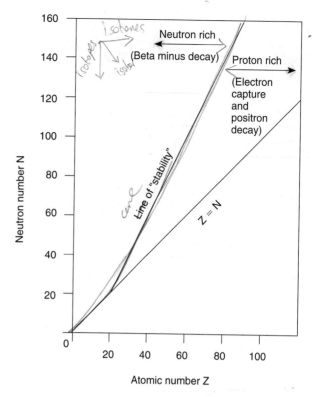

**Fig. 1-3**    Ratio of neutrons to protons. For low atomic number elements the two are roughly equal (Z = N). With increasing atomic number the relative number of neutrons increases. Stable nuclear species tend to occur along the line of "stability."

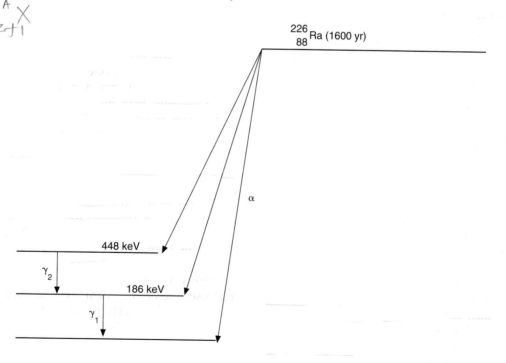

**Fig. 1-4**    Simplified decay scheme for radium-226. Decay is by alpha particle emission to the daughter product radon-222. The emission of an alpha particle results in a decrease in atomic number of 2 and a decrease in atomic mass of 4.

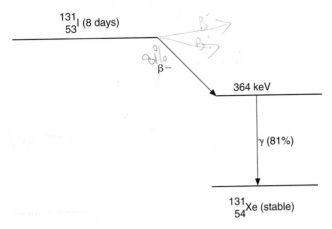

**Fig. 1-5**    Simplified decay scheme for iodine-131. Decay is by negatron emission. In negatron or beta minus decay the atomic mass does not change (isobaric transition). The atomic number increases by 1. The daughter, xenon-131, has one more proton in the nucleus.

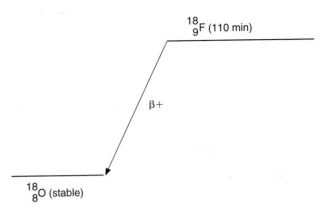

**Fig. 1-6**    Simplified decay scheme of fluorine-18 by positron emission. The daughter product, oxygen-18, has one fewer proton in the nucleus. Positron decay is another example of an isobaric transition without change in atomic mass between parent and daughter.

process its name. The term *negatron* is used to distinguish negative electrons from positive electrons, or *positrons*. Negatron decay is also called *beta decay*.

The N/P ratio decreases as a result of negatron decay, and this mode of decay could be predicted to occur in neutron-rich nuclei. That is, it occurs in nuclei with more neutrons than stable species in the respective part of the atomic chart. For example, stable iodine has a mass number of 127 (53 protons, 74 neutrons). By comparison, I-131 has 78 neutrons. This is a higher number than stable iodine, and I-131 undergoes beta decay (Fig. 1-5).

The transition energy in negatron decay is given off in the form of kinetic energy of the beta particle, the energy in the antineutrino, and the energy in any associated gamma radiation. The maximum kinetic energy ($E_{max}$) that a beta particle can have is a physical constant of the decay process. Beta particles are emitted with a continuous spectrum of energies lower than the maximum. The mean kinetic energy of beta particles ($E_\beta$) is approximately one third of the maximum ($E_\beta = \frac{1}{3} E_{max}$). For beta particles with less than the maximum kinetic energy, the energy is shared between the beta particle and the antineutrino.

Again, a decay scheme can have more than one pathway from the parent to the daughter. For many radionuclides decaying by negatron decay, beta particles with different maximum kinetic energies are given off. Because the total transition energy must be the same for each pathway, the energy of associated gamma radiation is also correspondingly different. For example, the decay scheme for I-131 presented in Fig. 1-5 illustrates only one pathway from parent to daughter, the one of most interest and importance in clinical practice. In reality, there are beta particles given off

with six different energies and there are 19 different gamma rays. However, the most abundant gamma ray, with an energy of 364 keV, occurs in 81% of transitions.

A number of beta-emitting radionuclides have been used in clinical nuclear medicine. I-131, the first radionuclide of importance in medicine, is still used. The disadvantage of beta emitters is the high radiation dose received by the patient from the beta particles. For radioiodine-131 this disadvantage becomes an advantage when the radionuclide is used in the therapy for thyroid cancer and hyperthyroidism.

## Positron Decay and Electron Capture

As the name implies, in *positron decay* a positive electron or positively charged beta particle is ejected from the nucleus. This results in a decrease in the atomic number between the parent and the daughter nuclei and an increase in the N/P ratio. Positron decay occurs in nuclides that are neutron poor, with N/P ratios lower than those occurring on the line of stability. Positron decay is illustrated in Fig. 1-6 for fluorine-18. The transition energy is embodied in the kinetic energy of the positrons and any associated gamma rays. For positrons given off with less than maximum kinetic energy, the energy difference is in subatomic particles called neutrinos. In both negatron and positron decay the neutrinos (or antineutrinos) carry away a substantial portion of the transition energy. The likelihood of neutrinos reacting in soft tissue is small, and the energy in neutrinos is not important in calculating radiation dosimetry for clinical applications.

The minimum transition energy required for positron decay is 1.02 MeV, which is the energy equivalent of the

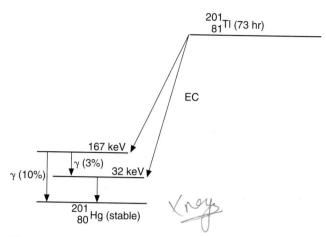

**Fig. 1-7** Thallium-201 decay by electron capture *(EC)* to mercury-201. The daughter nucleus has one fewer proton than the parent.

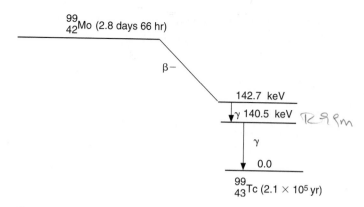

**Fig. 1-9** Simplified decay scheme of molybdenum-99 by negatron emission to technetium-99.

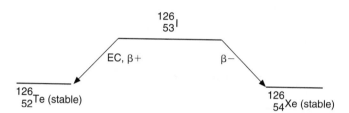

**Fig. 1-8** Iodine-126 undergoes decay through multiple processes. The diagram indicates decay by electron capture and by the emission of both positrons and negatrons.

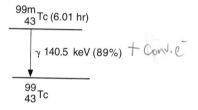

**Fig. 1-10** Isomeric transition of technetium-99m to technetium-99.

mass of two electrons. In unstable nuclei where the maximum available transition energy is less than 1.02 MeV, decay of neutron-poor radionuclides is by electron capture (Fig. 1-7). In *electron capture* an electron from one of the orbital shells (typically close to the nucleus) is incorporated into the nucleus, converting a proton into a neutron. The captured electron is usually from the K shell. The resulting vacancy is filled by transition of an electron from a shell farther from the nucleus. The energy released from this electron transition appears either as characteristic x-radiation or as the kinetic energy of an Auger electron.

Some radionuclides decay by multiple modes, including electron capture, positron decay, and negatron decay (Fig. 1-8). The likelihood of electron capture increases as the available transition energy decreases. The probability of electron capture also increases with increasing atomic number.

## Isomeric Transition and Internal Conversion

No radionuclide undergoes true radioactive decay just by the emission of gamma radiation. However, in some decay schemes there are intermediate species with

measurable half-lives that exist in a *metastable* state. The concept of metastability is arbitrary. Most gamma rays are emitted almost immediately ($10^{-12}$ seconds) after the primary decay process, whether it be alpha decay, negatron decay, positron decay, or electron capture. When the intermediate excited state lasts longer than $10^{-9}$ seconds, the term *metastable* is used and an *m* is placed after the mass number to indicate the phenomenon. The transition from the metastable state to the ground state is *isomeric* because the atomic number does not change.

The most important example of a metastable state in nuclear medicine practice is technetium-99m, which occurs in the decay of molybdenum-99 to technetium-99 (Figs. 1-9 and 1-10). The metastable state for Tc-99m has a half-life of 6 hours; this allows ample time for the separation of the metastable species from the parent radionuclide and its subsequent use for clinical imaging procedures. Tc-99m is attractive from a radiation safety or health physics standpoint because it is essentially a pure gamma emitter not associated with primary particulate radiations. Its use as a radiolabel is associated with favorably low radiation dosimetry.

The energy released in isomeric transitions may be used to dislodge an orbital electron instead of being emitted as a gamma ray. This process is called *internal conversion* (Fig. 1-11). The kinetic energy of the electron (conversion electron) is equal to the difference between the gamma ray energy and the binding energy of the electron. The internal conversion process reduces the number of usable, detectable gamma photons for imaging. It also results in a higher radiation dose to the patient because the conversion electron is absorbed in tissue close to its site of origin. In the "decay" of Tc-99m a 140-keV gamma ray is given off 89% of the time and internal conversion accounts for most of the remaining transitions.

### Gamma Ray Emission

As discussed previously, many radioactive decay processes result in the release of gamma rays or gamma photons. These are ionizing electromagnetic radiations that originate in the excited, unstable atomic nucleus. They have discrete energies defined by the decay scheme for the respective radionuclide. Gamma rays occur over a wide range of energies. Those most useful in conventional single-photon nuclear medicine applications have energies between approximately 80 and 400 keV. Modern nuclear medicine imaging equipment has been optimized for this energy range. Photons with energies below 80 keV present difficulties because of their relatively high attenuation in tissue and their scattering properties. Also, they are less reliably local-

ized by standard imaging devices because of the smaller amount of total energy available in the detection process. Gamma rays with energies significantly higher than 400 keV are progressively more difficult to image with conventional gamma cameras. The detection efficiency in gamma camera systems is less at higher energies. Spatial resolution is also lost through difficulty in collimating high-energy photons.

The 511-keV photon from positron-negatron annihilation is a special case. These photons form the basis for single- and dual-photon positron emission tomography (PET). These techniques are discussed in later chapters.

### Characteristic Radiation and Auger Electrons

When an orbital electron is removed from its shell, it leaves a vacancy that is rapidly filled by a free electron or an electron from a shell farther from the nucleus. In this process the "cascading" electron gives up energy as it fills in the vacancy and becomes more tightly bound. Most often the energy that is given up by the electron is emitted in the form of electromagnetic radiation.

The electromagnetic radiations that arise in the process of filling a vacancy are called *characteristic radiations* or *characteristic x-rays* where applicable because their energy is uniquely defined by the difference in the binding energy of the donor shell and the shell where the vacancy is being filled (that is, the x-ray

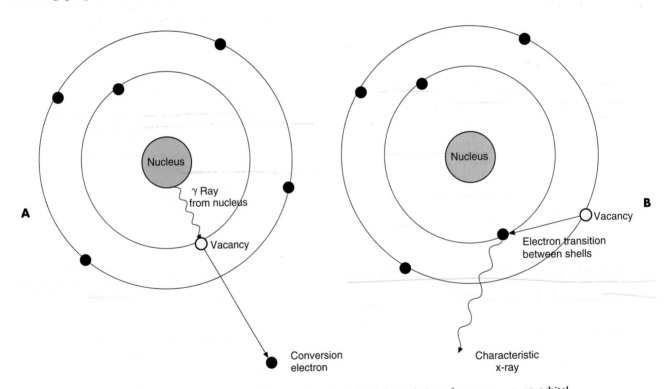

**Fig. 1-11    A,** Process of internal conversion. Instead of the emission of a gamma ray, an orbital electron is ejected from its shell. **B,** A characteristic x-ray is then given off as a consequence of the electron vacancy's being filled.

energy is "characteristic" of the respective transition) (Fig. 1-11). In some applications of radionuclides, detection of characteristic x-rays is the primary means of forming the image or measuring the amount of radioactivity. An example of this is myocardial perfusion imaging with thallium-201 (Tl-201). The most abundant photons used for imaging are actually characteristic x-rays from mercury-201, the daughter product of Tl-201 decay.

An alternative process to the emission of characteristic radiation is the ejection of another electron by the energy released in filling a given vacancy. An electron ejected in this way is termed an *Auger electron* (Box 1-2).

## TERMINOLOGY, UNITS, AND MATHEMATICS OF RADIOACTIVE DECAY

### Units of Radioactivity

Two systems for expressing decay or disintegration rates are in widespread use and are potentially confusing. The more widely used system historically was based on the *curie.* This unit was based on the disintegration rate of 1 gram of radium and was defined as $3.7 \times 10^{10}$ disintegrations per second (dps) (Box 1-3). It is now known that the disintegration rate of 1 gram of radium is slightly different than 1 curie, but the quantitative definition has been widely used throughout the world. Most medical diagnostic applications involve amounts of radioactivity in the microcurie ($3.7 \times 10^4$ dps) or millicurie ($3.7 \times 10^7$ dps) range.

An alternative to the curie in the international system (SI) of units is the becquerel (Bq), which is equal to 1 dps. The relationship between the curie and the becquerel is straightforward if somewhat confusing to those used to the older term. One millicurie equals 37 million Bq, or 37 MBq. Both terminology systems are used widely in the literature (Table 1-2). However, the SI system is increasingly preferred.

### Half-Life and Decay Constant

The mathematics of radioactive decay follow from direct physical measurements. The fundamental empirical observation determined early in the history of work

with radionuclides is that the number of atoms undergoing decay during any finite period of time is proportional to the number of radioactive atoms in the sample. This can be written:

$$\frac{-dN_t}{dt} \alpha N_t$$

where $N_t$ is the number of radioactive atoms in the sample at time *t*. The term $dN_t/dt$ is mathematical notation expressing the change in the number of radioactive atoms over a short interval. The negative sign in the equation denotes that the number of radioactive atoms decreases over time.

For any given radioactive species the equation may be rewritten as:

$$\frac{-dN_t}{dt} = \lambda N_t$$

The term $\lambda$ is the constant of proportionality and is a mathematical constant for each radionuclide. It is also called the *decay constant* and has units of 1/time.

---

**Box 1-3  Conversion of International System (SI) and Conventional Units of Radioactivity**

**CONVENTIONAL UNIT**

1 curie (Ci) = $3.7 \times 10^{10}$ disintegrations per second (dps)

**SI UNIT**

1 becquerel (Bq) = 1 dps

**CURIES → BECQUERELS**

1 Ci = $3.7 \times 10^{10}$ dps = 37 GBq
1 mCi = $3.7 \times 10^7$ dps = 37 MBq
1 $\mu$Ci = $3.7 \times 10^4$ dps = 37 KBq

**BECQUERELS → CURIES**

1 Bq = 1 dps = $2.7 \times 10^{-11}$ Ci = 27 pCi
1 MBq = $10^6$ dps = $2.7 \times 10^{-5}$ Ci = 0.027 mCi
1 GBq = $10^9$ dps = 27 mCi

---

**Table 1-2  Conversion from centimeter-gram-second (CGS) system to international system (SI) units**

| | CGS unit | SI unit | Conversion factor |
|---|---|---|---|
| Work | erg | joule (J) | $10^7$ |
| Radioactivity | curie (Ci) | becquerel (Bq) | $3.7 \times 10^{10}$ |
| Radiation absorbed dose | rad | gray (Gy) | 100 |
| Radiation exposure | roentgen (R) | coulomb/kg | $2.58 \times 10^{-4}$ |
| Roentgen equivalent man | rem | sievert (Sv) | 100 |

The last equation can be rearranged and integrated and provides the classic equation:

$$N_t = N_0 e^{-\lambda t}$$

The term $N_0$ represents the number of radioactive atoms at time $t = 0$, and $e$ is Euler's number (Box 1-1). The equation says in words that the number of radioactive atoms at any later point in time is equal to the product of the original number times an exponential factor that takes into account the rate of decay and the length of time after the initial measurement. Because the activity of the sample is proportional to the number of atoms in that sample, the equation can be rewritten as:

$$A_t = A_0 e^{-\lambda t}$$

where $A$ indicates activity in either curies or becquerels. The decay curve plotted on standard coordinates with time on the $x$-axis and activity on the $y$-axis for a radioactive sample shows an exponentially decreasing function that approaches but never reaches zero. On semilog graph paper the function is a straight line (Fig. 1-12).

From the preceding fundamental equations it is possible to derive the concept of physical half-life, which turns out to be a more intuitive and useful way of describing radioactive decay than using the decay constant. The *half-life* is simply defined as the time required for the number of radioactive atoms in a sample to decrease by exactly one half or 50%. Mathematically the value of the half-life can be derived from the above equations by substituting $\frac{N}{2}$ and $T_{1/2}$ on the two sides respectively as follows:

$$\frac{N_0}{2} = N_0 e^{-\lambda T_{1/2}}$$

$$\frac{1}{2} = e^{-\lambda T_{1/2}}$$

Because $e - 0.693 = \frac{1}{2}$, this equation can be simplified to yield:

$$\lambda T_{1/2} = 0.693$$
$$T_{1/2} = \frac{0.693}{\lambda}$$

From the preceding equations it is apparent that the decay constant and the physical half-life have reciprocal units of time. The half-life can be expressed in seconds, minutes, hours, days, or years. Radionuclides with long physical half-lives have smaller values for the decay constant. That is, the longer the physical half-life, the smaller the fraction of the radioactive atoms that undergoes disintegration in any given unit of time. From a practical standpoint, most radionuclides used in clinical nuclear medicine must have half-lives of hours or days. This permits shipping from the manufacturing site to the hospital, preparation of the radiopharmaceutical, and imaging. Use of shorter lived agents is feasible in institutions with radionuclide production facilities such as cyclotrons or special accelerators.

In certain cases radionuclides are obtained from "generator" systems, and the practical limitation is then the half-life of the parent compound. For example, the half-life of Tc-99m is 6 hours. The half-life of its parent, molybdenum-99 (Mo-99), is 2.7 days (Figs. 1-9 and 1-10). The Mo-99/Tc-99m generator system provides the dual advantage of a longer lived parent, which permits commercial distribution and prolonged on-site availability, while the short half-life of the Tc-99m daughter reduces radiation exposure to the patient compared with longer lived agents.

### Mean Life

The concept of the mean life of a radionuclide is useful in thinking about radiation dosimetry. The mean life is given as:

$$\bar{t} = \frac{1}{\lambda}$$

or

$$\bar{t} = 1.44 T_{1/2}$$

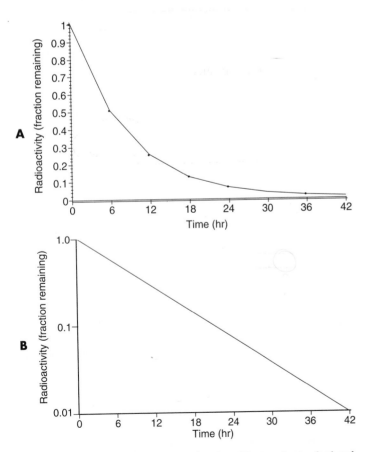

**Fig. 1-12**   Decay plot for technetium-99m on, **A,** standard and, **B,** semilog graphs.

The concept of mean life is more difficult to understand intuitively than the concept of physical half-life but may be thought of as the average length of time of the radioactive atoms in a sample before they undergo disintegration. Another way of thinking about mean life is to imagine extrapolating the decay curve to infinity. The mean life is the point on the time axis where half the area under the curve is on each side.

## Biological Half-Life and Effective Half-Life

An important concept in determining radiation exposure to patients is the *biological half-life* and the corollary concept, *effective half-life*. The term *biological half-life* is used to describe the biological clearance of the radionuclide from a particular tissue or organ system. Thus the actual half-life or *effective half-life* of a radiopharmaceutical in a biological system is dependent on both the physical half-life and the biological clearance. Because physical decay and biological clearance occur simultaneously in parallel, the relationship between them and the effective half-life is given by:

$$\frac{1}{T_{\frac{1}{2}eff}} = \frac{1}{T_{\frac{1}{2}p}} + \frac{1}{T_{\frac{1}{2}b}}$$

Rearranging terms, this becomes:

$$T_{\frac{1}{2}eff} = \frac{T_{\frac{1}{2}b} \times T_{\frac{1}{2}p}}{T_{\frac{1}{2}b} + T_{\frac{1}{2}p}}$$

The concept of biological half-life is not as mathematically clear-cut as the physical half-life. It can vary among subjects and does not necessarily follow a regular exponential process. For example, the biological half-time of radioactivity in the bladder is determined by the time at which a patient chooses to void. The half-time of xenon-133 in the lung during pulmonary ventilation studies is determined by the rate and depth of respiration and by the presence of pulmonary disease. Nonetheless, the term biological half-life is useful in thinking about the amount of exposure the patient actually receives during a nuclear medicine procedure.

## INTERACTIONS OF RADIATION WITH MATTER

### Negatrons (Beta Particles)

Negatrons, or beta particles, cause ionization in tissues by electrostatic interactions with orbital electrons. They give up energy through a series of such interactions along a tortuous path. As a rule of thumb, the maximum penetration of beta particles in soft tissue in centimeters is equal to the maximum kinetic energy of the negatron in megaelectron volts divided by 2. Thus the radiation dose delivered by negatrons in soft tissue is relatively close to their source. For example, the maximum kinetic

energy of the most abundant beta particle in the decay of I-131 is 0.606 MeV. The majority of the radiation dose delivered in I-131 therapy is within 0.3 cm of the location of the nucleus undergoing decay.

### Positrons

Positrons also give up their kinetic energy through electrostatic ionizations. As the positron approaches thermal energy, it undergoes *annihilation* by combining with a negatively charged electron (Fig. 1-13). Two gamma photons are given off, 180° apart. Each has an energy of 0.511 MeV, the energy equivalent of positron-electron mass. This unique phenomenon of annihilation radiation 180° apart is the basis for PET.

### Gamma Rays and X-Rays

Gamma rays and x-rays are attenuated in tissues through three processes. Photons can be completely absorbed by the *photoelectric effect* or in *pair production*. They can also undergo scattering or deflection from their original path by the *Compton effect* or *Compton-scattering* phenomenon, in which photons give up part of their original energy.

**Pair production**   Pair production requires a photon with a minimum energy of 1.02 MeV. The photon energy is converted into one negative and one positive electron. Because the energy required is greater than the photon energies used in medical imaging, this form of attenuation is not important in nuclear medicine.

**Photoelectric absorption**   Photoelectric absorption occurs when the total energy of an x-ray or gamma ray photon is transferred to an orbital electron (Fig. 1-14, *A*). The photon must possess energy greater than the binding energy of the electron. The electron is displaced from its orbit or shell and is either lifted to a higher shell or ejected from the atom (Fig. 1-14, *B*). Ejected electrons are termed *photoelectrons*.

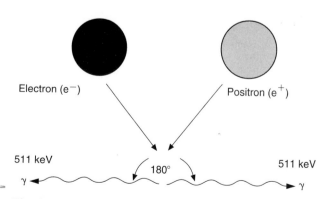

**Fig. 1-13**   In positron annihilation the mass of a positron and an electron is converted to energy in the form of two photons. The photons each have an energy of 0.511 MeV and are given off 180° apart.

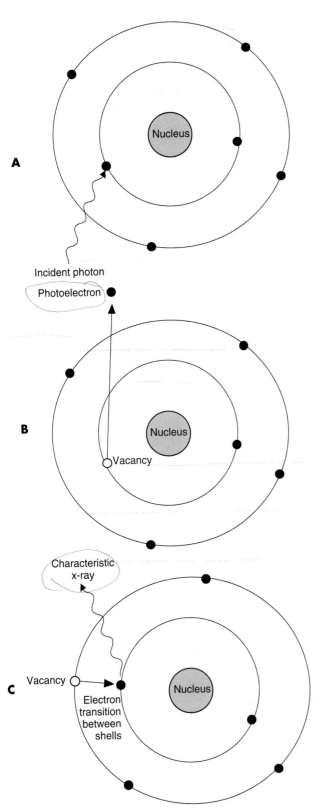

**Fig. 1-14**   **A,** In the photoelectric absorption process an incident photon interacts with an orbital electron. **B,** The electron is ejected from its shell, creating a vacancy. The electron is either ejected from the atom or moved to a shell farther from the nucleus. **C,** The orbital vacancy is filled by the transition of an electron from a more distant shell. A characteristic x-ray is given off as a consequence of this transition.

As a consequence of the photoelectric interaction, an electron cascade occurs to fill the vacancy, with the subsequent emission of characteristic x-rays or Auger electrons (Fig. 1-14, *C*). Photoelectric absorption is most likely to occur when the photon energy is just above the electron binding energy. The kinetic energy of the photoelectron is equal to the difference between the energy of the incident photon and the electron binding energy.

For a given absorbing material, as photon energy increases, the likelihood of a photoelectric event decreases. The photoelectric interaction is important in soft tissues up to an energy of approximately 50 keV. Radionuclides with associated photon energies lower than 50 keV are less desirable for clinical applications because of the high absorption of these photons in soft tissue owing to photoelectric interaction.

Although photoelectric absorption is undesirable in body tissues, it is fundamental to the detection of ionizing radiation. In both nuclear medicine and roentgenography the creation of images depends on energy absorption in a detecting medium through the photoelectric interaction. For this reason imaging systems typically are high-density, high-Z materials such as inorganic crystals, in which the likelihood of photoelectric absorption is high.

**Compton scattering or Compton effect**   In Compton scattering a photon interacts with a weakly bound outer shell electron. Instead of being completely absorbed as in the photoelectric interaction, in the Compton process the photon is deflected from its original direction and continues to exist but at lower energy (Fig. 1-15). The energy difference is transferred to the recoil electron as kinetic energy. Compton scattering is the dominant mode of gamma ray and x-ray interaction in soft tissues between 30 keV and 30 MeV.

Because the Compton-scattered photon gives up energy in the interaction, its wavelength increases. The formula for this is:

$$\Delta\lambda = 0.0243(1 - \cos \varnothing)$$

where $\Delta\lambda$ is the change in wavelength and the angle $\varnothing$ is the angle through which the photon is scattered. The angle of scatter can be minimal or up to 180° (backscatter).

The significance of Compton scattering in nuclear imaging is that scattered photons reaching the imaging detector must be discriminated against and not allowed to form part of the image. Because Compton-scattered photons give up part of their energy, one way to discriminate against them is through setting an "energy window" for acceptance of events in the detector. However, photons scattered through a relatively narrow angle lose only small amounts of energy and may not be effectively excluded by pulse height analysis and the setting of an energy window. Thus Compton-scattered

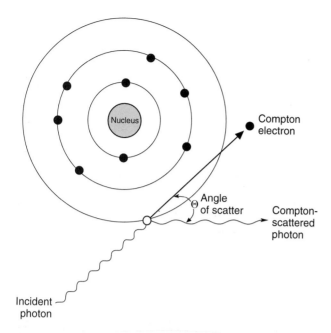

**Fig. 1-15** In the Compton scatter process an incident photon interacts with an outer or loosely bound electron. The photon gives up a portion of its energy to the electron and undergoes a change in direction at a lower energy.

photons contribute to the loss of spatial resolution in nuclear medicine images. The problem is progressively worse for lower energies because the lower the original photon energy, the less the change in energy for a given scattering angle.

## STATISTICS OF RADIOACTIVE DECAY

The time of decay of any single unstable radioactive nucleus is unpredictable and is not influenced by the decay of other nuclei or the physical or chemical environment of the nucleus. Because radioactive decay is random, the actual observed number of nuclei undergoing decay in any given period is subject to statistical uncertainty; this is a practical problem in clinical nuclear medicine. In any setting where a quantitative measurement is required such as determining the amount of radioactivity in a radiopharmaceutical to be given to the patient or in a blood sample used in calculating a physiologic parameter or performing quality control of nuclear instrumentation, estimates of statistical certainty are necessary.

Radioactive decay follows *Poisson statistics* or the Poisson probability law. The Poisson probability density function is similar but not identical to the gaussian or normal probability density function. Curves expressing the Poisson and gaussian probability density functions

are more closely matched as the number of observed events is increased.

For data obeying the Poisson probability distribution, the standard deviation (SD) is given by:

$$SD = \sqrt{r}$$

where $r$ is the true mean. Because the true mean is usually estimated from an average of a number of individual measurements, the estimated standard deviation is:

$$SD(est) = \sqrt{r}\,(est)$$

Expressing standard deviation as a fraction or a percentage is often useful. The *fractional standard deviation* is simply $1/\sqrt{r}$. The *percent fractional standard deviation* (% SD) is the fractional standard deviation $\times$ 100. For example, if 2500 counts are recorded in a picture element or "pixel" in an image, the fractional standard deviation of the measurement is $1/\sqrt{2500} = 0.02$. The percent fractional standard deviation is 2%. This can also be expressed in the equation:

$$\%SD = \frac{100}{\sqrt{n}}$$

where $n$ is the number of counts observed.

Calculation of standard deviation is useful in determining the number of counts to obtain in the measurement of a radioactive sample or in a scintigraphic image for statistical certainty. The larger the number of counts, the lower the percent fractional or relative standard deviation and the greater the ability to distinguish a true difference in the amount of radioactivity in two different samples. Likewise, in imaging, the greater the number of counts per pixel, the more likely that observed differences in the image actually represent true differences in the amount of activity between two locations in the image.

### SUGGESTED READINGS

Chandra R: Nuclear medicine physics: the basics, ed 4, Baltimore, 1998, Williams & Wilkins.

Hendee WR: *Medical radiation physics*, ed 3, St Louis, 1992, Mosby.

Johns HE, Cunningham JR: *The physics of radiology*, ed 4, Chicago, 1983, Thomas Books.

Powsner RA, Powsner ER: *Essentials of nuclear medicine physics*, Malden, Mass, 1998, Blackwell Science.

Sorenson JA, Phelps ME: *Physics in nuclear medicine*, ed 2, Philadelphia, 1987, WB Saunders.

Weber DA, Eckerman KF, Dillman LT, Ryman JC: *MIRD: radionuclide data and decay schemes*, New York, 1989, Society of Nuclear Medicine.

# Radiation Detection and Instrumentation

Detection of radioactivity is fundamental to the practice of nuclear medicine. The amount and type of radioactivity being administered to patients must be measured and documented, and the areas in which people work must be monitored to ensure safety to both health care personnel and patients. Radioactivity emanating from the patient must be detected to allow the temporal and spatial localization necessary to create scintigraphic images. The common denominator in all of the devices used in contemporary nuclear medicine practice for calibration of administered dosages, area monitoring, and imaging is the conversion of energy in the form of ionizing radiation into electrical energy. In modern imaging equipment these electronic signals are often recorded and processed by dedicated nuclear medicine computer systems. Nuclear medicine imaging devices, including the gamma scintillation camera, can be thought of as specialized radiation detection devices, highly modified and adapted to record the temporal and spatial localization of radioactivity in the patient.

## RADIATION DETECTION

### Ionization Chambers, Proportional Counters, and Geiger-Müller Counters

One important approach to radiation detection is the use of an ionization chamber. The generic design concept is a gas-filled chamber with positive and negative electrodes, at opposite sides of the chamber or in a concentric cylinder geometry. A potential difference is created between the two electrodes, but no current flows in the absence of exposure of the chamber to radiation. The interaction of ionizing radiation with the gas in the chamber creates positive and negative ions, which move to the electrodes, producing an electrical current.

The basic concept of the ionization chamber is extremely versatile; specialized devices have been designed for a wide variety of applications. For example, the problem of detecting alpha and beta radiation is quite different from that of detecting gamma radiation because of differences in both their power of penetrating different materials and their likelihood of interaction with matter. In addition, the problem of surveying a wide area to determine the presence or absence of radiation is quite different from the problem of accurately calibrating the millicuries of activity to be administered to a patient. Three of the important subtypes of ionization chamber with nuclear medicine applications are the basic ionization chamber, the proportional counter, and the Geiger-Müller counter.

**Basic ionization chambers** The voltage difference between the electrodes in the basic ionization chamber is calibrated to be just high enough to "harvest" all of the ions from the sensitive volume of the chamber, but not high enough that the ions in the chamber are accelerated to the point of creating additional secondary ionizations. As a result of this voltage calibration strategy, the current produced in any single event is very small and not measurable with any accuracy. Rather, the ionization chamber is used to measure the total current resulting from multiple events over a certain integration time in a given radiation detection setting.

A number of devices routinely used in nuclear medicine clinics operate on the principle of the ionization chamber. Radiation survey meters such as the cutie-pie, some pocket dosimeters, and radionuclide dose calibrators are all examples of specialized basic ionization chambers. The survey meters are typically calibrated to provide units of exposure such as milliroentgens per hour. Dose calibrators are set up to provide readings in the units of radioactivity used in clinical practice. Many laboratories now express these units in becquerels in response to a mandate from the U.S. Food and Drug Administration to use the international system as soon as possible; other laboratories have retained the Ci, mCi, and μCi convention. The amount of energy converted to electrical current per unit of radioactivity is unique for each radionuclide, and radionuclide dose calibrators must be calibrated for the radionuclide to be measured.

**Proportional counters** The main difference between a proportional counter and the basic ionization chamber is greater applied voltage between the electrodes in the former. The higher voltage results in secondary ionizations in the sensitive volume of the chamber. The term *gas amplification* describes this phenomenon. Gas amplification can result in increased ionization by a factor of $10^3$ to $10^6$. The resulting current pulse is large enough to be measured individually and is proportional to the energy originally deposited in the gas chamber. Typically an inert gas such as helium or argon is used. The name of the device is based on the proportionality of total ionization to the total energy of the ionizing radiation. Proportional chambers do not

have wide applicability in clinical nuclear medicine. They are used in research to detect alpha and beta particles.

**Geiger-Müller counter** In the Geiger-Müller counter the voltage is increased even higher than in the proportional chamber application. Because of the high voltage, the initial ionization causes an "avalanche" of secondary ionizations, so that the gas is essentially completely ionized. This mode of operation of an ionization chamber allows detection of individual events, but not their energy (i.e., pulse counting). Another important characteristic of the Geiger-Müller counter is detector dead time. Because the gas in the chamber is completely ionized, it takes a significant amount of time to become ready for the next event. Thus Geiger-Müller counters are not useful in the presence of large amounts of radioactivity. They are good for detecting low levels of activity and are widely used as area survey meters and area monitors. They are valuable in detecting radiation contamination.

## Scintillation Detectors: Thallium-Activated Sodium Iodide Crystals

Gas-filled ionization chambers of the kinds described in the preceding section are not very sensitive to x-rays and gamma rays because of the low likelihood of ionizing interactions. The "stopping power" of gas is low. In current practice, thallium-activated sodium iodide crystals (NaI [Tl]), are used as the detector medium for single-photon imaging systems. These crystals are optically transparent and have sufficient stopping power for sensitive detection of gamma rays (Table 2-1).

As noted earlier, an important common denominator of many types of radiation detectors is the conversion of the energy in ionizing radiation to electrical energy. Scintillation detector systems have an interesting conversion process. Gamma rays or x-rays enter the sodium iodide crystal and impart energy to valence electrons during photoelectric and Compton interactions. The

| Table 2-1 | Half-value layers of selected radionuclides | | | | |
|---|---|---|---|---|---|
| | | | **Half-value layer (cm)** | | |
| Radio-nuclide | Energy (keV) | | Lead | Water (soft tissue) | NaI |
| Tc-99m | 140 | | 0.028 | 4.50 | 0.265 |
| Tl-201 | 70 | | | 3.85 | 0.048 |
| | | Pb x-rays | 0.0005 | | |
| | 81 | | | 4.08 | 0.069 |
| I-131 | 364 | | 0.220 | 6.35 | 1.500 |

imparted energy raises the electrons into the conduction band of the crystal lattice. The energy difference between the valence band and the conduction band is on the order of a few electron volts. As the electrons give up energy in the transition back from the conduction band to the valence band, photons of light are given off. The light photons have a spectrum of energies, but for sodium iodide crystals the spectrum peaks at a wavelength of 4150 Å, or approximately 3 eV. The energy conversion efficiency in the NaI (Tl) crystal is approximately 13%. The remaining energy is dissipated in the crystal in the form of molecular motion or heat. The scintillation decay time or length of time for the scintillation event is approximately 1 $\mu$sec ($10^{-6}$ seconds).

Thallium-activated sodium iodide crystals have become the preferred scintillation detector in nuclear medicine applications for a number of reasons. The crystals are relatively inexpensive and afford great flexibility in size and shape. The stopping power of the sodium iodide crystals is good for the energy range used in clinical nuclear medicine for single-photon applications (i.e., 70 to 365 keV) (Table 2-1). The thallium impurities in the sodium iodide crystal provide "activation centers" or luminescence centers that offer "easier" pathways for the return of the electrons from the conduction band of the crystal to the valence bands of atoms requiring electrons for electrical neutrality. Only a small amount of thallium impurity (0.1 to 0.4 mole %) is required in the sodium

iodide crystal lattice to achieve the desired effect of making the scintillation process more efficient. The conversion efficiency of 13% is relatively high, and the crystals are internally transparent to the light photons so that they reach the photocathodes. The disadvantages of sodium iodide crystals are their fragility and their highly hydroscopic nature, necessitating hermetically sealed containers. In most applications the crystal is sealed on all sides by a thin aluminum canister except on the photomultiplier tube side, which is covered by a quartz window to allow the scintillation photons to escape and reach the photomultiplier tubes.

The next step in the detection process is the interaction of the light photons arising in the crystal with the photocathode of a photomultiplier tube (Fig. 2-1). In the typical sodium iodide detector system, whether it is a simple probe or a gamma scintillation camera, the crystal is optically coupled to the photocathode by a light guide or light pipe to ensure the efficiency of light collection. The light photons dislodge electrons from the photocathode. These electrons are then accelerated by a series of electrodes (dynodes) in the photomultiplier tube. With each acceleration the number of electrons is increased. The electrons are collected at the anode or collector of the photomultiplier tube. The multiplication factor is on the order of 3 to 6 per dynode stage and up to several million overall. The resulting voltage pulse from the photomultiplier tube is then available for further pro-

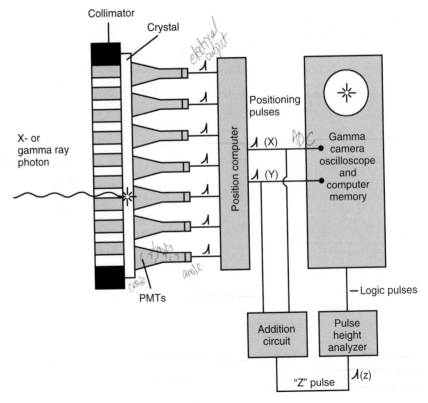

**Fig. 2-1**   Simplified schematic of gamma scintillation camera. The diagram shows a photon reaching the crystal through the collimator and undergoing photoelectric absorption. The photomultiplier tubes (*PMTs*) are optically coupled to the NaI (Tl) crystal. The electrical outputs from the respective photomultiplier tubes are further processed through positioning circuitry to calculate *x, y* coordinates and through addition circuitry to calculate the Z pulse. The Z pulse passes through the pulse height analyzer. If the event is accepted, it is recorded spatially in the location determined by the *x, y* positioning pulses.

cessing. This processing may take the form of amplification followed by pulse analysis to determine either the energy deposited in the crystal (pulse height analysis) or the spatial location of the event (position analysis) in the case of gamma scintillation cameras.

A key point to understand in the scintillation detection process is that proportionality is maintained at each step. That is, the number of light photons given off in the NaI (Tl) crystal is proportional to the energy deposited in the crystal from the x-ray or gamma ray. The number of electrons dislodged from the photocathode is proportional to the number of light photons, and the electrical output of the photomultiplier tube is proportional to the number of electrons dislodged from the photocathode. Thus the height of the electrical pulse coming from the photomultiplier tube is proportional to the energy of the radiation absorbed in the crystal. This allows different radionuclides with different energies to be distinguished from one another by pulse height analysis. It also permits a distinction between primary photons and photons that have undergone Compton scatter events before detection. Compton-scattered photons are less energetic than the primary photons and have lower pulse heights. Recognizing Compton-scattered photons is critical in imaging applications of scintillation detection because only primary photons are desired to create the image.

## Other Detection Devices

A host of other radiation detection devices are used in nuclear medicine and radiology. These include photographic film, which is used in personnel film badges; semiconductors; thermoluminescent and ultraviolet fluorescent detection devices; and other chemical detectors useful for measuring cumulative radiation effects over a long period. They are not discussed here.

## GAMMA RAY SPECTROMETRY AND PULSE HEIGHT ANALYSIS

The energies and relative abundance of the ionizing radiations given off by each radionuclide are physical constants. The proportionality between the energy of a gamma ray and the output of the electrical pulse from the photomultiplier tube provides a means for distinguishing between gamma rays (or x-rays) of different energies. However, the spectrum of recorded energies is more complex than would be predicted from the decay scheme because of Compton and photoelectric interactions both outside the NaI (Tl) scintillation detector and within the crystal. Recognizing the consequences of these interactions is important to the optimal use of counting and imaging instrumentation.

By convention the energy spectra from x-ray and gamma ray detection are plotted with energy on the x-axis and the relative number of events is plotted on the y-axis (Fig. 2-2). The important relationships in gamma spectra are illustrated here for technetium-99m (Tc-99m) because it is the most commonly used radionuclide in clinical practice.

## Photopeak

In a perfect detecting system and with the complete absorption of the 140-keV gamma rays of Tc-99m in the detector, a single line would be recorded on the energy spectrum at exactly 140 keV. In practice the 140-keV photopeak is recorded as a bell-shaped curve centered at 140 keV (Fig. 2-2). The gaussian distribution of recorded events is due to the statistical nature of the radiation detection process. Each step in the conversion of ionizing radiation to electrical current is subject to statistical fluctuation. Light photons are given off in the scintillation crystal with equal but random probability in all directions. Slightly different numbers of light photons impinge on the photocathodes between different absorption events. The number of electrons dislodged is also subject to statistical fluctuation, as is the electron amplification at each dynode stage in the photomultiplier tube.

The energy resolution of a detecting system can be expressed by the spread in the photopeak. A frequently used measure is full width at half maximum (FWHM). This is defined as the energy range encompassed by the bell-shaped curve halfway down from the apex of the photopeak (Fig. 2-2). A typical gamma scintillation

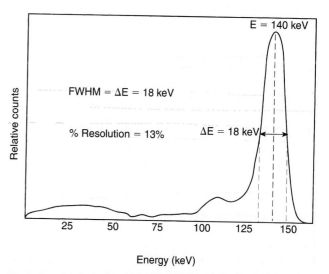

**Fig. 2-2** Spectrum for technetium-99m in air. The figure illustrates the concept of full width at half maximum (FWHM). For the particular detector system illustrated the FWHM is 18 keV. The energy resolution of the detector system for Tc-99m is 13%.

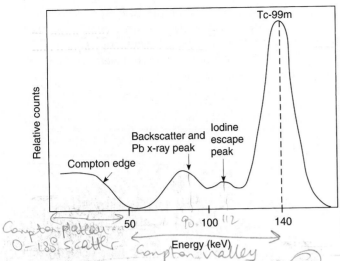

**Fig. 2-3**   Energy spectrum for technetium-99m in air for a gamma scintillation camera with the collimator in place. Note the iodine escape peak at approximately 112 keV. The 180° backscatter peak at 90 keV merges with the characteristic x-ray peaks for lead (Pb). The Compton edge is at 50 keV.

camera might have an FWHM equal to 14 keV for detecting Tc-99m. This can also be expressed as a percentage of the photopeak energy, and the detector would be said to have an energy resolution of 10% (14/140). The narrower the peak, the better the energy resolution of the detector, and the greater the ability to distinguish gamma rays with energies close to each other. *The photofraction is the fraction of total counts in the entire spectrum within the photopeak.*

**Iodine escape peak**   Photoelectric interactions occurring close to the edge of the sodium iodide crystal may result in the "escape" of iodine K–characteristic x-rays from the crystal. When this happens, the corresponding x-ray energy of approximately 28.5 keV is not deposited in the crystal and will result in a small peak on the energy spectrum at 112 keV (i.e., 140 keV − 28 keV) (Fig. 2-3). This peak, referred to as the *iodine escape peak,* can be observed with a Tc-99m source in air but is typically not observed in vivo because of the relatively much larger contribution from Compton-scattered photons from the patient in the recorded energy spectrum.

**Compton valley, edge, and plateau**   Not every photon entering an NaI (Tl) crystal undergoes photoelectric absorption. If a primary photon undergoes a Compton scatter interaction in the crystal with subsequent escape of the scattered photon, a smaller voltage pulse will be detected than those composing the photopeak. If the 140-keV gamma rays from technetium are used as the example, the maximum energy transferred to a recoil electron in the crystal occurs at the largest scattering angle (180°) and is 50 keV. This energy is referred to as the *Compton edge.* The energy from 0 to

50 keV is called the *Compton plateau* or *continuum* and corresponds to the energy deposited by photons that scatter from 0° to 180° before escaping the crystal (Fig. 2-3). The portion of the energy spectrum between the Compton edge and the photopeak is the *Compton valley.* Some gamma rays undergo multiple Compton scatter events before escaping from the detector crystal. These may be recorded in the region of the Compton valley. The energy relationships obviously differ for each radionuclide with differing photopeak energy.

**Backscatter peak**   Another peak resulting from Compton scattering occurs when primary gamma photons undergo 180° scattering outside the detector and are then completely absorbed. The scattering can take place either in front of the detector or behind it if a gamma ray has initially passed completely through the crystal without being scattered or absorbed. From the previous section, it is apparent that for Tc-99m the backscatter peak occurs at 90 keV (140 keV − 50 keV) (Fig. 2-3).

**Lead characteristic x-ray peak**   In most nuclear medicine applications, scintillation detectors are used in conjunction with lead collimators. The 140-keV primary photons of technetium are energetic enough to interact with the K shell electrons of lead. The resulting K-characteristic x-rays are in the range of 75 and 88 keV and are readily seen in the energy spectrum.

**Coincidence or sum peaks**   The likelihood of two separate events taking place simultaneously in the sodium iodide crystal increases with the amount of radiation present. If two events occur close enough in time, the detector system may record them as a single event. Two primary photons from Tc-99m that are detected in coincidence will appear at 280 keV on the energy spectrum. However, every combination of events is possible. That is, a primary photon can be detected in coincidence with a scattered photon of any energy or a lead characteristic x-ray, and so forth. For many detecting systems the ability to discriminate or resolve different discrete energies decreases with increasing amounts of radiation exposure because the likelihood of coincidence events increases with increasing event rate.

**Compton scatter in the patient**   The biggest single cause of degradation of clinical images is Compton scatter in the patient and the inability of imaging systems to completely discriminate primary from Compton-scattered photons. For the gamma scintillation camera, up to 35% of recorded events or even more are due to Compton-scattered photons. The energy spectrum for Tc-99m photons undergoing one scattering event in the patient ranges from 90 keV (i.e., 180° scattering angle) to just under the energy of the primary photon, 140 keV (Fig. 2-4). In Tc-99m spectra obtained with radioactivity in the patient, the lower limb of the primary photopeak merges into the events owing to Compton scatter-

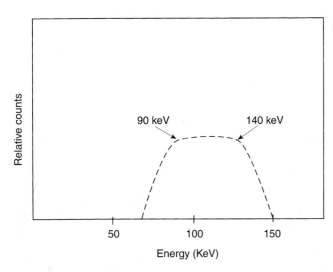

**Fig. 2-4** Nominal Compton scatter spectrum in soft tissue for single scattering events. Note that Compton-scattered photons have energy less than 140 keV but can be recorded above this level because of the imperfect energy resolution of the gamma camera.

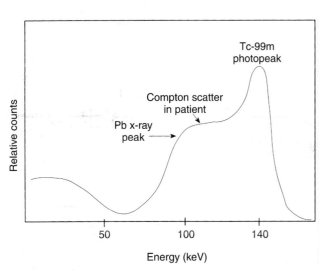

**Fig. 2-5** Observed energy spectrum from a gamma scintillation camera with the technetium-99m activity in the patient. Note the loss of definition of the lower limb of the Tc-99m photopeak. This spectrum can be thought of as a sum of the spectra in Figs. 2-3 and 2-4. This spectrum illustrates the difficulty of discriminating against Compton-scattered photons using pulse height analysis.

ing in the patient. This in turn merges with the lead K–characteristic x-ray peak (Fig. 2-5).

## IMAGING INSTRUMENTATION

The original instruments available for medical applications of radionuclides were handheld Geiger-Müller devices and simple scintillation probe systems. These systems did not allow spatial localization of radioactivity

emanating from the body but did provide a means of crude overall counting. Early clinical applications in nuclear medicine were aimed at calculating the percentage uptake of radioiodine in the thyroid gland with these simple radiation detector systems.

### Rectilinear Scanners

In the 1950s probe systems were adapted into electromechanical devices called *rectilinear scanners*. The geometric field of view of the probe was focused or restricted through the application of collimating devices, and the probes were mounted on mechanical transport systems to systematically traverse back and forth over an organ of interest. The original probe systems used calcium tungstate crystals, which rapidly gave way to sodium iodide crystals for the radiation detection step. By the 1960s rectilinear scanning systems were available with 3-, 5-, and 8-inch-diameter detectors.

### Gamma Scintillation Cameras

Rectilinear scanners have been displaced by the gamma scintillation camera invented by Hal Anger and also known as the Anger camera. The gamma camera offers far more flexibility than the rectilinear scanner and has been developed into a sophisticated series of imaging devices that permit dynamic and tomographic imaging, as well as conventional static planar imaging.

The major components of the gamma scintillation camera are illustrated in Fig. 2-1. Perhaps the easiest way to understand the way gamma cameras work is to follow a photon through the radiation detection and spatial localization process, beginning with the origin of photons in the patient.

**The patient as a source of photons**   Ideally the flux of photons arriving at a radiation detector would be proportional to the number of photons emitted in the respective part of the body being imaged. This assumption would be valid only if the body part were a point source of radiation in air. This is clearly never the case in clinical practice, and a number of factors cause distortion of the photon flux reaching the gamma camera.

One may think of "good" photons as primary photons arising in the organ of interest and emitted parallel to the axis of the collimator field of view. These are the photons desired for creating the scintigraphic image. Good photons are reduced in number by absorption and scatter, which decreases the information available for creating the image (Fig. 2-6). In the clinical applications in nuclear medicine, many potentially useful photons are absorbed or scattered before they reach the detector.

Unwanted primary photons can arise from background radioactivity in tissues in front of or behind the structure of interest (Fig. 2-6). These primary photons

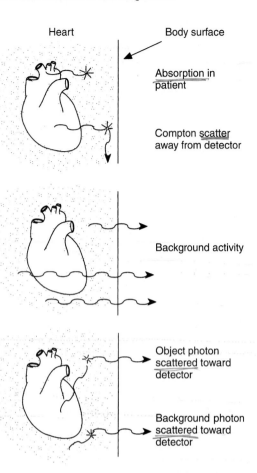

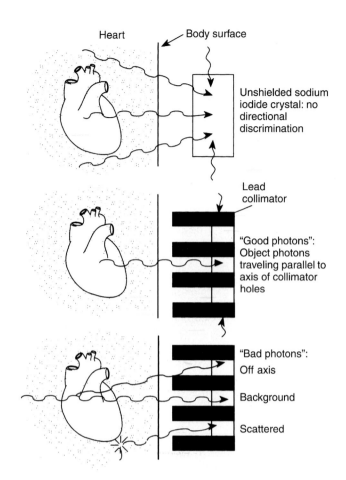

**Fig. 2-6**   The patient as a source of photons. The top drawing illustrates absorption and scattering of primary photons in the body. These never reach the detector. The middle drawing demonstrates background activity arising from in front of, behind, and beside the organ of interest. The bottom drawing illustrates object and background photons scattered toward the detector.

**Fig. 2-7**   Interaction of photons arising in the patient with the detector and a simplified parallel hole collimator. The collimator provides *directional* discrimination for primary and scattered photons. It does not eliminate either background or scattered photons that travel toward the detector within the geometric acceptance field of view of the collimator. "Good" photons are primary (unscattered) photons that originate in the object and travel parallel to the axis of the collimator field of view. All other photons (i.e., background, scattered, off axis) are undesirable in the image.

can travel directly to the detector and are then indistinguishable from photons arising in the body part of interest. They may be thought of as "bad" photons because they reduce image contrast and may distort quantitative data analysis. Background activity produced by primary photons is hard to correct. One major advantage of single-photon emission computed tomography (SPECT) is the increase in image contrast resulting from reduction in this kind of background activity superimposed on object activity.

Another source of bad photons is primary photons arising from the organ of interest, which travel "off axis" toward the detector. Radiation is given off isotropically (i.e., with equal probability in all directions), and only a small fraction of the total emitted photons are useful for forming the image. A principal function of collimators is to absorb off-axis photons (Fig. 2-7).

Compton scatter is a third source of bad photons (Figs. 2-6 and 2-7). Photons originating in or adjacent to the organ of interest can undergo scattering and subse-

quently travel toward the detector. Photons that undergo Compton scattering in the patient lose some of their energy and can be partially discriminated against by using pulse height analysis. However, this ability is far from perfect. For example, a 140-keV photon scattered through a 30° angle retains an energy of 135 keV. This energy would be accepted in a typical 20% energy window used for clinical imaging with Tc-99m.

**Collimators**   The collimator is the first part of the gamma scintillation camera potentially encountered by the photon after it leaves the patient (Fig. 2-1). The purpose of the collimator is to define the geometric field of view of the crystal and specifically to define the desired direction of travel of gamma rays allowed to reach the crystal (Fig. 2-7). The collimator discriminates against unwanted photons only on the basis of their direction of travel. The collimator does not distinguish

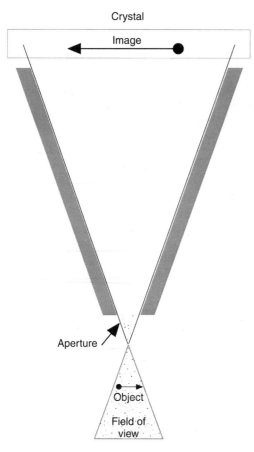

**Fig. 2-8** Pinhole collimator. The image is inverted. The image is magnified if the distance from the aperture to the object is smaller than the distance from the aperture to the gamma camera crystal. The object is minified if its distance from the aperture exceeds the aperture-to-crystal distance. Spatial resolution and count rate sensitivity are inversely affected by aperture diameter.

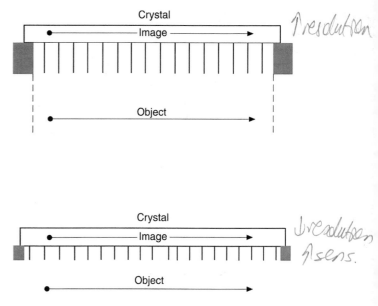

**Fig. 2-9** Two parallel hole collimators. The upper collimator with *longer* septa is designed to achieve higher resolution. Septal *thickness* and energy rating are the same.

between primary and scattered photons or among photons of different energies. The pulse height analyzer is used to discriminate against scattered photons and other photons of unwanted energy that reach the detector.

Collimators for gamma scintillation cameras are available in four basic types. These are the pinhole, parallel hole, converging, and diverging.

*Pinhole collimators*   The geometric behavior of a pinhole collimator is similar to that of a pinhole camera (Fig. 2-8). Beyond the focal point the field of view increases with distance and the image is inverted. The principal use of the pinhole collimator is in thyroid and parathyroid imaging. In this application it offers the advantage of image magnification when the aperture-object distance is shorter than the distance from the detector to the aperture. The geometric magnification allows the resolution of objects smaller than the intrinsic resolution of the gamma camera. This is particularly valuable for thyroid imaging, in which lesions as small as

3 to 5 mm may be resolved. The pinhole collimator also offers flexibility in patient positioning and is useful in obtaining oblique views of the thyroid. Pinhole collimators have been used to magnify small structures in pediatric patients.

The major disadvantage of the pinhole collimator is poor count rate sensitivity. The usual pinhole aperture diameter is 3 to 6 mm. Any increase in this size to increase count rate results in a corresponding decrease in spatial resolution.

*Parallel hole collimators*   The parallel hole collimator is the workhorse collimator in daily nuclear medicine practice (Fig. 2-9). Typically such collimators consist of lead foil with thousands of parallel holes or channels uniformly distributed. A number of terms are used to further characterize parallel hole collimators. The term *low-energy collimator* is used conventionally to refer to collimators designed for photons of the energy of Tc-99m (140 keV) or lower. *Medium-energy collimators* are designed for radionuclides with gamma emissions lower than 400 keV, such as gallium-67 (Ga-67) (multiple photopeaks at 93, 185, 300, and 395 keV). Although the principal gamma ray from iodine-131 (I-131) (364 keV) falls in this energy range, the presence of several higher energy photons (>600 keV) in the decay scheme results in significant degradation and septal penetration artifacts when I-131 is used with medium-energy collimators. *High-energy collimators* have been designed for I-131. These collimators have thicker septa than low-energy collimators. More recently special collimators made of tungsten or other high-Z material have been fabricated for imaging the 511-keV photons of positron emitters.

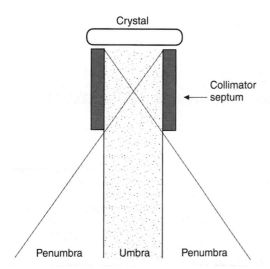

**Fig. 2-10**  Detail geometry of a single-hole collimator. The field of view increases with distance from the collimator face.

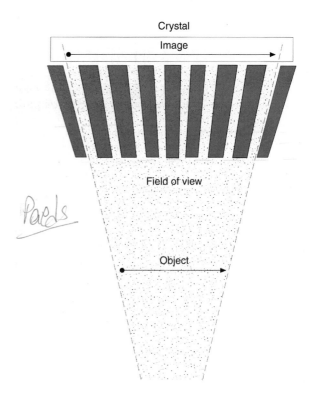

**Fig. 2-11**  Converging hole collimator. Objects are magnified.

Among low-energy collimators, designs are optimized for either sensitivity or resolution. For a given hole size and septal thickness, the thicker the collimator (i.e., the longer the holes), the higher the spatial resolution and the lower the sensitivity. Longer holes of equal diameter have a smaller acceptance angle, resulting in a loss of count rate sensitivity but an improvement in geometric or spatial resolution (Fig. 2-9).

One useful way to think about parallel hole collimators is to look in detail at the geometry and characteristics of an individual hole. Conceptualized in this way, the field of view of each hole becomes larger with increasing distance from the collimator face (Fig. 2-10). Fields of view from adjacent holes begin to overlap, and geometric resolution is degraded. For this reason the organ of interest should be positioned as close to the collimator surface as possible because that is where the resolution is best. Unlike with pinhole collimators, image size is not affected by collimator-to-source distance with parallel hole collimators.

The physics of collimator design and response is complex. In essence a trade-off occurs between spatial resolution and count rate sensitivity, and there is also a need to avoid excessive septal penetration. The need to minimize septal penetration defines the choice of septal thickness for a given energy (Table 2-1). The rule of thumb in collimator design is that less than 10% of recorded events should be due to septal penetration. The off-axis photons reaching the scintillation crystal by septal penetration degrade spatial resolution. However, thicker septa reduce sensitivity and observed count rate.

*Converging and diverging hole collimators*  Converging hole collimators are used to magnify the image geometrically (Fig. 2-11). They are applied especially in pediatric nuclear medicine, where they have partially replaced pinhole collimators for this purpose. Fan beam and cone beam collimators used in SPECT are special adaptations of converging collimators that optimize use of the detector surface area.

Diverging collimators were popular before large-field-of-view cameras became available (Fig. 2-12). They permit a larger area of the body to be imaged than is possible with a parallel hole collimator. For example, a lung scan of a large patient is not feasible with a gamma camera having a standard 10-inch-diameter field of view but is readily accomplished with a diverging hole collimator.

The main drawback of converging and diverging collimators is distortion of the image. This occurs because each portion of the organ of interest is magnified or minified to a different extent, depending on the distance between the respective location and the collimator.

In addition to the primary collimator designs a number of specialty use collimators have been described. Parallel slant hole collimators have found application in nuclear cardiology. Some nuclear medicine physicians favor a 30° caudal angulation for separating the left atrium from the left ventricle in radionuclide ventriculography. Rotating slant hole collimators and multiple-pinhole collimators have been used for limited angle emission computed tomography.

**Gamma ray detection: the sodium iodide crystal**  Modern gamma scintillation cameras use thallium-activated sodium iodide crystals as the radiation detector

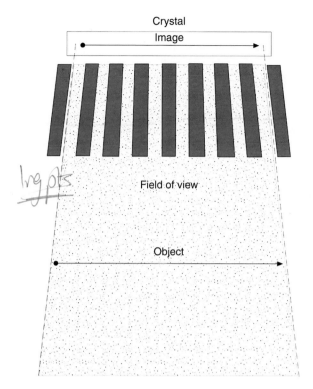

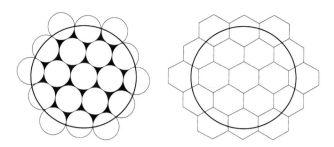

**Fig. 2-13** Circular (*left*) and hexagonal (*right*) photomultiplier tubes. The tubes are arrayed in a hexagonal configuration so that the distance from each tube to all of its nearest neighbors is identical. The switch from round to hexagonal tubes allows more complete coverage of the gamma camera crystal.

sodium iodide crystal was optically coupled to a hexagonal array of 19 3-inch-diameter photomultiplier tubes (Fig. 2-13).

For each event two kinds of signal processing are performed. First the output from all of the photomultiplier tubes is summed for the purpose of pulse height analysis. This summed pulse is typically referred to as the Z pulse and is used to determine whether the detected event is within the desired energy range and should be accepted into the formation of the image or whether it is of lower or higher energy and should be discriminated against and rejected (Fig. 2-1).

Simultaneously the output of each photomultiplier tube is looked at in a different way. Each tube may be thought of as having $x$ and $y$ coordinates in a cartesian plane with the center of the central photomultiplier tube being the origin. Each photomultiplier tube then can be thought of as contributing either a positive or a negative value for $x$ and $y$ positioning. The photomultiplier tubes closest to the event collect the greatest number of light photons, with lesser contributions from more remote tubes. The logic circuitry of the camera is used to compute the most likely coordinates of the event location in the crystal by adding together all of the $x$ and $y$ pulses from the 19 photomultiplier tubes (Fig. 2-1).

**Image recording**  If the Z pulse indicates that a primary photon has been absorbed, an unblanking signal is sent to the image-recording device. On original cameras the recording system was an oscilloscope with a Polaroid camera or 35-mm camera attachment. The $x$ and $y$ positioning signals provided the deflection coordinates for the cathode ray tube (CRT), and the event was recorded on film as a single flash of light from the screen. A typical image was created by recording 100,000 to 1 million individual events.

In contemporary practice most scintigraphic images are recorded on dedicated computer systems. An analog-to-digital converter is used to convert the $x$, $y$ positioning signals into digital coordinates to be stored in computer memory.

**Fig. 2-12**  Diverging hole collimator. Objects are minified.

(Fig. 2-1). The desired event in the camera crystal is the complete photoelectric absorption of a primary photon that reached the crystal by traveling parallel to the geometric axis of the collimator field of view from its origin in the organ of interest in the patient. The likelihood of a photoelectric interaction and complete energy absorption in the sodium iodide crystal is greater at low energies and decreases at higher energies as Compton scatter becomes more likely (Table 2-1).

As discussed in the section on radiation detection, the gamma ray energy is converted to light energy in the crystal. For every 140-keV technetium photon completely absorbed, approximately 4200 light photons are emitted, with an average energy of 3 eV. One of the limitations of lower energy gamma rays, including those from Tc-99m, is the limited number of light photons available for subsequent event localization. Higher energy photons potentially provide more light photons and better statistical certainty for event localization. This is counterbalanced by the greater likelihood of an initial Compton scatter event in the crystal before a terminal photoelectric interaction. When multiple scattering events occur in the crystal before complete energy absorption, spatial resolution is reduced.

**Signal processing and event localization**  The breakthrough concept in the design of the gamma scintillation camera is the use of an array of photomultiplier tubes behind the crystal for event localization. In the first commercial gamma camera a 10-inch-diameter

## Characteristics of Modern Gamma Scintillation Cameras

The original commercial gamma cameras had 10- to 12-inch-diameter crystals with a thickness of ½ inch. These cameras were designed in an era when I-131 (364 keV) was the most important radionuclide.

In the ensuing 25 years, crystal size and shape have changed. Large-field-of-view cameras with 15-inch-diameter fields of view have become the standard. Square and rectangular sodium iodide crystals have been developed for special applications, including SPECT and whole body imaging.

A series of changes in the original gamma camera design has been aimed at improving spatial resolution. Crystal thickness in many cameras is now ¼ inch. This crystal thickness is more suited to studies with lower energy radionuclides, such as Tc-99m and thallium-201. For Tc-99m with a 140-keV principal photon energy the loss in sensitivity between ½- and ¼-inch thickness is only 6% (Table 2-1), while the spatial resolution is improved by 20%. For Tl-201 there is virtually no loss of sensitivity and the same 20% improvement in spatial resolution. However, for studies using gallium (93, 185, 300, 394 keV), indium-111 (172, 247 keV), or I-131 (364 keV), a better compromise may be a ⅜-inch-thick crystal.

The advent of single-photon PET with the use of a modified gamma camera for SPECT imaging of fluoride-18 has rekindled interest in thicker crystals. The detection efficiency for 511-keV photons increases from ~12% for ⅜-inch NaI (Tl) crystals to ~18% for ½-inch crystals. Single-photon PET also requires heavier collimation to reduce septal penetration by 511-keV photons. Materials such as tungsten and even gold have more stopping power than lead and have been used in collimator fabrication. Even so, more septal penetration occurs in single-photon PET imaging than in other gamma camera applications.

The number of photomultiplier tubes used in gamma cameras has been increased. The first step was to reduce tube diameter from 3 inches to 2 inches, which permitted use of 37 photomultiplier tubes for a standard-field-of-view camera. Large-field-of-view cameras are available with 55, 61, 75, and even 91 tubes. Another advance in photomultiplier tubes is the hexagonal photocathode, which allows the tubes to cover the crystal completely without leaving gaps between them (Fig. 2-13). Light pipes have been replaced with direct coupling of the photomultiplier tubes to the crystal. The collection of more light photons reduces the statistical uncertainty in the $(x, y)$ event localization logic circuitry.

An area that has received major attention over the years is field uniformity. The basic problem is that each photomultiplier tube behaves slightly differently and may drift in its performance over time. Field uniformity was not a major problem before SPECT but is now critical to prevent artifacts in SPECT images.

In addition to slight differences in photomultiplier tube response, subtle differences occur in the crystal itself and in the efficiency of the optical coupling of the photomultiplier tubes with the crystal. For this reason the energy spectrum that is collected from any one photomultiplier tube is different from all the other tubes (Fig. 2-14). The observed energy spectrum from the overall camera is made up of a sum of the slightly different spectra from each tube. This could be dramatically demonstrated in older cameras by setting an asymmetrical pulse height analyzer window over a photopeak to accentuate the differences in tube performance.

Although vendors have tried a number of approaches to match the performance characteristics of the photomultiplier tubes, problems persist. The current approach is to use computer correction of the response across the crystal. In effect, after the camera system is manufactured and tuned as well as possible, its actual performance relative to a known radioactive source energy and its imaging geometry are empirically mapped and correction factors are established for each small area of the detector.

The ZLC system introduced by Siemens a number of years ago is illustrative of attempts to correct for spatial variation in energy response and for small nonlinearities. The Z signals are corrected by empirically measuring a $128 \times 128$ energy response matrix. Each Z signal is then corrected by a factor, $\Delta Z$, obtained for its respective pixel location in the matrix before the pulse reaches the pulse height analyzer. The corrected pulse $(Z + \Delta Z)$ is then analyzed. Each event is energy corrected on the fly during image acquisition.

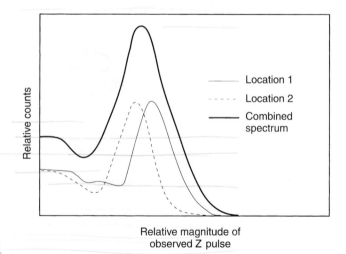

**Fig. 2-14** The slightly offset spectra from two different photomultiplier tubes or locations in the gamma camera crystal and the combined spectrum. Especially in older gamma scintillation cameras, a wide energy acceptance window was necessary to encompass the variations in response across the crystal.

For linearity correction a rectilinear grid is imaged and a 4k × 4k lookup table of correction factors for spatial localization is created. Each event is positioned in the image based on ΔX and ΔY correction factors corresponding to the observed location of the event.

More recently, several strategies for automatic and active photomultiplier tube adjustment have been introduced. In one system, light-emitting diodes of known output are used to measure and fine-tune photomultiplier tube response as often as 10 times per second. This is advantageous for applications in which the camera head is rotating, since photomultiplier tube performance can be affected by changes in alignment to the earth's magnetic field (Fig. 2-15). Each gamma camera vendor has taken a different approach to the energy response and spatial localization problems. The unifying theme is increasing sophistication in making corrections event by event.

In the best contemporary cameras the recording of each event is corrected separately for location and energy. This kind of event-by-event correction permits the use of asymmetrical windows. The advantage of an asymmetrical window offset to the high side of the photopeak is reduction in scattered photons accepted in the image. However, unless energy correction is performed properly, the response across the image will vary depending on photomultiplier tube response. Events in areas of lower output tubes will be underrepresented in the image, while events in areas with higher output tubes will be overrepresented (Fig. 2-16). Further

advances from commercial vendors have led to automatic tuning systems and on-line adjustment systems for photomultiplier and overall system response.

The past 15 years has seen an explosion in the number and kinds of gamma cameras on the commercial market. Mobile cameras, whole body imaging systems, and cameras adapted to special nuclear cardiology applications are available, as are camera systems with multiple detector heads for SPECT and whole body imaging.

## Gamma Camera Quality Control

Gamma scintillation cameras are complex devices with physical, mechanical, and electronic components. Malfunction or breakage of any of these can be catastrophic to system performance and may not be recognized from a review of clinical images. For these reasons a number of comprehensive and sophisticated procedures have been developed over the years to ensure adequate camera performance. The ones used most often in routine clinical practice are summarized in Box 2-1. In addition to these the National Electrical Manufacturers Association has developed a comprehensive set of tests to measure camera performance.

**Field uniformity** One fundamental parameter that requires daily assessment is the uniformity of response of the gamma camera across its entire field of view (Fig. 2-17). A source of radioactivity of appropriate energy is used to test the camera response. Measurements made with the collimator in place are referred to as *extrinsic,*

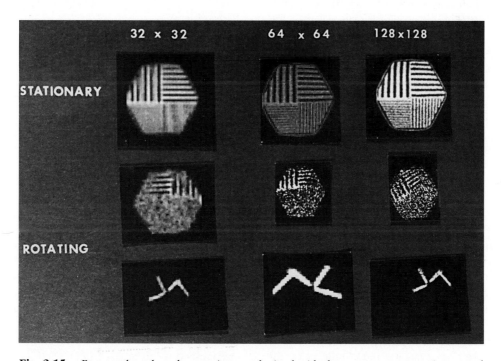

**Fig. 2-15**   Four-quadrant bar phantom images obtained with the gamma camera stationary and during rotation. Note the degradation in bar phantom resolution in this early generation rotating SPECT system. (Courtesy K.A. McKusick, MD, and John Hergenrother, CNMT, Massachusetts General Hospital, Boston.)

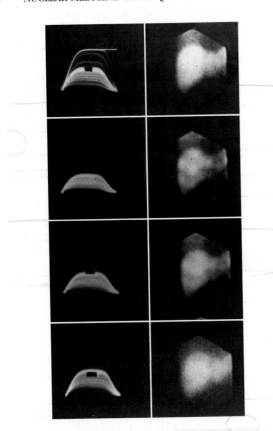

**Fig. 2-16** Multiple images from the same subject obtained with different window settings. The left-hand panel of images illustrates the energy spectrum coming from the patient. The location of the energy window is indicated by the black rectangle superimposed over the spectral lines. The top panel illustrates a symmetrical window centered at the photopeak. The middle two panels illustrate the energy window offset to the high side, and the lower panel illustrates the energy window offset to the low side. Note the loss of homogeneity in the liver in the two middle images with a geometric pattern of hot and cold areas owing to the location pattern of the photomultiplier tubes. Scatter is decreased, as indicated by the lower counts coming from the region of the heart, but the images are grossly misleading. On the bottom panel the image is degraded by excessive scatter and loss of spatial resolution. Note the blurring of the liver margin. (Courtesy K.A. McKusick, MD, and John Hergenrother, CNMT, Massachusetts General Hospital, Boston.)

and those made with the collimator off are referred to as *intrinsic.*

The specific method for assessing field uniformity varies widely. For example, a uniform disk or flood source in a phantom can be used to measure extrinsic field uniformity. With this approach the radioactive source is placed at or on the surface of the gamma camera collimator. To measure intrinsic field uniformity a point source of radioactivity is positioned at the center of the crystal at a distance of 5 feet or more from the uncollimated crystal face. Typically, 1000k to 5000k counts are obtained to evaluate field uniformity for planar imaging.

For extrinsic field uniformity testing, most laboratories use either a phantom filled with a uniform solution

## Box 2-1   Gamma Camera Quality Control Summary

| PARAMETER | COMMENT |
|---|---|
| **Daily** | |
| Uniformity check | Flood field; intrinsic (without collimator) or extrinsic (with collimator) |
| Window setting | Confirm energy window setting relative to photopeak for each radionuclide used |
| **Weekly** | |
| Spatial resolution | Requires a "resolution" phantom (PLES, four-quadrant bar, orthogonal hole) and standardized protocol |
| Linearity check | Qualitative assessment of bar pattern linearity |
| **Periodic (biannually or when a problem is suspected)** | |
| Collimator performance | High count flood with each collimator |
| Energy registration | For cameras with capability of imaging multiple energy windows simultaneously |
| Count rate performance and count rate linearity | More important in cameras with "count skimming" or "count addition" correction circuitry |
| Energy resolution | Easiest in cameras with built in multiple-channel analyzers |
| Sensitivity | Count rate performance per unit of activity |

of Tc-99m or a permanent disk source of uniformly distributed cobalt-57 (Co-57; $T_{1/2}$ 270 days, 122 keV). The standard practice is to obtain a flood image with each camera every day before it is used for clinical studies. In laboratories where obtaining the daily flood image with the collimator in place is more practical, obtaining an intrinsic flood image weekly is still useful, and vice versa for laboratories that routinely acquire flood images without the collimator in place.

The image obtained in the field uniformity examination should be carefully inspected. A well-tuned camera with proper photomultiplier tube and correction circuitry performance should provide a flood image with a highly uniform appearance or only minor mottling with slightly increased intensity in regions corresponding to photomultiplier tubes (Fig. 2-17). Photomultiplier tube drift or even the failure of a photomultiplier tube can be recognized as an area of decreased activity (Fig. 2-18). Cracked crystals are readily identified, and even damage to a collimator can be detected. The soft lead in collimators is often protected by a covering but can still

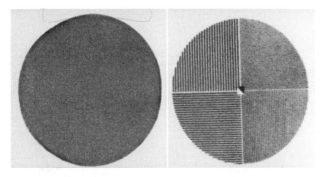

**Fig. 2-17**   Images of the flood source (*left*) and a four-quadrant bar phantom (*right*) from a well-tuned gamma scintillation camera with the collimator off. The flood image shows slight mottling but no focal or localized areas of increased or decreased activity within the center of the field of view. The slightly increased activity along the rim is a common characteristic of gamma cameras seen on intrinsic flood images. The smallest bars are partially discernible on the bar phantom image. They have a spacing of 3 mm. The bar images show good linearity.

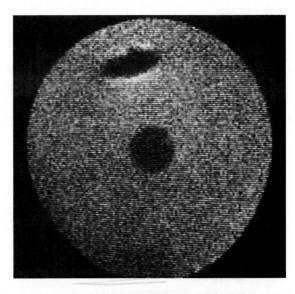

**Fig. 2-18**   Flood image from a camera with a nonfunctioning central photomultiplier tube and a crystal defect. (Courtesy K.A. McKusick, MD, and John Hergenrother, CNMT, Massachusetts General Hospital, Boston.)

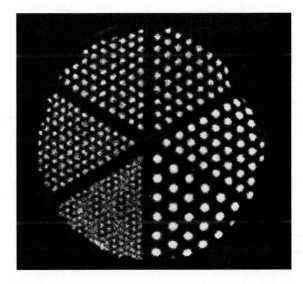

**Fig. 2-19**   Moiré patterns are present in the three triangles on the left in an image of a "hot spot" phantom. The distortion is especially marked in the lower left triangle.

be subject to denting, with bending and distortion of the septa.

**Spatial resolution and linearity**   The four-quadrant bar phantom is probably the most commonly used phantom for evaluating linearity and spatial resolution (Fig. 2-17). Some authorities recommend performing this procedure daily, but with modern cameras a weekly assessment is sufficient.

The phantom is positioned on the collimator face so that the center of the four-quadrant pattern corresponds to the center of the camera. A uniform Tc-99m flood source is then placed on the bar phantom. Four images are obtained at sequential 90° rotations between positions. Care must be taken not to position the bars on the collimator in such a way that an interference or moiré pattern occurs (Fig. 2-19).

Modern gamma scintillation cameras have excellent spatial resolution. When the spatial resolution check is made without the collimator in place, it is difficult to find a four-quadrant bar phantom with small enough bar spacing. An alternative is the parallel-line equal-spacing bar phantom. When this device is used, two images are necessary. Because signals from the photomultiplier tubes are processed through two essentially independent positioning circuits ($x$ and $y$), degradations can occur in a selective direction. Yet another alternative is the orthogonal hole test pattern. It is designed so that only a single image is required. Regardless of the phantom chosen, when trouble is suspected, the procedure should be repeated with and without the collimator.

In a properly functioning camera, all groups of bars in the bar phantom pattern should appear straight and parallel (Fig. 2-17). Some distortion is typically seen at the edge of the field of view. When the study is acquired on an analog CRT with direct film recording, it is

important to calibrate the dot size and confirm the dot shape first.

The spatial resolution of gamma cameras is often expressed as the full width at half maximum (FWHM) of a line spread function. A line spread function is obtained by first imaging a narrow line source of radioactivity on the collimator (extrinsic) or crystal face (intrinsic) and then determining a count profile or histogram perpendicularly across it. This histogram is called the *line spread function*. In an imaging system with perfect spatial resolution the line spread function would have a single spike corresponding to the radioactive line source. In practice a bell-shaped curve is seen.

FWHM is simply the distance encompassed by the curve halfway down from its peak. This is the same kind of measurement previously discussed for describing energy resolution. By analogy the narrower the peak, the better the spatial resolution and therewith the ability to resolve objects close to each other. In modern gamma cameras, intrinsic resolution (collimator off) approaches 3-mm FWHM or less.

## Clinical Use of the Gamma Scintillation Camera

Applying the gamma scintillation camera to clinical procedures requires the development of imaging protocols that define the diagnostic purpose, the radiopharmaceutical to be used, patient preparation, and the imaging sequence. These issues are discussed in the organ system chapters for the major scintigraphic studies. The protocols include selection of collimator, the timing of image acquisition after radiopharmaceutical administration, the time per image or the number of counts to be recorded, and the actual images or views to be obtained.

### Window Setting

A quality control issue sometimes overlooked in the clinical application of gamma cameras is the setting of the energy window. The most common approach is to use a symmetrical window centered at the energy peak of the radionuclide label being used in the imaging procedure. For Tc-99m the most common recommendation is to use a 20% window centered at 140 keV. The acceptance range for this window is 126 to 154 keV. In gamma cameras with energy correction circuitry, setting an asymmetrical window to reduce Compton scatter may be possible. Using a narrower window of 10% or 15% for higher resolution imaging may also be desirable. These approaches should be undertaken with caution for older gamma cameras because of the problem of nonuniform response across the crystal, which is discussed in some detail in a previous section.

The most conservative approach is to confirm the window setting for each radionuclide used during the course of a day and then to reconfirm the window setting before imaging each patient. Setting the energy window ("peaking in the camera," "setting the peak") should be done with a radioactive source in air and *not* by using radioactivity in the patient. The spectrum from the patient includes scatter that can shift the perceived location of the photopeak.

Fig. 2-16 illustrates four different window settings for the same patient. The top image was obtained with the optimal setting for the camera being used. The bottom three panels illustrate energy windows offset to the high and low sides of the photopeak, with consequent degra-

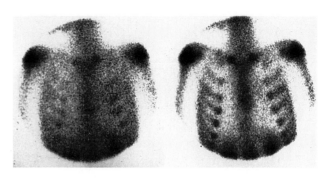

**Fig. 2-20** The image on the left was obtained with a 20% window set at 122 keV, the energy of the cobalt-57 flood source. The image quality is dramatically improved in the image on the right, which was obtained at the correct window setting for technetium-99m.

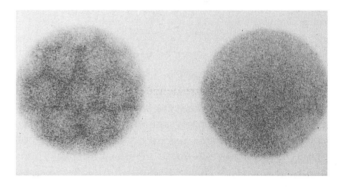

**Fig. 2-21** Gallium-67 flood images obtained using multiple photopeaks. In the left-hand panel are artifacts in the flood image caused by spatial misregistration. The properly registered image on the right shows good uniformity. (Courtesy John Hergenrother, CNMT, Massachusetts General Hospital, Boston.)

dation of image quality. False positive and false negative interpretations may occur because of artifacts and loss of resolution, respectively, with incorrect window settings. Occasionally the window is inadvertently left at the setting for a Co-57 flood source (122 keV). Fig. 2-20 illustrates the degradation of image quality in a Tc-99m diphosphonate bone study resulting from this.

Another practical problem of window setting occurs in cameras that image multiple photopeaks simultaneously. Care must be taken to ensure that the image data from the different photopeaks are correctly registered together on the clinical image. Fig. 2-21 illustrates incorrect *(left)* and correct *(right)* multipeak registration for a Ga-67 flood image.

## COMPUTERS IN NUCLEAR MEDICINE

Computers in nuclear medicine were a curiosity until the development of multiframe gated blood pool imaging in the mid-1970s. Subsequently the computer has be-

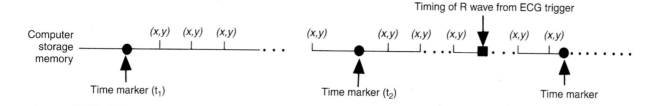

(x,y) = coordinates of each individual scintillation

**Fig. 2-22**    List mode data acquisition.

come a primary image acquisition and processing device and is frequently used for image management and to control film formatting, in addition to its integral role for dynamic studies and SPECT.

## Creation of the Digital Image

The *x* and *y* pulses generated in the gamma scintillation camera logic circuitry define event location. In older cameras these pulses are in analog form and must be converted to digital form for computer processing. To accomplish this, an analog-to-digital converter is interposed between the gamma camera and the computer. Some modern cameras convert the (*x, y*) signals to digital form within the camera's own electronic circuitry. The Z pulse is used in computer data acquisition to indicate that a particular event should be accepted for storage.

Two fundamentally different modes are used to acquire and store digitized data: list (serial) mode and frame (histogram) mode. In the list mode approach each pair of digitized (*x, y*) position signals is stored separately and sequentially in computer memory. The "list" is simply a line of data flowing into computer memory. If time information is desired, additional time markers are inserted into the list. Physiological signals such as the R wave on the ECG can also be recorded (Fig. 2-22).

The list mode approach offers great flexibility. For example, data from each cardiac cycle can be analyzed separately. If a particular beat was due to a dysrhythmia, the data from that beat can be excluded from the desired data from normal sinus beats. Alternatively, data from beats caused by particular types of dysrhythmias can be analyzed separately. The major disadvantage of list mode is that it requires a large amount of computer memory. It also requires additional time to process data into an image format after acquisition is complete.

In the alternative histogram or frame mode of data acquisition the digitized (*x, y*) pairs are used to locate the picture element to which they belong. The image may be thought of as a grid or matrix superimposed on the analog data (Fig. 2-23). The *x* and *y* numbers determine

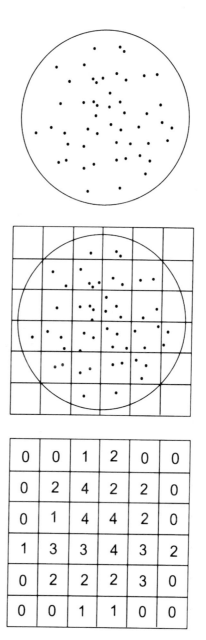

**Fig. 2-23**    Analog image *(top)* has 6 × 6 matrix superimposed *(middle)*. The number of events (dots) in each pixel is recorded to create the digital matrix *(bottom)*.

which matrix element encloses the location of the original event. At the end of data collection, rather than having discrete information on each event, each matrix location has a number corresponding to the total events accumulated throughout the imaging period.

Frame mode is much more sparing of computer memory and has the further advantage that the data are immediately ready for display or analysis, without post-processing or formatting. Physiological signals can still be used to control data collection as in multigated cardiac studies. However, once recorded, data from dysrhythmic beats cannot be excluded.

The larger the matrix, the better the potential spatial resolution but the longer the time required to achieve adequate counting statistics in each pixel. Most studies in current practice are obtained in a $64 \times 64$ or $128 \times 128$ matrix.

## Data Analysis

Computer recording of image data greatly facilitates quantitative analysis. Specific types of analyses are discussed in the respective organ system chapters. A recurring requirement in data analysis is the definition of a "region of interest." These regions can be defined by the computer operator or through the use of automated region of interest definition programs. The latter are often used to define the area of the left ventricle in calculating ejection fractions.

The computer can make various calculations on the pixels in regions of interest. In most applications the total count within the region is of greatest value. This kind of data analysis allows calculation of quantitative parameters such as the left ventricular ejection fraction or the percentage of the total glomerular filtration rate attributable to the left versus the right kidney.

## Data Display and Formatting

Clinics with contemporary computer systems frequently use them to archive image data and to control image-formatting devices such as laser printers. The advantages of using the computer for this purpose rather than using analog imaging or recording directly from the gamma camera CRT are that images may be windowed and centered to provide the optimum gray scale after the fact and that the same image data may be viewed with and without secondary image processing, including background subtraction or contrast enhancement. The computer is invaluable for looking at dynamic data. This is most important for viewing the beating heart in nuclear cardiology, but it also has value in performing time lapse photography for other applications such as localizing the site of bleeding in gastrointestinal bleeding detection studies or assessing biliary dynamics during hepatobiliary imaging studies.

## SUGGESTED READINGS

Chandra R: *Nuclear medicine physics: the basics,* ed 4, Baltimore, 1998, Williams & Wilkins.

Hendee WR: *Medical radiation physics,* ed 3, St Louis, 1992, Mosby.

Johns HE, Cunningham JR: *The physics of radiology,* ed 4, Chicago, 1983, Thomas Books.

Powsner RA, Powsner ER: *Essentials of nuclear medicine physics,* Malden, Mass, 1998, Blackwell Science.

Sorenson JA, Phelps ME: *Physics in nuclear medicine,* ed 2, Philadelphia, 1987, WB Saunders.

Weber DA, Eckerman KF, Dillman LT, Ryman JC: *MIRD: radionuclide data and decay schemes,* New York, 1989, Society of Nuclear Medicine.

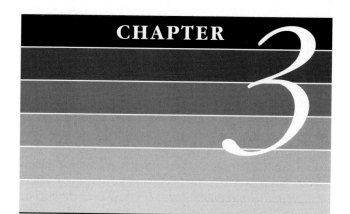

# CHAPTER 3

# Single-Photon Emission Computed Tomography and Positron Emission Tomography

## RADIONUCLIDE TOMOGRAPHY

Conventional or planar radionuclide imaging suffers a major limitation in loss of object contrast as a result of background radioactivity. In the conventional planar image, radioactivity underlying and overlying an object is superimposed on radioactivity coming from the object. The fundamental goal of tomographic imaging systems is a more accurate portrayal of the distribution of radioactivity in the patient, with improved definition of image detail. The Greek *tomo* means "to cut"; tomography may be thought of as a means of "cutting" the body into discrete image planes. Tomographic techniques have been developed for both single-photon and positron tomography.

Rectilinear scanners with focused collimators represent a crude type of tomography; the count rate sensitivity is greatest in the collimator focal plane, and therefore more weight is given to radioactivity arising in that plane than in planes superficial or deep to it. However, this is not "true" tomography because out-of-plane radiation still contributes to the image.

Restricted angle or longitudinal (frontal) tomography shares the phenomenon of the rectilinear scanner; in-plane data are kept in focus, with blurring of out-of-plane data. Restricted angle or longitudinal tomography is analogous to conventional x-ray tomography, in which the relative positions of the film and x-ray source remain constant for the desired image plane but move relative to each other in the overlying and underlying planes, blurring the out-of-plane structures.

A number of restricted angle systems enjoyed a vogue in the late 1970s and early 1980s. These included the seven-pinhole collimator system, pseudorandom coded aperture collimator systems, and various kinds of rotating slant hole collimator systems. These approaches have given way to rotating gamma camera systems for single-photon tomography.

The rotating systems offer the ability to perform true transaxial tomography. The most important characteristic is that only data arising in the image plane are used in the reconstruction or creation of the tomographic image. Rotational single-photon emission computed tomography (SPECT) shares this feature with x-ray computed tomography (CT) and positron emission tomography (PET). This is an important characteristic because it offers a higher image contrast than with tomographic systems that merely blur the out-of-plane data.

## SINGLE-PHOTON EMISSION COMPUTED TOMOGRAPHY

With use of conventional radiopharmaceuticals, SPECT allows true three-dimensional image acquisition and display. Reconstruction of cross-sectional slices has traditionally used filtered backprojection, the same methodology used for CT.

### Instrumentation

The most common approach to rotational SPECT is to mount one or more gamma camera heads on a special rotating gantry. Original systems used a single head, but now systems with two, three, and even four heads are commercially available. In particular, two-headed systems that allow flexibility in orientation between the heads have become popular. For body imaging the heads are typically arrayed 180° apart, and they can be placed at right angles for cardiac applications (Fig. 3-1).

Multiple heads are desirable because they allow more data to be collected in a given period. Rotational SPECT is "photon poor" compared with x-ray CT, and it is desirable both to collect as many counts as possible and to complete imaging within a reasonable time because of radiopharmaceutical pharmacokinetics and limits of the patient's ability to remain still. Thus a study of Tl-201 distribution in the heart should be accomplished before significant redistribution occurs.

In addition to the special gantry that permits camera head rotation, modifications have been necessary for rotational SPECT. Photomultiplier tube performance can be affected by gravitational and magnetic fields. These change depending on rotational angle, and subtle alterations in photomultiplier tube energy response can degrade images. Magnetic shielding of photomultiplier tubes reduces this problem.

Rotational SPECT has highlighted the need to improve every aspect of gamma camera system performance. Flood field nonuniformities are translated as major artifacts in tomographic images because they distort the data obtained from each view or projection. Desirable characteristics for SPECT are an intrinsic spatial resolution (FWHM) of 3 mm, linearity distortion of 1 mm or less, uncorrected field uniformity within 3%, and corrected field uniformity within 1%.

All contemporary rotational SPECT systems have on-line uniformity and energy correction. Nonlinearities in photomultiplier tube energy response degrade both gamma camera energy resolution and spatial resolution. Degraded energy resolution is devastating, since 35% or more of recorded events can represent Compton-scattered photons. Poor energy resolution degrades the ability to reject scattered photons on the basis of pulse height analysis. It also degrades spatial resolution through decreased accuracy of determining $x$ and $y$ event localization coordinates.

### Image Acquisition

Box 3-1 summarizes factors that must be considered in performing rotational SPECT. In addition to standard gamma camera quality control, confirmation is needed that the axis of rotation corresponds to the center of the matrix in the computer. Incorrect alignment results in a blurring of the image or poorer resolution and can even produce ring artifacts in the SPECT images.

**Collimator selection**    Collimator selection is generally limited to those supplied by the system vendor. As discussed previously, for a given septal thickness and

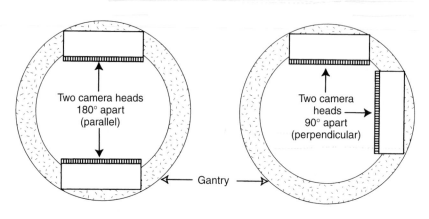

**Fig. 3-1**    Two configurations for dual-headed SPECT systems.

hole diameter, collimators with longer channels have higher resolution and lower sensitivity. Even though SPECT is relatively photon poor, collimator selection should favor higher resolution whenever possible. This means selecting the high-resolution collimator over a high-sensitivity or general purpose collimator for studies using Tc-99m. The multiheaded systems permit the operator to trade the improved count rate sensitivity for improved resolution by using ultra-high-resolution collimators.

Two special collimator options are available for imaging the brain: angled collimators allow the camera head to be maintained closer to the patient, and special fan beam and cone beam collimators permit more of the camera crystal to be used for radiation detection. The fan and cone beam collimators are similar in geometry to converging collimators and have the effect of magnifying the object being imaged when it is placed proximal to the focal point of the respective collimators. The resulting geometric distortion of the image data must be taken into account during image reconstruction.

**Orbit** The orbit selected depends on the organ of interest and on whether the system being used offers a noncircular orbit capability. The ideal orbit keeps the gamma head as close to the organ of interest as possible because for parallel hole collimators the resolution is best at the face of the collimator. Much imaging is still done using circular orbits, but contemporary systems permit the use of elliptical orbits and customized orbits that better approximate body contours (Fig. 3-2). Orbit selection attempts to minimize the distance between the camera head and the object being imaged.

**Arc of acquisition, angular sampling, and matrix size** The choice of angular sampling interval and arc of acquisition depend on the clinical application and collimator selection. For body imaging applications the arc of acquisition is typically a full 360°. For studies with

Tc-99m-labeled agents it is often feasible to use a high-resolution collimator and to acquire data in a $128 \times 128$ matrix with an angular increment of 3° or a total of 120 angular projections. If these studies are performed with a general purpose or lower resolution collimator, a $64 \times 64$ matrix is typically selected with an angular sampling increment of 6° for a total of 60 angular projections or 4° for a total of 90 angular projections. These combinations of sampling increment, matrix size, and collimator selection "balance" the resolution of the respective parameters. For imaging of tumors and infections with gallium-67 (Ga-67) or indium-111 (In-111) tracers, a $64 \times 64$ matrix is selected with a 6° angular sampling increment. (Note that in some SPECT systems 64, 96, or 128 angular projections are used. For simplicity this discussion refers to 60, 90, and 120 projections only.)

The merits of 180° versus 360° rotation for cardiac studies have been debated in the literature. A minimum arc of 180° is necessary for true transaxial tomography. Proponents of the 180° approach argue that because the heart is close to the anterior chest wall, the best data are

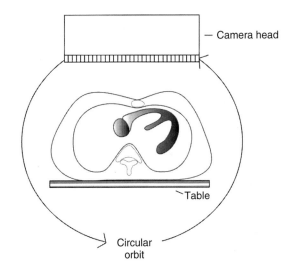

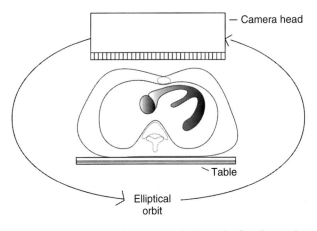

**Fig. 3-2** Circular orbit *(top)* and elliptical orbit *(bottom).*

---

**Box 3-1    Image Acquisition Issues for Rotational Single-Photon Emission Computed Tomography**

Center of rotation check
Collimator selection
Energy window selection
Orbit
Matrix size
Angular increment—number of views
180° versus 360° rotation
Time per view
Total examination time
Patient factors

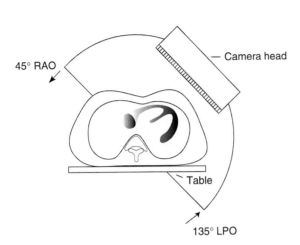

**Fig. 3-3**   The 180° arc frequently used for cardiac imaging.

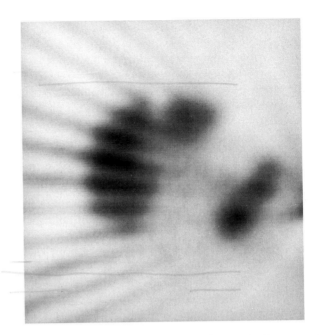

**Fig. 3-4**   Degraded SPECT image of the liver and spleen caused by focal activity at the injection site included in the field of view during imaging. The starburst artifact is due to backprojection of the hot spot activity across the image. In this case the degree of activity in the injection site could not be accommodated in the reconstruction algorithm.

available by imaging in a 180° arc typically spanning 135° left posterior oblique to 45° right anterior oblique (Fig. 3-3). The use of 180° arcs for cardiac SPECT is widely accepted in clinical practice and has won the day for cardiac imaging when attenuation correction is not used.

Another question is whether to use continuous data acquisition or "step and shoot" acquisition. Continuous acquisition has the advantage of not wasting time during movement of the camera head from one angular sampling position to the next. However, the data are blurred by the motion artifact of the moving camera head. The resultant trade-offs between sensitivity and resolution favor step and shoot acquisition for most clinical applications. Exceptions are applications with rapidly changing tracer distribution and when determination of overall tracer concentration is more important than spatial resolution.

**Imaging time**   Most clinical protocols require a total imaging time between 15 and 30 minutes. Correspondingly the time per projection is usually between 15 and 30 seconds, but as much as 40 to 60 seconds may be needed for relatively photon-poor studies with Ga-67 and In-111.

**Patient factors**   A major limitation in data acquisition time is the ability of the patient to remain still throughout the imaging procedure. Within accepted limits for dosimetry and radiation exposure, the larger the administered dosage, the more counts available. Although clinically accepted limits for administered radioactivity should never be exceeded, the radiation risk versus benefit must take into account the likelihood of obtaining a diagnostic quality image. The goal of obtaining higher counting statistics is meaningless if the patient

moves, causing data between the different angular sampling views to be misregistered. Attempts to correct for motion have been made by registering data after acquisition using fiducial markers or other data manipulations, but in practice this is cumbersome.

Patient compliance is improved by taking time during setup to position the patient comfortably. For scans of the head the patient's arms can be in a natural position at the sides. For rotational SPECT studies of the heart, thorax, abdomen, or pelvis the arms are typically raised out of the field of view so that they do not interfere with the path of photons toward the detector. In all applications it is important to keep the injection site out of the field of view to prevent artifacts resulting from residual or infiltrated activity (Fig. 3-4).

## Image Reconstruction

Each commercially available SPECT system takes a somewhat different and proprietary approach to the image reconstruction process. The most common approach to SPECT reconstruction has been filtered backprojection. Reconstruction is accomplished either in the spatial domain or in the frequency domain after Fourier transformation of the raw data. All approaches to reconstruction use mathematical filters that alter the raw data to facilitate tomographic image creation. Although reconstruction of SPECT images is highly analytical, it is also an art, since different observers prefer different

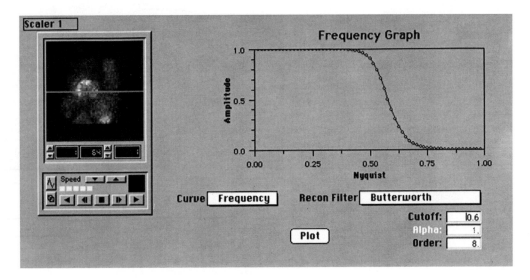

**Fig. 3-5** Frequency graph of image profile data corresponding to the cursor in the image on the left after Fourier transformation. The frequencies are scaled as a fraction of Nyquist. Their frequencies could also be scaled in terms of cycles per pixel or cycles per centimeter. Nyquist 1.00 corresponds to 0.5 cycle/pixel.

characteristics in the final images that are determined by operator-adjustable parameters, including filtering.

Before a discussion of the image reconstruction process, the following terms should be defined.

**Spatial domain** The spatial domain is the one in which we live. Its terminology is that of counts per pixel, and measurements of pixel size are in millimeters or centimeters.

**Fourier transformation and frequency domain** The French mathematician Fourier demonstrated that any continuous function, such as projection profiles, in the spatial domain can be approximated within an arbitrarily determined value by a series of trigonometric functions. This process is known as *Fourier transformation*. After Fourier transformation the data are said to reside in the *frequency domain*, reflecting the periodicity of trigonometric functions. Fig. 3-5 is a frequency graph of image data after Fourier transformation. One *cycle* of a periodic function is the interval from peak to peak (Fig. 3-6). High-frequency phenomena have short cycles and vary rapidly, and low-frequency phenomena have longer cycles. The distance between maximum and minimum values in a periodic function is termed the *amplitude* (Fig. 3-6).

The advantage of working with image data in the frequency domain is the relative simplicity of the mathematical manipulations once the data have been transformed. Less computing power and computational time are required than to perform reconstructions on the raw data in the spatial domain. As computing power is becoming less expensive, this relative advantage is

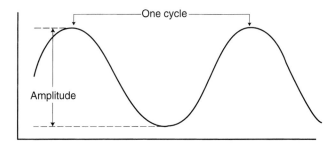

**Fig. 3-6** A periodic function. One cycle is the distance from peak to peak. Amplitude is the distance from peak to trough.

fading, and more computations may be done in the spatial domain in the future.

**Angular projection (view)** The term *angular projection,* or view, refers to the standard planar images obtained at each angle of SPECT acquisition. The SPECT raw data set typically has 60 to 120 angular projections, corresponding to angular increments between 6° and 3°, respectively. Fig. 3-7 illustrates the detector in two sampling positions.

**Projection profile (slice profile)** The angular projections exist in the computer as either $64 \times 64$ or $128 \times 128$ matrices. A projection profile, also referred to as a slice profile, represents the data in one row of the matrix. The raw data for a given tomographic slice come from all the projection profiles corresponding to that slice in the angular projection views. Thus a study with 60 angular projections yields 60 projection profiles as the input data for reconstruction of each tomographic image (Fig. 3-8).

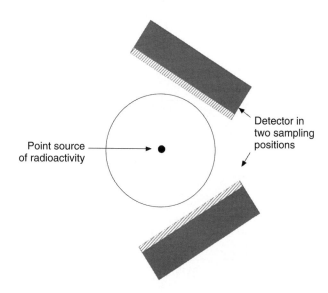

**Fig. 3-7** Point source of radioactivity with the detector illustrated in two sampling positions. Typically 60 to 120 sampling positions are used for SPECT.

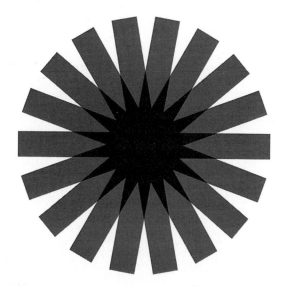

**Fig. 3-9** Star artifact resulting from simple backprojection. The star results from the multiple summations in the areas of intersection of the backprojected rays.

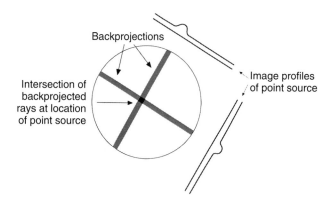

**Fig. 3-8** Simplified drawing of backprojection for two rays obtained at different sampling angles. The respective counts for the rays are projected for each pixel along their paths. Note the summation at the point of intersection.

**Ray sum** The value of each pixel in a projection profile is called the *ray sum*. It is equal to the total activity recorded from the corresponding ray perpendicular to the camera face in the plane of interest.

**Nyquist frequency** The Nyquist frequency is the highest frequency that can be resolved in the image based on the resolution characteristics of the imaging system and the parameters selected for data acquisition. For SPECT the Nyquist frequency is equal to 0.5 cycle/pixel (1 Nyquist = 0.5 cycle/pixel). The Nyquist frequency can also be expressed in cycles per centimeter. Thus for an acquisition matrix with 6 mm pixels the Nyquist frequency would equal approximately 0.8 cycle/cm (0.5 cycle/pixel = 0.5 cycle/0.6 cm = 0.8 cycle/cm). The Nyquist frequency is an important consideration in the design and selection of filters used in the tomographic reconstruction process.

**Backprojection** The concept of backprojection is fundamental to the reconstruction of tomographic images from the raw data. Backprojection takes the line data from the projection profiles and projects it back into a two-dimensional (tomographic) image. In simple backprojection in the spatial domain the count values or ray sums in each pixel of the projection profiles corresponding to a given tomographic slice are first redistributed equally along the corresponding rays (Fig. 3-8). The distribution is made equal along the ray because there is no way of telling from what depth the counts originated. In simple backprojection these recorded values for each ray from all sampling angles are added together at their intersections in the tomographic image plane. That is, at each pixel in the tomographic image plane, rays from all of the angular projections intersect, and the count value given to the pixel is the sum of the values assigned to all the rays intersecting at that point (Fig. 3-8). "Hot spots" are associated with high count values in the backprojected rays intersecting at their corresponding location. Cold spots do not contribute to counts in the individual ray projections, and the cumulative value of the corresponding summation is less.

If one performs only simple backprojection, it is obvious that satisfactory tomographic images are not obtained. Reconstructing a point source results in a "star" artifact with exaggerated borders of the point source itself and starburst ray artifacts emanating from it (Fig. 3-9).

**Filters** To solve the problem of the star artifact that arises from simple backprojection and also to address issues of background and noise, image data are "filtered." The filters are mathematical functions designed for enhancement of desired characteristics in the image, such as elimination of the star artifact, background subtraction, edge enhancement, and suppression of statistical noise. *Low-pass filters* selectively let through low frequencies and filter out high frequencies in the data; the opposite applies for *high-pass filters.* Background activity, including the star artifact, resides in the low-frequency portion of the spectrum. Statistical noise exists at all frequencies but becomes dominant at higher frequencies.

In diagrams of filter functions in the frequency domain, the amplitude is plotted on the *y*-axis and the frequency is plotted on the *x*-axis (Fig. 3-10). The frequencies and amplitudes under the filter function are "passed" by the filter. Since Fourier series are by definition infinite, a *cut-off* frequency is also defined for practical purposes and is typically equal to the Nyquist frequency. This makes sense because frequencies higher than the Nyquist frequency cannot contribute additional information to the image. Restricting the filter function to a cut-off frequency simplifies the calculations.

*Ramp filters*   As the name implies, the ramp filter has the shape of a straight line extending up from the origin when graphed in frequency space (Fig. 3-10). By inspecting the area under the curve one can see that ramp filters are high-pass filters. Ramp filters are applied in filtered backprojection reconstruction algorithms to suppress the star artifact and low-frequency noise. They also eliminate low frequencies from the signal.

*Other filters*   While the ramp filter takes care of the star artifact and low-frequency background, other filters are used to suppress high-frequency noise. Many of these filters have been named after their inventors, and such names as Butterworth, Hamming, Hanning, and Hann are frequently seen in the literature (Fig. 3-10). These low-pass filters eliminate higher frequency noise components. Too little filtering of high-frequency noise results in images with excessively grainy texture. Too much filtration of high-frequency data results in oversmoothing of images with loss of edge definition (Fig. 3-11). Areas where radioactivity concentrations change rapidly, such as the borders of organs, are represented in the high-frequency data, and oversmoothing blurs borders.

The Butterworth filter is particularly flexible because it allows the operator to select two defining parameters, the *cut-off frequency* and the *order.* The cut-off frequency is sometimes called the power of the filter and as described previously is the maximum frequency that a filter will pass. For the Butterworth filter the *order* is a parameter that controls the shape or slope of the filter.

**Reconstruction in the frequency domain**   With the foregoing concepts in hand, it is possible to describe the entire reconstruction process as it applies to filtered backprojection in frequency space or the frequency domain (Fig. 3-12). First, the individual projection profiles undergo Fourier transformation into frequency space. The transformed profiles are filtered with a ramp

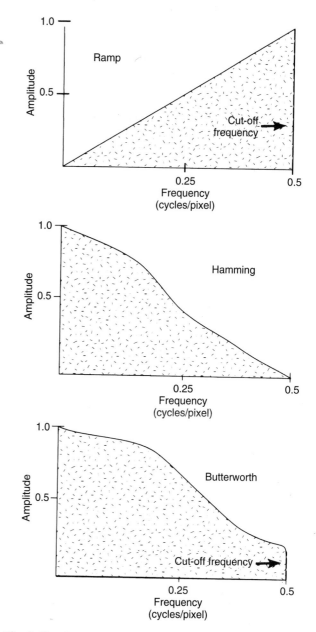

**Fig. 3-10**   Ramp, Hamming, and Butterworth filters. The ramp filter is a "high-pass" filter designed to reduce background activity and the star artifact. Hamming and Butterworth filters are "low-pass" filters designed to reduce high-frequency noise.

filter and other selected filters. (The order in which the filters are applied varies among SPECT systems, but the purpose is the same.) The filtered profiles are then summed from all projection angles akin to backprojection. Finally an inverse Fourier transform is applied to the data to create the reconstructed image in the spatial domain. Alternatively, the inverse Fourier transformation can be performed after filtration and the backprojection accomplished in the spatial domain.

**Other reconstruction techniques**   With the availability of increasing computer power, iterative methods are being explored for the reconstruction of SPECT and

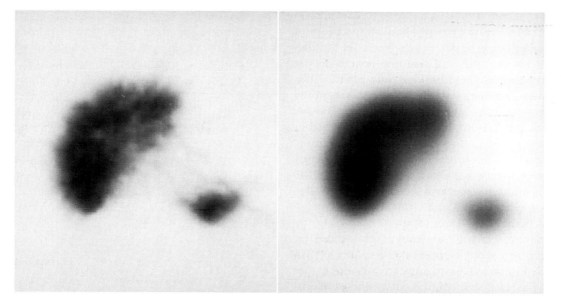

**Fig. 3-11**    Effect of different filters on the appearance of SPECT liver and spleen images. The filter on the left has resulted in excessive noise texture in the image. The filter on the right has oversmoothed the image, with loss of detail.

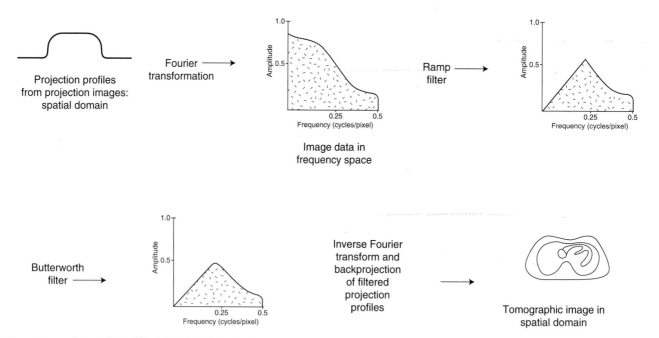

**Fig. 3-12**    Steps in filtered backprojection reconstruction for SPECT.

other tomographic images. In the iterative approach an initial set of tomograms is reconstructed. This three-dimensional data set is then used to create a new set of projection images. If the reconstruction process were perfect, the reprojection images would be identical to the initial projection images. Since this is not the case, the difference between the original projection and the reprojection based on tomographic reconstruction is used as input for another iteration of reconstruction.

This process can go on as long as is practical or until there is no further convergence between the reprojection views based on the tomographic data and the initial projection images.

Iterative reconstruction techniques offer the flexibility to include corrections for system performance (e.g., scatter correction and resolution degradations) and are finding use in various approaches to attenuation correction.

## Attenuation Correction

A special problem of SPECT imaging is the attenuation of radioactivity in tissue. Radiations arising deeper within the subject are attenuated to a greater extent than more superficial activity. Evidence is increasing that certain studies such as myocardial perfusion imaging benefit from attenuation correction. There are two fundamentally different approaches to the problem, both designed to create an image attenuation correction matrix. The value of each pixel in the attenuation correction matrix represents the correction factor that should be applied to the corresponding data in the reconstructed image.

For solid organs, such as the liver, in which an assumption of near uniform attenuation can be made, an analytical or mathematical approach such as the Chang algorithm can be used. After the object is initially reconstructed, an outline of the body part is made on the computer for each tomographic slice. From this outline the depth and therefore the appropriate correction factor for each pixel location can be computed.

The theoretical attenuation coefficient for Tc-99m in soft tissue is 0.15 per centimeter. (This applies only to "good" geometry, that is, a point source with no scatter into the ray. The observed value for Tc-99m in the abdomen is 0.12 per centimeter and in the brain is 0.13 per centimeter.) Thus, at a depth of 7 cm in a liver SPECT study, almost 60% of the corresponding activity is attenuated. The observed count value would have to be multiplied by a factor of 2.5 ($0.4 \times 2.5 = 1$) to correct for attenuation.

The major limitation of the analytical approach occurs when multiple types of tissue, each with a different attenuation coefficient, are in the field of view. Cardiac imaging is the most important example. The soft tissues of the heart and thorax are surrounded by the air-containing lungs and the bony structures of the thorax. In this setting a transmission scanning approach is used for attenuation correction. In essence a CT scan of the thorax is obtained, using a radionuclide source rather than an x-ray tube. Innumerable specific techniques have been described that use sheet sources of radioactivity, moving line sources, and arrays of line sources.

The transmission SPECT scan can be obtained either separately or simultaneously with the diagnostic SPECT scan. In the simultaneous approach a radionuclide such as gadolinium-153 (Gd-153) or cobalt-57 (Co-57) is used with a separate energy window set for the appropriate photopeak. The high-energy photopeak of Gd-153 is roughly 100 keV, and the energy of Co-57 is 122 keV. For studies using Tc-99m, correction for cross-talk caused by downscatter from the 140-keV photons is done first and then the radionuclide transmission CT image is reconstructed using the kinds of SPECT reconstruction techniques described previously. This image is then normalized and scaled for the difference between the energy of the transmission source and the 140-keV photon energy of Tc-99m. The resulting image is an attenuation map of the thorax that can be applied pixel by pixel to correct for the effects of attenuation.

It is hoped that this approach will address two lingering problems with cardiac SPECT. For men, scans often show spuriously decreased activity in the inferior wall, possibly resulting from attenuation by overlapping organs beneath the diaphragm. For women, overlying breast tissue can significantly distort SPECT data by differential attenuation.

## Image Reformatting: Transaxial, Sagittal, Coronal, and Oblique Views

A particular advantage of gamma camera rotational SPECT is that a volume of image data is collected at one time. This permits the acquisition of multiple tomographic slices simultaneously and the registration of the data between planes. Interslice filtering is also used to reduce artifacts in reformatted data. In addition to the standard transaxial images, other image planes that have special relevance to the organ of interest can be reconstructed.

The resorting or reformatting approach is particularly valuable in cardiac imaging (Fig. 3-13). The orientation of the heart varies among patients. The heart usually has a horizontal orientation in shorter subjects and a more vertical orientation in taller ones. Ideally, image planes both perpendicular and parallel to the long axis of the heart would be available. This is readily accomplished with a volume data set. The computer operator defines the geometry of the long axis of the heart. The computer is programmed to resort the data to create cardiac long-axis and short-axis planes oblique to the transaxial slices. The optimum angulation is highly variable among patients, reflecting the differing orientation of the heart.

A useful strategy is to reproject the tomographic data as a sequence of planar images having the same fields of view as the original angled sampling images. Viewing the reconstructed projection images in cinematic mode gives an excellent three-dimensional display of the data. An additional advantage of using the reconstructed data is that overlying structures can be removed before the data are reprojected and selected features in the data can be emphasized. For example, in Tc-99m pyrophosphate imaging of the heart the ribs can be subtracted from the three-dimensional data set before the data are reprojected. The ribs no longer obscure the cardiac activity. Another advantage of using reprojection rather than tomographic images is that this techniques provides a better overall orientation of the heart in the chest.

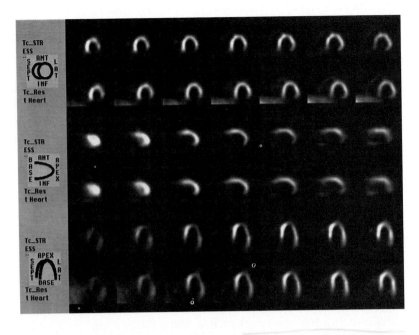

**Fig. 3-13** Cardiac SPECT images from a Tc-99m sestamibi study illustrating the ability to reformat data into multiple planes. The top two rows are short-axis views obtained perpendicular to the long axis of the left ventricle. The middle two rows are horizontal long-axis images, and the bottom two rows are vertical long-axis images. The patient has a large fixed perfusion defect involving the inferior wall of the left ventricle. The ability to reformat the data allows more precise and accurate localization of abnormalities.

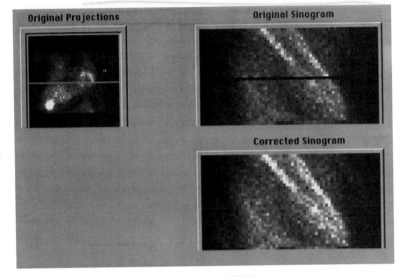

**Fig. 3-14** Sinogram from a myocardial perfusion study. The sinogram corresponds to the level of the cursor in the image on the left. Note the regular progression in the data across the projection profiles, indicating stability and lack of unwanted movement of the heart from one projection view to the next.

A maximum intensity projection scan (MIPS) can be created by reprojecting the hottest point along each particular ray for any given projection. These MIPS images emphasize areas of abnormally increased accumulation while providing a better overall orientation of the abnormality to the skeleton than do individual tomographic slices. Looking at individual transaxial tomograms can be confusing without knowing a lesion's location relative to surrounding structures.

## Quality Assurance

The projection data from all SPECT scans should be inspected before image reconstruction. Excessive patient motion degrades the quality of SPECT scans because of misregistration of data in the different angular projections. Patient motion can be assessed in a number of ways. When the angular unprocessed projections are viewed in a cinematic closed loop display, excessive patient motion is readily detected as a flicker or discontinuity in the display. Some laboratories use radioactive marker sources placed on the patient to assess motion. Another approach is to view a sinogram of a slice. Sinograms are constructed by placing the projection profiles for a given tomographic slice in a stack. The borders of the sinogram should be smooth, and interslice changes in intensity should be small; any discontinuity indicates motion of the patient (Figs. 3-14 and 3-15). Only up-and-down motion can be corrected.

Rotational SPECT requires maximum performance from the gamma camera. All standard quality control procedures are observed, as well as several additional

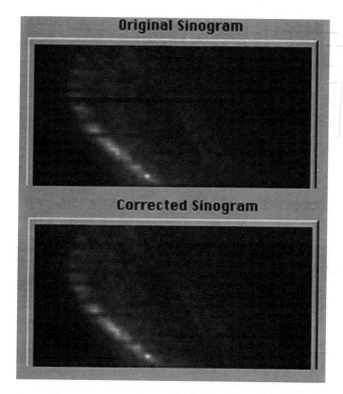

**Fig. 3-15**   Sinogram illustrating multiple gaps in the sequential profile data. Compare these discontinuities with the regular progression of data in Fig. 3-14. The discontinuities indicate unwanted motion of the object from one sampling position to the next.

| PARAMETER | COMMENT |
|---|---|
| **Box 3-2   Selected Quality Assurance Issues in Single-Photon Emission Computed Tomography** | |
| Center of rotation | Center of rotation should match center of image matrix in the computer; look for horizontal shift on $x$-axis |
| Pixel size | $x$ and $y$ dimensions should be equal; any change in pixel size requires recalibration of attenuation correction factors |
| Uniformity | Counts of 3 million for routine intrinsic and extrinsic uniformity checks; 30 million for input for uniformity correction |
| Spatial resolution and linearity | Weekly per usual gamma camera quality control |
| Detector head alignment | Camera face parallel to axis of rotation |
| Head matching | Alignment of multiple heads for correct event localization |

points (Box 3-2). The alignment of the detector, gantry, and imaging table is critical. In transaxial rotation the basic assumption is that the face of the collimator is truly parallel to the axis of rotation. If it is off axis, the tilted field of view of the collimator will result in misregistered data. Similarly, for multihead cameras the detector heads must be aligned with each other for correct registration of data.

Another fundamental assumption is that the center of rotation corresponds to the center of the image matrix in the computer. If the center of rotation is offset, it manifests first as degradation in resolution and, if severe enough, as ring artifacts in the reconstructed images.

The gamma camera–computer interface is particularly important in rotational SPECT. The pixel size must be carefully calibrated. Attenuation correction depends on depth estimates, and a change in pixel size will change distance and therefore attenuation correction factors. Pixel size is adjusted by the setting of the analog-to-digital converters and should be checked in both the $x$ and $y$ dimensions. Pixel width should be identical in the $x$ and $y$ directions. The $y$-axis determines slice thickness, and a difference in $x$ and $y$ pixel dimensions will create problems in reformatting image data into oblique planes. The importance of the center of rotation is discussed in

the preceding paragraph. A shift in the performance of the analog-to-digital converters can result in movement of the center of rotation.

Field uniformity corrections are critical in SPECT imaging. Detector nonuniformity results in bull's-eye or ring artifacts. The usual 1 million to 5 million count flood image obtained for planar imaging is inadequate for uniformity correction in SPECT imaging. For large-field-of-view cameras and a $64 \times 64$ matrix, 30 million counts are acquired or roughly 10,000 counts per pixel in the image to achieve the desired relative standard deviation of 1%. This can also be written as:

$$\frac{SD}{N} \times 100\% = 1\%$$

Acquiring this number of counts requires a significant amount of time. The temptation to use very large amounts of radioactivity should be avoided because high count rates can also result in degraded performance of gamma camera electronics and in the recording of spurious coincidence events. Conservatively, the correction floods should be obtained at 20,000 counts/sec or less. The radioactivity in the flood itself must have a uniformity within 1%. Water-filled sources are subject to problems of incomplete mixing and introduction of air bubbles, as well as bulging of the container. For these reasons Co-57 sheet sources are more convenient and more reliable than water-filled sources.

## SINGLE-PHOTON EMISSION COMPUTED TOMOGRAPHY AT 511 KEV; "SINGLE-PHOTON POSITRON EMISSION TOMOGRAPHY"

In the past several years the feasibility of imaging positron-emitting radionuclides with SPECT systems has been widely explored. The use of this approach has been established with greatest applicability to studies of the heart and certain tumors using fluorine-18 fluoro-deoxy-glucose (F-18 FDG).

Special high-energy collimators have been fabricated and are commercially available for most SPECT systems. These collimators have thick septa to absorb off-angle and scattered photons, but they reduce the sensitivity for photon recording.

The clinical utility of "single-photon PET" is under active investigation. F-18 FDG studies of the myocardium are clearly feasible. Current experience also indicates a reasonable level of efficacy for tumor imaging, but there are limitations in visualizing smaller lesions. Simultaneous dual-tracer imaging with F-18 FDG and Tc-99m sestamibi is described in Chapter 5.

Systems incorporating coincidence detection circuitry have been developed for dual-headed SPECT devices. This approach aims to replace the special heavy 511-keV collimators with "electronic" collimation, which results in significant improvements in count rate sensitivity. Spatial resolution is also improved when coincidence detection is used.

## POSITRON EMISSION TOMOGRAPHY

PET is a kind of tomography made possible by the unique fate of positrons. When positrons undergo annihilation by combining with negatively charged electrons, two 511-keV gamma rays are given off in opposite directions 180° apart. In contrast to SPECT imaging, which detects single events, in PET imaging two detector elements on opposite sides of the subject are used to detect paired annihilation photons (Fig. 3-16).

### Instrumentation

Instrumentation for PET has undergone several generations of development. Early systems had a single ring with multiple detectors and generated a single tomographic section at a time. Each detector in the ring was typically paired with multiple other detectors on the opposite side of the detector ring. These detectors or this arc of detectors is selected to encompass the field of view of the object or organ being imaged (Fig. 3-17).

Multiple-ring systems were rapidly developed. Early

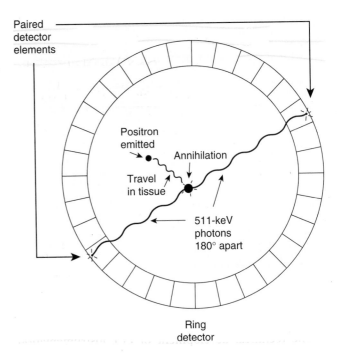

**Fig. 3-16**   PET ring detector. After emission, positrons travel a short distance in tissue before the annihilation event. The 511-keV protons are given off 180° apart.

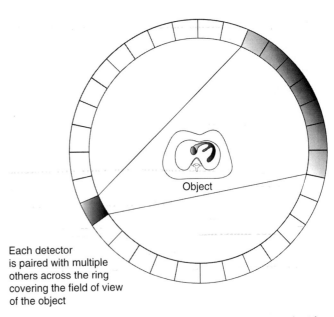

**Fig. 3-17**   In the PET tomograph, each detector is paired with multiple detectors on the opposite side of the ring to create an arc encompassing the object. This multiple-pairing strategy increases the sensitivity of the device.

systems with three to eight rings of detectors typically had septa inserted between the tomographic planes to shield the detectors from cross-talk from activity arising outside of the plane of interest. These multiple-ring systems with septa inserted between the tomo-

**Table 3-1   Characteristics of positron emission tomography detector materials**

| Material | Density | Effective Z | Delay time (nsec) |
|---|---|---|---|
| Bismuth germanate oxide (BGO) | 7.13 | 74 | 300 |
| Barium fluoride (BaF₂) | 4.89 | 54 | <1 |
| Cesium fluoride (CsF) | 4.64 | 53 | 3 |
| Leutetium oxyorthosilicate (LSO) | 7.40 | 66 | 40 |
| Sodium iodide (NaI [T1]) | 3.67 | 50 | 230 |

graphic planes are often referred to as "two-dimensional" systems.

The technical development of PET instrumentation has now reached the point that systems have as many as 32 rings of detectors with the capability of creating a simultaneous tomographic section for each ring and an additional section between each pair of rings for a total of 63 simultaneously acquired tomographic images. Contemporary systems have retractable septa between the planes and with the septa retracted are referred to as "three-dimensional" systems. This design greatly increases system sensitivity. The concept of pairing each detector with multiple detectors on the opposite side of the ring has been retained with these systems and extended to pairings between different rings.

**Gantry size**   Similar to the history of x-ray, CT, and magnetic resonance imaging, the first PET scanners were designed for head imaging. The early PET systems had a typical diameter of 60 cm. Current systems are suitable for head and body imaging, and the typical diameter is 100 cm.

**Detector materials**   The density and effective atomic number, Z, for NaI (Tl) crystals are not ideal for "stopping" or detecting the 511-keV gamma rays used in PET imaging. Bismuth germanate (BGO) is approximately twice as dense, with an effective Z of 74, compared with an effective Z of 50 for NaI (Tl). BGO detectors have been used extensively in PET imaging applications for this reason. Other detector materials that have found application include cesium fluoride and barium fluoride. These have much faster resolution than BGO but are not as dense (Table 3-1).

A new detector material, leutetium orthosilicate, has been evaluated. It combines the high density of BGO with far better time resolution and superior light yield. This material shows promise as the detector material of choice for the future.

**Coincidence detection**   Special circuitry in the PET tomograph allows detection of coincidence events from the two gamma ray photons given off by a single positron annihilation event. The coincidence window is on the order of 10 nsec. Thus, when events are registered in paired detectors within 10 nsec of each other, they are accepted as true coincidence events. If a recorded event is not matched by a paired event within the coincidence time window, the data are discarded. This approach effectively provides "electronic collimation" to define the tomographic image planes. By not having to physically collimate the detector elements, PET tomographs offer much higher sensitivity than would otherwise be the case.

One of the problems in the coincidence approach is the presence of paired random events that appear to the detection circuitry as paired annihilation photons (Fig. 3-18). As the amount of radioactivity in the field of view increases and the count rate increases, the number of falsely recorded paired random events also increases. Paired random events are two photons arising from two different positron annihilation events and are therefore not useful in reconstructing the true location of tracer distribution.

**Spatial resolution**   The spatial resolution of modern PET tomographs is excellent. Specialized experimental devices approach 1.5-mm resolution (full width half measure [FWHM]) as measured by a line source in air. Resolution under clinical scanning conditions is superior in PET compared with SPECT. Resolution for clinical studies is in the 4- to 6-mm FWHM range with high-end contemporary PET scanners.

The ultimate spatial resolution of PET is limited by two physical phenomena related to positrons and their annihilation. First, positrons are given off at different kinetic energies. Energetic positrons such as those given off in the decay of oxygen-15 (O-15), Ga-68, and rubidium-82 (Rb-82) may travel several millimeters in tissue before undergoing annihilation (Fig. 3-16). Thus the detected location of the annihilation event is some distance from the actual location of the radionuclide. This travel in tissue degrades the ability to truly localize the biodistribution of the radioactive agent in the patient.

The second phenomenon limiting resolution is the noncolinearity of the annihilation photons. In addition to the energy equivalent of the rest mass of two electrons, the annihilation event incorporates residual kinetic energies of the positron and the negative electron with which it combines. This results in a small deviation from true colinearity along a single ray (Fig. 3-18). The angle by which the gamma rays depart from the theoretical 180° colinearity results in a 2- to 3-mm spatial uncertainty in event localization for head and body ring detectors used clinically.

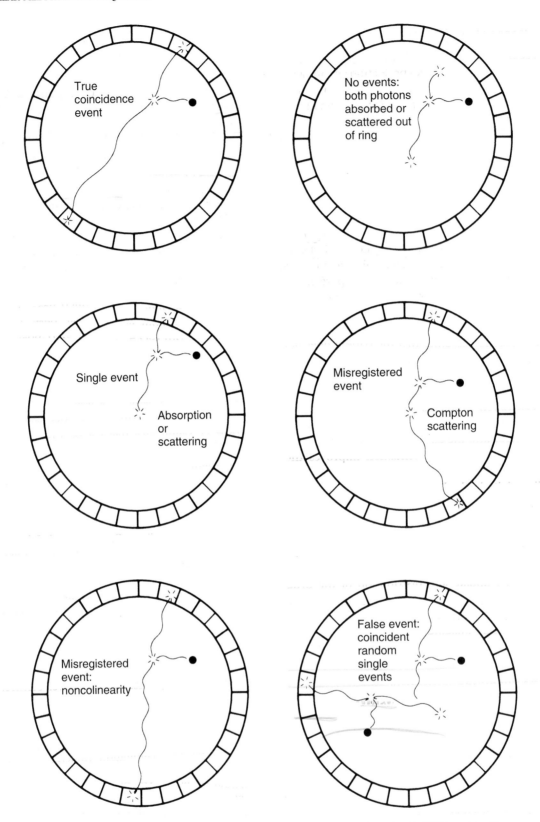

**Fig. 3-18**    The different possibilities in positron decay and event detection in PET imaging. The wanted event is a true coincidence event. Single events are easily rejected but contribute to processor dead time. Misregistered events caused by noncolinearity are difficult to discriminate. "False events" may be incorrectly accepted if the two photons are intercepted in paired detectors.

## Image Reconstruction

Image reconstruction in PET uses many of the same principles as SPECT. Filtered backprojection and iterative reconstruction algorithms have both found application. In three-dimensional systems, cross-plane information is incorporated into the "in-plane" or "direct plane" data.

**Attenuation correction and quantitative analysis** A unique and important characteristic of PET is the ability to correct for attenuation of the 511-keV gamma rays in tissue. The basis of this ability is the fact that attenuation and therefore coincidence detection of positron annihilation are independent of the location along a given ray between opposite detectors. Since the total amount of tissue traversed by the two photons is a constant for each ray, the correction factor for each coincidence line can be determined empirically by performing a transmission scan. The observed count rate obtained along each ray during the actual scan is corrected by dividing it by the attenuation factor. This approach to attenuation correction assumes that the patient does not move between the transmission scan and the emission scan. Techniques for performing simultaneous emission and transmission scanning have been developed to eliminate the registration problems. The transmission scan must have sufficient counting statistics to avoid introducing statistical error into the data.

The ability to correct for attenuation improves the quality of PET images and permits absolute quantification of radioactivity in the body. Quantitative analysis is the basis for numerous metabolic, perfusion, and biodistribution measurements. For example, a therapeutic drug can be radiolabeled with a positron-emitting radionuclide. With knowledge of the specific activity of the radiolabeled drug and the ability to correct for attenuation, the absolute uptake and distribution of the drug can be quantitatively measured. Box 3-3 summarizes several of the important quantitative measurements used in applications of PET imaging.

---

### Box 3-3   Selected Quantitative Measurements by Positron Emission Tomography

Regional (absolute) radionuclide localization
pH
Blood flow
Blood volume
Oxygen extraction fraction
Oxygen metabolism
Glucose metabolism
Receptor binding and occupancy

---

## Comparison of Positron Emission Tomography and Single-Photon Emission Computed Tomography

The advantages of PET are superior sensitivity and resolution and a far greater flexibility of incorporating positron labels into biomolecules. PET scanners are considerably more expensive than SPECT systems and also require the presence of an on-site cyclotron for a full range of applications.

SPECT has significant cost advantages. SPECT systems are smaller and easier to place within hospitals. SPECT has a singular advantage in being applicable to the most commonly performed procedures in nuclear medicine, including myocardial perfusion imaging with either thallium-201 (Tl-201) or Tc-99m and oncological imaging with Ga-67 citrate.

### SUGGESTED READINGS

Celler A, Sitek A, Stoub E, et al: Multiple line source array for SPECT transmission scans: simulation, phantom and patient studies, *J Nucl Med* 39:2183-2189, 1998.

Chandra R: *Nuclear medicine physics: the basics,* ed 5, Baltimore, 1998, Williams & Wilkins.

Freeman LM, Blauflox MD, editors: The coming age of PET (part 1), *Semin Nucl Med,* vol 28, 1998.

Freeman LM, Blaufox MD, editors: The coming age of PET (part 2), *Semin Nucl Med,* vol 28, 1998.

Hichwa RD: Production of PET radioisotopes and principles of PET imaging. In Henkin RE, editor: *Nuclear medicine,* St Louis, 1996, Mosby, pp 279-291.

Patton JA, Rollo FD: Basic physics of radionuclide imaging. In Freeman LM, editor: *Freeman and Johnson's clinical radionuclide imaging,* ed 3, New York, 1984, Grune & Stratton.

Patton JA, Turkington TG: Coincidence imaging with a dual-head scintillation camera, *J Nucl Med* 40:4432-4441, 1999.

Phelps ME, Mazziotta JC, Schelbert HR, editors: *Positron emission tomography and autoradiography: principles and application for the brain and heart,* New York, 1986, Raven Press.

Powsner RA, Powsner ER: *Essentials of nuclear medicine physics,* Malden, Mass, 1998, Blackwell Science.

Reivich M, Alavi A, editors: *Positron emission tomography,* New York, 1985, Alan R Liss.

Rollo FD, editor: *Nuclear medicine physics, instrumentation and agents,* St Louis, 1977, Mosby.

Simmons GH: *The scintillation camera,* New York, 1988, Society of Nuclear Medicine.

Sorenson JA, Phelps ME: *Physics in nuclear medicine,* ed 2, Philadelphia, 1987, WB Saunders.

Votaw JR: The AAPM/RSNA physics tutorial for residents: physics of PET, *Radiographics* 15:1179-1190, 1995.

Yester MV: Theory of tomographic reconstruction. In Henkin RE, editor: *Nuclear medicine,* St Louis, 1996, Mosby, pp 222-231.

*- Drug Interactions.*
*- Paed. dosing.*

The richness of diagnostic capability in nuclear medicine rests largely on the diversity of available radiopharmaceuticals. In some sense the "best" radiopharmaceuticals are those that truly portray the physiological or pathological system under investigation. The historical term *tracer* is a rather good one because it implies the ability to study or follow a process without disturbing the process. Radiopharmaceuticals have the highly desirable property that they do not perturb function, unlike some other types of diagnostic drugs, including iodinated x-ray contrast media, that have profound physiological effects when administered intravascularly.

Most radiopharmaceuticals are a combination of a radioactive component that permits external detection and a biologically active moiety or drug component that is responsible for biodistribution. For a few agents, such as the radioactive inert gases, the radioiodines, gallium-67 (Ga-67), and thallium-201 (Tl-201), the radioactive atoms themselves confer the desired localization properties and a larger chemical component is not required.

Box 4-1 summarizes some of the important mechanisms of localization for radiopharmaceuticals used in clinical practice. Understanding the mechanism or rationale for the use of each agent is critical to understanding the normal and pathological findings demonstrated scintigraphically. There is great flexibility in designing radiopharmaceuticals for specific diagnostic purposes because both naturally occurring molecules and synthetic molecules can be radiolabeled.

Radiopharmaceuticals for each major clinical application are considered in detail in chapters on the respective organ systems. This chapter presents some of the general principles of radiopharmaceutical production, radiolabeling, quality assurance, and dispensing.

## Box 4-1   Mechanisms of Radiopharmaceutical Localization

| MECHANISM | APPLICATIONS OR EXAMPLES |
|---|---|
| Compartmental localization | Blood pool imaging, direct cystography |
| Passive diffusion (concentration dependent) | Blood-brain barrier breakdown, glomerular filtration, cisternography |
| Capillary blockade (physical entrapment) | Arterial perfusion imaging |
| Physical leakage from a luminal compartment | Gastrointestinal bleeding, detection of urinary tract or biliary system leakage |
| Metabolism | Glucose, fatty acids |
| Active transport (active cellular uptake) | Hepatobiliary imaging, renal tubular function, thyroid and adrenal imaging |
| Chemical bonding and adsorption | Skeletal imaging |
| Cell sequestration | Splenic imaging (heat-damaged red blood cells), white blood cells |
| Receptor binding and storage | Numerous applications in positron emission tomography, adrenal medullary imaging |
| Phagocytosis | Reticuloendothelial system imaging |
| Antigen/antibody | Tumor imaging |

**Combined Mechanisms**

| | |
|---|---|
| Perfusion and active transport | Myocardial imaging |
| Active transport and metabolism | Thyroid uptake and imaging |
| Active transport and secretion | Hepatobiliary imaging, salivary gland imaging |

## TERMINOLOGY: RADIOPHARMACEUTICALS, RADIOCHEMICALS, AND RADIONUCLIDES

The terminology in nuclear pharmacy can be confusing. The term *radionuclide* refers only to the radioactive atoms. When a radionuclide is combined with a chemical molecule to confer desired localization properties, the combination is referred to as a *radiochemical*. The term *radiopharmaceutical* is reserved for radioactive materials that have met legal requirements for administration to patients or subjects. This often necessitates the addition of stabilizing and buffering agents to the basic radiochemical and in the United States requires approval by the Food and Drug Administration (FDA) before an agent is acceptable for routine clinical use.

The term *carrier-free* implies that a radionuclide is not contaminated by either stable or radioactive nuclides of the same element. The presence of carrier material can influence biodistribution and efficiency of radiolabeling. The term *specific activity* refers to the radioactivity per unit weight (mCi/mg). Carrier-free samples of a radionuclide have the highest specific activity. "Specific activity" should not be confused with *specific concentration*, which is defined as activity per unit volume (mCi/ml).

## Design Characteristics of Radiopharmaceuticals

Certain characteristics are desirable in the design of radiopharmaceuticals. Regarding the radioactive label, these include gamma emissions of suitable energy and abundance for external detection. Energies between 100 and 200 keV are ideal for the gamma camera. The effective half-life should be long enough for the intended application, and ideal radiolabels do not emit particulate radiations. The specific activity should be high. Technetium-99m (Tc-99m) is popular as a radiolabel because it closely matches these desirable features.

Regarding the pharmaceutical component, desirable characteristics include suitable biodistribution for the intended application and absence of toxicity or secondary effects. The overall radiopharmaceutical should not dissociate in vitro or in vivo, should be readily available or easily compounded, and should have a reasonable cost.

## PRODUCTION OF RADIONUCLIDES

All radionuclides in clinical use today are produced either in nuclear reactors or in cyclotrons or other types of accelerators. Naturally occurring radionuclides have long half-lives and are heavy, toxic elements; they include uranium, actinium, thorium, radium, and radon. They have no clinical role in diagnostic nuclear medicine.

Bombardment of medium–atomic weight nuclides with low-energy neutrons in nuclear reactors results in neutron-rich radionuclides that typically undergo beta minus decay. This reaction is referred to as *neutron activation.* Since the daughter product is the same element, the radioactive and stable atoms cannot be separated, typically resulting in a low–specific activity product with significant *carrier* from the original target material. Neutron activation of molybdenum-98 (Mo-98) was the original production method used to obtain Mo-99 for Mo-99/Tc-99m generator systems.

Neutron bombardment of enriched uranium-235 (U-235) results in fission products in the middle of the atomic chart. For example, Mo-99 is now obtained through such a fission reaction. The uncontrolled release of radioactive iodines in atomic bomb explosions and during accidents at nuclear power plants is a well-known phenomenon that can also be used for production purposes under controlled conditions in a nuclear reactor.

Proton bombardment of a wide variety of target nuclides in cyclotrons or other special accelerators produces proton-rich radionuclides that undergo positron decay or electron capture. Tables 4-1 and 4-2 summarize the production source and physical charac-

**Table 4-1  Physical characteristics of single-photon radionuclides used in clinical nuclear medicine**

| Radionuclide | Principal mode of decay | Physical half-life | Principal photon energy (keV) and abundance | Production method |
|---|---|---|---|---|
| Molybdenum-99 | Beta minus | 2.8 days | 740 (12%) 780 (4%) | Reactor |
| Technetium-99m | Isomeric transition | 6 hr | 140 (89%) | Generator (molybdenum-99) |
| Iodine-131 | Beta minus | 8 days | 364 (81%) | Reactor |
| Iodine-123 | Electron capture | 13.2 hr | 159 (83%) | Accelerator |
| Gallium-67 | Electron capture | 78.3 hr | 93 (37%) 185 (20%) 300 (17%) 395 (5%) | Accelerator |
| Thallium-201 | Electron capture | 73.1 hr | 69-83 (Hg x-rays) 135 (2.5%) 167 (10%) | Accelerator |
| Indium-111 | Electron capture | 2.8 days | 171 (90%) 245 (94%) | Accelerator |
| Xenon-127 | Electron capture | 36 days | 172 (26%) 203 (7%) 375 (17%) | Accelerator |
| Xenon-133 | Beta minus | 5.2 days | 81 (37%) | Reactor |
| Cobalt-57 | Electron capture | 272 days | 122 (86%) | Accelerator |

**Table 4-2  Physical characteristics of positron-emitting (dual-photon) radionuclides used in nuclear medicine**

| Radionuclide | Physical half-life (min) | Positron energy (MeV) | Range in soft tissue (mm) | Production method |
|---|---|---|---|---|
| Carbon-11 | 20 | 0.96 | 4.1 | Accelerator |
| Nitrogen-13 | 10 | 1.19 | 5.4 | Accelerator |
| Oxygen-15 | 2 | 1.73 | 7.3 | Accelerator |
| Fluorine-18 | 110 | 0.635 | 2.4 | Accelerator |
| Gallium-68 | 68 | 1.9 | 8.1 | Generator (germanium-68) |
| Rubidium-82 | 1.3 | 3.15 | 15.0 | Generator (strontium-82) |

teristics of commonly used radionuclides in clinical nuclear medicine practice.

## RADIONUCLIDE GENERATORS

One of the practical issues faced in nuclear medicine is the desirability of using relatively short-lived agents (hours versus days or weeks) and at the same time the need to have radiopharmaceuticals delivered to hospitals or clinics from commercial sources. One way around this dilemma is the use of radionuclide generator systems. These systems consist of a longer-lived parent and a shorter-lived daughter. With this combination of half-lives, the generator can be shipped from a commercial vendor and the daughter product will still have a reasonable half-life for clinical applications. Although a number of generator systems have been explored over the years (Table 4-3), the most important generator is the Mo-99/Tc-99m system, which is ubiquitous in the practice of clinical nuclear medicine (Table 4-4).

## MOLYBDENUM-99/TECHNETIUM-99m GENERATOR SYSTEMS

The historical production method for Mo-99 was a neutron activation reaction on Mo-98:

$$Mo\text{-}98 \ (n,\gamma) \rightarrow Mo\text{-}99$$

This production method results in low specific activity, requiring a large ion exchange column to hold both the desired Mo-99 and the carrier Mo-98 left over from the target material. The low–specific activity column resulted in low specific concentrations of Tc-99m pertechnetate from generator elution because of the larger volume of eluant needed for complete removal of the Tc-99m activity.

Mo-99 is now produced by the fission of U-235. (The product is often referred to casually as "fission moly.") The reaction is:

$$U\text{-}235 \ (n,fission) \rightarrow Mo\text{-}99$$

After Mo-99 is produced in the fission reaction, it is chemically purified and passed on to an anion exchange column composed of alumina ($Al_2O_3$) (Table 4-4). The column is typically adjusted to an acid pH to promote binding. The positive charge of the alumina binds the molybdate ions firmly.

The loaded column is placed in a lead container with tubing attached at each end to permit column elution. Commercial generator systems are autoclaved, and the elution dynamics is quality controlled before shipment. Alternatively, systems may be aseptically assembled from previously sterilized components.

### Generator Operation and Yield

Fig. 4-1 illustrates the relationship between Mo-99 decay and the ingrowth of Tc-99m. Maximum buildup of Tc-99m activity occurs at 23 hours after elution. This is convenient, especially if sufficient Tc-99m activity is available to accomplish each day's work. Otherwise the generator can be eluted, or "milked," more than once a day. Partial elution is also illustrated in Fig. 4-1. Fifty percent of maximum is reached in approximately 4½ hours, and 75% of maximum is available at 8½ hours.

| Table 4-3 | Radionuclide generator systems and parent and daughter half-lives | | | |
| --- | --- | --- | --- | --- |
| **Parent** | **Parent's half-life** | **Daughter** | **Daughter's half-life** | |
| Molybdenum-99 | 66 hr | Technetium-99m | 6 hr | |
| Rubidium-81 | 4.5 hr | Krypton-81m | 13 sec | |
| Germanium-68 | 270 days | Gallium-68 | 68 min | |
| Strontium-82 | 25 days | Rubidium-82 | 1.3 min | |
| Tin-113 | 115 days | Indium-113m | 1.7 hr | |
| Yttrium-87 | 3.3 days | Strontium-87m | 2.8 hr | |
| Tellurium-132 | 3.2 days | Iodine-132 | 2.3 hr | |

| Table 4-4 | Molybdenum-99 (Mo-99)/technetium-99m (Tc-99m) generator systems | |
| --- | --- | --- |
| | **Parent (Mo-99)** | **Daughter (Tc-99m)** |
| **RADIONUCLIDES** | | |
| Half-life | 66 hr | 6 hr |
| Mode of decay | Beta minus | Isomeric transition |
| Daughter products | Tc-99m Tc-99 | Tc-99 |
| Principal photon energies* | 740 keV 780 keV | 140 keV (89%) |
| **GENERATOR FUNCTION** | | |
| Composition of ion exchange column | $Al_2O_3$ | |
| Eluant | Normal saline (0.9%) | |
| Time from elution to maximum daughter yield | 23 hr | |

*The decay scheme for Mo-99 is complex, with over 35 gamma rays of different energies given off. The listed energies are those used in clinical practice for radionuclidic purity checks.

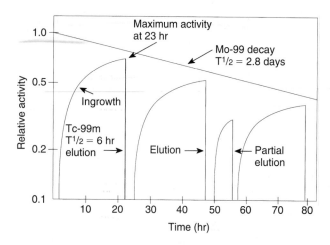

**Fig. 4-1** Decay curve for molybdenum-99 and ingrowth curves for technetium-99m illustrating successive elutions, including a partial elution. Relative activity is plotted on a logarithmic scale, accounting for the straight line of Mo-99 decay.

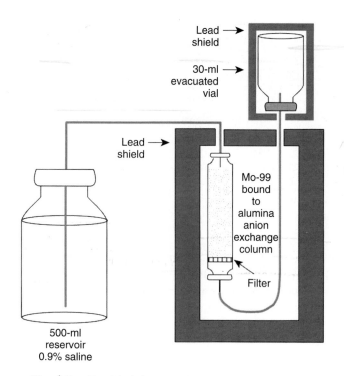

**Fig. 4-2** Simplified drawing of a "wet" generator system.

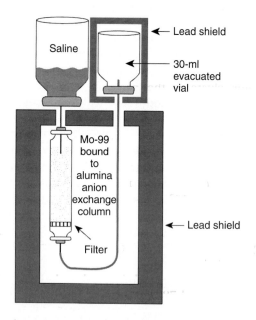

**Fig. 4-3** Simplified drawing of a "dry" generator system.

Although greatest attention is paid to the rate of Tc-99m buildup, it should also be remembered that Tc-99m is constantly decaying, with buildup of Tc-99 in the generator. Generators received after commercial shipment or generators that have not been eluted for several days have significant carrier Tc-99 in the eluate. Because the carrier Tc-99 behaves chemically in an identical fashion to Tc-99m, it can adversely affect radiopharmaceutical labeling. Many labeling procedures require the reduction of Tc-99m from a +7 valence state to a lower valence state. If the eluate contains sufficient carrier Tc-99, complete reduction may not occur, with resultant poor labeling and undesired radiochemical contaminants in the final preparation.

There are two basic types of generator systems with respect to elution. "Wet" systems are provided with a reservoir of normal saline (0.9%) (Fig. 4-2). Elution is accomplished by placing a special sterile vacuum vial on the exit or collection port. The vacuum vial is designed to draw the appropriate amount of saline across the column.

In "dry" systems a volume-calibrated saline charge is placed on the entry port and a vacuum vial is placed on the collection port (Fig. 4-3). The vacuum draws the saline eluant out of the original vial, across the column, and into the elution vial. Elution volumes are typically in the range of 5 to 20 ml. Elutions can be performed for add-on or emergency studies that come up in the course of a day (Fig. 4-1).

From Fig. 4-1 it is obvious that the amount of Tc-99m activity available from a generator decreases each day as a result of decay of the Mo-99 parent. In practice the 2.8-day half-life of Mo-99 allows generators to be used for 2 weeks, although many larger nuclear medicine operations require two generator deliveries per week.

## Quality Control

Although generators are rigorously quality controlled before commercial shipment, it is important that each laboratory perform quality control steps each time the generator is eluted (Table 4-5). These quality control steps are good medical practice and are necessary to meet various regulations and guidelines of the federal

**Table 4-5    Purity checks: molybdenum-99 (Mo-99)/technetium-99m (Tc-99m) generator systems**

| | Problem | Standard |
|---|---|---|
| Radionuclidic purity | Excessive Mo-99 in eluant | <0.15 $\mu$Ci Mo-99/ mCi Tc-99m *at time of dosage administration* |
| Chemical purity | Al$^2$O$_3$ from generator ion exchange column in elution | <10 $\mu$g/ml (fission generator) (aurin tricarboxylic acid spot test) |
| Radiochemical purity | Reduced oxidation states of Tc-99m (i.e., +4, +5, or +6 instead of +7) | 95% of Tc-99m activity should be in +7 oxidation state |

**Table 4-6    Physical decay of technetium-99m**

| Time (hr) | Fraction remaining |
|---|---|
| 0 | 1.000 |
| 1 | .891 |
| 2 | .794 |
| 3 | .708 |
| 4 | .631 |
| 5 | .532 |
| 6 | .501 |
| 7 | .447 |
| 8 | .398 |
| 9 | .355 |
| 10 | .316 |
| 11 | .282 |
| 12 | .251 |

Tc-99m physical half-life = 6.02 hours.

government and the Joint Commission on Healthcare Organizations (JCAHO).

**Radionuclidic purity**    The only desired radionuclide in the Mo-99/Tc-99m generator eluate is Tc-99m. Any other radionuclide in the sample is considered a radionuclidic impurity and is undesirable, since it will result in additional radiation exposure to the patient without clinical benefit.

The most common radionuclidic contaminant in the generator eluate is the parent radionuclide, Mo-99. Tc-99, the daughter product of the isomeric transition of Tc-99m, is also present but is not considered an impurity or contaminant. Although Tc-99 can be a problem from a chemical standpoint in radiolabeling procedures, it is not a problem from a radiation or health standpoint and is not tested for as a radionuclidic impurity. The half-life of Tc-99 is $2.1 \times 10^5$ years. It decays to ruthenium-99, which is stable.

The amount of Mo-99 in the eluate is subject to limits set by the Nuclear Regulatory Commission (NRC) and must be tested on each elution. Perhaps the easiest and most widely used approach is to take advantage of the energetic 740- and 780-keV gamma rays of Mo-99 with dual counting of the specimen. In brief, the generator eluate is placed in a lead container carefully designed so that all of the 140-keV photons of technetium are absorbed but approximately 50% of the more energetic Mo-99 gamma rays can penetrate. Adjusting the dose calibrator to the Mo-99 setting provides an estimate of the number of microcuries of Mo-99 in the sample. The unshielded sample is then measured on the Tc-99m setting, and a ratio of Mo-99 to Tc-99m activity can be calculated.

The NRC limit is 0.15 $\mu$Ci of Mo-99 activity per 1 mCi of Tc-99m activity in the *administered* dose (Table 4-5).

Because the half-life of Mo-99 is longer than that of Tc-99m, the ratio actually increases with time. This is rarely a problem, but if the initial reading shows near maximum Mo-99 levels, either the actual dose to be given to the patient should be restudied before administration or the buildup factor should be computed mathematically. From a practical standpoint the Mo-99 activity may be taken as unchanged and the Tc-99m decay calculated (Table 4-6). With modern generators, breakthrough is rare but unpredictable. When it does occur, Mo-99 levels can be far higher than the legal limit.

**Chemical purity**    Another routine quality assurance step is to measure the generator eluate for the presence of the column packing material, Al$^2$O$_3$. For fission generators the maximum alumina concentration is 10 $\mu$g/ml. Aurin tricarboxylic acid is used for colorimetric spot testing. The color reaction for a standard 10 $\mu$g/ml sample of alumina is compared with a corresponding sample from the generator eluate. Acceptable levels are present if the color is less intense than the color of the standard. The comparison is made visually and qualitatively. No attempt is made to measure the alumina concentration quantitatively. Aluminum levels in excess of this limit have been shown to interfere with the normal distribution of certain radiopharmaceuticals such as Tc-99m sulfur colloid (increased lung activity) and technetium–methylene diphosphonate (Tc-MDP) (increased liver activity).

**Radiochemical purity**    The expected valence state of Tc-99m, as eluted from the generator, is +7 in the chemical form of pertechnetate (TcO$_4^-$). The clinical use of sodium pertechnetate as a radiopharmaceutical and the preparation of Tc-99m-labeled pharmaceuticals, typically from commercial kits, are predicated on the +7 oxidation state. The *U.S. Pharmacopeia* (USP) standard

**Table 4-7   Measures of pharmaceutical purity**

| Parameter | Definition | Example issues |
|---|---|---|
| Chemical purity | Fraction of wanted versus unwanted chemical in preparation | Amount of alumina breakthrough in Mo-99/Tc-99m generator eluate |
| Radiochemical purity | Fraction of total radioactivity in desired chemical form | Amount of bound versus unbound Tc-99m in Tc-99m diphosphonate |
| Radionuclidic purity | Fraction of total radioactivity in the form of desired radionuclide | Ratio of Tc-99m versus Mo-99 in generator eluate; I-124 in an I-123 preparation |
| Physical purity | Fraction of total pharmaceutical in desired physical form | Correct particle size distribution in Tc-99m MAA preparation; absence of particulate contaminates in any agent that is a true solution |
| Biological purity | Absence of microorganisms and pyrogens | Sterile, pyrogen-free preparations |

for the generator eluate is that 95% or more of Tc-99m activity be in this +7 state. Reduction states at +4, +5, or +6 may be present and are detected by various thin-layer chromatography systems. In practice, problems with radiochemical purity of the generator eluate are infrequently encountered but should be considered if kit labeling is poor. The different measures of pharmaceutical purity are summarized in Table 4-7.

## TECHNETIUM CHEMISTRY AND RADIOPHARMACEUTICAL PREPARATION

Tc-99m has become the most commonly used radionuclide because of its ready availability, the favorable energy of its principal gamma photon, its favorable dosimetry with lack of primary particulate radiations, and its nearly ideal half-life for many clinical imaging studies. However, technetium chemistry is challenging. In most labeling procedures technetium must be reduced from the +7 valence state. In current practice the reduction is usually accomplished with stannous ion.

The actual final oxidation state of technetium in many radiopharmaceuticals is either unknown or subject to debate. A number of technetium compounds are che-

lates, and others are used on the basis of their empirical efficacy without complete knowledge of how technetium is being complexed in the final molecule. One exception to the need to reduce technetium from the +7 oxidation state is in the preparation of Tc-99m sulfur colloid ($Tc_2S_7$).

The details of individual technetium radiopharmaceuticals are discussed in the chapters on individual organ systems and include key points in preparation and the recognition of in vivo markers of radiopharmaceutical impurities. Box 4-2 summarizes the major Tc-99m-labeled agents that are used clinically.

The introduction of stannous ion for reducing technetium in radiolabeling procedures was a major breakthrough in nuclear medicine. Commercial kits contain a reaction vial with the appropriate amount of stannous ion, the nonradioactive pharmaceutical to be labeled, and other buffering and stabilizing agents. The vials are typically flushed with nitrogen to prevent atmospheric oxygen from interrupting the reaction. Fig. 4-4 illustrates the sequence of steps in a sample labeling process. In brief, sodium pertechnetate is drawn into a syringe and assayed in the dose calibrator. After the proper Tc-99m activity is confirmed, the sample is added to the reaction vial. The amount of Tc-99m activity added for each respective product is determined by the number of patient doses desired in the case of a multidose vial, an estimate of the decrease in radioactivity due to decay between the time of preparation and the estimated time of dosage administration, and the in vitro stability of the product. The completed product is labeled and kept in a special lead-shielded container until it is time to withdraw a sample for administration to a patient. Each patient dose is individually assayed before being dispensed.

Excessive oxygen can react directly with the stannous ion, leaving too little reducing power in the kit. This can result in unwanted free Tc-99m pertechnetate in the preparation. A less common problem is radiolysis after kit preparation. The phenomenon is seen when high amounts of Tc-99m activity are used. The kit preparations are usually designed so that multiple doses can be prepared from one reaction vial.

## QUALITY ASSURANCE OF TECHNETIUM-99m-LABELED RADIOPHARMACEUTICALS

The difficult nature of technetium chemistry highlights the importance of checking the final product for *radiochemical purity.* This term is defined as the percentage of the total radioactivity in a specimen that is in the specified or desired radiochemical form. For example, if 5% of the Tc-99m activity remains as free

Box 4-2 Technetium-99m (Tc-99m) Radiopharmaceuticals

| AGENT | APPLICATION* |
|---|---|
| Tc-99m sodium pertechnetate | Meckel's diverticulum detection, salivary gland scintigraphy, thyroid gland scintigraphy |
| Tc-99m sulfur colloid (filtered) | Liver and spleen scintigraphy (RES), gastrointestinal bleeding detection, bone marrow scintigraphy |
| Tc-99m sulfur colloid | Lymphoscintigraphy |
| Tc-99m pyrophosphate | Acute myocardial infarction detection (skeletal scintigraphy) |
| Tc-99m diphosphonate | Skeletal scintigraphy |
| Tc-99m macroaggregated albumin (MAA) | Pulmonary perfusion scintigraphy, peripheral and regional (e.g., liver); arterial perfusion scintigraphy |
| Tc-99m red blood cells | Radionuclide ventriculography, gastrointestinal bleeding detection, hepatic hemangioma detection |
| Tc-99m human serum albumin | Blood pool imaging (e.g. radionuclide ventriculography) |
| Tc-99m pentetate (diethylenetriamine-pentaacetic acid [DTPA]) | Renal and urinary tract scintigraphy, lung ventilation (aerosol), (glomerular filtration rate), (brain scintigraphy) |
| Tc-99m mercaptoacetyltriglycine (MAG$_3$) | Renal scintigraphy |
| Tc-99m glucoceptate | Renal scintigraphy |
| Tc-99m dimercaptosuccinic acid (DMSA) | Renal cortical scintigraphy |
| Tc-99m hepatic iminodiacetic acid (HIDA) and derivatives | Hepatobiliary scintigraphy |
| Tc-99m sestamibi | Myocardial perfusion scintigraphy, breast imaging |
| Tc-99m tetrofosmin | Myocardial perfusion scintigraphy |
| Tc-99m teboroxime | Myocardial perfusion scintigraphy |
| Tc-99m exametazine | Cerebral perfusion scintigraphy, white blood cell labeling |
| Tc-99m bicisate | Cerebral perfusion scintigraphy |
| Tc-99m arcitumomab | Monoclonal antibody for colorectal cancer evaluation |
| Tc-99m apcitide | Acute venous thrombosis imaging |

*Parentheses indicate less common applications.

pertechnetate in a radiolabeling procedure, the radiochemical purity would be stated as 95%, assuming no other impurities. Each radiopharmaceutical has a specific radiochemical purity to meet USP or FDA requirements, typically 90%. Causes of radiochemical impurities include poor initial labeling, radiolysis, decomposition, pH changes, light exposure, or presence of oxidizing or reducing agents.

For many agents the presence of a radiochemical impurity can be recognized by altered in vivo biodistribution. However, intercepting the offending preparation before administration to a patient is obviously desirable. A number of systems have been developed to assay radiochemical purity. The basic approach is to use thin-layer chromatography. Many commercial products and variations are available. In brief, radiochromatography is accomplished in the same manner as conventional chromatography, by spotting a sample of the test material at one end of a strip. A solvent is then selected for which the desired radiochemical and the potential contaminants have known migration patterns. The presence of the radiolabel provides an easy means of quantitatively measuring the migration patterns. In vivo, radiochemical impurities contribute to background activity or other unwanted localization and degrade image quality.

For soluble technetium radiopharmaceuticals the presence of free pertechnetate and the presence of insoluble, hydrolyzed reduced technetium moieties are tested. For example, free pertechnetate migrates with the solvent front in a paper and thin-layer chromatography system using acetone as the solvent, whereas Tc-99m diphosphonate and hydrolyzed reduced technetium remain at the origin (Fig. 4-5). For selective testing of hydrolyzed reduced technetium, a silica gel strip is used with saline as the solvent. In this system both free pertechnetate and Tc-99m diphosphonate move with the solvent front and, again, hydrolyzed reduced technetium stays at the origin (Fig. 4-5). This combination of procedures allows measurement of each of the three components. Chromatography systems have been worked out for each major technetium-labeled radiopharmaceutical.

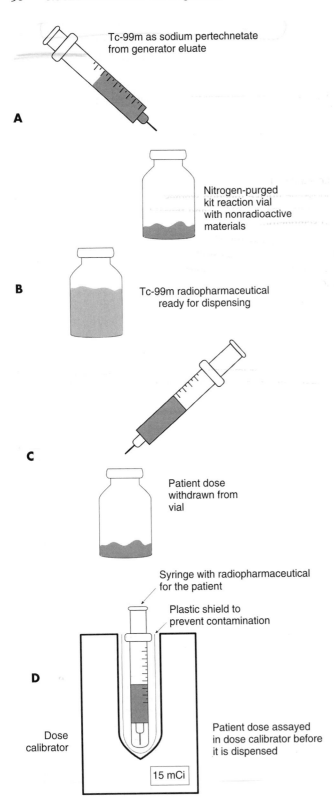

Fig. 4-4   Selected steps in the preparation of a technetium-99m-labeled radiopharmaceutical. **A,** Tc-99m as sodium pertechnetate is added to the reaction vial. **B,** Tc-99m radiopharmaceutical is ready for dispensing. **C,** The patient dose is withdrawn from the vial. **D,** Each dose is measured in the dose calibrator before it is dispensed.

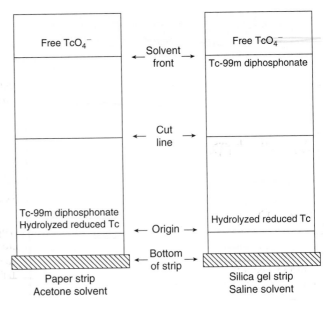

Fig. 4-5   Two-part radiochromatography system for the quality control of technetium-99m diphosphonate.

Elaborate systems are available to "read" the chromatography strips. Chromatographic scanners provide detailed strip chart recording of radioactivity distribution. In practice, the easiest way to perform chromatography is simply to cut the chromatography strip into two pieces that can be counted separately.

Chromatography is something of an art form, and a number of common pitfalls must be avoided. Inadvertently immersing the chromatography strip into the solvent past the location of the sample spot results in less migration than expected. Also, if spots are not allowed to dry before being used with organic solvents, spurious migration patterns will occur. On the other hand, excessive delay before starting the chromatogram can result in reoxidation of the technetium in the sample; again, spurious results will be encountered.

## OTHER SINGLE-PHOTON AGENTS

### Radioiodines

Radioiodine-131 as sodium iodide was the first radiopharmaceutical of importance in clinical nuclear medicine. It was used exclusively for studies of the thyroid gland for several years in the late 1940s (Box 4-3). Subsequently I-131 was used as the radiolabel for a wide variety of radiopharmaceuticals, including human serum albumin, macroaggregated albumin, and a number of different antibodies, as well as agents for the kidney (hippuran) and multiple agents for adrenal scintigraphy (metaiodobenzylguanidine and labeled cholesterol derivatives). The disadvantages of I-131 include relatively

## Box 4-3   Radiopharmaceuticals for Single-Photon Imaging (Non-Tc-99m)

| AGENT | APPLICATION |
|---|---|
| Tl-201 thallous chloride | Myocardial perfusion scintigraphy |
| Ga-67 gallium citrate | Inflammatory disease detection |
| | Tumor imaging |
| Xe-133 xenon (inert gas) | Pulmonary ventilation scintigraphy |
| Xe-127 xenon (inert gas) | Pulmonary ventilation scintigraphy |
| Kr-81m krypton (inert gas) | Pulmonary ventilation scintigraphy |
| I-131 sodium iodide | Thyroid scintigraphy |
| | Thyroid iodine uptake function studies |
| | Treatment of hyperthyroidism and thyroid cancer |
| I-123 sodium iodide | Thyroid scintigraphy |
| | Thyroid iodine uptake function studies |
| I-131 hippuran | Renal imaging and function studies |
| I-123 hippuran | Renal imaging and function studies |
| In-111 white blood cells | Inflammatory disease detection |
| In-111, I-131, labeled antibodies, proteins, and peptides | Wide variety of receptor binding and tumor localization studies |
| I-123 iodoamphetamine | Cerebral perfusion scintigraphy |
| I-131, I-123 metaiodobenzylguanidine (MIBG) | Adrenal medullary imaging, neural crest tumor detection |
| I-131 NP-59 (6β iodomethyl-19—norcholesterol) | Adrenal cortical scintigraphy |
| In-111 pentetreotide | Somatostatin receptor imaging |
| In-111 capromabpendetide | Monoclonal antibody for prostate Ca evaluation |
| Sm-153 lexidronan | Bone palliation |
| Sr-89 chloride | Bone palliation |
| In-111 satumomabpendetide | Monoclonal antibody for colorectal and ovarian cancer evaluation |

high principal photon energy (364 keV), long half-life (8 days), and the presence of beta particle emissions. Radioiodine-131 remains an important agent in nuclear medicine practice for the treatment of hyperthyroidism and differentiated thyroid cancer. It also continues to be used for selected diagnostic applications, including antibody labeling and the labeling of adrenal agents.

The quality control of radioiodinated pharmaceuticals is important to reduce unwanted radiation exposure to the thyroid gland. In nonthyroid imaging applications of I-131 as a radiolabel it is common practice to block the thyroid gland with Lugol's solution or SSKI to prevent thyroid accumulation of any iodine ion present as a radiochemical impurity or metabolite.

Whenever possible in contemporary practice, I-123 is substituted for I-131. It has a shorter half-life (Table 4-1), and its principal photon energy of 159 keV is better suited to imaging with the gamma scintillation camera. I-123 decays by electron capture, and the dosimetry is favorable compared with that of I-131. Two limitations to the use of I-123 are its relatively high expense and its limited availability owing to a short half-life of 13 hours. In some applications with radiolabeled antibodies and thyroid and adrenal scintigraphy, imaging over a period

of several days is desirable, which also represents a limitation of I-123 as compared with I-131.

### Indium-111

Another versatile label that has found a variety of applications in clinical nuclear medicine is indium-111 (Box 4-3). Its principal photon energies of 172 keV and 245 keV are favorable compared with I-131. The 2.8-day half-life of In-111 permits multiday sequential imaging, which is commonly used in the evaluation of inflammatory disease (In-111-labeled white blood cells) and in imaging with antibodies. In-111 pentetreotide (OctreoScan) is a new peptide agent that binds to somatostation receptors found in a variety of tumors of neuroendocrine origin.

### Gallium-67 Citrate

The discovery that Ga-67 citrate localizes in tumors and inflammatory conditions was fortuitous. Different radionuclides of gallium were initially under evaluation as bone scanning agents. Soft tissue uptake in a patient with Hodgkin's disease was noted incidentally and led to the recognition of gallium's utility as a tumor-imaging agent and subsequently its use in detecting areas of inflammation. In many respects Ga-67 does not have favorable properties for clinical imaging. For example, the most abundant photon has the lowest energy (Table 4-1). Until gamma cameras with the capability of imaging multiple photopeaks simultaneously became available, there was no ideal way to image Ga-67. In current practice it is common to bracket the lower three photopeaks (93 keV, 185 keV, 300 keV). Nonetheless, "downscatter" from the higher energies degrades the image data in the lower windows.

Other disadvantages of Ga-67 include slow clearance from background tissues, necessitating delayed imaging at 24, 48, and even 72 hours or more in some applications. Early excretion (<24 hours) through the kidneys and delayed excretion via the gut make imaging in the abdomen difficult. Care must be taken to interpret the scintigram with a full knowledge of how long after tracer administration the study was obtained. Laxatives may be required to clear confusing or obscuring activity from the colon.

### Thallium-201

Thallium-201 became clinically available in the mid-1970s as an agent for myocardial scintigraphy. Thallium behaves as a potassium analog, with high net clearance (~85%) in its passage through the myocardial capillary bed. This makes it an excellent marker of regional blood flow to viable myocardium. The major disadvantage of thallium as a radioactive imaging agent is the absence of an ideal photopeak for imaging. The gamma rays at 135 keV and 167 keV occur in low abundance (Table 4-1). In practice, the mercury x-rays are used. The ability of the gamma scintillation camera to discriminate scattered events from primary photons is suboptimal at their energy. Literally from the time of introduction of Tl-201 into clinical practice the nuclear medicine community has been interested in finding an alternative agent for myocardial perfusion imaging, preferably labeled with Tc-99m. Such agents are now available but have their limitations, as discussed in the chapter on cardiac imaging.

### Radioactive Inert Gases

The radioactive inert gases xenon and krypton are used for pulmonary ventilation imaging. Xenon-133 (Xe-133) is a convenient agent to maintain in inventory because of its 5.2-day half-life. The major disadvantage of Xe-133 is the relatively low energy of its principal photon (81 keV). This low energy dictates the performance of ventilation scintigraphy before Tc-99m perfusion scintigraphy or the use of cumbersome sub-

traction techniques. Nonetheless, Xe-133 is still the most commonly used agent because of its ready availability and relatively low price compared with the alternative agents.

Xe-127 is theoretically superior to Xe-133 because of its higher photon energies (Table 4-1). Because its photon energies are higher than those of Tc-99m, the ventilation portion of a ventilation-perfusion study can be performed after the locations of any perfusion defects are known. This allows the examination to be tailored to the findings in individual patients. The high cost of producing Xe-127 has kept it from wide use.

For practical purposes krypton-81m has never progressed beyond evaluation by a few dedicated clinical researchers. It has the potential advantage of allowing virtually continuous imaging. The short half-life of 13 seconds permits multiple views to be obtained without concern for retained activity.

A host of other radionuclides have been used over the years. The radionuclides summarized in Table 4-1 are the most important in current practice.

### RADIOPHARMACEUTICALS FOR POSITRON EMISSION TOMOGRAPHY

The physical characteristics of commonly used positron-emitting radionuclides are summarized in Table 4-2. Now many dozens of radiopharmaceuticals have been described for use in positron emission tomography (PET) (Box 4-4). Carbon, oxygen, and nitrogen are found ubiquitously in biological molecules. It is thus theoretically possible to radiolabel just about any molecule of biological interest. Fluorine-18 (F-18) has the advantage of a longer half-life than C-11, N-13, or O-15 and has had use as a label for the glucose analog F-18 fluorodeoxyglucose. This pharmaceutical has found widespread application in imaging of the brain, the heart, and a wide variety of tumors throughout the body. Tumors derive their energy from glucose metabolism, and the uptake of F-18 fluorodeoxyglucose is a marker of tumor metabolism and viability.

Rubidium-82 is available from a generator system with a relatively long-lived parent (strontium-82, $T_{1/2}$ = 25 days) (Table 4-3). Rubidium, like thallium, is a potassium analog and has been used for myocardial perfusion imaging. Its availability from a generator system obviates the need for an on-site cyclotron for production. One limitation of Rb-82 is the high energy (3.15 MeV) of its positron emissions. This high energy results in a relatively long average path in soft tissue before annihilation, degrading the ultimate spatial resolution available with the agent. This feature is shared to a lesser extent by O-15.

---

**Box 4-4    Selected Radiopharmaceuticals for Positron Emission Tomography**

**PERFUSION AGENTS**

Oxygen-15 carbon dioxide    $CO_2$
Oxygen-15 water    $H_2O$
Nitrogen-13 ammonia    $NH_3$
Rubidium-82 rubidium chloride    $Rb_{82}$

**BLOOD VOLUME**

Oxygen-15 carbon monoxide    $CO$
Carbon-11 carbon monoxide    $CO$
Gallium-68 EDTA    $GaEDTA$

**METABOLIC AGENTS**

Fluorine-18 sodium fluoride    $NaF$
Fluorine-18 fluorodexyglucose    $FDG$
Oxygen-15 oxygen    $O_2$
Carbon-11 acetate
Carbon-11 palmitate
Nitrogen-13 glutamate

**TUMOR AGENTS**

Fluorine-18 fluorodeoxyglucose    $FDG$
Carbon-11 methionine

**RECEPTOR-BINDING AGENTS**

Fluorine-18 spiperone
Carbon-11 carfentanil
Fluorine-18 fluoro-L-dopa
Carbon-11 raclopride

---

With the exception of Rb-82, the production of positron-emitting radionuclides and their subsequent incorporation into PET radiopharmaceuticals are expensive and complex, requiring a cyclotron or other special accelerator and relatively elaborate radiochemical-handling equipment. However, radiochemists and radiopharmacists are working to develop single-photon agents based on mechanisms first studied using positron emitters. For example, a number of single-photon-labeled receptor-binding agents and perfusion agents have been made available based on knowledge gained initially from PET radiopharmaceuticals. Interest is also growing in the use of F-18 fluorodeoxyglucose (FDG) supplied by regional pharmacies.

## DISPENSING RADIOPHARMACEUTICALS

### Normal Procedures

The dispensing of radiopharmaceuticals is under a series of exacting rules and regulations promulgated by the FDA and the NRC, as well as state boards of pharmacy and hospitals. In brief, radiopharmaceuticals are prescription drugs that cannot be legally administered without being ordered by an authorized individual. The nuclear medicine physician and the radiopharmacy are responsible for confirming the appropriateness of the request, ensuring that the correct radiopharmaceutical in the requested or designated amount is administered to the patient, and keeping records of both the request and the documentation of the dosage administration.

Before any material is dispensed, all appropriate quality assurance measures should be carried out. These are described in detail earlier in the chapter for the Mo-99/Tc-99m generator system and Tc-99m-labeled radiopharmaceuticals. For other agents the package insert or protocol for formulation and dispensing should be consulted to see what radiochromatography or other quality control steps must be performed before dosage administration. As a good standard of practice, quality control should always be performed even when not legally required.

Every dose should be physically inspected before administration for any particulate or foreign material, such as bits of rubber from the tops of multidose injection vials. Each dose administered to a patient must be assayed in a dose calibrator. The administered activity must be within ±10% of the prescription request.

### Special Considerations

**Pregnancy and lactation**  The possibility of pregnancy should be considered for every woman of child-bearing age referred to the nuclear medicine service for a diagnostic or therapeutic procedure. Pregnancy alone is not an absolute contraindication to performing a nuclear medicine study. For example, pulmonary embolism is encountered in pregnant women, and ventilation-perfusion scintigraphy is a safe procedure in this circumstance. The radiation dosage is kept at a minimum. Neither of the radiopharmaceuticals employed (Xe-133 or Tc-99m macroaggregated albumin [MAA]) crosses the placenta in considerable amounts. On the other hand, radioiodine does cross the placenta. The fetal thyroid develops the capacity to concentrate radioiodine at approximately the 10th to 12th week of gestation, and cases of cretinism caused by in utero exposure to radioiodine have been documented.

The management of women who are lactating and breast feeding an infant is another special problem. The need to suspend breast feeding is determined by the half-life of the radionuclide involved and the degree to which it is secreted in breast milk. Radioiodine is secreted, and conservatively, breast feeding should be terminated altogether or for at least 3 weeks after the administration of I-131 or I-125. The same recommendations hold for Ga-67 citrate and Tl-201 chloride.

For technetium-labeled radiopharmaceuticals that are cleared rapidly by the kidney or that stay in the blood pool (Tc-99m pentetate, Tc-99m-labeled red blood cells [RBCs], Tc-99m diphosphonate), there is little activity in breast milk, and nursing can resume after several hours. For other Tc-99m-labeled radiopharmaceuticals, nursing should be suspended for at least two half-lives (12 hours). In the United States it is usually practical simply to discontinue breast feeding if there is any question about exposure to the child.

**Dosage selection for pediatric patients**  A number of approaches have been proposed for scaling down the amount of radioactivity administered to children. There is no perfect way to do this because of the differential rate of maturation of body organs and the changing ratio of different body compartments to body weight. Empirically, body surface area correlates better than body weight for dosage selection. Various formulas and nomograms have been developed. Each laboratory should select a method and standardize its application.

An approximation based on body weight uses the formula:

$$\text{Pediatric dose} = \frac{\text{Patient weight (kg)}}{70 \text{ kg}} \times \text{Adult dose}$$

Another alternative is the use of Webster's rule:

$$\text{Pediatric dose} = \frac{\text{Age} + 1}{\text{Age} + 7} \times \text{Adult dose}$$

This formula is not useful for infants. Moreover, in some cases a calculated dose may not be adequate to obtain a diagnostically useful study and physician judgment must be used. For example, a newborn infant with suspected biliary atresia may require 24-hour delayed Tc-99m hepatobiliary iminodiacetic acid (HIDA) imaging, which is not feasible if the dose is too low. Therefore a minimum dose for each radiopharmaceutical should be established.

**Misadministration**  The definition and procedures for handling misadministrations of radiopharmaceuticals are set out in the Code of Federal Regulations (10 CFR-35). The code was revised in 1991, including the definition of a misadministration. (The code is under revision again at the time of this writing and the reader is advised to determine whether new regulations have been officially adopted.)

The occurrence of a misadministration as defined by NRC rules and regulations requires that specific administrative responses be performed by the respective radioactive material license holder in response to an incident. A misadministration is defined as a radiopharmaceutical dose administration involving at least one of the following:

1. The wrong patient
2. The wrong radiopharmaceutical
3. The wrong route of administration

4. The administered dose differing from the prescribed dose when involving:
   a. Diagnostic doses other than sodium iodide, and the patient effective dose equivalent exceeds 5 rem to the whole body or 50 rem to any individual organ
   b. Diagnostic doses of sodium iodide, when the administered dose differs by more than 20% from the prescribed dosage and that difference exceeds 30 μCi
   c. Therapeutic doses when the administered dose differs by more than 20% from the prescribed dosage

After the occurrence of a misadministration is recognized, regulations for reporting of the event and management of the patient should be followed. The details are determined in part by the kind of material involved and the amount of the adverse exposure of the patient. All misadministrations must be recorded locally and, where appropriate, reported to the NRC. Complete records on each event must be retained and available for NRC review for 10 years.

**Adverse reactions to diagnostic radiopharmaceuticals**  Adverse reactions to radiopharmaceuticals are much less common than adverse reactions to iodinated contrast media. Reactions are usually mild and, for the radiopharmaceuticals in use today, rarely fatal. The greatest concern is for agents containing human serum albumin. Also, preparations of Tc-99m-sulfur colloid have a gelatin stabilizer derived from animal protein. These agents can be associated with allergic reactions. Of concern in the future is the possibility of reactions caused by the development of human antimouse antibodies (HAMA) after repeated exposure to radiolabeled antibody imaging agents. The concern over the development of HAMA and potential adverse consequences has been a factor in the FDA's delay in granting approval for radiolabeled antibodies, although the precedent has been set.

## RADIATION ACCIDENTS (SPILLS)

In a busy nuclear medicine practice handling several dozen patient doses a day, as well as stock solutions of generator eluate, with most materials in liquid form, accidental spills of radioactive material occur from time to time. The spills are somewhat arbitrarily divided into minor and major categories, depending on the radionuclide and the amount spilled. For I-131, incidents involving activities up to 1 mCi are considered minor, and above that level major. For Tc-99m, Tl-201, and Ga-67, the threshold for considering a spill major is 100 mCi.

The basic principles of responding to both kinds of spills are the same. For minor spills people in the area are warned that the spill has occurred. Attempts are made to prevent the spread of the spilled material. Absorbent paper may be used to cover the spilled material if it is visibly identifiable. Minor spills can be cleaned up directly with an appropriate technique, including use of disposable gloves and remote handling devices. All contaminated material, including gloves and other objects, should be disposed of carefully. The area should be continually surveyed until the reading from a Geiger-Müller survey meter is at background levels. All personnel involved should also be monitored, including their hands, shoes, and clothing. The spill should be reported to the institution's radiation safety officer.

For major spills the area is cleared immediately. Attempts are made to prevent further spread with absorbent pads, and if possible the radioactivity is shielded. The room is sealed off, and the radiation safety officer is notified immediately. The radiation safety officer typically directs the further response, including determination of when and how to proceed with cleanup and decontamination.

In dealing with both minor and major spills, an attempt is made to keep radiation exposure of patients, hospital staff, and the environment to a minimum. There are no absolute guidelines that provide a definitive approach to every spill. The radiation safety officer must restrict access to the area until it is safe for patients and personnel.

## QUALITY CONTROL IN THE NUCLEAR PHARMACY

Selected quality control procedures for Tc-99m-labeled radiopharmaceuticals and for Mo-99/Tc-99m generator systems are described earlier in this chapter. Considerations of radiochemical and radionuclidic purity also apply to other single-photon agents and positron radiopharmaceuticals (Table 4-7). For example, radiochemical purity is a special concern with radioiodinated agents because of the potential for uptake of free radioiodine in the thyroid gland. Additional quality control procedures in the nuclear pharmacy are aimed at ensuring the sterility and apyrogenicity of administered radiopharmaceuticals. Quality control monitoring of the performance of the dose calibrator is also important to ensure that administered doses are within prescribed amounts.

### Sterility and Pyrogen Testing

Sterility implies the absence of living organisms (Table 4-7); *apyrogenicity* implies the absence of metabolic products such as endotoxins. Because many radiopharmaceuticals are prepared just before use, definitive testing before they are administered to the patient is impractical. This doubles the need for careful aseptic technique in the nuclear pharmacy.

Autoclaving is a well-known means of sterilization. It is useful for sterilizing preparation vials and other utensils and materials but is not useful for any of the radiopharmaceuticals employed in clinical practice. When terminal sterilization is required, various membrane filtration methods are used. Special filters with pore diameters smaller than microorganisms have been developed for this purpose. A filter pore size of 0.22 $\mu$m is necessary to sterilize a solution. This size traps bacteria, including small organisms such as *Pseudomonas*.

Sterility testing standards have been defined by the *United States Pharmacopeia* (USP). Standard media including thioglycollate and soybean casein digest media are used for different categories of microorganism, including aerobic and anaerobic bacteria and fungi.

Pyrogens are protein or polysaccharide metabolites of microorganisms or other contaminating substances that cause febrile reactions (Table 4-7). They can be present even in sterile preparations. The typical clinical syndrome is fever, chills, joint pain, and headache developing minutes to a few hours after injection. The pyrogenic reaction lasts for several hours and alone is not fatal.

The USP has established criteria for pyrogen testing. The historical method involved injecting pharmaceutical samples into the ear veins of rabbits while measuring their temperature response. The current USP test uses limulus amebocyte lysate (LAL). The test is based on the observation that amebocyte lysate preparations from the blood of horseshoe crabs become opaque in the presence of pyrogens. The LAL test is more reliable, more sensitive, and easier to perform than the rabbit test.

### Radiopharmaceutical Dose Calibrators

The dose calibrator is a key instrument in the radiopharmacy and is subject to quality control requirements. Four basic measurements are included: accuracy, linearity, precision or constancy, and geometry. All of these tests must be performed at installation and after repair.

**Accuracy** Accuracy is measured by using reference standard sources obtained from the National Institute of Standards and Technology. The test is performed annually, and two different radioactive sources are used. If the measured activity in the dose calibrator varies from the standard or theoretical activity by more than 10%, the device must be recalibrated.

**Linearity** The linearity test is designed to determine the response of the calibrator over a range of measured activities. A common approach is to take a sample of Tc-99m pertechnetate and sequentially measure it during radioactive decay. Because the change in activity with time is a definable physical parameter, any deviation in the observed assay value indicates equipment malfunction—nonlinearity. An alternative approach is to use precalibrated lead attenuators with sequential measurements of the same specimen. This test is performed quarterly.

**Precision or constancy**  The precision or constancy test is designed to measure the ability of the dose calibrator to repeatedly measure the same specimen over time. A long-lived standard such as barium-133, cesium-137, or cobalt-57 can be used. The test is performed daily, and observed values should be within 10% of the value for the reference standard.

**Geometry**  The geometric test is performed during acceptance testing of the dose calibrator. The issue is that the same amount of radioactivity contained in different volumes of sample can result in different measured or observed radioactivities. For a given dose calibrator, if readings vary by more than 10% from one volume to another, correction factors are calculated. For convenience the correction factors are based on the most commonly measured volume of material, which is typically determined from day-to-day clinical use of the dose calibrator.

## RADIATION DOSIMETRY

Exposure of the patient to radiation limits the amount of radioactivity that can be administered in the scintigraphic procedures performed in clinical nuclear medicine. In general, the exact radiation dose that an individual patient receives from a nuclear medicine procedure cannot be calculated. The amount of data necessary to calculate the actual radiation absorbed dose for a particular patient is not practical to acquire. It includes the percent localization of the administered dose in each organ of the body, the time course of retention in each organ, and the size and relative distribution of the organs in the body. Such information is obtained from biodistribution studies and pharmacokinetic studies in experimental animals during the development and regulatory approval process for a new radiopharmaceutical. For each radiopharmaceutical, estimates of radiation absorbed doses are made as part of the approval process and may be taken as "average" or nominal levels of exposure.

In brief, the radiation absorbed dose to any organ in the body depends on biological factors (percent uptake, biological half-life) and physical factors (amount and nature of emitted radiations from the radionuclide). Radiation doses are typically given in rads (radiation absorbed dose). One rad is equal to the absorption of 100 ergs per gram of tissue. The formula for calculating the radiation absorbed dose is:

$$D(r_{k \leftarrow} r_h) = \tilde{A}_h S(r_{k \leftarrow} r_h)$$

The formula states that the absorbed dose in a region $k$ resulting from activity from a source region $h$ is equal to the cumulative radioactivity given in microcurie-hours in the source region ($\tilde{A}$) times the mean absorbed dose per unit of cumulative activity in rads per microcurie-hour ($S$). The cumulative activity is determined from experimental measurements of uptake and retention in the different source regions. The mean absorbed dose per unit of cumulative activity is based on physical measurements and is determined by the kind of radiations emanating from the radionuclide being used.

The total absorbed dose to a region or organ is the sum of the contributions from all source regions around it and from activity within the target organ itself. For example, a calculation of the absorbed dose to the myocardium in a Tl-201 scan must take into account contributions from radioactivity localizing in the myocardium and from radioactivity in the lung, blood, liver, gut, kidneys, and general background soft tissues. The percentage uptake and the biological behavior of Tl-201 are different in each of those tissues. The amount of radiation reaching the myocardium is also different, depending on the geometry of the source organ and its distance from the heart. The formula is applied separately for each source region, and the individual contributions are summed.

Factors that affect the dosimetry between patients include the amount of activity administered originally, the biodistribution in one patient versus another, the route of administration, the rate of elimination, the size of the patient, and the presence of pathological processes. For example, for radiopharmaceuticals cleared by the kidney, radiation exposure is greater in patients with renal failure. Another commonly encountered example is differing percentage uptakes of radioiodine in the thyroid depending on whether a patient is hyperthyroid, euthyroid, or hypothyroid.

Estimates of radiation absorbed dose for each major radiopharmaceutical are provided in tabular form in the organ system chapters. The tables indicate the absorbed dose per unit of administered activity for selected organs.

## SUGGESTED READINGS

Chilton HM, Witcofski RL: *Nuclear pharmacy: an introduction to the clinical application of radiopharmaceuticals,* Philadelphia, 1986, Lea & Febiger.

Kowalsky RJ, Perry JR: *Radiopharmaceuticals in nuclear medicine practice,* Norwalk, Conn, 1987, Appleton & Lange.

Ponto JA: The AAPM/RSNA physics tutorial for residents: radiopharmaceuticals, *Radiographics* 18:1395-1404, 1998.

Saha GB: *Fundamentals of nuclear pharmacy,* New York, 1998, Springer.

Simpkin DJ: The AAPM/RSNA physics tutorial for residents: radiation interactions and internal dosimetry, *Radiographics* 19:155-167, 1999.

Swanson DP, Chilton HM, Thrall JH: *Pharmaceuticals in medical imaging,* New York, 1990, Macmillan.

# CLINICAL SCINTIGRAPHY

# Cardiovascular System

Heart disease is the leading cause of death in the United States. Acute myocardial infarction (MI) claims over 600,000 lives per year and may strike without warning. Millions more people are at risk because of underlying coronary artery disease (CAD). Several nuclear imaging procedures are valuable in the diagnosis and management of heart disease, and collectively nuclear cardiology procedures are the most commonly performed studies in nuclear medicine, constituting about 40% of the total for the entire field.

This chapter is divided into four principal sections that address myocardial perfusion imaging (status of the myocardium and coronary perfusion), radionuclide ventriculography (status of heart function), cardiac positron emission tomography, and infarct-avid imaging (detection of acute myocardial infarction [MI]).

The clinical utility of radiotracer studies of the heart must always be considered in the context of other cardiac diagnostic procedures, including echocardiography, contrast angiography, electrocardiography (ECG), and measurement of serum enzymes. The value of the scintigraphic studies comes largely from their noninvasiveness and their accurate portrayal of a wide range of functional and metabolic parameters.

## MYOCARDIAL PERFUSION IMAGING

The single most frequent application of nuclear cardiology is the assessment of myocardial perfusion. The original radiopharmaceutical of clinical importance for this application was thallium-201 chloride. Three technetium-99m-labeled agents have now been approved by the Food and Drug Administration (FDA) for clinical application, and several PET pharmaceuticals are available for perfusion imaging, including rubidium-82, also approved by the FDA. The diagnosis of CAD remains a common application of myocardial perfusion scintigraphy, but it is increasingly being used for diagnosis of acute MI, risk stratification after infarction, and assessment of viable myocardium versus scar in patients with chronic coronary disease.

There are numerous major and subtle differences among the different radiopharmaceuticals for myocardial perfusion imaging. However, the integrative concept is that the scintigram depicts two sequential events. First, tracer must be delivered to the myocardium. Second, a viable, metabolically active myocardial cell must be present to localize the tracer. Thus the scintigram may be thought of as a map of regional myocardial perfusion to viable myocardial tissue. If a patient has a decrease in relative regional perfusion, as is seen in hemodynamically significant CAD, or a loss of cell viability, as is seen in MI, a photon-deficient lesion is depicted scintigraphically. All diagnostic patterns in the many diverse applications of myocardial perfusion scintigraphy follow from these simple observations.

### Pharmaceuticals for Perfusion Imaging

**Thallium 201-chloride**  Potassium is the major intracellular cation. Sodium-potassium homeostasis is main-

---

### Box 5-1  Thallium-201: Summary of Physical Characteristics and Dosimetry

**PHYSICAL CHARACTERISTICS**

| | |
|---|---|
| Mode of decay | Electron capture |
| Physical half-life | 73 hr |

| **Principal Radiations** | **Abundance** |
|---|---|
| 135 keV gamma | 2.7% |
| 167 keV gamma | 10.0% |
| 69-83 keV mercury x-rays | 95.0% |

**DOSIMETRY***
| Organ | Rads/mCi |
|---|---|
| Heart | 0.5 |
| Liver | 0.55 |
| Kidneys | 1.2 |
| Testes | 0.5 |
| Ovaries | 0.5 |
| Total body | 0.2 |

*Data from product information for thallous chloride-201, DuPont Co, Billerica, Mass.

---

tained as an energy-dependent process involving the Na, K-ATPase pump. It is logical to consider potassium or a potassium analog for myocardial perfusion imaging, and indeed, radionuclides of potassium, cesium, and rubidium have been evaluated. None is suitable for single-photon imaging. Rubidium-82 is discussed later in the section on PET pharmaceuticals.

Thallium is a member of the III A series in the Periodic Table and behaves in its organ and tissue distribution much like potassium, although it is not a true potassium analog in a chemical sense. Thallium-201 (Tl-201) has a physical half-life of 73 hours. It decays by electron capture to mercury-201. The photons available for imaging are mercury K-alpha and K-beta characteristic x-rays in the range of 69 to 83 keV (95% abundant) and thallium gamma rays of 167 keV (10% abundant) and 135 keV (3% abundant) (Box 5-1).

*Mechanism of localization and pharmacokinetics* One of the principal advantages of Tl-201 for myocardial perfusion imaging is its high extraction fraction during transit through the myocardial capillary bed. Approximately 88% of thallium is extracted in the first pass through the coronary circulation under conditions of normal flow. At very high flow rates the percent efficiency of extraction decreases, and at very low flow rates the percent extraction increases. However, over a wide range of flow rates the extraction is proportional to relative regional perfusion.

Blood clearance after intravenous (IV) injection of Tl-201 is rapid, with only 5% to 8% of the dose in blood 5 minutes after injection. Peak uptake in the myocardium occurs 10 to 20 minutes after injection. In normal subjects approximately 5% of the administered dose localizes in the myocardium. The scintigraphic images obtained early after injection reflect the blood flow conditions at the time of tracer administration.

After initial uptake has occurred, thallium undergoes "redistribution" in the body. A dynamic changing equilibrium of Tl-201 exists between the myocardium and vascular pool. After initial uptake, Tl-201 leaves the myocardium and is partially replaced by circulating Tl-201 from the systemic pool, which is also undergoing constant recirculation and redistribution. Thus several hours after initial tracer administration the scintigraphic images depict an equilibrated pattern. This is the basis of the "stress-redistribution" imaging strategy that has been used in the detection of CAD and is discussed more fully later in the chapter. Cold defects seen on early images may represent areas of significantly decreased flow or areas of myocardial scar without viable cells to fix the tracer. Defects on delayed or reinjection images depict scar. Areas demonstrating equilibration or "fill-in" of activity represent viable myocardium rendered ischemic during exercise. Some nuclear medicine departments prefer Tl-201 over the Tc-99m-labeled perfusion agents because they believe Tl-201 is superior for detecting viable myocardial tissue under conditions of very low flow, as may be seen in hibernating myocardium.

**Technetium-99m sestamibi** Tc-99m sestamibi is a member of a chemical family referred to as isonitriles; its chemical name is hexakis 2-methoxyisobutyl isonitrile. The radiopharmaceutical Tc-99m sestamibi is a monovalent cation in which Tc-99m is surrounded by six isonitrile ligands. Tc-99m sestamibi is prepared from a kit and requires boiling to effect labeling.

Tc-99m sestamibi diffuses passively out of the blood and apparently localizes in mitochondria on the basis of their negative electrical potentials. The extraction fraction for Tc-99m sestamibi in the coronary circulation is similar to Tc-99m tetrofosmin and lower than that of either Tc-99m teboroxime or Tl-201 (Table 5-1). At resting flows the extraction is approximately half that of Tl-201. The maximum extraction decreases with increasing flow but remains proportional to flow. As with Tl-201, Tc-99m sestamibi underestimates flow at very high flows and overestimates flow at low flows. Radiation dosimetry is favorable because of the Tc-99m label (Table 5-2).

*Pharmacokinetics* Tc-99m sestamibi is cleared from the blood fairly rapidly, with less than 5% of activity remaining in the blood at 10 minutes. Uptake in myocardium is also rapid but is somewhat obscured by activity in the lung and liver in the time immediately after tracer administration. However, the clearance half-time of Tc-99m sestamibi from the myocardium is long, in excess of 5 hours. Minimal recirculation or redistribution

**Table 5-1  Comparison of technetium-99m (Tc-99m) teboroxime against Tc-99m sestamibi and Tc-99m tetrofosmin**

|  | Tc-99m teboroxime | Tc-99m tetrofosmin, Tc-99m sestamibi |
|---|---|---|
| Myocardial extraction | >Thallium-201 | <Thallium-201 |
| Myocardial clearance | $T_{1/2}$ ~5-10 min | $T_{1/2}$ >5 hr |
| Imaging time after injection | 1-2 min | 15-30 min (stress) 30-90 min (rest) |
| "Redistribution" | Nil owing to uptake; differential regional washout may cause myocardial scintigraphic appearance to change | Slight; differential regional washout may cause myocardial scintigraphic appearance to change |

**Table 5-2  Dosimetry for technetium (Tc-99m) tetrofosmin, Tc-99m sestamibi, and Tc-99m teboroxime**

|  | Tc-99m tetrofosmin* (rad/mCi) | Tc-99m sestamibi† (rad/mCi) | Tc-99m teboroxime‡ (rad/mCi) |
|---|---|---|---|
| Heart wall | 0.02 | 0.02 | 0.02 |
| Liver | 0.01 | 0.02 | 0.06 |
| Kidneys | 0.04 | 0.07 | 0.02 |
| Gallbladder | 0.12 | 0.07 | 0.10 |
| Urinary bladder | 0.06 | 0.07 | 0.03 |
| Upper colon | 0.08 | 0.18 | 0.12 |
| Lower colon | 0.06 | 0.13 | 0.09 |
| Testes | 0.01 | 0.01 | 0.01 |
| Ovaries | 0.03 | 0.05 | 0.04 |
| Total body | — | 0.02 | 0.02 |

*Adapted from Amersham Healthcare package insert.
†Adapted from DuPont Radiopharmaceutical Division package insert.
‡Adapted from Squibb Diagnostics package insert.

of Tc-99m sestamibi occurs after initial uptake in the heart, a time window of several hours after tracer administration is available for imaging. Progressive clearance of liver and lung activity with excretion of the tracer through the kidneys and via the biliary system results in better myocardium-to-background activity ratios at 60 to 120 minutes than immediately after tracer administration. In current practice, imaging is initiated from 30 to 90 minutes after tracer administration for resting studies (Table 5-1). Imaging may be started at 15 minutes for exercise stress studies because the heart/

lung and heart/liver ratios are higher than when tracer is given at rest.

**Technetium-99m tetrofosmin**    Tc-99m tetrofosmin [6,9-bis (2-ethoxyethyl)-3, 12-dioxa-6, 9-diphospha-tetradecane] is a second-generation Tc-99m-labeled myocardial imaging agent and a member of the diphosphine chemical class. Tc-99m tetrofosmin is lipophilic and, like Tc-99m sestamibi, localizes in mitochondria. Tc-99m tetrofosmin is prepared from a kit and has the advantage over Tc-99m sestamibi of not requiring boiling.

*Pharmacokinetics*    Tc-99m tetrofosmin is cleared rapidly from the blood with less than 5% of activity remaining in the circulation at 5 minutes after injection. Uptake in the myocardium is also rapid and on the same order as Tc-99m sestamibi, with roughly 1.2% of the injected dose in the myocardium at 5 minutes after injection. Tc-99m remains in the heart with little evidence of recirculation or redistribution. Again, similar to Tc-99m sestamibi, this provides a window of several hours after tracer administration in which to accomplish imaging. Heart/lung and heart/liver ratios increase with time because of physiological background clearance. However, heart/liver ratios are somewhat higher for Tc-99m tetrofosmin, and earlier imaging times are often used. After stress injections, imaging at 10 to 15 minutes is feasible; some departments begin at 5 minutes. Rest studies are typically started 30 minutes after injection.

**Technetium-99m teboroxime**    Technetium-99m teboroxime is a neutral lipophilic agent from a class of compounds referred to as boronic acid adducts of technetium dioxime (BATO). Tc-99m teboroxime is avidly extracted from the blood. The extraction fraction is higher than that for Tl-201 (Table 5-1). At resting flow rates the extraction is 90% or better. The extraction fraction decreases with increasing flow but remains proportional to flow, so that the regional uptake and distribution of Tc-99m teboroxime constitute a suitable marker of regional myocardial perfusion.

*Pharmacokinetics*    The myocardial uptake and blood clearance of Tc-99m teboroxime are very rapid. The dominant component of blood clearance has a half-life of less than 1 minute. Myocardial clearance or washout is also extremely rapid, with a half-time on the order of 5 to 10 minutes for the major component. Early regional washout appears to be proportional to regional flow. After initial clearance from the blood the tracer is metabolized into complexes that do not show uptake in the myocardium. Therefore significant redistribution does not occur with Tc-99m teboroxime.

Rapid myocardial uptake and clearance dictate a narrow window for imaging, between 2 and 6 minutes. During this time window the tracer distribution in the myocardium reflects relative regional perfusion.

*Clinical applications*    Use of Tc-99m teboroxime for evaluating cardiac interventions attracted some initial

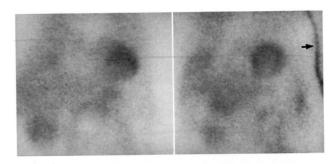

**Fig. 5-1**    Anterior *(left)* and left anterior oblique *(right)* thallium-201 scintigrams in a patient with a large apical and inferior myocardial infarction. The tracer was injected with the patient at rest. Note the retention of thallium in a vein in the left arm *(arrow)*. Note also the uptake in the lung, liver, and other abdominal viscera.

interest. For example, the rapid clearance of Tc-99m teboroxime from the myocardium makes it a potentially ideal agent for assessing the effects of thrombolytic therapy. However, this agent is no longer commercially available and is not used in current practice.

## Imaging Protocols

**Thallium-201 chloride**    Ideally, the patient should have fasted for 4 hours or more to reduce uptake in the abdominal viscera; other special considerations for stress studies are discussed later in the chapter. Direct intravenous injection is desirable to prevent drug-drug interactions and to minimize loss of tracer activity caused by adsorption to IV tubing or adherence to venous structures exposed to medication (Fig. 5-1). The package insert dosage recommendation is 1 to 2 mCi (33 to 74 MBq). However, this recommendation was based on the economics of Tl-201 when it was first approved by the FDA and not on either intrinsic radiation safety factors or ideal amounts for imaging. Most laboratories use 2 to 3.5 mCi (75 to 120 MBq) (Box 5-2).

Several choices are available for setting the energy window of the gamma camera. In one approach a 20% to 25% window is centered at 80 keV. This window encompasses the K-beta series of mercury-201 x-rays. This asymmetrical window setting on the mercury x-rays eliminates inclusion of scatter from the K-beta series into the energy range of the K-alpha series and also reduces the contribution from lead characteristic x-rays generated by interactions in the collimator. The lead K-alpha series x-rays are in the 73- to 75-keV range. Thus, while using the entire mercury x-ray range to increase counting rates is tempting, the spatial resolution in the image is significantly degraded if this is done. Nevertheless, many clinics use a symmetrical window to include all of the mercury x-rays (69 to 83 keV). Even with modern correction circuitry this improves field uniformity and

---

**Box 5-2  Thallium-201 Myocardial Imaging: Protocol Summary**

**PATIENT PREPARATION AND FOLLOW-UP**

Patients should ideally fast for 4 hr beforehand
Electrocardiographic leads should be moved out of field of view

**DOSAGE AND ROUTE OF ADMINISTRATION**

2 to 3.5 mCi (75 to 120 MBq) thallium-201 as thallium chloride
Intravenous administration, with the patient upright if possible

**TIME OF IMAGING**

10 min after radiopharmaceutical administration

**PLANAR IMAGING**

Use a low-energy, general purpose, parallel hole collimator and a 20% to 25% window centered at 80 keV (can also use a second 20% window at 167 keV, if available)
Obtain anterior, 35° left anterior oblique (LAO) 70° LAO, and left lateral views for 10 min each
For rest-redistribution studies, repeat the same views 2 to 4 hr later

**SPECT IMAGING ACQUISITION PARAMETERS**

Use a general all-purpose collimator and a 20% window centered at 80 keV
Patient position: supine, left arm raised
Rotation orbit: circular or elliptical
Matrix: 64 × 64 word mode
Arc and framing: 64 views, 180° (45° RAO, 135° LPO), 20 seconds per view

**SPECT RECONSTRUCTION PARAMETERS***

Filter: Butterworth; cutoff 0.5 and order 8
Attenuation correction: yes, if available
Reconstruction technique: filtered backprojection
Images: transaxial, short axis, horizontal long axis, and vertical long axis

*Choice of SPECT acquisition and reconstruction parameters is highly influenced by the equipment used. Protocols for available SPECT cameras and computers should be established in each nuclear medicine unit.

---

also improves counting statistics. If the gamma camera has an option for multiple windows, a second 20% window can be centered at 167 keV. This will increase the counting statistics by 10%.

Imaging is begun 10 minutes after injection for both poststress studies and resting studies. For planar imaging a standard-field-of-view camera or large-field-of-view camera with a low-energy, high-resolution or all-purpose collimator is used. A minimum of three and preferably four views are obtained in the anterior, 35° to 40° left anterior oblique (LAO), 60° to 70° LAO, and left lateral projections. Mobile gamma cameras are typically used in the emergency room and at the patient's bedside in the coronary care unit for imaging in the diagnosis of acute myocardial infarction.

Each view is obtained for 300,000 counts (standard-field-of-view camera) to 500,000 counts (large-field-of-view camera). Two alternatives are to obtain the anterior view first and subsequent views for the same length of time, or to image in each projection for a fixed length of time, typically on the order of 8 to 10 minutes.

Tl-201 imaging is most commonly performed as a SPECT study. However, the relatively low count rates and suboptimal energy of the available photons make Tl-201 SPECT less satisfactory, at least esthetically, than SPECT studies obtained with one of the Tc-99m-labeled myocardial perfusion agents.

**Technetium-99m sestamibi and technetium-99m tetrofosmin**  High-quality imaging with Tc-99m sestamibi or Tc-99m tetrofosmin can be accomplished with either planar or SPECT techniques (Box 5-3). For planar imaging a dose of 10 mCi provides a sufficient count rate for imaging with a high-resolution collimator. For rest studies imaging is begun 60 to 90 minutes after tracer administration. Between 750,000 and 1 million counts are obtained per image, with anterior, 35° to 40° and 60° to 70° LAO, and lateral views obtained. The high count rate afforded by the Tc-99m-labeled agents also permits the use of ECG gated image acquisition. The same computer program is used as for radionuclide ventriculography. The advantage of gated imaging is that the function of the myocardium may be evaluated by assessing wall motion and wall thickening. Some of the advantages and disadvantages of the Tc-99m-labeled agents are summarized in Box 5-4.

Up to 30 mCi of Tc-99m sestamibi or Tc-99m tetrofosmin may be used for SPECT imaging. The time delay after tracer administration is the same as for planar imaging. Gated SPECT is also feasible with these agents, especially if multiheaded SPECT systems are used. A few laboratories take advantage of the high count rate available from the 10- to 30-mCi dose to perform first-pass radionuclide ventriculography. With this approach right and left ventricular function and myocardial perfusion can be assessed with a single dose of radiopharmaceutical. It does add to procedure complexity and is not commonly performed in practice.

Techniques have been developed to perform Tc-99m stress/rest procedures either as a 1-day study or on 2 different days (Box 5-2). Since Tc-99m sestamibi and Tc-99m tetrofosmin have long biological halftimes in the myocardium, studies on the same day require the use of a smaller initial dose followed by a larger dose. Different laboratories choose to do either the stress portion or the resting portion of the procedure first. The initial study is

---

## Box 5-3   Technetium-99m Sestamibi and Technetium-99 Tetrofosmin Imaging: Protocol Summary

**PATIENT PREPARATION**

Standard preparation and precautions for stress studies

**DOSE AND ROUTE OF RADIOPHARMACEUTICAL ADMINISTRATION**

10 to 30 mCi (370 to 1110 MBq) for single dose
Intravenous administration

**IMAGING PROTOCOL—PLANAR STUDIES**

Use a high-resolution collimator and a 20% window centered at 140 keV

Begin imaging at 60 to 90 min after tracer injection for rest studies

Begin imaging at 15 to 30 min after tracer injection for stress studies

Obtain anterior, 30° to 40° left anterior oblique (LAO), and 70° LAO views

Obtain 750,000 to 1 million counts per view

Consider electrocardiographic gating to evaluate questionable lesions

For single-day rest and stress studies give 10 mCi at rest and image at 30 to 60 min

Wait 4 hours and give 20 mCi with repeat imaging at 15 to 30 min

**IMAGING PROTOCOL—SPECT**

1-Day rest/stress imaging
   Rest: 8 to 10 mCi Tc-99m sestamibi or Tc-99m tetrofosmin; imaging begun at 30 to 90 min
   Stress: 20-30 mCi Tc-99m sestamibi or Tc-99m tetrofosmin; imaging begun at 15 to 30 min
2-Day rest/stress or stress/rest imaging: 25 mCi Tc99m sestamibi or Tc-99m tetrofosmin

**SPECT Acquisition Parameters**

Patient position: supine, left arm raised (180° arc)
Rotation: counterclockwise
Matrix: $64 \times 64$ word mode
Image/arc combination: 64 views (180°, 45° right anterior oblique, 135° left posterior oblique)

**SPECT Reconstruction Parameters***

Interslice filter
Convolution filter: Butterworth
   Rest: cutoff = 0.6, order = 0.8
   Stress: cutoff = 0.6, order = 0.8
Attenuation correction: yes, if available
Oblique angle reformatting: yes, vertical and horizontal long axis, short axis
Gated SPECT
   ECG synchronized data collection: R wave trigger
   8 Frames/cardiac cycle

---

*Choice of SPECT acquisition and reconstruction parameters is highly influenced by the equipment used. Protocols should be established in each nuclear medicine unit for available cameras and computers.

---

## Box 5-4   Advantages and Disadvantages of Using Technetium-99m Sestamibi/Tetrofosmin Rather Than Thallium-201 Chloride for Myocardial Perfusion Imaging

**ADVANTAGES**

Higher count rates; SPECT and gated SPECT
Higher energy photons; fewer attenuation artifacts
Simultaneous assessment of perfusion and function; gated SPECT
First-pass assessment of right and left ventricular function

**DISADVANTAGES**

No redistribution
Lung uptake not diagnostic
Less extraction at hyperemic flows
Less sensitive than Tl-201 for viability assessment (rest-redistribution)

accomplished with 10 mCi Tc-99m sestamibi or Tc-99m tetrofosmin, and the second study is performed 3 to 4 hours later using 20 to 30 mCi. The image interpreter must take into account residual activity just as with reinjection thallium imaging. Another approach is to combine Tc-99m sestamibi or Tc-99m tetrofosmin with Tl-201 for a dual tracer study. If thallium is used first for the resting procedure, its lower energy does not interfere with subsequent imaging of Tc-99m, since the higher energy photons (167 keV) from Tl-201 have low abundance (10%).

**SPECT imaging**   For SPECT imaging a general all-purpose collimator is used with Tl-201 and a high-resolution collimator is used for the Tc-99m-labeled agents (Box 5-3). The details of image acquisition are dictated by the SPECT system employed. Variations include continuous versus discontinuous data acquisition, length of acquisition, arc length, and shape of orbit. In current practice, laboratories with single-head cameras and most with two-headed cameras use a 180° arc length from a 45° right anterior oblique (RAO) position to a 135° left posterior oblique (LPO) position. Also a 180° arc is preferable only with Tl-201 because of attenuation artifacts from the spine if a full 360° acquisition is obtained. Another advantage of the 180° arc is that the patient has to hold the left arm up only during data acquisition. Imaging is typically completed within 20 to 25 minutes to minimize internal redistribution of Tl-201 during the imaging sequence. Patient movement because of discomfort is a major source of image degradation in cardiac SPECT and dictates as short an imaging time as possible.

Noncircular orbits or body-contoured arc paths are desirable in theory to keep the camera head as close to the body surface as possible, since spatial resolution is degraded the farther the camera head is from the organ of interest. However, in practice, a circular orbit with the heart in the center of rotation is the most common approach.

The high counts available with Tc-99m sestamibi and Tc-99m tetrofosmin offer the opportunity to add ECG-synchronized SPECT to myocardial perfusion imaging protocols (Box 5-3). An important advantage of gating is the ability to replay sequential gated images in a cinematic display to assess regional wall motion. Gated SPECT also creates the possibility of calculating left ventricular ejection fractions, measuring wall thickening, and more accurately analyzing tracer distribution. It also permits three-dimensional display of the myocardium.

The cardiac cycle is typically divided into eight frames. Data collection is triggered from the R-wave of the ECG with arrhythmic beats filtered out of the data collection cycle. Gated images have proportionately fewer counts per image based on the number of frames obtained per cardiac cycle, but the higher count rates available with the Tc-99m-labeled agents and the use of multiheaded detector systems make gated studies quite feasible.

## Appearance of the Normal Myocardial Perfusion Scintigram

**Thallium-201** Tl-201 scintigrams obtained in normal subjects after tracer injection at rest should demonstrate uniform uptake of thallium throughout the left ventricular myocardium (Fig. 5-2). The right ventricle is typically not seen on planar studies at rest but can be seen with SPECT. Visualization is significant in cases of right ventricular hypertrophy (Fig. 5-3). In normal subjects the myocardium may appear thinner at the apex than in other portions of the ventricle. This pattern of apical thinning should not be misinterpreted as a pathological defect. The valve planes also demonstrate absence of uptake, giving the heart a horseshoe or U-shaped appearance on long-axis SPECT views and on steep oblique and lateral planar views (Figs. 5-2 and 5-4). The heart has a ring or doughnut appearance on

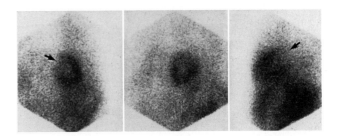

**Fig. 5-2**   Anterior, left anterior oblique, and left lateral views of a thallium-201 study obtained at rest in a normal subject. Uptake of thallium is uniform throughout the myocardium. Absence of tracer uptake in valve planes *(arrows)* gives the heart a horseshoe appearance on the anterior and left lateral views.

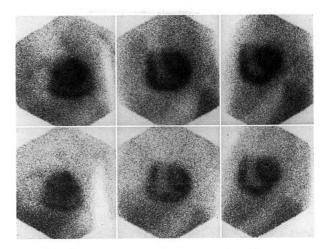

**Fig. 5-3**   Rest *(top)* and redistribution *(bottom)* thallium scintigrams in a patient with severe lung involvement by scleroderma. Note right ventricular hypertrophy and enlargement of the right ventricular cavity. The thickness and intensity of uptake in the right ventricular myocardium are equal to or greater than the thickness and intensity of uptake in the left ventricular myocardium. This appearance is characteristic of conditions causing right-sided pressure overload.

short-axis SPECT views and a variably circular or ellipsoidal appearance on LAO planar views, depending on the patient's habitus and the axial orientation of the heart in the chest. Decreased uptake in the septum on more posterior short-axis SPECT views near the base is due to the membranous septum and should not be mistaken for an abnormality (Fig. 5-4). Some lung uptake is usually noted. Significant lung uptake may be seen in heavy smokers, patients with underlying lung disease, and patients in congestive heart failure (Fig. 5-1).

Myocardial perfusion scintigrams with Tl-201 obtained immediately after exercise or pharmacological stress intervention are strikingly different from those obtained at rest (Fig. 5-5). The target-to-background ratio is typically better. Right ventricular activity is frequently seen. During exercise, blood flow is diverted from the splanchnic bed, and less tracer activity should be seen in the liver and other abdominal structures. Assessing the degree of uptake in the liver is useful as an internal quality control check on the adequacy of exercise. Poorly exercised subjects will demonstrate higher than expected liver activity. SPECT studies reflect these differences as well (Fig. 5-4).

On delayed Tl-201 redistribution images and reinjection images the overall appearance of the myocardium is

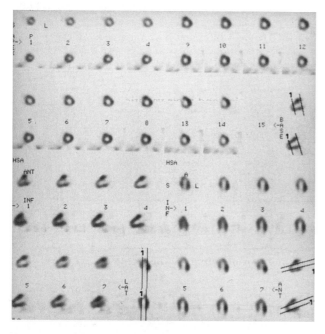

**Fig. 5-4**    Normal stress thallium study with SPECT imaging and typical computer-generated display. The top two rows for each slice orientation are the immediate poststress images, and the bottom two rows are the delayed images. Short-axis *(top four rows)*, vertical long-axis *(bottom left)*, and horizontal long-axis views are typically used for interpretation.

similar in normal subjects to the appearance with tracer injected at rest. The myocardium-to-background ratio is usually decreased, and significantly more activity is seen in the liver and other abdominal structures than on stress images (Fig. 5-5).

Thallium is taken up in all cellular, metabolically active tissues in the body with the exception of the brain. It does not cross the normal blood-brain barrier. Activity on resting studies is normally seen in the liver (Fig. 5-2) and gastrointestinal (GI) tract but to a lesser extent than with the Tc-99m agents. Other structures accumulating significant thallium that may occasionally be in the field of view are the thyroid and salivary glands, the kidneys, and skeletal muscle.

**Technetium-99m sestamibi and technetium-99m tetrofosmin**    Studies obtained with tracer given at rest demonstrate uniform uptake in the left ventricular myocardium in the same patterns described above for Tl-201. However, the right ventricle is often seen by both planar and SPECT imaging. Significant lung and liver activity is present right after injection and, as noted above, heart/lung and heart/liver ratios improve over time so that imaging is delayed for 30 to 90 minutes. Variable and often significant bowel activity may obscure the inferior wall of the heart. Since the count rate is higher and high-resolution collimators are used, images obtained with the Tc-99m agents often appear crisper than with Tl-201 (Figs. 5-6 and 5-7). SPECT studies typically provide excellent visualization of the myocardium in normal subjects (Fig. 5-7).

Differences between rest and stress studies obtained in normal subjects with the Tc-99m-labeled agents are less striking than those with Tl-201. The heart/lung and

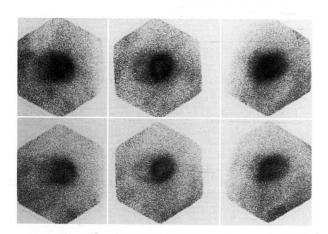

**Fig. 5-5**    Normal stress thallium study with planar imaging. Immediate poststress *(top)* and 3-hour delayed *(bottom)* thallium-201 scintigrams in a normal subject. The left ventricular myocardium-to-background ratio is excellent. Right ventricular uptake is clearly visible. On the immediate poststress images little activity is seen in the region of the liver or other abdominal viscera. Some increase in these areas is seen on the delayed images. There are no abnormal defects in the myocardial tracer uptake.

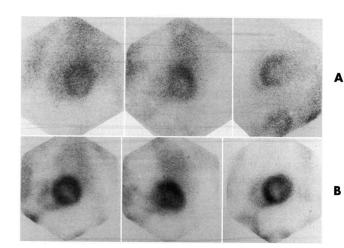

**Fig. 5-6**    Comparison of, **A,** thallium-201 scintigraphy and, **B,** technetium-99m sestamibi scintigraphy in the same patient after stress. Although the myocardium is well visualized with both agents, the count rate available with Tl-201 is less than with Tc-99m sestamibi and the target-to-background ratio is lower. Some attenuation artifact caused by interposition of the diaphragm and subdiaphragmatic structures can be seen on the lateral view. The effect is greater on the Tl-201 examination.

heart/liver ratios are higher, but the overall appearance of the myocardial uptake is the same. The Tc-99m offers a higher count rate with superior visualization of the myocardium and fewer extenuation artifacts. SPECT studies in normal subjects demonstrate excellent visualization of the myocardium in all image planes (Fig. 5-7).

Two special problems in imaging the left ventricular myocardium have been described. First, in some women the overlying soft tissue of the breast causes attenuation of activity from the heart. This reduces the overall number of counts available for creating the image and can also result in spurious defects, especially along the lateral heart border. Images of women should be carefully inspected for breast attenuation artifacts. A breast binder can be used to flatten the tissue and hold the breast in the same position between poststress and rest imaging. Reimaging with the breast held out of the field of view may be necessary.

The second artifact is interposition of the diaphragm and subdiaphragmatic viscera between the gamma camera and the heart on the left lateral view with the patient supine. Activity from the inferior and posterior lateral walls of the left ventricle can be attenuated, causing a spurious photon-deficient defect. In planar imaging the diaphragmatic artifact is minimized by placing the patient in the right lateral decubitus position, which causes the left hemidiaphragm to move down. These are more significant problems for studies obtained with Tl-201 than with Tc-99m agents because of the lower energy of the photons (Box 5-4). In Fig. 5-6 the greater attenuation artifact obtained with thallium *(A)* than with Tc-99m sestamibi *(B)* can be seen.

## Diagnosis of Coronary Artery Disease

A recurrent theme in nuclear medicine and in this book is the ability to extend the diagnostic capability of a nuclear imaging procedure by applying an interventional maneuver to alter organ function, often while testing functional reserve. Cardiac interventions in the form of various stress tests are the cornerstone of the diagnosis of CAD, and exercise stress testing in conjunction with ECG monitoring was used for many years before nuclear perfusion imaging was introduced. Box 5-5 summarizes the important indications and contraindications for stress testing.

The number of different approaches to cardiac exercise stress testing and their variations can be confusing. The rationale for all exercise stress testing in CAD is the same: to unmask critical CAD by increasing cardiac work and oxygen demand. Thus the physiological rationale for the different exercise stress tests is the same, but the diagnostic endpoint is different, depending on the parameter(s) the test is designed to measure (Box 5-6).

With the traditional treadmill stress test, myocardial ischemia is detected by characteristic changes on the ECG caused by alterations in electrolyte flux across the ischemic cell membrane. The ischemic cell membrane

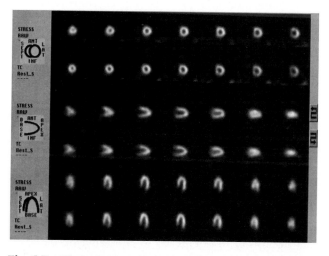

**Fig. 5-7** Normal stress and rest technetium-99m sestamibi SPECT images. Note the excellent visualization of the left ventricular myocardium. The more posterior short-axis views *(top rows, far right)* demonstrate decreased uptake in the region of the membranous septum.

---

### Box 5-5  Indications for and Contraindications to Stress Testing

**INDICATIONS**

Diagnosis of chest pain syndromes
Evaluation of known coronary artery disease; location and extent of ischemia
Assessment of medical therapy
Assessment after percutaneous transluminal coronary angioplasty or coronary artery bypass grafting
Evaluation and prognosis post myocardial infarction
Evaluation of myocardial reserve
Preoperative evaluation for major noncardiac surgery
Guide to rehabilitation therapy
Screening high-risk patient populations

**CONTRAINDICATIONS**

Acute myocardial infarction
Unstable angina
Life-threatening cardiac arrhythmia
Acute inflammatory disease of the heart; myocarditis, valvulitis, pericarditis
Critical aortic stenosis
Pulmonary edema/congestive heart failure
Pulmonary embolism
Excessive arterial hypertension
Serious intercurrent noncardiac illness
Unwilling patient
Inability to provide informed consent

---

**Box 5-6   Rationale and Endpoint Measures in Exercise Testing**

**RATIONALE**

Physical exercise increases cardiac workload; increased work increases myocardial oxygen demand

Normal coronary arteries dilate and flow increases

Stenotic vessels do not dilate; flow reserve is limited; myocardial ischemia is induced

**MANIFESTATIONS OF MYOCARDIAL ISCHEMIA**

Electrocardiogram: Ion flux across cell membrane is impaired by ischemia; electrical activity also changes and is manifest as ST segment depression on electrocardiogram

Myocardial perfusion imaging: Relative decrease in regional flow is manifest as relative photon-deficient area on scintigram

Radionuclide ventriculography: Contraction of ischemic myocardium is decreased and manifest as either segmental wall motion abnormalities or a fall in global parameters, including ejection fraction, or both

---

**Box 5-7   Reasons for Failing to Achieve Adequate Exercise**

Poor general conditioning, low exercise tolerance

Poor motivation

Arthritis, other musculoskeletal problems

Lung disease

Peripheral vascular disease

Medications (beta-blockers, calcium channel blockers)

Angina

Arrhythmia

Cardiac insufficiency

---

will not sustain a normal exchange of sodium and potassium. The classic ECG change is depression of the ST segment. On myocardial scintigrams, exercise-induced ischemia is manifested as a decrease in relative regional blood flow, which in turn is seen on the scintigram as a segmental photon-deficient or cold area. On exercise or stress radionuclide ventriculograms, myocardial ischemia is detected by deterioration in regional myocardial wall motion and global ventricular function compared with the rest state. Ischemic myocardium does not contract normally. The hallmark of ischemia is the development of an exercise-induced regional wall motion abnormality. Also, the normal functional response to exercise is an increase in left ventricular ejection fraction. With significant myocardial dysfunction resulting from segmental ischemia, the ejection fraction fails to increase or may even decrease in response to exercise-induced ischemia.

One of the important principles of all interventions is that the degree of stress must be sufficient to unmask underlying abnormalities. For cardiac stress testing by exercise, the adequacy of exercise is judged by how much the heart has to work. The blood pressure and heart rate provide an indication of the external work of the heart. They are monitored throughout exercise and recorded. Typically, patients achieving >85% of the age-predicted maximum heart rate (220 − age = maximum predicted heart rate) are considered to have achieved adequate exercise to meet the rationale for exercise stress testing. A "double product" is often calculated—the heart rate times the systolic blood pressure. A double product greater than 25,000 is another frequently used indicator of the adequacy of exercise.

As simple as the preceding principle may seem, failure to achieve adequate exercise is probably the most common reason for false negative stress tests. A number of the reasons for failure to achieve adequate exercise are summarized in Box 5-7. In many stress-testing laboratories, less than half of patients tested achieve adequate stress. This is always recorded as a qualification on the stress test report. That is, a negative test in the face of inadequate exercise or minimal exercise has much less significance than a negative test when adequacy criteria have been met.

Healthy subjects have tremendous coronary flow reserve, such that blood flow may be three to five times greater during exercise because normal vessels can dilate. However, flow reserve across a fixed mechanical stenosis is limited. If exercise is vigorous enough, myocardium in the watershed of a coronary artery with a hemodynamically significant stenosis can become ischemic. Lower blood flow to such an area than to surrounding normally perfused myocardium results in the delivery and localization of less Tl-201 or Tc-99m. This is seen on the scintigram as a cold defect in the poorly perfused area.

Coronary stenoses of up to 90% may not be associated with any observable perfusion abnormality or symptoms under resting conditions, and what percentage of stenosis actually constitutes a hemodynamically critical lesion has been the subject of much study and debate. Factors such as the length or irregularity of a stenosis are clearly important in addition to circumferential narrowing. When the sensitivity of myocardial perfusion imaging is assessed against cardiac catheterization as the gold standard, the criteria that were used are important to know. Most angiographic laboratories consider a coronary stenosis of 70% or greater to be significant, based on the rapid fall-off of flow reserve augmentation ability above this level.

## Technique for Exercise Stress

The patient is prepared in the same way for the scintigram as for a standard treadmill exercise test. The

---

**Box 5-8  Cardiac Drugs That May Interfere with Stress Testing and Recommended Withdrawal Interval**

**EXERCISE**

| | |
|---|---|
| Beta-blockers | 72 hr |
| Calcium channel blockers | 48-72 hr |
| Nitrates (long acting) | 12 hr |

**PHARMACOLOGICAL**

Aminophylline
Caffeine

---

**Box 5-9  Indications for Terminating a Stress Test**

Patient's request
Inability to continue owing to fatigue, dyspnea, or faintness
Chest pain
Syncope, blurred vision
Pallor, diaphoresis
Ataxia
Claudication
Ventricular tachycardia
Atrial tachycardia or fibrillation
Onset of second- or third-degree heart block
ST segment depression >3 mm
Decrease in systolic blood pressure
Increase in systolic blood pressure above 240 mm Hg or diastolic above 120 mm Hg

---

patient should fast before the test, and at the discretion of the attending physician cardiac medication should be withdrawn. Box 5-8 summarizes some of the more important types of cardiac drugs and the length of time before exercise testing that they should be withdrawn to minimize residual effects. In some cases discontinuing the medications will not be possible. If so, this must be noted in the report, since medication effects from beta-blockers can prevent achievement of maximum heart rate and nitrates or calcium channel blockers may mask or prevent cardiac ischemia. A negative test while the patient is taking cardiac medications may augur well for the clinical course but is moot diagnostically. In some cases medications are deliberately continued to assess adequacy of drug therapy in blocking ischemia.

In addition to a standard 12-lead ECG baseline evaluation and continuous monitoring during the treadmill test, an IV line with keep-open solution is placed so that it will not interfere with exercise. When the patient is judged to have achieved maximal exercise or peak patient tolerance, the selected radiopharmaceutical is injected and flushed through the IV line. For Tl-201 imaging, many laboratories use 3 to 3.5 mCi and in current practice may split the dose between an injection during stress and a reinjection at rest. The procedure is discussed in detail below. For imaging with Tc-99m sestamibi or Tc-99m tetrofosmin the dose depends on which protocol is being used (Box 5-3).

After tracer injection the patient is asked to maintain exercise for another 30 to 90 seconds if possible. This ensures that the initial uptake of tracer in the heart will reflect the perfusion pattern at peak stress. Early discontinuation of exercise may result in a tracer distribution reflecting perfusion at submaximal rather than maximal exercise levels.

At one time with Tl-201 imaging, it was recommended that imaging be started immediately to detect ischemic lesions that might "fill in" in the first minutes after initial tracer uptake. This unusual occurrence often represented low-grade stenosis. Most nuclear medicine departments now wait 10 minutes to begin imaging with

Tl-201 to allow the position of the heart to stabilize in the chest. Immediately after maximal exercise, patients are breathing deeply. The lungs are fully expanded, and the diaphragm is down. As the patient returns to baseline, the diaphragm comes up in the chest and the heart moves cephalad. This "cardiac creep" is particularly bad when it occurs during SPECT imaging, since the position of the heart is slightly different in each of the angular views obtained sequentially during imaging. A compromise to avoid missing an area of mild ischemia with Tl-201 is to obtain a single planar image for 10 minutes while the patient's breathing stabilizes. The 40° LAO is the single best view from the standpoint of sensitivity of lesion detection. A SPECT study or standard multiview imaging then follows immediately. This is not an issue with the Tc-99m-labeled agents because imaging is delayed anyway to allow more background clearance.

Although radiologists and nuclear medicine specialists do not commonly perform the stress portion of the myocardium perfusion stress study, they should know the indications for terminating exercise. A brief summary is provided in Box 5-9. Most of the indications for stopping exercise are manifestations of ischemia.

**Thallium-201 reinjection imaging** Beginning in the late 1970s and for over a decade thereafter, the most common protocol for stress Tl-201 imaging was immediate poststress imaging followed by redistribution imaging 3 to 4 hours later. These delayed images are supposed to depict the baseline or equilibrated perfusion pattern. However, this approach does not always demonstrate baseline resting perfusion and it overestimates the number of fixed myocardial defects (Fig. 5-8). In some patients imaging delayed up to 24 hours after tracer injection shows further redistribution. To avoid the need for these delayed images, an alternative strategy is to administer a second injection of tracer, typically 1 mCi, at the time of redistribution imaging (Fig. 5-8). Some nuclear

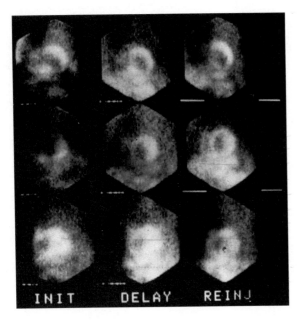

**Fig. 5-8**    Initial poststress images reveal extensive defects in the septum and inferior wall. After a several hour delay *(middle column)*, extensive defects remain. Following reinjection *(right column)*, all areas of the myocardium demonstrate some degree of uptake. The difference between the delay and reinjection images is most striking in the septum. (Courtesy of H. William Strauss, M.D., Stanford University.)

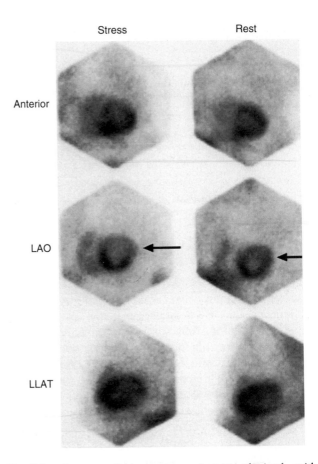

**Fig. 5-9**    Stress and rest planar images obtained with technetium-99m tetrofosmin. A large area of decreased tracer uptake that can be seen in the anterolateral wall on the poststress image represents essentially normal tracer uptake at rest. This is best seen in the left anterior oblique view *(arrows)*. This pattern indicates exercise-induced ischemia and coronary artery disease. *LAO,* Left anterior oblique; *LLAT,* left lateral.

**Table 5-3    Diagnostic patterns: myocardial perfusion imaging after stress testing**

| Pattern on immediate poststress images | Pattern on resting delayed or reinjection images | Diagnosis |
| --- | --- | --- |
| Normal | Normal | Normal |
| Defect(s) | Normal | Transient ischemia |
| Defect(s) | Defect (unchanged) | Prior infarct with scar* |
| Defect(s) | Some normalization with areas of persistent defect | Transient ischemia and scar* |
| Normal | Defect | "Reverse" redistribution |

*Delayed* Tl-201 imaging without reinjection may overestimate the presence and amount of infarcted area because of incomplete redistribution.

medicine departments perform the reinjection earlier than the usual 3- to 4-hour delay for redistribution imaging. However, early reinjection leads to overestimation of scar and underestimation of the number of viable segments. Many institutions are exploring studies with combined thallium- and technetium-labeled myocardial perfusion agent to streamline the examination.

The rationale for reinjection imaging comes from the observation that 15% to 35% of ischemic segments do not fill in or normalize by 3 to 4 hours. If delayed imaging is relied on for distinguishing scar and ischemia, myocardial

scar will be overestimated and the number of patients with stress-induced ischemia will be underestimated. This is a serious error because it is the patients with transient ischemia who may benefit from surgery or angioplasty and who are at risk for ischemia-induced cardiac dysrhythmia and sudden death. A relationship exists between the degree of stenosis and the rate of equilibration. Areas of severe narrowing appear to fill in more slowly.

## Diagnostic Patterns in Coronary Artery Disease

A diagnostic schema is presented in Table 5-3 that uses the appearance of the scintigrams on the immediate poststress studies and the resting delayed (reinjection) images to characterize myocardial perfusion as (1) normal (Figs. 5-4, 5-5, and 5-7) (no defects noted on either image set), (2) having evidence of transient ischemia (Figs. 5-9 and 5-10) (cold defects on poststress images that fill in or reverse on delayed images), or (3) having evidence of

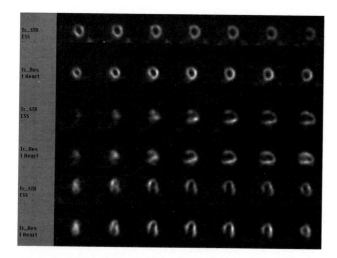

Fig. 5-10    SPECT images at stress and rest obtained with technetium-99m sestamibi. A large area of decreased tracer uptake in the anterior wall is best seen on the long-axis views. The defect substantially fills in on the resting images *(middle rows)*. As in Fig. 5-9, this pattern indicates exercise-induced ischemia and coronary artery disease.

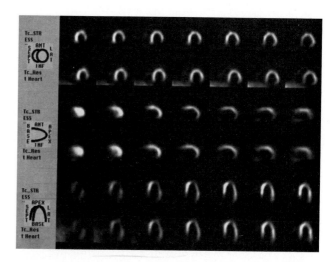

Fig. 5-12    SPECT images obtained at stress and rest in a patient with a history of prior myocardial infarction. A large fixed defect involving the inferior wall of the heart is visible and can best be seen on the short-axis and vertical long-axis views. No substantial change in the scintigraphic appearance is noted between the poststress and rest images.

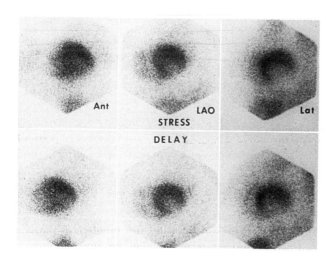

Fig. 5-11    Planar thallium-201 scintigrams after stress *(top row)* and with a 2-hour delay *(bottom row)* reveal a fixed inferoapical defect. Essentially no fill-in is seen between the two sets of images. The ventricular cavity is slightly larger on the initial images, a common finding in patients with coronary artery disease. Fixed defects are indicative of myocardial scarring, most commonly resulting from prior infarction.

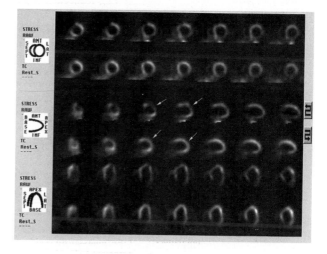

Fig. 5-13    SPECT images obtained at stress and rest with technetium-99m sestamibi reveal a large defect in the anterior wall best seen on the vertical long-axis views *(arrows)* that substantially fills in between the stress and rest images. A second fixed defect is present in the inferior wall and is best seen on the short-axis views *(short-axis images immediately above the arrows)*. This pattern of both fixed and transient defects is indicative of combined myocardial ischemia and scarring in a patient with multivessel disease.

prior infarction (Figs. 5-11 and 5-12) (defects that remain "fixed" between the image sets). Patients may have a combination of fixed and transient defects (Fig. 5-13). The patterns apply to both planar and SPECT imaging. Box 5-10 defines several important terms used to characterize the myocardium.

After initial assessment of the presence or absence of defects, a complete evaluation of the Tl-201 or Tc-99m stress study includes assessment of the size, location,

severity, and when possible likely vascular distribution of the visualized abnormalities (Figs. 5-14 and 5-15). Box 5-11 summarizes the scintigraphic patterns associated with the major vessels. A variety of computer-based methods to define defect size are in use and are discussed in the following paragraphs.

Perfusion defects caused by CAD are more common distally than at the base of the heart. In deciding whether a given abnormality is a true perfusion defect, the diag-

## Box 5-10   Common Terms Used to Describe the Status of the Myocardium

| TERM | DEFINITION AND SCAN APPEARANCE |
| --- | --- |
| Myocardial ischemia | Oxygen supply below normal metabolic requirements usually due to inadequate circulation of blood as a result of coronary artery disease; ischemic myocardium appears photon deficient on perfusion scintigrams |
| Myocardial infarction | Necrosis of myocardial tissue, most commonly as a result of coronary occlusion; appears photon deficient on perfusion and metabolic imaging studies |
| Transmural infarction | Necrosis involves all layers from endocardium to epicardium; high sensitivity for detection by perfusion imaging |
| Subendocardial infarction | Necrosis involves only muscle adjacent to endocardium; lower sensitivity for detection on perfusion imaging |
| Myocardial scar | Late result of infarction; appears photon deficient scintigraphically |
| Hibernating myocardium | Viable but chronically ischemic myocardium with down regulation of contractility; reversible with restoration of blood flow; photon deficient by perfusion imaging with positive uptake by FDG metabolic imaging |
| Stunned myocardium | Myocardium with persistent contractile dysfunction despite restoration of perfusion after a period of ischemia; usually improves with time; normal or somewhat decreased uptake by perfusion imaging, positive uptake by FDG metabolic imaging |

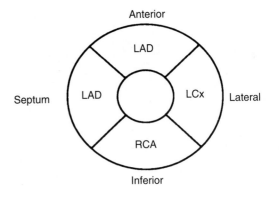

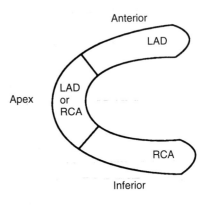

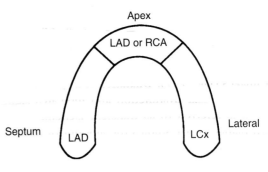

**Fig. 5-14**   Usual correlation of myocardial wall segments and vascular supply as seen on short-axis, vertical long-axis, and horizontal long-axis SPECT views. *LAD*, Left anterior descending artery; *LCx*, left circumflex branch; *RCA*, right coronary artery.

nostician's confidence goes up if the defect is seen on more than one view. Certainty also increases with lesion size and the degree or severity of photon deficiency.

Although the actual anatomy of the coronary circulation varies in its details, the distribution of the major vessels is reasonably predictable (Figs. 5-14 to 5-16). The left anterior descending coronary artery serves most of the septum and the anterior wall of the left ventricle. The left circumflex coronary artery serves the lateral and posterior walls. The right coronary artery serves the right ventricle, the inferior portion of the septum, and

portions of the inferior wall of the left ventricle. The apex may be perfused by branches from any of the three main vessels. Defects in more than one coronary artery distribution area point to multiple vessel disease. Poor uptake and slow Tl-201 washout are secondary signs of multiple-vessel disease.

In addition to the location, severity, and size of perfusion abnormalities in the myocardium, other factors should be assessed. Stress-induced dilatation of the left ventricular cavity is readily detected by comparing the images immediately after exercise with the delayed

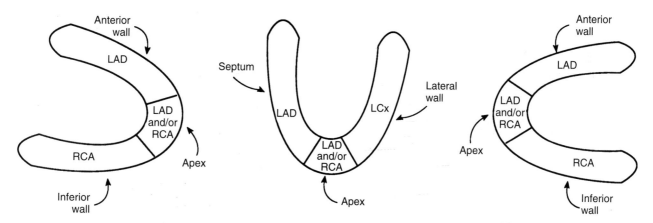

**Fig. 5-15** Usual relationship between left ventricular wall segments and vascular supply as seen on anterior, left anterior oblique, and left lateral thallium-201 or technetium-99m planar images. *LAD,* Left anterior descending artery; *LCx,* left circumflex branch; *RCA,* right coronary artery.

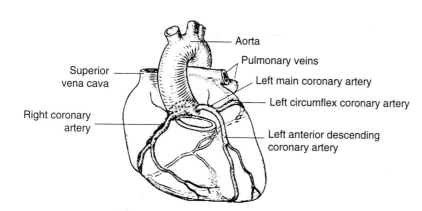

**Fig. 5-16** Simplified drawing of the distribution of the main coronary arteries. Note the correlations with the wall segments for SPECT (Fig. 5-14) and planar (Fig. 5-15) images.

rest images (Fig. 5-17). Dilatation is a secondary indicator of ventricular dysfunction and indicates significant CAD. It is referred to as transient ischemic dilatation.

On planar Tl-201 studies the amount of lung activity should be carefully scrutinized. In normal subjects lung background activity should be minimal. In patients with left ventricular failure, increased left ventricular end-diastolic pressure, and increased pulmonary capillary wedge pressure, lung uptake can be striking. Exercise-induced Tl-201 uptake indicates ischemia-induced dysfunction and is a sign of multivessel disease. The ratio of lung activity to myocardial activity should be well below 0.5. Ratios at or above this level are abnormal and are secondary indicators of left ventricular dysfunction and possibly CAD. Lung uptake is not a useful secondary sign of heart disease when either Tc-99m sestamibi or Tc-99m tetrofosmin is used because these agents are normally taken up in the lung to a higher degree than Tl-201.

**Reverse redistribution** "Reverse redistribution" is a relatively uncommon but vexing scintigraphic pattern. Reverse redistribution is defined as a pattern of worsening of a perfusion defect or the development of a new

### Box 5-11 Summary of Scintigraphic Patterns for Specific Vascular Distributions

| VESSEL | SCINTIGRAPHIC PATTERNS ASSOCIATED WITH STENOSIS AND OBSTRUCTION |
|---|---|
| Left anterior descending artery | Defects in septum, anterior wall, apex |
| Left circumflex artery | Defects in lateral wall, posterior wall, posterior inferior wall, apex |
| Right coronary artery | Defects in inferior wall, posterior inferior wall, right ventricular wall |
| Left main coronary artery | Defects in anterior wall, septum, posterolateral wall |
| Multiple-vessel disease | Defects in multiple vascular distributions, ventricular enlargement in response to exercise or pharmacological stress, increased lung uptake of Tl-201 |

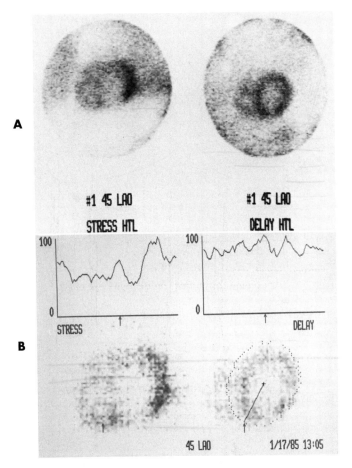

A

B

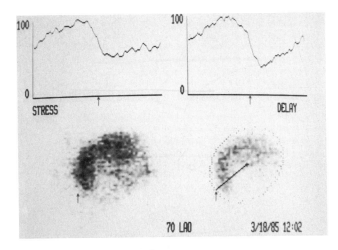

**Fig. 5-18** Quantitative analysis of a fixed defect using the circumferential profile technique. Note the failure of the curve on the right of the arrow to demonstrate significant normalization between stress and delay.

**Fig. 5-17** **A,** Planar poststress image in the left anterior oblique view reveals marked decrease in thallium-201 uptake in the septum and inferior wall with dilatation of the left ventricular cavity. The delayed image reveals essentially complete normalization of myocardial uptake and reduction in left ventricular cavity volume. **B,** Quantitative analysis from the poststress and delayed images using a circumferential profile technique. The maximum value along each of 60 rays emanating from the center of the left ventricle is calculated and plotted clockwise as a histogram. The arrow on the image corresponds to the arrow on the x-axis of the histogram. Note the lower histogram values in the areas representing the inferoapical wall *(to the right of the arrow)* and the septum *(to the left of the arrow)* on the stress image. These areas demonstrate significant fill-in on the delayed image with corresponding normalization of the histogram values.

defect on Tl-201 redistribution images compared with immediate poststress images. Some patients with severe coronary artery disease and collateral vessels demonstrate the reverse redistribution pattern, probably because of differential washout between normal and diseased areas. Unfortunately, the presence of reverse redistribution does not always indicate CAD and the finding should be viewed with caution, especially when patients have a low pretest probability of CAD, because the sign is neither sensitive nor specific.

Reverse redistribution is now also clearly recognized in patients after myocardial infarction, especially after successful thrombolytic therapy with patency of the infarct-related artery. The mechanism may be an imbalance in tracer delivery (perfusion) versus the ability of stunned myocardium to retain the tracer, leading to a differential high rate of washout from the infarct zone compared with periinfarct myocardial tissue.

Reverse redistribution has also been reported in a variety of conditions, including after coronary artery surgery and transplantation and in such diverse disorders as Wolff-Parkinson-White syndrome, Chagas' disease, sarcoidosis, and Kawasaki disease.

The term *reverse redistribution* has also been applied to studies with Tc-99m sestamibi and Tc-99m tetrofosmin. In the case of these agents, which demonstrate minimal true "redistribution," the phenomenon is really one of differential washout. That is, a new or worsening defect on delayed images is created in a tissue zone having faster washout. The diagnostic implications are probably the same as for Tl-201.

## Quantitative Analysis

A number of techniques have been described for quantitative analysis of myocardial perfusion scans obtained by both planar imaging and SPECT. These typically make use of a data set derived from normals that provides a reference for the expected range of relative regional uptake and rates of washout. In one approach a circumferential profile histogram is created from the patient's scintigram and compared with a reference standard (Figs. 5-17 and 5-18).

In another approach a polar map is created from the short-axis SPECT tomograms. The circumferential profiles are presented in a two-dimensional "bull's-eye" display. The display is generated by polar mapping of nested sets of circumferential profiles obtained from the short-axis SPECT views, starting at the apex, which is depicted at the center of the display (Fig. 5-19).

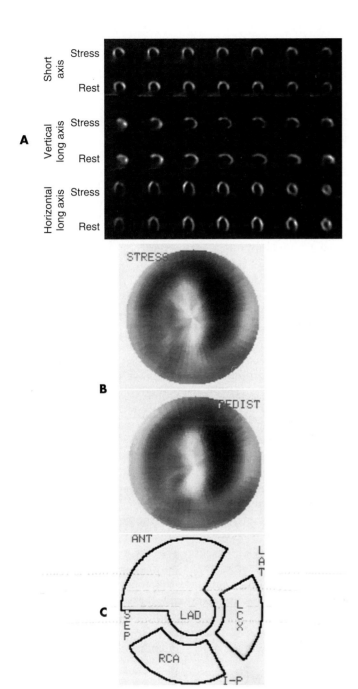

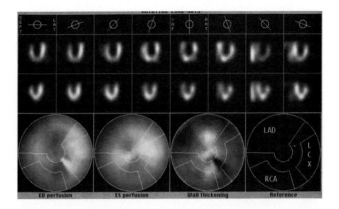

**Fig. 5-20** In addition to end-diastolic and end-systolic perfusion, the bull's eye display can be used to portray wall thickening on gated SPECT studies. The top row of images represents end-systole and the bottom row end-diastole. An area of relatively diminished tracer uptake inferolaterally corresponds with decreased wall thickening *(dark area)* on the bull's eye display.

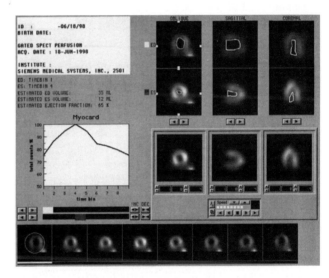

**Fig. 5-21** Gated SPECT perfusion scan in a normal subject. Estimated ejection fraction is 65%.

**Fig. 5-19** **A,** Stress and rest SPECT images obtained with technetium-99m sestamibi reveal a large fixed defect in the inferior wall best seen on the short-axis and vertical long-axis images *(middle rows)*. The patient also has transient abnormalities involving the anterior wall and apex. **B,** Corresponding "bull's-eye" display. Uptake in the region of the left circumflex artery is normal corresponding to the lateral wall. Uptake is essentially absent inferiorly and somewhat diminished anteriorly. **C,** Correlation of vascular distributions. The redistribution bull's eye display reveals no significant change inferiorly and some fill-in in the anterior wall area.

For Tl-201, washout criteria can be used but the degree of initial stress and therefore uptake of thallium in the heart directly affect the rate of washout. Higher levels of exercise are associated with more rapid washout. After adequate exercise a 30% to 40% decrease in thallium activity should occur by 3 hours after tracer injection in normal subjects. Patients with CAD demonstrate both less uptake and slower washout. However, slower washout associated with lower levels of exercise can be misinterpreted as abnormal on quantitative analysis.

A number of new approaches to quantitative analysis are being applied to gated SPECT studies obtained with the Tc-99m agents. Measures of regional perfusion at end-diastole and end-systole and estimates of wall thickening are calculated from regions of interest placed systematically around the myocardium (Fig. 5-20). Estimates of ejection fraction can be obtained by measuring the change in size of the left ventricular cavity through the cardiac cycle (Figs. 5-21 and 5-22).

Quantitative analysis of gated SPECT myocardial perfusion imaging has been extended to three-dimensional

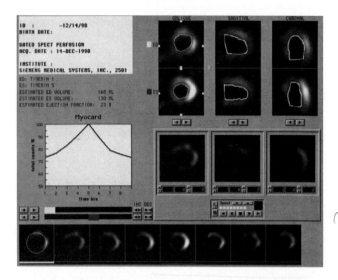

**Fig. 5-22**  Gated SPECT scan in a patient with significant coronary artery disease. Decreased tracer uptake is seen in multiple wall segments. The left ventricular cavity is dilated with an estimated end-diastolic volume of 168 ml. The ejection fraction is calculated at 23%.

reconstructions of the data. Fig. 5-23, *A,* demonstrates a largely fixed defect in the inferior and apical walls. Fig. 5-23, *B,* shows the area of defect in a series of three-dimensional displays. The left set of images compares the patient's data to a reference data set, and the right set compares poststress with rest testing. The fixed nature of the defect is readily apparent.

Fig. 5-24, *A,* demonstrates a reversible defect in the anterior wall with extension to the apex. The three-dimensional images in Fig. 5-24, *B,* demonstrate the defect versus the normal reference data set *(left)* and clearly demonstrate the reversibility *(right).*

The merits of the various quantitative analysis techniques continue to be debated in the literature. Some of the pitfalls in using the approach include problems of misregistering the patient's study with the reference data set, use of data sets generated from other laboratories on equipment different from that used in the patient's examination or on different patient populations, and lack of uniformity in the amount of exercise or stress achieved. Nonetheless, the use of quantitative methods is increasing and likely to become a standard practice.

### Sensitivity and Specificity

The accuracy of stress myocardial perfusion imaging to diagnose CAD has been studied in literally dozens of medical centers around the world. Reported sensitivities range from 60% to 95%. Specificity is variably reported as 50% to 90%. These wide ranges in reported accuracy are due in part to differences in study populations. If patients with known multiple-vessel disease and prior MI

are included in the study population, the sensitivity observed will be predictably high. On the other hand, if only younger subjects with suspected but not yet proven disease are studied, the sensitivity will be lower. Also, if the sensitivity is reported only for patients achieving adequate exercise, the sensitivity will be higher than if it is reported for all patients combined.

Specificity is an even greater problem. In many institutions the decision to perform cardiac catheterization and coronary arteriography is based on the myocardial perfusion scan. If only patients with abnormal or equivocal myocardial perfusion scans are sent to the catheterization laboratory, the specificity stress of myocardial scintigraphy in the "proven" population will be predictably low because most people with normal studies will not have the gold standard test. Other than observer and test performance, causes of false positive examinations for CAD include cardiomyopathy, valvular heart disease, and myocarditis.

It is extremely important to determine in the materials and methods sections of an article exactly what patient population was studied, if the results of patients achieving adequate versus inadequate exercise were included, and whether patients with prior MI were included. In patients achieving adequate exercise and without prior MI or known CAD, a reasonable estimate of sensitivity is 85% to 90%. A figure for specificity is more difficult because patients with normal myocardial perfusion scans typically do not undergo arteriography. SPECT and quantitative analysis may increase observer confidence but have not been shown convincingly to improve overall study accuracy.

An interesting observation in following patients over time is that people with normal stress perfusion scans, even if the results are false negatives based on anatomical angiographic criteria, have a better prognosis than those with scintigraphic evidence of ischemia. The myocardial perfusion scan is a physiological test, and the ultimate gold standard is the outcome of the patient.

### Alternatives to Leg Exercise

One of the major attractions of the combined myocardial perfusion scan–ECG stress test is the ease with which the nuclear medicine procedure is grafted onto the standard treadmill examination. The clinical information on exercise tolerance and the information from the ECG itself are valuable to the cardiologist, in addition to the information gained from the scintigraphic study. However, many patients are unable to achieve levels of exercise adequate to meet the underlying rationale of the exercise stress test. Cardiologists and nuclear medicine physicians have sought alternatives that might be applied in such patients.

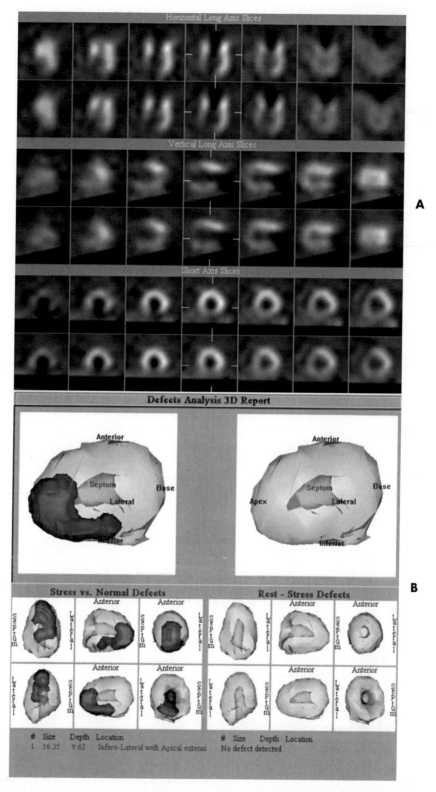

**Fig. 5-23    A,** SPECT images of a patient with a large fixed defect involving the apex. (In this display the apex is at the bottom of the image on the horizontal long-axis slices and to the left on the vertical long-axis slices.) The fixed defect is seen on all three slice orientations. **B,** Three-dimensional quantitative analysis of the images from **A** reveal the large apical and inferior defect when the stress scintigrams are compared with a normal data set *(left images).* The fixed nature of the scintigraphic defect is illustrated on the right. No differences are detected between the rest and stress views. (Courtesy of T. Yasuda, M.D., Massachusetts General Hospital.)

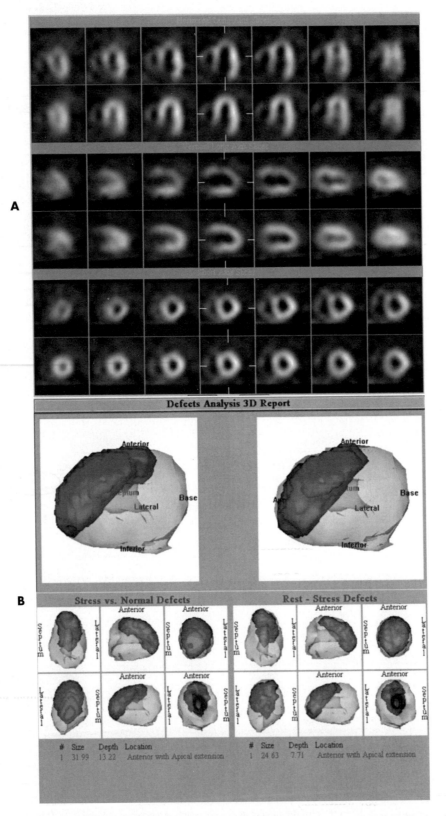

**Fig. 5-24**   **A,** SPECT images at stress and rest in a patient with a large transient defect involving the anterior wall. The defect is best seen on the vertical long-axis *(middle row)* and short-axis views. The rest images are normal. **B,** Three-dimensional quantitative analysis of the images in **A** reveals the large stress-induced defect when the patient's images are compared with a normal reference data set *(left images)*. The transient nature of the defect is illustrated in the images on the right where the rest and stress images from the patient are compared. The three-dimensional quantitative analysis provides an excellent demonstration of the extent of abnormality. (Courtesy of T. Yasuda, M.D., Massachusetts General Hospital.)

A number of alternative approaches are summarized in Box 5-12. Some of these have enjoyed brief popularity, including cold pressor testing. Other techniques such as isometric handgrip exercise have become useful as adjuncts in pharmacological stress testing. Provocative testing with ergonovine has been used in patients with suspected Prinzmetal's angina. Ergonovine provokes coronary spasm that may not be elicited during standard exercise testing or other stress testing. This is certainly not a common indication and is somewhat dangerous because the antidote for ergonovine-induced coronary spasm is intracoronary nitroglycerin.

**Dipyridamole and adenosine pharmacological stress testing**    The most important alternative to leg exercise is pharmacological stress testing with dipyridamole or adenosine. Both these agents are potent coronary vasodilators capable of causing a threefold to fourfold increase in flow in normal coronary arteries. They achieve this effect in basically the same way. Dipyridamole is an inhibitor of adenosine deaminase and thus acts by augmenting the effect of endogenous adenosine. In experience to date, both agents appear equal in their utility for diagnosing CAD (Fig. 5-25).

Adenosine has the advantage of a very short plasma half-life. If symptoms develop, no antidote to the adenosine is necessary. Infusion is simply terminated. The action of dipyridamole is more prolonged. Side effects include chest pain (angina), nausea and vomiting, dizziness, headache, shortness of breath, and a drop in blood pressure. In clinical experience approximately 20% to 25% of patients undergoing dipyridamole pharmacological stress testing experience chest pain. Chest pain may not be ischemic, although it may be secondary to coronary steal. ECG changes retain their specificity. Chest pain usually resolves when the infusion is stopped, especially if adenosine is the testing agent. The antidote is IV aminophylline (125 to 250 mg), which may have to be repeated. ST segment depression is noted in approximately 10% of cases. When using dipyridamole, some laboratories routinely administer 50 mg of aminophylline after tracer uptake is complete. In severe cases of angina, sublingual nitroglycerin is also administered.

The technical details for dipyridamole and adenosine protocols are significantly different because of their

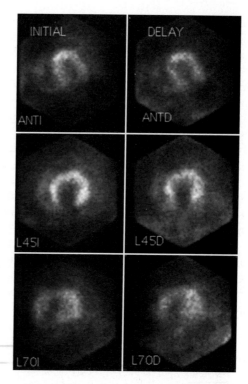

**Fig. 5-25**    Planar images of a patient undergoing a dipyridamole pharmacological stress study with thallium-201. A large fixed defect involves the inferoapical wall of the left ventricle.

## Box 5-13    Dipyridamole Perfusion Scintigraphy: Protocol Summary

| TIME FROM START OF INFUSION (MIN) | PROTOCOL |
| --- | --- |
|  | Obtain baseline ECG and blood pressure; report at 1-min intervals |
| 0-4 | Administer dipyridamole 0.14 mg/kg/min for 4 min intravenously |
| 7-9 | Inject myocardial perfusion agent intravenously at 7 to 9 min from *start* of infusion |
| 12 | Begin imaging at 12 min (5 min after tracer) |
| 10-12 (optimal) | Administer 75 to 100 mg aminophylline *slowly* by intravenous injection to reverse effects of dipyridamole |

different half-times of pharmacological effect. With dipyridamole a "keep-open" IV line is started with 0.9% saline. The drug is infused at 0.14 mg/kg/min for 4 minutes (Box 5-13). The selected tracer is injected IV 7 to 9 minutes after the start of infusion. Imaging is then begun 12 to 15 minutes after the start of infusion. During the infusion and the interval before radiotracer injection, some departments also have the patient perform mild exercise such as handgrip isometric exercise or walking in place to augment the effect. Injection is ideally performed with the patient standing or sitting to minimize splanchnic activity.

The protocol for adenosine is 140 μg/kg/min for 6 minutes. The selected tracer is injected 3 minutes after the start of the adenosine infusion. Imaging is begun 5 minutes after tracer administration.

Since both dipyridamole and adenosine are antagonized by methylxanthines, drugs containing methylxanthines (such as theophylline) should be discontinued if possible for the time of study. Also, caffeine in coffee, tea, or soft drinks can antagonize dipyridamole and adenosine, and patients should fast before the study and imaging. These agents are contraindicated in patients with bronchospastic disease (asthma, chronic obstructive pulmonary disease).

The diagnostic criteria are the same as with stress-rest studies (Table 5-3). However, abdominal activity is commonly greater after pharmacological stress than after exercise studies.

The dipyridamole and adenosine protocols are also used with PET agents.

**Dobutamine pharmacological stress imaging** Dobutamine is a synthetic catecholamine that acts on both alpha- and beta-adrenergic receptors and has both inotropic and chronotropic properties that increase cardiac workload. In normal coronary arteries dobutamine infusion results in increased perfusion. In the face of significant stenosis, coronary flow does not increase in response to dobutamine. Thus the differential effect of dobutamine in normal versus diseased arteries is the rationale for its use in myocardial perfusion imaging. The reported accuracy of dobutamine thallium scintigraphy is high with a sensitivity in the range of 90% and specificity of 85%.

The major limitation to the use of dobutamine is the common occurrence of side effects, including chest pain, and the inability of a significant percentage of patients to tolerate the maximum required dose. It is considered a second-line pharmacological agent. Nonetheless, for selected patients unable to exercise or patients with contraindications to dipyridamole-adenosine scintigraphy, dobutamine is an alternative.

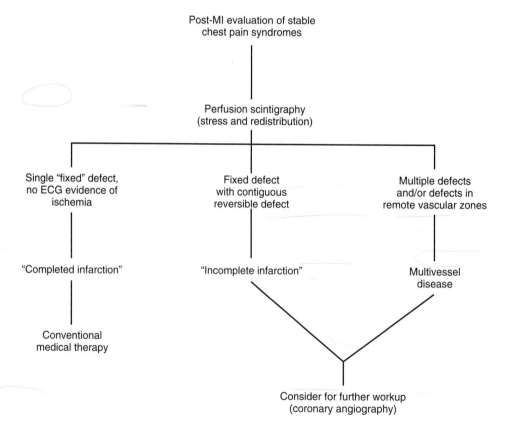

**Fig. 5-26** Diagnostic scheme illustrating the incorporation of perfusion scintigraphy into one approach for stratifying risk after myocardial infarction. *MI*, Myocardial infarction; *ECG*, electrocardiographic.

## Other Applications of Myocardial Perfusion Imaging

**Stress testing for risk stratification after myocardial infarction**   Another important application of stress myocardial perfusion imaging is in the management and risk stratification of patients after acute MI (Fig. 5-26). In some medical centers post-MI patients are routinely studied before hospital discharge. The combined results of a treadmill ECG and a treadmill or dipyridamole stress myocardial perfusion scan have become central to clinical decision making.

As indicated in the decision tree, if patients have a single fixed defect (or no defect) and no ECG evidence of ischemia after adequate exercise, they are treated conservatively. If the postinfarction myocardial perfusion stress study demonstrates a reversible component contiguous to the site of infarction and a reversible or fixed defect remote from the infarct, residual ischemia or multivessel disease is highly likely. Patients with these findings are at much greater risk for subsequent cardiac events and death and warrant more aggressive management. The decision tree does not pertain to patients with

unstable angina or other clinical manifestations of cardiac dysfunction such as congestive heart failure.

**Assessment of coronary artery bypass surgery and angioplasty**   Follow-up stress myocardial perfusion imaging after coronary artery bypass graft (CABG) surgery or angioplasty provides an objective assessment of therapeutic effect on the coronary circulation. Successful surgery or angioplasty results in the elimination of transient defects caused by exercise-induced ischemia (Fig. 5-27). Surgery and angioplasty have no effect on scarred areas, and fixed defects should appear unchanged. If a patient has an infarction as a result of the therapeutic intervention, a previously transient defect may be converted into a fixed defect or an entirely new defect may occur as a result of the injury. Imaging should be delayed 6 weeks or more because some preintervention defects may persist if the scan is done too soon.

When symptoms recur, as they do in a significant percentage of patients, the early posttherapy study serves as a useful baseline. The development of new or recurrent disease is readily detected on repeat stress imaging.

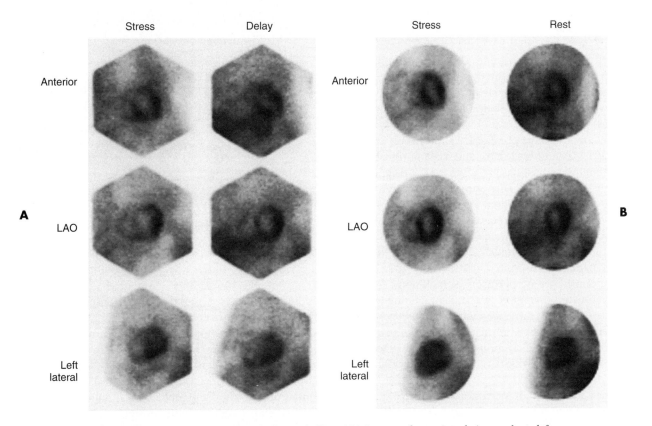

**Fig. 5-27**   **A,** Stress and delayed planar thallium-201 images of a patient being evaluated for coronary artery bypass graft surgery. The poststress images reveal significantly decreased uptake in the anterior wall and septum. In addition, lung uptake is abnormally increased, a secondary indicator of coronary artery disease. The poststress perfusion abnormality has significantly normalized at the time of delayed imaging as is best seen on the left anterior oblique view. **B,** After coronary artery bypass graft surgery the poststress Tl-201 study is essentially normal. Note the improved target-to-background ratio and the absence of abnormal lung uptake. *LAO,* Left anterior oblique.

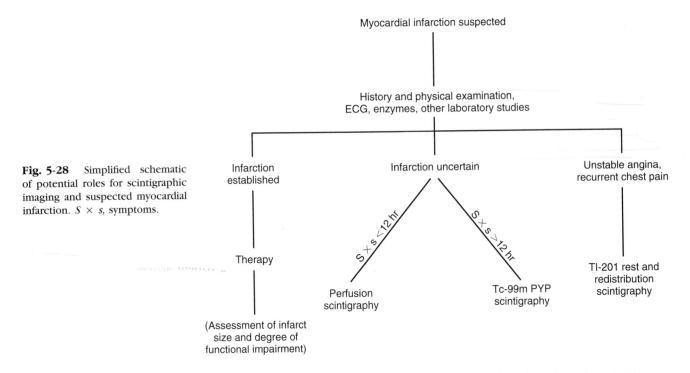

**Fig. 5-28**  Simplified schematic of potential roles for scintigraphic imaging and suspected myocardial infarction. $S \times s$, symptoms.

## DIAGNOSIS OF ACUTE MYOCARDIAL INFARCTION

Studies obtained at rest are used to diagnose acute MI, determine infarct size (or, alternatively, residual mass of viable myocardium), and assess the results of therapeutic interventions such as angioplasty and thrombolysis (Fig. 5-28).

The major advantage of myocardial perfusion imaging with Tl-201, Tc-99m sestamibi, and Tc-99m tetrofosmin over Tc-99m pyrophosphate imaging for the diagnosis of MI is that the study is positive immediately post infarction. Areas of completed infarction are completely cold or photon deficient (Figs. 5-1 and 5-29). Areas of periinfarct ischemia and edema also demonstrate diminished or absent tracer uptake.

When patients are imaged immediately after infarction, the sensitivity of perfusion scintigraphy is high, probably greater than 90% for transmural infarctions. This high sensitivity decreases with time as the periinfarct edema and ischemia resolve. By 24 hours after the acute event, smaller infarctions may not be detectable and the overall sensitivity is much lower, on the order of 60%.

A major limitation of perfusion scintigraphy in the diagnosis of acute MI is the inability to distinguish new from old lesions. Patients with sufficiently large healed infarctions resulting in scar formation may demonstrate cold defects indefinitely. In some cases, without the benefit of a baseline scan for comparison, a cold defect in the presence of new chest pain is moot. A conservative approach is to treat the patient as having had an acute MI until other tests, such as ECG, serum enzyme

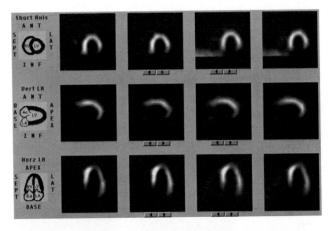

**Fig. 5-29**  Resting study of a patient with suspected acute myocardial infarction. The large defect involving the inferior wall of the heart is compatible with infarction.

determinations, or Tc-99m pyrophosphate scan, rule in or rule out this occurrence.

Another limitation is the difficulty of distinguishing defects caused by severe ischemia in a patient with angina from defects associated with true infarctions. Delayed imaging may help distinguish ischemia from infarction if the cold defect seen initially fills in. In occasional patients with unstable angina, rest and redistribution or delayed Tl-201 scintigraphy (12 to 24 hours) can be used to detect the ischemic tissue (Fig. 5-30). Such a patient may be thought of as undergoing a natural stress test, and the patterns of early and delayed distribution have much the same significance as they do on a formal stress test. The Tc-99m agents require a second injection when angina has remitted to differen-

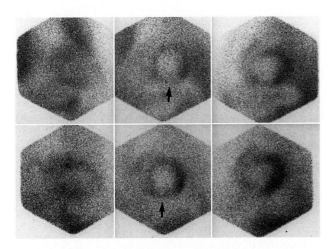

**Fig. 5-30**    "Rest-rest" thallium-201 scintigrams in a patient with acute chest pain. The top row illustrates decreased uptake in the septum, apex, and anterior wall. The lung shows marked uptake, compatible with congestive heart failure. On the delayed follow-up images *(bottom row)*, tracer has accumulated to a variable degree in all areas of abnormality. The inferoapical defect on the left anterior oblique view has filled in almost completely *(arrows)*. This pattern of initial abnormality with normalization at delayed imaging is compatible with ischemia rather than acute myocardial infarction.

tiate scar from ischemia. This also illustrates the potential for making a false positive diagnosis of MI in patients with acute chest pain.

Inasmuch as half or even two thirds of patients admitted to coronary care units (CCUs) are subsequently found not to have sustained an acute MI, perfusion imaging to triage for CCU admission appears useful. Indeed, this approach has had strong proponents over the past decade and a half but has not been generally accepted in practice.

### Prognosis After Myocardial Infarction

The long-term prognosis of patients after MI has been a subject of intense interest clinically. Traditional evaluation has included assessment of Killip classification, location of infarction, presence of congestive heart failure, history of prior infarction, and left ventricular ejection function. The size of the defect as demonstrated by myocardial perfusion scintigraphy is now well established as a predictor of patient outcome. This confirms the links that would be expected between infarct size, left ventricular function, and long-term prognosis.

### Assessment of Thrombolytic Therapy

Myocardial perfusion scintigraphy can be useful in assessing thrombolytic therapy, and a number of approaches have been described. Before thrombolytic therapy, thallium scintigraphy can be used to demonstrate the ischemic areas of the heart and the watershed distal to the coronary thrombosis. After successful clot lysis

with reestablishment of perfusion, a perfusion scintigram is used to document the degree of reperfusion.

Although the preceding paradigm seems straightforward, several pitfalls must be recognized. The most important is that the full significance of thallium accumulation as a predictor of long-term viability has not been established. Similarly, persistently diminished tracer activity may be due to edema and hemorrhage rather than failure to recanalize the affected vessel. Follow-up imaging 1 or 2 weeks after thrombolysis may be necessary to make the distinction in both cases.

Tc-99m sestamibi and Tc-99m tetrofosmin offer unique advantages in assessing thrombolytic therapy, since they are not redistributed but remain fixed for many hours in the myocardium. An initial dose may be given at the time a patient arrives at the hospital, but imaging can be delayed until the patient is stabilized or even until after thrombolytic therapy is given. The initial dose is used to document the amount of myocardium at risk. A second dose is then used to determine the effectiveness of therapy. Reduction in defect size correlates with vessel patency and better prognosis after MI.

In patients undergoing thrombolysis, myocardial perfusion studies are performed under resting conditions as discussed previously. After recovery, stress imaging is useful to determine outcome and detect any areas of residual exercise- or stress-induced ischemia.

### Stunned Myocardium

The term *stunned* myocardium has been used to describe abnormal but still viable myocardium in the immediate postocclusion phase after infarction (Box 5-10). Tissue in the affected watershed distal to a lysed thrombus may be viable and may accumulate Tl-201 or the Tc-99m-labeled myocardial perfusion agents in the time immediately after reperfusion. The uptake of tracer indicates viability, but the myocardial segment may be akinetic (stunned) and may or may not survive in the long run. If it does survive, wall motion will improve.

The concept of stunned myocardium should not be confused with *hibernating* myocardium, which refers to severe, chronically ischemic tissue that is viable but appears cold on conventional Tl-201 or Tc-99m perfusion imaging and nonfunctional on ventriculography or echography (Box 5-10). PET imaging with F-18 FDG has been shown to detect such tissue and correctly indicate its viability and is discussed further in that section of the chapter.

### POSITRON EMISSION TOMOGRAPHY OF THE HEART

Positron emission tomography (PET) affords superior spatial resolution compared with single-photon imaging and also offers the use of a wide variety of physiologically, biochemically, and metabolically useful radiopharmaceuticals. PET is available in a limited number of institutions but provides a horizon for the future of nuclear cardiology. PET studies of the heart can now also be accomplished using specially modified gamma scintillation cameras with high-energy collimators and appropriately shielded camera heads or newly available dual-headed coincidence sysems.

## Pharmaceuticals for Positron Emission Tomography

The three most important radiopharmaceuticals for study of the heart are rubidium-82 (Rb-82), nitrogen-13 (N-13) ammonia, and F-18 FDG. Rb-82 is obtained from a strontium-rubidium generator. N-13 and F-18 are obtained from cyclotron production. Rb-82 and N-13 ammonia are myocardial perfusion agents. FDG is a marker of myocardial glucose metabolism. The fatty acid C-11 palmitate is less commonly used but adds the dimension of studying fatty acid metabolism.

**Rubidium-82 chloride**    In the strontium-82/Rb-82 generator system, the half-life of the Sr-82 parent is 25 days. This is a favorable half-life that from a practical standpoint means that facilities using Rb-82 for myocardial perfusion imaging need to receive only one generator system per month to perform PET studies and no on-site cyclotron or specialized pharmaceutical production facilities are required.

The half-life of Rb-82 is 76 seconds. This very short half-life allows the performance of multiple sequential studies before and after the kinds of pharmacological interventions ordinarily used in PET myocardial perfusion imaging for the diagnosis of CAD. Rb-82 is a monovalent cation and analog of potassium. Like potassium and thallium, Rb-82 is taken up into the myocardium by active transport through the Na,K-ATPase pump. The extraction of Rb-82 is somewhat lower than that of N-13 ammonia and also demonstrates a reduction at higher flow rates. As with N-13 ammonia, the relative extraction and localization of Rb-82 are proportional to blood flow and a useful basis for myocardial perfusion imaging.

*Technique*    Rb-82 is infused over 30 to 60 seconds. Between 30 and 50 mCi is given intravenously, and imaging is begun after a short time is allowed for arterial clearance. Imaging can be accomplished within 5 minutes, and the short-half life of Rb-82 allows sequential studies within 10 minutes.

In the diagnosis of CAD a second study is typically performed after administration of either a vasodilator (dipyridamole, adenosine) or an inotropic-chronotropic agent (dobutamine). The protocols for these agents are the same as described previously for single-photon myocardial perfusion imaging. Because of its high cost

the rubidium generator requires a large patient volume to be practical.

**Nitrogen-13 ammonia**    At physiological pH the major form of ammonia is $NH_4^+$. This moiety is extracted by the myocardial cells at a level of 70% to 80% at normal coronary flow rates. The extraction of ammonia is an energy-dependent process that is not fully understood. As noted with many other perfusion tracers, the extraction efficiency of ammonia drops at higher rates of flow but N-13 ammonia provides a useful map of regional myocardial perfusion over a range of flow rates. The N-13 label remains fixed in the heart with a longer biological residence time than Rb-82 because ammonia is metabolically changed to glutamine.

*Technique*    Since the physical half-life of N-13 is 10 minutes, this agent must be produced in a cyclotron on site. Patients are given 15 to 20 mCi of N-13 ammonia intravenously, and imaging is typically begun 5 minutes after tracer injection, although the long biological half-life in the myocardium offers some flexibility in this regard. As with Rb-82, studies under baseline conditions and after pharmacological stress are used in the diagnosis of CAD.

**Fluorine-18 fluorodeoxyglucose**    FDG is a marker of myocardial glucose metabolism. Its principal use in practice is in combination with a perfusion tracer to assess myocardial viability. Under normal conditions 85% of the energy needs of the heart are met through fatty acid metabolism. Areas of ischemia switch preferentially to glucose metabolism and demonstrate increased uptake of FDG.

Blood clearance of FDG is multicompartmental and takes much longer than the perfusion agents. Imaging is typically begun 45 to 60 minutes after tracer injection to allow blood and soft tissue background clearance.

The physical half-life of F-18 is 1.8 hours (110 minutes). In the myocardial cell FDG is phosphorylated to FDG-6-phosphate. No further metabolism takes place, and the radiolabel stays in the myocardial cell over a prolonged period.

The state of glucose metabolism in the body highly influences the amount of FDG taken up in the heart. Different strategies involving glucose loading and even administration of insulin have been used to promote better FDG uptake. Fig. 5-31 was obtained in a study of a diabetic subject. Initial uptake of FDG was poor. After insulin injection, uptake increased. A common clinical approach is to wait until 1 hour after administering a glucose load before injecting the radiopharmaceutical. The glucose load elicits an insulin response that increases cellular glucose uptake. The typical dose is 5 to 10 mCi of FDG.

**Carbon-11 palmitic acid**    Fatty acids supply the majority of the heart's metabolic requirements at rest under normal circumstances. The rationale for using radiola-

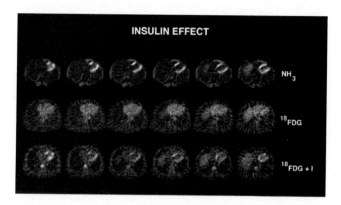

**Fig. 5-31**    Nitrogen-13 ammonia images *(top row)* and two sets of fluorine-18 fluorodeoxyglucose images of a diabetic subject. The N-13 ammonia images reveal a large perfusion defect at the cardiac apex. The initial F-18 FDG images show essentially no myocardial uptake *(middle row)*. After insulin administration, FDG accumulates in the myocardium and reveals a matched defect at the apex.

beled fatty acids is that myocardial metabolism of these agents is sensitive to ischemia.

Simple imaging with C-11 palmitate gives information similar to the perfusion agents. Myocardial time-activity curves of C-11 palmitate reflect fatty acid metabolism. A combination of lower than normal uptake and delayed clearance indicates myocardial ischemia. The added complexity of measuring time-activity curves has resulted in less widespread use of C-11 palmitate than of the other agents described. C-11 requires an on-site cyclotron because of its short half-life.

## Diagnosis of Coronary Artery Disease

The two PET perfusion agents, Rb-82 and N-13 ammonia, are used most commonly for the diagnosis of CAD. Because tomographic imaging is sensitive to motion artifacts and the time from tracer injection to imaging is short with both of these agents, pharmacological stress without adjunctive physical exercise is used for the stress portion of the study. After baseline studies are obtained under resting conditions, one of the pharmacological agents is administered to challenge coronary flow reserve. The protocols are the same as in single-photon imaging and are described previously. The timing of injection of the PET pharmaceutical is synchronized with the administration of the pharmacological agent and the desired delay after injection before the onset of imaging.

As noted, PET imaging offers superior spatial image resolution and typically excellent target-to-background ratios. Otherwise, the scintigraphic appearance of the heart and diagnostic criteria for Rb-82 and N-13 ammonia studies are the same as the appearance and findings on perfusion scans obtained with Tl-201 or one of the Tc-99m-labeled perfusion agents. Normal subjects

should have homogeneous uptake of the tracer throughout both the left and right ventricular myocardium. Patients with hemodynamically significant coronary artery disease but no ischemia at rest demonstrate normal visualization of the myocardium at rest with the appearance of perfusion defects after pharmacological stress. Patients with resting ischemia (hibernating myocardium) demonstrate perfusion defects, even on baseline studies, that may become worse after pharmacological stress. Areas of prior myocardial infarction appear cold on both baseline and poststress images.

The reported sensitivity of PET in the diagnosis of CAD is on the order of 95%. The specificity reported in the early literature is also 95% or better. The specificity should be regarded with caution, since early reports under clinical research protocols frequently use normal volunteers to determine specificity, which is very different from determining specificity in a more broadly chosen cross section of patients with and without CAD.

## Detection of Myocardial Viability and Prediction of Posttreatment Functional Improvement with Combined Perfusion and Fluorine-18 Deoxyglucose Imaging

One of the vexing problems with perfusion imaging with either single-photon agents or PET agents is the ultimate inability to distinguish myocardial segments with markedly diminished perfusion from scarred segments. It is now recognized that 20% to 40% of defects that appear to be "fixed" by conventional Tl-201 stress-rest perfusion imaging may actually represent such severely ischemic areas.

Functional imaging methods including echocardiography, gated blood pool ventriculography, or gated SPECT also fail to make the distinction between severe ischemia and scar because the severely ischemic segments typically demonstrate reduced or absent contractility. These segments are "hibernating" in a functional and metabolic sense.

The combination of perfusion imaging and metabolic imaging with FDG is of great benefit in correctly diagnosing and assessing the potential therapeutic outcome in patients with severely ischemic or hibernating myocardium (Table 5-4). The rationale for using FDG is that severely ischemic myocardium switches from fatty acid metabolism selectively to glucose metabolism. Perhaps counterintuitively, FDG uptake can actually be greater in the ischemic areas than in the remainder of the myocardium.

In normal subjects, perfusion and FDG activity are uniform and matched (Fig. 5-32). The combination of a photon-deficient area by perfusion imaging that demonstrates FDG uptake is the scintigraphic hallmark of

**Table 5-4    Diagnostic patterns for combined positron emission tomography perfusion and FDG imaging**

|  | Perfusion (NH₃, Rb) | Glucose metabolism (FDG) |
|---|---|---|
| Normal myocardium | + | + |
| Ischemic myocardium (severe, chronic) | Absent or decreased | + |
| Necrotic myocardium or scar | Absent | Absent |

*FDG*, Fluorodeoxyglucose; *NH₃*, ammonia; *Rb*, rubidium; +, present.

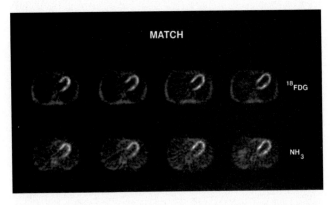

**Fig. 5-32**    Fluorine-18 fluorodeoxyglucose and nitrogen-13 ammonia positron emission tomography in a normal subject. The uniform uptake of both tracers is concordant with a normal appearance of the heart.

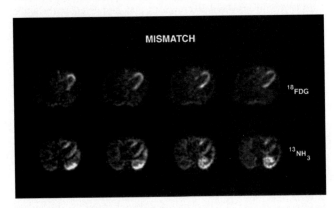

**Fig. 5-33**    Fluorine-18 fluorodeoxyglucose and nitrogen-13 ammonia studies reveal a mismatch or discordant pattern. On the N-13 ammonia perfusion study, uptake is decreased anteroapically. The same area demonstrates good uptake by FDG. This pattern indicates diminished perfusion to an area of viable myocardium. Prognosis for functional improvement after coronary artery bypass grafting is good with this pattern.

severely ischemic or hibernating myocardium (Fig. 5-33). The presence of FDG indicates myocardial viability. Completely infarcted or scarred areas do not accumulate FDG. In areas of flow-metabolism mismatch the functional prognosis following revascularization is very good, with an average of 80% of such segments demonstrating contractile improvement after coronary artery bypass surgery.

The combination of matched flow and FDG abnormalities is indicative of myocardial scarring (Fig. 5-34). This matched pattern of abnormal flow and glucose indicates a low likelihood of improved function after therapeutic intervention with only an average of 15% of such segments demonstrating contractile improvement after coronary artery bypass grafting.

The detection and distinction of severely ischemic (hibernating) myocardium from scarred areas are crucial to clinical management. Patients with viable but severely ischemic myocardium have better survival and event outcomes from surgical revascularization than from medical management. Patients with only myocardial scarring and no ischemia do not benefit from revascularization surgery. Some may be candidates for cardiac transplantation.

## Combined Technetium-99m Sestamibi and Fluorine-18 Deoxyglucose Imaging

Many patients who are candidates for coronary artery bypass surgery have experienced myocardial infarctions, have multivessel disease, and have abnormal left ventricular function. Since the likelihood of benefit from revascularization of scarred tissue is low, studying such patients with combined perfusion and metabolic imaging preoperatively is valuable to assess prognosis and to guide decision making about surgical versus medical management.

With contemporary gamma cameras modified for single-photon PET imaging and the use of two energy windows, a simultaneous combination of Tc-99m sesta-

mibi or Tc-99m tetrofosmin perfusion imaging and FDG metabolic imaging is possible. One advantage of doing simultaneous imaging is that the data from the two radiopharmaceuticals are perfectly registered, allowing optimal comparison of the respective uptake patterns. This elegant approach uses the same diagnostic criteria described previously. Areas demonstrating diminished Tc-99m activity with normal or increased FDG represent ischemic but viable tissue and have a high likelihood of functional recovery after revascularization. Areas of matched perfusion and metabolic abnormality are unlikely to improve (Figs. 5-35 and 5-36).

Patients undergoing evaluation for cardiac transplantation can also be studied in a combined perfusion and FDG metabolism protocol. If the poor function of the heart can be shown to result from multiple areas of chronically ischemic but viable (hibernating) tissue, coronary artery bypass grafting is probably a better option than cardiac transplantation. On the other hand,

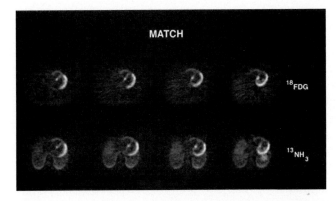

**Fig. 5-34** Fluorine-18 deoxyglucose and nitrogen-13 ammonia studies reveal concordant or matched abnormalities in the region of the septum and apex. The pattern of matched abnormalities indicates myocardial scar with absence of perfusion and metabolism.

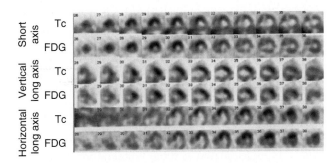

**Fig. 5-36** Simultaneous combined technetium-99m perfusion imaging and fluorine-18 fluorodeoxyglucose metabolic imaging reveal matched abnormalities in the inferior wall of the left ventricle. This pattern of matched abnormalities is indicative of myocardial nonviability. (Courtesy of Tsunehiro Yasuda, M.D., Department of Radiology, Massachusetts General Hospital, Boston.)

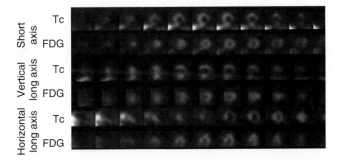

**Fig. 5-35** Combined technetium-99m sestamibi and fluorine-18 fluorodeoxyglucose imaging reveals a mismatched or discordant pattern. Tc-99m perfusion imaging shows a large inferoapical defect that corresponds with normal uptake of FDG. This pattern is indicative of ischemic but viable myocardium. (Courtesy of Tsunehiro Yasuda, M.D., Department of Radiology, Massachusetts General Hospital, Boston.)

if there is just diffuse abnormality without evidence of hibernating myocardium in the face of extremely poor global function, coronary bypass grafting is unlikely to improve pump function. Given the high cost, risk, and morbidity of cardiac transplantation, studying all candidates with perfusion-metabolic PET imaging or combined single-photon perfusion and PET metabolic imaging seems reasonable.

## RADIONUCLIDE VENTRICULOGRAPHY

The goal of radionuclide ventriculography is to evaluate global and regional ventricular function. Techniques are available to study both the right and left ventricles and may be categorized as either first-pass studies, in which all data collection occurs during the initial transit of a tracer bolus through the central

circulation, or equilibrium studies, in which data are collected over many cardiac cycles using gating and a tracer that remains in the blood pool. The principal advantages of radionuclide ventriculography over contrast ventriculography are the noninvasiveness of the nuclear imaging procedure, the ability to study all cardiac chambers simultaneously, and the ability to make repeated measurements over time or before and after an intervention.

### Radiopharmaceuticals

**Blood pool agents** The pharmaceutical of choice for equilibrium gated blood pool imaging is technetium-99m-labeled red blood cells (Tc-99m RBCs). Labeling may be accomplished by any of three approaches—an in vivo approach, a modified in vivo approach, and an in vitro approach.

The original in vivo approach is the simplest. Cold stannous pyrophosphate is reconstituted with saline and injected directly intravenously. The dose is 15 µg/kg body weight. After 15 to 30 minutes, Tc-99m pertechnetate is also administered by direct intravenous injection. The pertechnetate diffuses across the RBC membrane, where it is reduced by the stannous ions administered previously. The Tc-99m label binds to the beta chain of hemoglobin.

Although the in vivo technique is simple, the labeling yield is less than ideal, on the order of 80% but frequently as low as 60% to 65%. Tc-99m activity not labeled to RBCs can contribute to background activity and also reduces the number of counts available from the cardiac blood pool. In some cases the labeling fails dramatically owing to drug-drug interactions or other causes of poor labeling (Box 5-14). Special care is taken not to inject through heparinized intravenous tubing. For these reasons many laboratories have adopted either the modified in vivo approach or the in vitro approach. Excessive gastric, thyroid, and soft tissue background activity suggests poor labeling with free Tc-99m pertechnetate.

In the modified in vitro approach, cold stannous pyrophosphate is again administered directly intravenously. After the 15- to 30-minute wait for equilibration of stannous ion in RBCs, 3 to 5 ml of blood is withdrawn through an intravenous line into a shielded syringe containing Tc-99m pertechnetate and a small amount of either acid-citrate-dextrose (ACD) solution or heparin. The blood is incubated at room temperature for at least 10 minutes. The syringe is agitated periodically, and the syringe contents are reinjected into the patient. The syringe is left attached to the intravenous line during the procedure so that the entire system is closed with respect to the patient's circulation. The labeling efficiency increases to approximately 90% in the modified in vivo approach.

In the in vitro approach, blood is first withdrawn from the patient and added to a reaction vial containing cold stannous chloride. The stannous ion diffuses across the RBC membrane. After incubation, sodium hypochlorite is used to oxidize excess extracellular stannous ion to prevent extracellular reduction of Tc-99m pertechnetate. A sequestering agent can also be added to remove extracellular stannous ion. Radioactive labeling is then accomplished by adding sodium pertechnetate. Tc-99m pertechnetate crosses the RBC membrane and is reduced by stannous ion in the cell. The mixture is incubated for 20 minutes before reinjection. Labeling efficiency is on the order of 95% or greater. This approach is somewhat less convenient than the in vivo approaches but has the advantage of the highest labeling efficiency. It is also less subject to drug-drug interference to labeling and to problems of excessive or deficient stannous ion. A simple in vitro kit is commercially available.

Another potential agent is Tc-99m-labeled human serum albumin (Tc-99m HSA). This agent is also typically prepared from a kit by adding Tc-99m pertechnetate containing human serum albumin and a reducing agent. The advantage of Tc-99m HSA is that it may be prepared ahead of time for administration of multiple doses. This facilitates studies in the cardiac care unit and whenever urgency is required. Labeling efficiency is on the order of 90% for commercial kits, and satisfactory images of the blood pool can be obtained. A disadvantage of Tc-99m HSA is greater uptake in the liver with less activity available in the blood pool. The agent is also contraindicated in patients with histories of allergy to human albumin.

*Pharmacokinetics* One of the advantages of using Tc-99m-labeled RBCs is that they circulate in the blood pool with essentially the half-life of the radiolabel. It is feasible to obtain multiple sequential studies during an interventional maneuver, and it is possible to reimage using the same dosage. By comparison, Tc-99m HSA demonstrates a progressive leakage from the intravascular space resulting in higher background. Less than half of the original activity is available in the blood pool 4 hours after tracer administration. This still makes it feasible to perform multiple acquisitions during an interventional procedure such as stress ventriculography.

**First-pass agents** All of the agents just described may be administered by a bolus technique for first-pass imaging of the central circulation. Several other agents labeled with Tc-99m have also been used for first-pass imaging. If only a single study is anticipated, Tc-99m as sodium pertechnetate may be used. The disadvantage of this approach is high residual background activity if multiple studies are required, as in stress ventriculography. Tc-99m sulfur colloid has the advantage of rapid clearance from the circulation, which offers the ability to perform multiple studies in succession. Similarly, Tc-99m DTPA has been used, although its blood clearance is less rapid than that of sulfur colloid. As discussed previously, some institutions perform a first-pass study with one of the Tc-99mm-labeled myocardial

---

### Box 5-14   Causes of Poor Technetium-99m Red Blood Cell Labeling

| | |
|---|---|
| Drug-drug interactions | Heparin, doxorubicin, methyldopa, hydralazine, iodinated contrast media, quinidine |
| Circulating antibodies | Prior transfusion, transplantation, some antibiotics |
| Too little stannous ion | Insufficient to reduce Tc (VII) |
| Too much stannous ion | Reduction of Tc (VII) outside of red blood cell before cell labeling |
| Carrier Tc-99 | Buildup of Tc-99m in the Mo-99/Tc-99m generator due to long interval between elutions |
| Too short an interval for "tinning" | Not enough time for stannous ion to penetrate the red blood cells before addition of Tc-99m |
| Too short an incubation time | Not enough time for reduction of Tc (VII) |

perfusion agents in conjunction with the perfusion study.

## Acquisition Techniques

**First-pass studies** First-pass studies are obtained by injecting a compact bolus of a suitable radiopharmaceutical intravenously. If a peripheral injection is used, the Oldendorf technique or a variation thereof is employed. The arm is held in a neutral position, and a medial vein in the basilic system is used at the antecubital fossa. Use of veins in the cephalic system should be avoided, if possible, to prevent "hang-up" of the bolus at the thoracic inlet. Injections directly through central catheters placed in the superior vena cava provide the most compact boluses. A jugular venous access approach is also sometimes used for interventional studies.

Details of data acquisition depend on the computer system used. Data may be acquired either in rapid frame mode or in list mode, with or without ECG gating. Whichever approach is used, the goal is to obtain 16 to 30 frames per second while the bolus passes through the central circulation. In most patients the total data acquisition time required is on the order of 30 seconds or less. In patients with congestive heart failure, bolus transit is delayed and, conservatively, first-pass imaging is carried out for 60 seconds.

The patient may be placed in any position. Typically a right anterior oblique view at 20° to 30° angulation is chosen (Fig. 5-37). This view best separates the right atrium and the right ventricle and is also one of the standard views of the left ventricle used during cardiac catheterization. It is suitable for both quantitative and qualitative analysis of biventricular function.

The major advantage of the first-pass approach is that data are collected rapidly over very few cardiac cycles. Therefore ventricular function can be measured at peak stress during exercise ventriculography or other inter-

vention. Right ventricular function is also easier to measure than on equilibrium gated blood pool studies, in which overlap usually occurs between the right and left ventricles in the RAO view and between the right atrium and the right ventricle in the LAO view.

The major disadvantage of the first-pass or first-transit approach is that counting statistics are low in each frame because of the count rate limitations of gamma scintillation cameras. Also, even with tracers that clear the blood, only a limited number of repeated measurements or views is possible. In current practice, equilibrium gated blood pool studies are performed much more frequently than first transit studies. A creative new approach made possible by the availability of Tc-99m-labeled myocardial perfusion agents is to obtain a first-transit ventriculogram and then obtain the myocardial perfusion image in a conventional manner.

**Equilibrium gated blood pool studies** The limited counting statistics available during any one cardiac cycle and the desirability of linking phases of the cardiac cycle to image data underlie the equilibrium gated blood pool approach to radionuclide ventriculography (RNV) (Box 5-15). In this approach ECG leads are placed on the patient and a gating signal that triggers the R wave of the

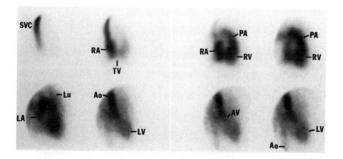

**Fig. 5-37** First-pass radionuclide angiogram. Cardiac structures are sequentially visualized as the bolus passes through the right side of the heart into the lungs and then returns to the left side. *Ao,* Aorta; *AV,* aortic valve; *LA,* left atrium; *Lu,* lung; *LV,* left ventricle; *PA,* pulmonary artery; *RA,* right atrium; *RV,* right ventricle; *SVC,* superior vena cava; *TV,* tricuspid valve.

---

> ### Box 5-15  Equilibrium Gated Blood Pool Ventriculography: Protocol Summary
>
> **PATIENT PREPARATION AND PRECAUTIONS**
> Establish that patient is in normal sinus rhythm (less than 5% to 10% premature ventricular contractions)
>
> **DOSAGE AND ROUTE OF TRACER ADMINISTRATION**
> Tc-99m red blood cells 10-20 mCi (370-740 MBq)
> Intravenous administration
>
> **IMAGING PROTOCOL**
> Use a low-energy, general purpose or high-sensitivity collimator and a 15% to 20% window centered at 140 keV
> Obtain 10° right anterior oblique (or anterior), mid–left anterior oblique (LAO) (best septal), and left lateral views. Consider additional views (e.g., left posterior oblique) if clinical conditions warrant
> Use the gamma camera persistence oscilloscope to determine the optimum LAO position for separating left and right ventricular activity
> Obtain a minimum of 16 frames per cardiac cycle, and use a frame duration of 50 msec or less
> Obtain 250k counts per frame for studies performed at rest (10-inch field-of-view camera)
> Obtain 100k counts per frame in the optimum LAO view for studies obtained during an intervention (10-inch field-of-view camera)

ECG is sent to the nuclear medicine computer system (Fig. 5-38). The R wave is a useful marker because it occurs at the end of diastole and the beginning of systole. It is the largest electrical signal in the normal ECG and therefore is not only useful from a timing standpoint, but also relatively easy to detect.

The cardiac cycle is divided into 16 to 24 frames in typical commercially available computer systems (Fig. 5-39). Individual frame duration is approximately 40 to 50 msec. This frame rate is a compromise between optimal temporal and statistical data sampling. Enough frames are needed to catch the peaks and valleys of the cardiac cycle (temporal sampling), but too many frames reduce counting statistics available in any single frame (statistical sampling).

During each heartbeat data are acquired sequentially into the frame buffers spanning the cardiac cycle. With imaging of more than 100 to 300 cardiac cycles, sufficient counting statistics are obtained for valid quantitative analysis and reasonable spatial resolution. Studies at rest are obtained for 250,000 counts per frame. Studies obtained during exercise or other intervention are often obtained for somewhat fewer counts per frame to capture the peak effect of the stress (Box 5-15).

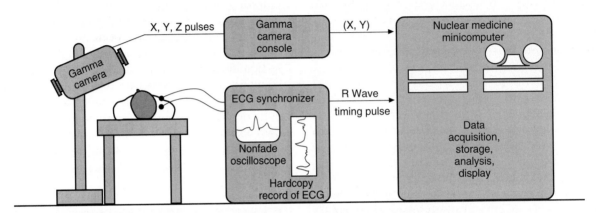

**Fig. 5-38**   R wave gated radionuclide ventriculography acquisition. A special electrocardiographic synchronizer or gating device depicts the R wave and sends a timing pulse to the nuclear medicine computer system. This timing pulse is used to sort incoming scintillation events into a sequence of frames that spans the cardiac cycle.

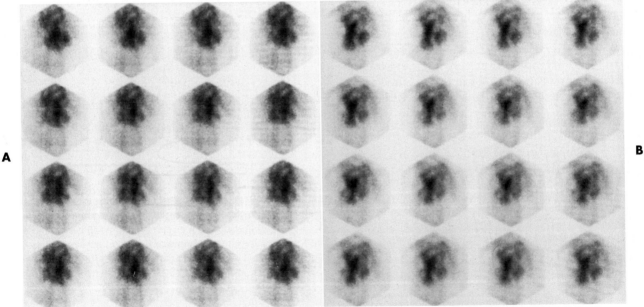

**Fig. 5-39**   **A,** R wave gated radionuclide ventriculograms in, **A,** the anterior and, **B,** the 45° left anterior oblique views. In this study the cardiac cycle was divided into 16 frames. Note the change in size and count density of the cardiac chambers through the cardiac cycle.

The underlying assumption of R-wave gating is the presence of normal sinus rhythm so that data are added together from corresponding segments of the cardiac cycle over the entire time of the study (Fig. 5-40). Any significant dysrhythmia degrades the quality of the data and reduces the accuracy of quantitative analysis.

A rhythm strip should be obtained for every patient before the injection of a radioactive tracer to determine suitability for examination. For example, rapid atrial fibrillation with an irregular ventricular response is a contraindication to the study (Fig. 5-40). Up to 5% to 10% premature ventricular contractions (PVCs) can be tolerated. Recording a beat histogram throughout the study is also useful (Fig. 5-41). Other problems with gating include spurious signals from skeletal muscle activity, giant T waves triggering the gating device, and artifacts from pacemakers. The pacemaker signal itself is usually a reliable trigger for gating, and high-quality studies of patients with pacemakers may be obtained.

Special computer techniques may be used to filter data from premature contractions and postextrasystolic beats, but these increase the time needed to perform a study. By the same token, elegant gated list mode data acquisition techniques have been developed to analyze separately the normal sinus beat, the premature contraction, and the postextrasystolic beat.

For studies at rest, multiple views are obtained to provide the most comprehensive evaluation of regional ventricular wall motion. These views include a shallow 10° RAO, a 30° to 60° LAO, and an LPO (Fig. 5-42). The exact angulation for the LAO view is determined empirically by moving the head of the gamma camera. The LAO angle that best separates the activity in the left and right ventricles is selected to facilitate calculation of the left ventricular ejection fraction and other quantitative and functional parameters. For studies obtained during exercise stress testing or other forms of stress intervention, the gamma camera head is left in the optimal LAO view, again to facilitate quantitative analysis of ejection fraction and other parameters.

Protocols for obtaining exercise RNVs vary widely among institutions. Some departments measure the left ventricular ejection fraction at each stage of a graded exercise program designed to recapitulate graded treadmill stress. Other departments obtain a baseline study and a single stress study during peak exercise. Exact

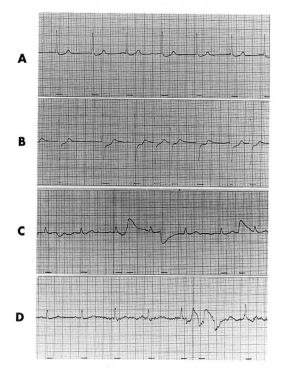

**Fig. 5-40**    Electrocardiographic rhythm strips obtained from patients referred for gated radionuclide ventriculography. **A,** Desired normal sinus rhythm. **B,** Excessive premature ventricular contractions or, **C,** atrial fibrillation with irregular ventricular response degrades image quality. **D,** Skeletal muscle artifacts can trigger the gating pulse in patients undergoing exercise.

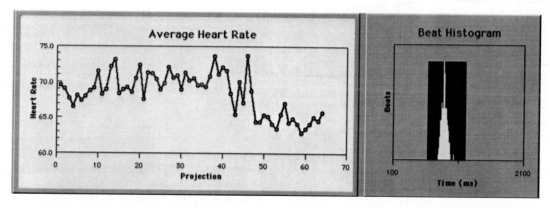

**Fig. 5-41**    Beat histogram depicts the number of recorded beats for each observed cardiac cycle length. These data were actually from a gated myocardial perfusion scan but illustrate the point that heart rate and therefore beat length vary significantly during data collection.

exercise protocols are typically customized to the physical condition of the patient.

In addition to exercise stress, a number of alternatives have been proposed, including cold pressor testing, handgrip isometric exercise, atrial pacing, and pharmacological stress. Unlike the success of pharmacological intervention for myocardial perfusion imaging, none of the alternatives to leg exercise have proved equal to leg exercise studies.

## Data Analysis and Study Interpretation

**Qualitative analysis**    Comprehensive analysis and interpretation of RNVs require both qualitative and quantitative assessments (Box 5-16). Wall motion is typically analyzed by observing the RNV in a repetitive cinematic closed loop display on the computer screen. Wall motion is inferred from "shrinkage" of the ventricular activity from diastole to systole. Failure of activity to

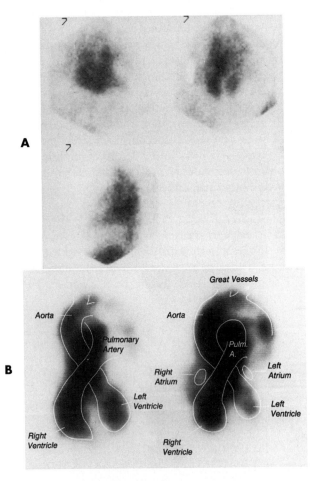

**Fig. 5-42**    **A,** End-diastolic images from a gated radionuclide ventriculogram. Anterior *(top left),* left anterior oblique *(top right),* and left posterior oblique *(bottom)* views are the most commonly obtained. **B,** Drawings over left anterior oblique end-diastolic *(left)* and end-systolic *(right)* frames, indicating position and relationships of major structures.

diminish or clear along the ventricular periphery is an indication of abnormal wall motion. Septal contraction is inferred from seeing the photon-deficient area between the right ventricular and left ventricular blood pools thicken during systole.

Complete absence of wall motion is termed *akinesis.* Abnormal areas demonstrating residual but diminished contraction are said to be *hypokinetic.* Areas demonstrating paradoxical wall motion—that is, an actual outward bulge during systole—are termed *dyskinetic.* If motion is still present but delayed compared with adjacent segments, the term *tardokinesis* is used.

In normal subjects all wall segments should contract, with the greatest excursion seen in the left ventricular free wall and apex. Areas of ventricular scar are typically akinetic or dyskinetic. Areas of ventricular ischemia are akinetic or hypokinetic with exercise. Tardokinesis may be the result of ischemia or conduction abnormalities such as bundle-branch block.

The complete qualitative or visual analysis of the RNV includes an assessment of cardiac chamber size for all four cardiac chambers, assessment of regional wall motion and overall biventricular performance, and assessment of any extracardiac abnormalities such as aortic aneurysms or pericardial effusions that are in the detector's field of view. Accurate qualitative assessment requires some experience. The computer controls can be used to vary the speed of the cinematic closed loop display, which can be a visual cue for detecting more motion abnormalities. Only portions of the ventricles not overlapped by other cardiac structures should be assessed on any given view. For example, on the anterior or shallow RAO view the right ventricle usually overlaps the septum and inferior wall of the left ventricle.

In addition to visual analysis of regional wall motion, attempts have been made to use quantitative and functional or parametric images to detect abnormalities in regional wall motion. For example, regions of interest may be flagged along the ventricular perimeter to

---

### Box 5-16    Functional Parameters Determined on Equilibrium Blood Pool Ventriculograms

Wall motion assessment (regional and global)
End-diastolic and end-systolic ventricular volume
Stroke volume
Cardiac output
Ejection fraction (left and right ventricles)
Regurgitant fraction (stroke index ratio)
Ventricular filling and emptying rates (dV/dt) (peak and average)
Cardiac shunt quantitation

calculate regional ejection fractions. Fourier phase analysis and other parametric image analysis techniques are described in the following section.

### Quantitative data analysis

*Ejection fraction* The most frequently calculated quantitative parameter of ventricular function is the left ventricular ejection fraction (Box 5-15). This is defined as the fraction of the left ventricular end-diastolic volume expelled during contraction. The principle underlying the calculation is that the net left ventricular count rate at each point in the cardiac cycle is proportional to ventricular volume. The net ventricular counts are determined by flagging a region of interest over the left ventricle for each frame (Fig. 5-43) of the cardiac cycle and a background region, typically taken as a crescent adjacent to the left ventricular apex (Fig. 5-44). The background region of interest should not overlap activity emanating from the spleen. A background-corrected ventricular time-activity curve is then generated (Fig. 5-43). End-

diastole is taken as the frame demonstrating the highest counts, and end-systole the frame with the fewest counts.

Ejection fraction is calculated as follows:

$$\text{Ejection fraction} = \frac{\text{End diastolic count (net)} - \text{End systolic count (net)}}{\text{End diastolic count (net)}}$$

The average ejection fraction in normal subjects is on the order of 0.65, with a range of 0.55 to 0.75. Many nuclear medicine departments use 0.50 as a cutoff for normal. (These fractions are also frequently given as percentages.) The accuracy of the ejection fraction calculation by RNV is considered very good and better than that of nonnuclear techniques such as cardiac echo. Numerous studies have demonstrated good correlation with contrast-enhanced left ventriculography.

The time-activity curve should be inspected in each case as a quality control measure. Theoretically, the count values at the beginning and end of the curve should be identical. In practice, the trailing frames in late diastole usually have fewer counts, owing to slight variations in the length of the cardiac cycle, even in patients with normal sinus rhythm (Fig. 5-45). In patients with frequent PVCs the fall-off in counts at the end of the curve is much greater. In atrial fibrillation with an irregular ventricular response a marked fall-off may occur because cardiac cycles of widely varying length are being added together. Quantitative analysis of gated data in cases with major dysrhythmias is not accurate. On cine display a fall-off in counts in later frames is seen as a flicker.

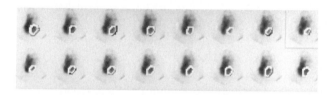

**Fig. 5-43** Calculation of the left ventricular ejection fraction defines a region of interest over the left ventricle in each frame of the cardiac cycle.

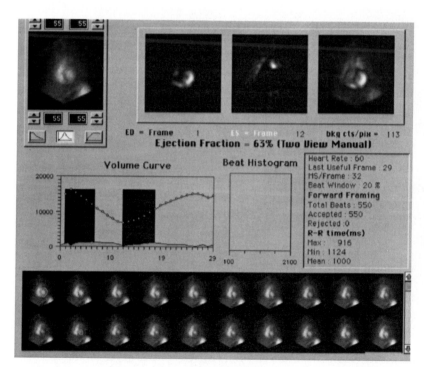

**Fig. 5-44** Composite computer-generated display from the analysis of the gated radionuclide ventriculogram. The sequential left anterior oblique views are displayed across the bottom. The end-diastolic and end-systolic regions of interest are indicated, along with the crescent-shaped background region of interest adjacent to the left ventricle at end-systole *(bottom row, second image from right).* The three parametric images in the upper right-hand corner represent ejection fraction (ES − ED), paradox (ES − ED), and amplitude. The ejection fraction of 63% is normal.

Numerous other quantitative parameters have been proposed for calculation from equilibrium gated blood pool examinations (Box 5-16; Fig. 5-46). None of these can be considered as well documented and validated as the left ventricular ejection fraction. Calculation of the right ventricular ejection fraction from equilibrium data is a problem because of overlap of chambers. Calculation of stroke volume and cardiac output requires correction of the left ventricular count rate for soft tissue attenuation. All proposed attenuation correction methods are subject to error. Use of quantitative parameters other than the left ventricular ejection fraction is reserved largely for research studies.

Rates of ventricular filling and emptying (dV/dt) (Figs. 5-44 and 5-45) have found some utility in assessing drug therapy. For example, calcium channel blockers used in

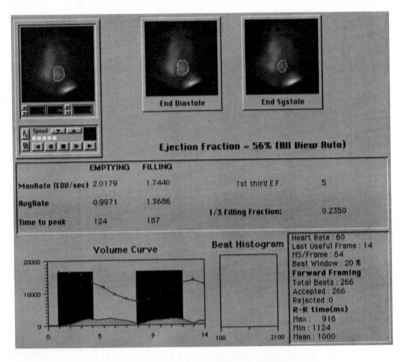

**Fig. 5-45** Small changes in beat length result in fewer counts being recorded in the trailing frames of late diastole. Note how the last data point in the volume curve is lower than the one adjacent to it and the trailing end of the volume curve is somewhat lower than the beginning.

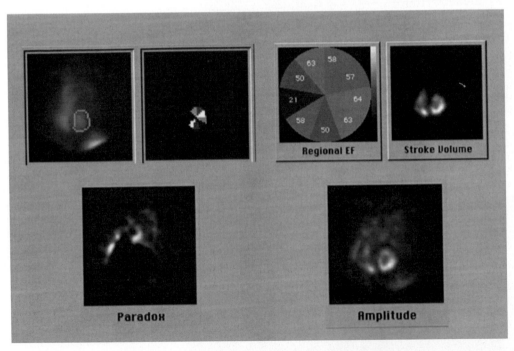

**Fig. 5-46** Calculation of regional ejection fractions from eight pie-shaped regions centered in the middle of the left ventricle. The stroke volume, paradox, and amplitude images are also illustrated.

the treatment of idiopathic hypertrophic subaortic stenosis facilitate myocardial relaxation and thereby more rapid diastolic filling. Again, the measurement is used primarily in clinical research and requires more than 24 frames per cycle for acquisition.

*Fourier phase analysis* Fourier phase analysis reduces four-dimensional data into a pair of two-dimensional images. These images portray cardiac contractility (amplitude) and contraction sequence (phase) (Fig. 5-47). Simplistically, each pixel in the cardiac image can be considered to have its own cycle, having an amplitude and a characteristic temporal relationship (i.e., phase) with respect to the R wave. The amplitude image simply portrays the maximum net count variation for each pixel during the cardiac cycle. The phase image portrays the relative time delay from the R wave to the start of the cardiac cycle for that individual pixel.

If the complete cardiac cycle is taken as encompassing 360°, the atria and ventricles are 180° "out of phase" normally (Fig. 5-47). Areas of the ventricle that contract slightly earlier in the cardiac cycle owing to the pattern of the electrical conduction down the septum and through the bundle branches are seen to be slightly out of phase with adjacent ventricular areas.

Wall motion abnormalities are portrayed on phase images as low-amplitude areas. Regions of paradoxical motion resulting from left ventricular aneurysms, for example, are 180° "out of phase" with the ventricle. Abnormal conduction patterns like those seen in Wolff-Parkinson-White syndrome or bundle-branch block cause affected areas to be slightly out of phase with adjacent portions of the ventricle owing to premature or delayed contraction.

Amplitude and phase maps are often displayed in color to highlight the temporal sequences of cardiac chamber emptying. A dynamic color display mode can be used to demonstrate the propagating wavefront that sweeps across the ventricle during contraction, linking pixels with similar phase angles together.

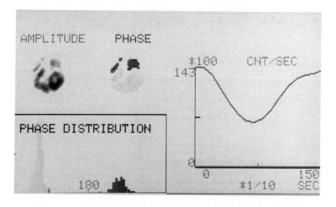

**Fig. 5-47**  In addition to the amplitude image that portrays cardiac contractility, the phase parametric image portrays the relative time of contraction for each pixel on the image. The atria and ventricles are 180° "out of phase" normally.

Although Fourier phase analysis is elegant, the studies require exceptionally well-synchronized data to be useful for localizing abnormal conduction pathways. Amplitude and phase images are often presented automatically as part of computer analysis packages and are useful for cueing the observer to areas of abnormal wall motion.

*Functional images*  Other functional images can also be created that are somewhat simpler to understand than Fourier phase analysis. The intensity of the computer display at each point in an image is determined by the number of scintigraphic events recorded at that point and in turn is proportional to the amount of radioactivity in the corresponding location. By subtracting the end-systolic image from the end-diastolic image point by point, a derived or functional image is created that portrays regional stroke volume. The stroke volume image may be further processed by dividing it point by point by the end-diastolic frame to create an "ejection fraction" image. In these images akinetic wall segments correspond to areas of diminished or absent intensity (Fig. 5-46).

In the paradox image the end-diastolic frame is subtracted from the end-systolic frame. In subjects with normal ventricular function this leaves a void. In patients with areas of paradoxical ventricular wall motion the systolic bulge is readily detected as an area of unsubtracted activity.

A complete analysis and interpretation of the RNV include a qualitative visual assessment of the cardiac chambers and great vessels to assess their size and relationships. Visual assessment of the dynamic cinematic display is also used to analyze regional wall motion. Quantitative analysis includes at a minimum calculation of the left ventricular ejection fraction. For specific applications other quantitative parameters such as left and right ventricular stroke volume ratios, cardiac output, ventricular volume, and rates of ventricular filling and emptying may be also be calculated but require more sophisticated analysis and in some cases more sophisticated data acquisition techniques.

## Clinical Applications

**Acute myocardial infarction**  The hallmark of acute MI on RNV is the development of a wall motion abnormality in the region of the infarct (Fig. 5-48) and a decrease in the global ejection fraction. The global left ventricular ejection fraction may be decreased even in patients without clinical manifestations of congestive heart failure or other hemodynamic indicators of infarction.

The prognosis of patients following acute MI is directly linked to the degree of functional impairment. In most series over 75% of patients with acute MIs have abnormal ejection fractions. The mean ejection fractions of those with uncomplicated infarcts is higher than in

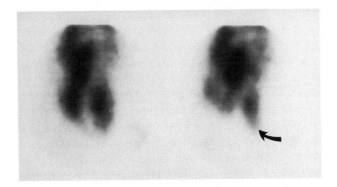

**Fig. 5-48**  Selected end-diastolic and end-systolic images for a patient with acute anteroapical myocardial infarction. The apex is akinetic *(arrow)*. The right ventricle and other portions of the left ventricle show good contraction.

those who also have left ventricular failure or overt pulmonary edema. Patients showing a serial decline in ejection fraction have a significantly higher risk of mortality in the early postinfarction period.

In patients with inferior infarctions the right ventricle should be carefully assessed in addition to the left ventricle. Right ventricular wall motion abnormalities may be seen in as many as 40% of patients with inferior infarctions. Right ventricular involvement is unusual in pure anterior infarctions. The finding of right ventricular involvement, particularly as an isolated or dominant finding, is significant in directing therapy. Therapy for right ventricular dysfunction includes volume loading to maintain left atrial filling pressure and thereby adequate left ventricular filling. Volume loading is usually contraindicated in left ventricular infarction.

Radionuclide techniques are frequently applied after the acute phase of infarction to determine the presence of residual disease and the degree of functional impairment. In contemporary practice, stress myocardial perfusion scintigraphy is more frequently employed for this purpose than exercise RNV. The goal of both examinations is to detect ischemia that indicates myocardial segments at risk for future events. Sudden death after MI, either immediate or delayed, is often due to arrhythmias arising from ischemic areas of the ventricle. Therefore the prognosis and management of patients not demonstrating postinfarction ischemia are significantly different from those of patients with residual ischemia.

**Coronary artery disease**  Many patients with CAD have no clinical manifestations and have normal ventricular function at rest. Exercise-induced myocardial ischemia can be detected with RNV. The hallmarks of ischemia are the development of a new wall motion abnormality during exercise stress testing that was not present at rest and an ejection fraction that fails to increase or even decreases in response to exercise (Box 5-17 and Fig. 5-49).

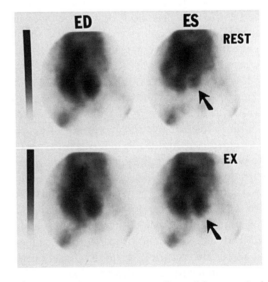

**Fig. 5-49**  Abnormal exercise radionuclide ventriculogram. Note the decreased emptying of the left ventricle in response to exercise *(arrows)*. *ED,* End diastolic; *ES,* end systolic; *EX,* exercise.

In patients able to achieve adequate levels of exercise the technique is highly sensitive, on the order of 90%, for the detection of CAD. The major limitations of the technique are the inability of a significant percentage of patients to achieve adequate levels of exercise and the nonspecificity of an abnormal ventricular functional response to exercise stress. In one series the overall sensitivity of RNV for CAD was 85%. In patients with chest pain, ST segment depression of at least 1 mm, or a pressure-rate product greater than 250,000, the sensitivity was 94%. Twenty-five percent of the patients failed to achieve adequate exercise, and the exercise RNV was abnormal in only 62%.

## Box 5-18    Causes of Abnormal Ventricular Functional Response to Exercise

Hemodynamically significant coronary artery disease
Cardiomyopathy
Myocarditis
Valvular heart disease
Pericardial disease
Drug toxicity
Prior surgery or injury

The question of specificity is complex. In selected normal volunteers the specificity is very high, approaching 100%. However, when the test is applied in a broader cross section of patients, including those with noncoronary heart disease as well as coronary heart disease, specificity drops and has been reported to be as low as 55%. In current practice the true sensitivity and specificity of noninvasive tests are difficult to assess because the results are used to guide selection of patients for cardiac catheterization. This selection bias tends to make noninvasive tests look more sensitive and less specific than they really are because patients with abnormal tests are more frequently referred for the reference standard of cardiac catheterization than patients with normal results.

A decade ago, exercise stress RNV and stress Tl-201 myocardial perfusion imaging were competitive as the procedures of choice for the diagnosis of CAD. Myocardial perfusion imaging is the clear winner in current practice. It is far easier to perform and is easily grafted onto a standard treadmill stress ECG examination.

Box 5-18 lists some conditions other than CAD that result in abnormal response to exercise. These are all potential causes of false positive, abnormal test results, lowering the specificity of exercise RNV for detecting CAD.

**Evaluation after coronary artery bypass graft surgery** Exercise RNV has been used to evaluate the functional outcome of CABG surgery. Since resting studies are frequently normal before CABG, the comparison of interest is the preoperative versus postoperative response to exercise stress. The literature consensus suggests that the majority of patients show improvement after surgery for both global ejection fraction and regional wall motion. Again, surgical efficacy can also be assessed with myocardial perfusion scintigraphy, and the ventriculographic approach has largely been replaced.

*Valvular heart disease* Patients with valvular heart disease may experience pressure overload, volume overload, or both. The response to pressure overload is con-

centric hypertrophy. The response to volume overload may be congestive heart failure, if it is acute, or dilation, if it is chronic and progressive. Radionuclide ventriculography allows assessment of ventricular size and ejection fraction. Because the ejection fraction is in part determined by preload, afterload, and heart rate, determination of the ejection fraction at rest cannot be used alone to assess myocardial contractility or functional reserve. Moreover, the diagnosis of CAD by RNV in patients with severe valvular abnormalities is problematic because abnormalities associated with valvular disease can cause both regional and global dysfunction.

The findings regarding chamber size and function on RNV are essentially as would be predicted from observations at cardiac catheterization. One useful measurement that is easier to determine with RNV than with contrast angiography is a calculation of stroke volume ratios for the left and right ventricles. With mitral insufficiency, for example, some of the blood is propelled antegrade and some regurgitates through the mitral valve during each left ventricular contraction. In normal subjects the stroke volume ratio between the ventricles should be 1.0, since all of the blood is propelled antegrade. Thus the stroke volume ratio provides a measure of the severity of regurgitation that can be followed sequentially and that has been shown to correlate with the clinical status of the patient.

The major limitation of the calculation of the stroke volume ratio from equilibrium blood pool studies is chamber overlap between the right and left ventricles and between the right ventricle and the right atrium. The exact level of the pulmonic valve is also difficult to establish in many cases. For these reasons most investigators have established an LV/RV ratio of 1.5 as the upper limit of normal, which is greater than the expected value of 1.0.

**Cardiomyopathy-myocarditis** Cardiomyopathies are a diverse group of disorders. They may be classified as congestive, hypertrophic, or restrictive. In congestive cardiomyopathies the ventricles are typically enlarged and dysfunctional. The global ejection fraction is decreased and wall motion is uniformly poor, except that the septal and anterior basal segments are frequently spared.

The hallmark of the hypertrophic cardiomyopathies is asymmetrical septal hypertrophy. Echocardiography is the diagnostic procedure of choice. The left ventricular chamber is typically small, and the ejection fraction is above normal. Diastolic filling is abnormal because of poor compliance of the hypertrophied myocardium. Diastolic filling rates have been measured with RNV to assess response to therapy. Many patients improve with calcium channel blocker therapy.

**Assessment of drug therapy** The role of RNV has been studied extensively to assess the therapeutic effects of cardiac drugs and the toxic effects of noncardiac drugs. Studies of cardiac therapeutic drugs are not used in routine clinical practice but are valuable in clinical research. Among the cardiac drugs studied by RNV in the literature are digitalis, nitroglycerin, aminophylline, propranolol and other beta blockers, isoproterenol, and calcium channel blockers. The functional outcome of thrombolytic therapy has been evaluated by RNV performed before and after thrombolysis.

Of perhaps more widespread applicability is the use of RNV to follow the cardiotoxic effects of noncardiac drugs. A well-studied drug in this regard is doxorubicin. Administration of doxorubicin (Adriamycin) in excess of 550 mg/m$^2$ results in cardiotoxicity in approximately one third of patients. However, in serial monitoring of drug response as little as 350 mg/m$^2$ may result in toxicity, and some patients can tolerate significantly more drug than a nominal 550 mg/m$^2$. It has been recommended that the drug be discontinued if the ejection fraction decreases more than 15% during therapy. Functional recovery after cessation of doxorubicin is poor. This is currently the most common medication for RNV.

**Pulmonary disease**  Most RNVs are obtained to assess left ventricular function. However, findings in the right side of the heart are characteristic in patients with cor pulmonale. Right ventricular enlargement is readily detected, and in virtually all patients judged to have cor pulmonale on other grounds the right ventricular ejection fraction is abnormal.

In patients with a new onset of dyspnea, the RNV can help differentiate left ventricular from pulmonary dysfunction. The demonstration of a normal left ventricular ejection fraction, wall motion, and chamber size strongly suggests a pulmonary etiology.

**Congenital heart disease**  Radionuclide ventriculography has not played a large role in the evaluation of patients with congenital heart disease. However, it is possible to detect shunts using the technique and to calculate shunt index ratios for both left-to-right and right-to-left shunts.

For left-to-right shunts the central circulation is studied using the first-transit technique. Early recirculation into the right ventricle is detected with a curve-fitting technique. In brief, the lung transit curve (Fig. 5-50, *A*) is modeled by a mathematical function called a gamma variate (Fig. 5-50, *B*). The contribution to the time-activity curve from recirculation is taken as the difference between the total area under the time-activity curve minus the area under the gamma variate fit (Fig. 5-50, *C*). This approach allows detection of shunts as small as 20%.

Right-to-left shunts may be detected with Tc-99m-labeled macroaggregated albumin. The ratio of tracer in the lung to tracer gaining access to the systemic circulation provides a measure of the severity of shunting. Right-to-left shunts are generally given as a relative

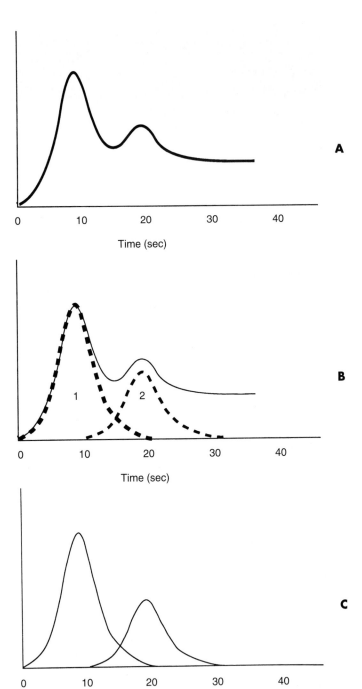

**Fig. 5-50**  **A,** Time-activity curve obtained from a region of interest over the lungs in a patient with a left-to-right shunt. The second peak is due to early recirculation of tracer through the left-to-right shunt. **B,** The relative contributions from the initial transit and the shunt are determined from a curve-fitting technique. **C,** Initial time-activity curve and the two mathematically fitted curves. The shunt ratio ($Q_p/Q_s$) is calculated from the areas under these curves.

contraindication to the use of macroaggregated albumin, owing to the theoretical risk of embolizing the capillary bed of the brain. In practice this has not been a problem, but great caution and care are needed in preparing the material and using this approach.

## INFARCT-AVID IMAGING

### Technetium-99m Pyrophosphate

Tc-99m-labeled pyrophosphate is prepared in the same way as the Tc-99m-labeled bone-imaging agents. Sodium pertechnetate from a generator is added to a vial containing pyrophosphate and stannous ion Sn (II) as the reducing agent. The Tc-99m forms a chelate with the pyrophosphate molecule. The labeling process is susceptible to the adverse effects of oxygen, with the potential for the formation of colloidal impurities and the reduction in labeling efficiency with the presence of free pertechnetate. Colloidal impurities are recognized because of excessive uptake in the liver, and free pertechnetate is recognized by uptake in the thyroid gland, salivary glands, and GI tract and by excessive vascular and soft tissue background activity. In clinical practice it is important to avoid introduction of air into multidose vials. As with the skeletal agents, the prepared radiopharmaceutical should be used within 2 or 3 hours.

In current practice most departments wait 3 to 4 hours after tracer administration to allow more complete clearance from the blood. Radioactivity retained in the circulation contributes to background activity in the cardiac blood pool. The blood pool activity can be confused with myocardial uptake, which could result in false positive interpretations of Tc-99m pyrophosphate images. A further delay to allow more complete clearance should be considered if background activity remains high 4 hours after injection.

**Mechanisms of localization**  After cell death in acute MI an influx of calcium occurs and various calcium phosphate complexes are formed. These microcrystalline deposits act as sites for Tc-99m pyrophosphate uptake. Some binding may also occur on denatured macromolecules. Also, the status of the periinfarction circulation is important in tracer uptake. Some residual blood flow is necessary to deliver the tracer to the infarct area and surrounding tissue. The tracer then diffuses into the necrotic tissue and is bound. The highest uptake of Tc-99m pyrophosphate is at the periphery of infarctions. In large infarctions, with neither direct flow nor diffusion to the central area, no tracer is delivered, and a characteristic ring or doughnut pattern is seen due to activity around the margin of the damaged area (Fig. 5-51).

Tc-99m pyrophosphate is an avid bone seeker. In normal subjects and in patients without MI the sternum and ribs should be clearly seen, with no focal or diffuse activity in the region of the heart. Faint residual activity is often seen in the cardiac blood pool.

**Technique**  Tc-99m pyrophosphate infarct-avid studies are most commonly performed in the cardiac care unit with a mobile gamma scintillation camera. Imaging is performed 3 to 4 hours after intravenous administration of 15 to 25 mCi (555 to 925 MBq). A high-resolution

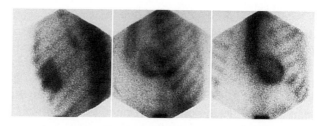

**Fig. 5-51**  Technetium-99m pyrophosphate scan in a patient with a huge anterior myocardial infarction. Uptake is greatest at the periphery of the infarct, producing a "doughnut" appearance on the left anterior oblique *(middle)* and anterior *(right)* views.

---

**Box 5-19  Technetium-99m Pyrophosphate Infarct-Avid Imaging: Protocol Summary**

**PATIENT PREPARATION AND FOLLOW-UP**

Electrocardiographic leads should be moved out of field of view

Frequent voiding to minimize radiation dose to bladder

**DOSAGE AND ROUTE OF ADMINISTRATION**

20 mCi (740 MBq) Tc-99m pyrophosphate
Intravenous administration

**TIME OF IMAGING**

3-4 hr after radiopharmaceutical administration (may be performed at 1 hr if clinically indicated)

**PROCEDURE**

Use a low-energy, high-resolution or general purpose, parallel hole collimator

Obtain the anterior view for 500k counts and record the length of time

Obtain 35° left anterior oblique (LAO), 70° LAO, and left lateral views for equal time

Consider SPECT if the patient can come to the nuclear medicine clinic

---

collimator should be used, and most departments acquire three or four views, including the anterior, 35° LAO, 70° LAO, and left lateral views. At least 500,000 counts are obtained. An alternative is the acquisition of a 500,000-count anterior view and subsequent imaging for the same length of time in the other views (Box 5-19).

The sensitivity for detecting MI is highest at 24 to 48 hours after acute infarction. Earlier or more delayed imaging may be indicated by the clinical situation. For patients who can be transported to the nuclear medicine department, SPECT imaging should be considered. This technique offers greater image contrast, allowing detection of smaller abnormalities and also more exact anatomical localization of infarct. In general the technique is used only when other clinical parameters are nondiagnostic.

A major limitation of Tc-99m pyrophosphate imaging for diagnosis of acute MI is the delay between the time of infarction and the time of scintigram positivity. Significant uptake becomes demonstrable at 12 hours after infarction. Maximum localization occurs at 48 to 72 hours. Thereafter uptake begins to diminish as the infarcted area heals. In uncomplicated cases the scintigram reverts to normal within 14 days.

If initial images reveal diffuse activity in the region of the heart, further delay can be helpful to allow more complete clearance of tracer from the blood pool. If a comparison of early and further delayed images shows a decrease in skeletal-to-heart activity, it suggests residual blood pool background. On the other hand, if the activity becomes more focal or increases relative to surrounding skeleton, it points to a myocardial etiology.

## Scintigraphic Patterns in Acute Myocardial Infarction

The classic scintigraphic pattern in MI is a focal area of increased tracer uptake corresponding to the affected region of the heart. Grading the degree of uptake is useful. One grading system assigns zero to a normal study, 1+ to faint uptake, possibly caused by residual blood pool activity, 2+ to uptake equal to rib intensity, and 3+ to uptake greater than rib intensity. The degree of diagnostic confidence increases with the relative grade of uptake and with focal versus diffuse activity.

In addition to the presence of an abnormality, a complete interpretation includes an assessment of location and size. Location is inferred from comparison of the relationship of the abnormal uptake to the expected location of the heart and the skeletal structures on the multiple views obtained from different angles or SPECT. Anterior infarctions are seen en face on the anterior view and project just behind the sternum on the lateral view (Fig. 5-52). Lateral wall infarcts appear as vertical curvilinear lesions on the anterior view (Fig. 5-53). With progressive obliquity the area of abnormality moves either closer to the sternum (anterolateral infarcts) or farther from the sternum (posterolateral infarcts). Inferior wall infarctions are concave upward and may have a characteristic "lazy 3" configuration if they involve the inferior portion of the septum and right ventricle.

As noted, large infarctions, most frequently in the anterior wall of the left ventricle, may exhibit a doughnut pattern of increased uptake resulting from absence of tracer in the center of the infarct area (Fig. 5-51). This pattern is associated with a poor clinical prognosis; it is typically seen only with quite large infarctions. Experimental data suggest that a minimum of 3 g of tissue must be infarcted for scintigraphic detection.

The sensitivity of Tc-99m pyrophosphate scintigraphy is high, on the order of 95%, for transmural or Q-wave

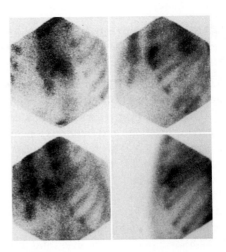

**Fig. 5-52**   Large anterior wall infarction. Note the convex anterior configuration on the lateral view *(bottom right)*.

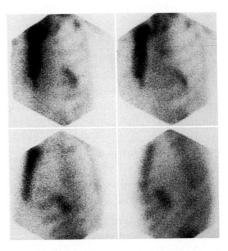

**Fig. 5-53**   Lateral wall infarction. Uptake is greater than rib uptake and not equal to sternal uptake.

infarctions. The sensitivity for subendocardial infarctions is difficult to establish but is significantly less, probably approximately 65% for planar Tc-99m pyrophosphate scintigraphy.

The true specificity of the study is difficult to establish because of the lack of an ideal reference standard for ruling out MI. In the early literature the specificity was reported to be over 90% in the majority of series.

Numerous potential causes of false positive Tc-99m pyrophosphate scans have been reported. Some of the more important are summarized in Box 5-20. False positive studies may result from diffuse activity in the cardiac blood pool that is misinterpreted as emanating from the myocardium. Uptake in areas of chest wall trauma, in skeletal muscle that is necrotic because of prior cardioversion, and in calcifications in or near the heart accounts for most false positive findings. Calcifications in the costal cartilage are occasionally associated with up-

## Box 5-20  Causes of False Positive Technetium-99m Pyrophosphate Infarct-Avid Studies

**FOCAL**

Old myocardial infarction (persistent positivity)
Calcification: valvular, pericardial
Ventricular aneurysm
Costal cartilage calcification

**DIFFUSE**

Myocarditis
Pericarditis
Cardiomyopathy
Amyloidosis
Radiation therapy
Persistent blood pool activity
Doxorubicin (Adriamycin) therapy

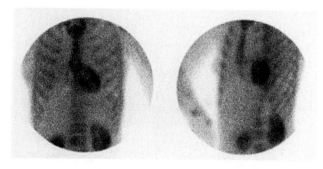

**Fig. 5-54**   Cardiac amyloidosis. Technetium-99m pyrophospate is taken up throughout the left ventricular myocardium. Subtle uptake can also be seen in the right ventricular myocardium.

## Box 5-21  Clinical Situations in Which Technetium-99m Pyrophosphate Scintigraphy May Have Clinical Utility

Suspected infarction in a patient with left bundle-branch block
Delay in diagnosis; enzymes past expected peak
After cardioversion
After major surgery or trauma
Subendocardial (non-Q-wave) infarction versus ischemia
Baseline electrocardiogram abnormal because of prior myocardial infarctions
Prior electrocardiogram not available
Right ventricular infarction

take. Old or chronic conditions with mature calcification take up less tracer than do evolving abnormalities.

Several conditions can result in diffusely increased myocardial uptake of Tc-99m pyrophosphate. The most dramatic is amyloidosis (Fig. 5-54). The tip-off to amyloid as the etiology is visualization of the entire myocardium, including the right ventricle, with quite good myocardium-to-background ratio. Myocarditis, postradiation injury, and doxorubicin cardiotoxicity are all reported causes of diffusely increased myocardial uptake.

Tc-99m pyrophosphate scintigrams may remain abnormal for weeks or months after an MI. Those that continue to show uptake for more than 3 months are called persistently abnormal. Patients in this category are at higher risk for future MIs and are more likely to have ongoing angina.

### Clinical Applications and Utility

The major limitation of Tc-99m infarct-avid scintigraphy is its delayed positivity after the onset of symptoms. In most patients the diagnosis is established from the history, physical examination, ECG, and serum enzyme determinations before the ideal time window for Tc-99m pyrophosphate imaging. The study is not a routine test in suspected acute MI.

The Tc-99m pyrophosphate study is used mainly when the diagnosis of MI is uncertain (Box 5-21). If diagnosis is delayed, serum enzyme levels and ECG changes may already have returned to normal. After surgery or major trauma a "spillover" into the MB fraction may occur, making serum creatine kinase isoenzyme levels difficult to determine. In patients with left bundle-branch block, Q waves can be difficult to assess;

the Tc-99m pyrophosphate study can add to the diagnostic certainty.

## OTHER RADIONUCLIDE TECHNIQUES FOR STUDYING THE HEART

A number of experimental radiopharmaceuticals have been used to study the heart. Fatty acids labeled with either single-photon or positron-emitting radiolabels have been studied. As noted earlier, 85% of the energy needs of the heart are normally met by fatty acid metabolism. It has been hoped that radiolabeled fatty acids could be used to measure this important metabolic parameter. Several radiolabeled fatty acids have yielded excellent images of the heart, but controversy remains regarding the significance of the metabolic information provided (Fig. 5-55). Metabolic turnover is inferred from the clearance pharmacokinetics in the myocardium.

Radioiodinated metaiodobenzylguanidine (MIBG) has been used to study the adrenergic status of the heart.

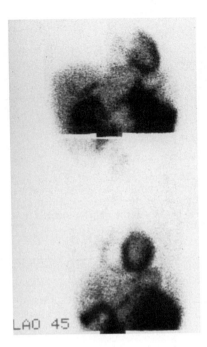

**Fig. 5-55** Iodine-123-labeled fatty acid imaging in a volunteer subject provides excellent visualization of the left ventricle and demonstrates some right ventricular uptake.

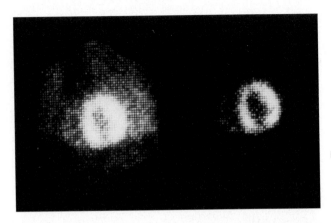

**Fig. 5-56** Myocardial scintigram obtained with iodine-131 metaiodobenzylguanidine in a normal volunteer subject. The tracer is taken up in presynaptic storage vesicles in the adrenergic nervous system. Cocaine abusers and diabetic patients with cardioneuropathy have decreased uptake.

The heart is richly innervated, and MIBG has been used to provide some interesting insights (Fig. 5-56). Uptake of MIBG is blocked in patients taking drugs, such as guanethidine and cocaine, that compete for uptake into the presynaptic storage vesicles of the adrenergic system. Decreased uptake is seen after MI and in diabetic patients with denervated hearts. Some patients with cardiomyopathies also have diminished or absent uptake. A clinical role has not been established for MIBG, although it is being used assess reinnervation after cardiac transplantation and to help determine prognosis in patients with dilated cardiomyopathy.

A recently approved agent that is interesting from a clinical standpoint is radiolabeled antimyosin antibody. The tracer localizes in areas of acute MI (Fig. 5-57). The Fab′ fragment is radiolabeled with In-111 or Tc-99m. The sensitivity for detecting acute MI is quite high, over 85% in reported series. A major disadvantage is the slow pharmacokinetics of antimyosin antibody, which means that optimum imaging cannot be accomplished for many hours after radiopharmaceutical administration because of high background activity. False positive studies may also be seen in patients with myocarditis. Antimyosin has been used to diagnose transplant rejection, myocarditis, and drug toxicity.

The heart continues to be a fertile ground for the development of new radiopharmaceuticals, again with both single-photon and positron labels. Metabolic, antibody-binding, and receptor-binding agents are under active development in laboratories around the world.

Anterior          45° LAO

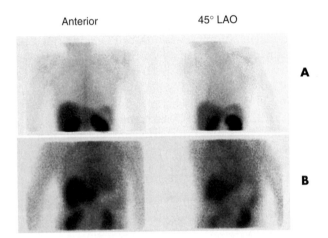

**Fig. 5-57** **A,** Imaging in a normal subject with indium-111-labeled antimyosin antibody demonstrates no abnormal uptake in the region of the heart. Uptake is intense in the liver, spleen, and kidneys. *LAO,* Left anterior oblique. **B,** In a subject with active myocarditis, uptake is significant throughout the left ventricle. (Courtesy of Tsunehiro Yasuda, M.D., Department of Radiology, Massachusetts General Hospital, Boston.)

## SUGGESTED READINGS

Arrighi JA, Soufer R: Reverse redistribution: is it clinically relevant or a washout? *J Nucl Cardiol* 5:195-201, 1998.

Bax JJ, Cornel JH, Visser FC, et al: Comparison of fluorine-18-FDG with rest-redistribution thallium-201 SPECT to delineate viable myocardium and predict functional recovery after revascularization, *J Nucl Med* 39:1481-1486, 1998.

Bonte FJ, Parkey RW, Graham KD, et al: A new method for radionuclide imaging of myocardial infarcts, *Radiology* 110:473, 1974.

Brady TJ, Thrall JH, Lo K, Pitt B: The importance of adequate exercise in the detection of coronary heart disease by radionuclide ventriculography, *J Nucl Med* 21:1125, 1980.

Braunwald E, Rutherford JD: Reversible ischemic left ventricular dysfunction: evidence for the "hibernating myocardium," *J Am Coll Cardiol* 8:1467, 1986.

Carbet JR, Ficaro EP: Clinical review of attenuation-corrected cardiac SPECT, *J Nucl Cardiol* 6:54-68, 1999.

DePuey G, Parmett S, Ghensi M, et al: Comparison of Tc-99m sestamibi and Tl-201 gated SPECT, *J Nucl Cardiol* 6:278-285, 1999.

Freeman LM, Blaufox MD, editors: Cardiovascular nuclear medicine, parts 1 and 2, *Semin Nucl Med,* vol 19, 1999.

Gerson MC, editor: *Cardiac nuclear medicine,* ed 3, New York, 1997, McGraw-Hill.

Gould KL, Westcott RJ, Albro PC, Hamilton GW: Non-invasive assessment of coronary stenoses by myocardial imaging during pharmacologic coronary vasodilation. II. Clinical methodology and feasibility, *Am J Cardiol* 4:279, 1978.

Guiberteau MJ, editor: *Nuclear cardiovascular imaging,* New York, 1990, Churchill Livingstone.

Hansen CL, Rastogi A, Sangrigoli R: On myocardial perfusion, metabolism and viability, *J Nucl Cardiol* 5:202-205, 1998.

Iskandrian AE, German G, VanDecker W, et al: Validation of left ventricular volume measurements by gated SPECT Tc-99m-labeled sestamibi imaging, *J Nucl Cardiol* 5:574-578, 1998.

Khaw A, Gold HK, Yasuda T, et al: Scintigraphic quantification of myocardial necrosis in patients after intravenous injection of myosin-specific antibody, *Circulation* 74:501, 1986.

Manrique A, Foraggi M, Vera P, et al: Tl-201 and Tc-99m MIBI gated SPECT in patients with large perfusion defects and left ventricular dysfunction: compression with equilibrium radionuclide angiography, *J Nucl Med* 40: 805-809, 1999.

Marcus ML, Schelbert HR, Skorton DJ, Wolf GL, editors: *Cardiac imaging,* Philadelphia, 1991, WB Saunders.

Merlet P, Pouillart F, Dubois-Rande J, et al: Sympathetic nerve alterations assessed with I-123-MIBG in the failing human heart, *J Nucl Med* 40:224-231, 1999.

Santana-Boado C, Candell-Riera J, Castell-Conesa J, et al: Diagnostic accuracy of technetium-99m-MIBI myocardial SPECT in women and men, *J Nucl Med* 39:751-755, 1998.

Schelbert HR: Current status and prospects of new radionuclides and radiopharmaceuticals for cardiovascular nuclear medicine, *Semin Nucl Med* 27:145, 1987.

Schwaiger M, Hutchins GD: Evaluation of coronary artery disease with positron emission tomography, *Semin Nucl Med* 21:210, 1992.

Silverman KJ, Becker LC, Bulkley BH, et al: Value of early thallium-201 scintigraphy for predicting mortality in patients with acute myocardial infarction, *Circulation* 61:996, 1980.

Soman P, Parsons RGN, Lahiri N, Lahiri A: The prognostic value of a normal Tc-99m sestamibi SPECT study in suspected coronary disease, *J Nucl Cardiol* 6:252-256, 1999.

Takeishi Y, Takahashi N, Fujiwara S, et al: Myocardial tomography with technetium-99m-tetrofosmin during intravenous infusion of adenosine triphosphate, *J Nucl Med* 39:582-586, 1998.

Tsui BMW, Frey EC, LaCroix KJ, et al: Quantitative myocardial perfusion SPECT, *J Nucl Cardiol* 5:507-522, 1998.

Zaret BL, Beller GA, editors: *Nuclear cardiology,* St Louis, 1999, Mosby.

# CHAPTER 6

# Skeletal System

The singular advantages of skeletal scintigraphy are its high sensitivity in detecting early disease of many types and its ability to survey the entire skeleton quickly, at reasonable expense. Most broadly, the uptake of skeletal seeking radiotracers depicts osteoblastic activity and regional blood flow to bone. Any medical condition that changes either of these factors in a positive or negative way can result in an abnormal skeletal scintigram.

The major limitation of skeletal scintigraphy is its nonspecificity. Any cause of altered bone formation will result in abnormal tracer localization. In the vast majority of cases the diagnostic significance of the scintigraphic findings comes from the clinical context and not the image findings alone.

In the constantly changing exercise of selecting the right imaging study for a given indication, skeletal scintigraphy has maintained its strong role in evaluating patients for metastatic disease. Magnetic resonance imaging (MRI) and, to a lesser extent, computed tomography (CT) have displaced skeletal scintigraphy in whole or in part in other applications, such as the diagnosis of osteonecrosis, osteomyelitis, and trauma, including stress fractures.

**Table 6-1  Characteristics of selected skeleton-seeking agents**

| Radionuclide | Physical half-life | Principal mode of decay | Principal photon energy (keV) | Usual dosage (mCi) |
|---|---|---|---|---|
| Strontium-85 | 65 days | Electron capture | 514 | 0.1-0.25 |
| Strontium-87m | 2.8 hr | Isomeric transition | 388 | 3-10 |
| Fluorine-18 | 1.8 hr | Positron | 511 | 3-10 |
| Technetium-99m MDP | 6 hr | Isomeric transition | 140 | 15-25 |

# RADIOPHARMACEUTICALS

The first clinically important radiopharmaceutical for skeletal imaging was strontium-85 (Table 6-1). This radionuclide is an analog of calcium and an avid bone seeker. Limitations of Sr-85 include higher than ideal gamma photon energy (514 keV) and a long half-life (65.1 days), resulting in a high radiation absorbed dose. Imaging had to be delayed for 2 days to allow background clearance. The tracer is also excreted partially in the gastrointestinal (GI) tract, which commonly necessitated cleansing enemas to remove background activity.

Strontium-87m enjoyed a brief vogue in the 1960s. This tracer is obtained from an yttrium-87 parent in an yttrium-87–strontium-87m generator system. Sr-87m has a short half-life (2.8 hours), decays by isomeric transition, and has a more favorable energy (388 keV) than Sr-85. Neither Sr-85 nor Sr-87m is used in current practice. The beta emitter, strontium-89, has been used to treat bone pain in the therapy for skeletal malignancy.

Fluorine-18 is an avid bone seeker and is an analog of the hydroxyl ion found abundantly in the calcium hydroxyapatite crystals of bone. Fl-18 was the agent of choice for skeletal imaging before the development of technetium 99m (Tc-99m)-labeled bone imaging agents. F-18 decays by positron emission (97%) and has a half-life of 1.8 hours (Table 6-1). The photons available for imaging have an energy of 511 keV. This tracer is enjoying a modest renaissance in institutions with cyclotrons and positron emission tomography (PET) scanners but is not widely available commercially.

The modern era of skeletal imaging began with the invention of Tc-99m-labeled polyphosphate in 1971. As discussed throughout this book, Tc-99m is a desirable label with its reasonable 6-hour half-life, 140-keV principal photon, and availability from the Mo-99–Tc-99m generator system. Rapidly after the description of Tc-99m polyphosphate, a family of Tc-99m label compounds were developed. In current practice the agents of choice are in the chemical class of diphosphonates (Fig. 6-1). These agents are characterized by the organic

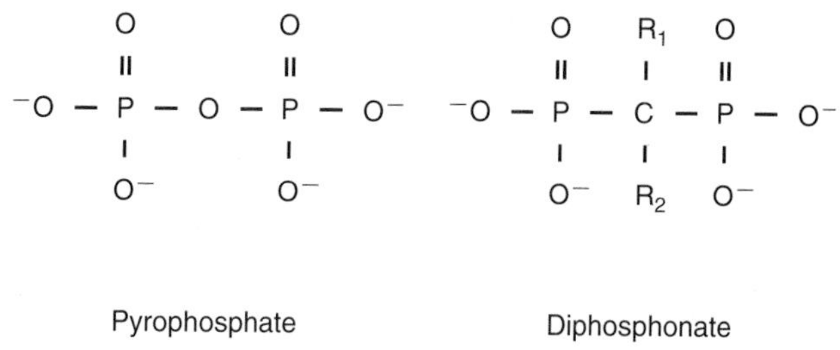

**Fig. 6-1**  Chemical structures of pyrophosphate and diphosphonate.

P – C – P structure. Subtleties of uptake and pharmacokinetics are controlled by the R groups attached to the central carbon atom. The diphosphonates are preferred over the closely related Tc-99m-labeled pyrophosphate radiopharmaceutical. The diphosphonates demonstrate superior clearance from the circulation and from background soft tissues because of less protein binding.

## Preparation of Technetium-99m-Labeled Bone-Imaging Agents

Tc-99m labeled bone agents are prepared by the addition of sodium pertechnetate ($NaTcO_4$) obtained from an Mo-99–Tc-99m generator system to a vial containing the respective diphosphonate (or pyrophosphate) compound and stannous ion, Sn(II), a reducing agent. Tc-99m forms a chelate with the diphosphonates. Successful labeling requires sufficient Sn(II) to reduce Tc(VII) to effect the chelation. If oxygen is allowed into the vial, Sn(II) is hydrolyzed, with the potential formation of colloidal impurities that can result in liver and other reticuloendothelial uptake in vivo, degrading images of the skeleton. Moreover, if the available Sn(II) is hydrolyzed, the labeling efficiency is compromised, resulting in free pertechnetate, which also degrades in vivo images by uptake in the soft tissues, thyroid gland, salivary gland, and stomach (Fig. 6-2). In clinical practice, air must be prevented from entering multidose vials and the radiopharmaceutical should be used within 2 or 3 hours of preparation.

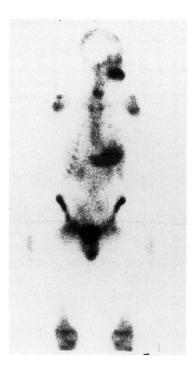

**Fig. 6-2** Free pertechnetate in the radiopharmaceutical preparation has resulted in uptake in the stomach, thyroid gland, and oropharynx. By the usual time of imaging at 2 to 4 hours after tracer administration, free pertechnetate has cleared from the salivary glands, accounting for the activity in the oropharynx and the absence of salivary activity.

## Pharmacokinetics After Intravenous Administration of Technetium-99m Diphosphonate

The Tc-99m-labeled skeletal radiopharmaceuticals are distributed rapidly throughout the extracellular fluid space (Fig. 6-3). Uptake in bone is also rapid, and by 2 to 6 hours after tracer injection represents approximately 50% of the injected dose. Net clearance from the body is via the kidneys, primarily by glomerular filtration. In patients with normal renal function, 50% to 60% of the injected dose is excreted in the urine within 24 hours. The skeleton–to–background tissue ratio improves with time, and the selection of imaging time is based on a compromise between clinical convenience, decay of the radiolabel, and target-to-background ratio. In practice, most nuclear medicine departments begin imaging 2 to 3 hours after tracer administration. By then the blood level is 3% to 5% of the injected dose.

### Mechanisms of Tracer Localization

The mechanism of radiostrontium and radiofluorine localization is straightforward. They are analogs, respectively, of calcium and hydroxyl ion and bind avidly to hydroxyapatite crystals in bone. The mechanism of uptake of the Tc-99m phosphorus–containing compounds is less well understood. For Tc-99m diphospho-

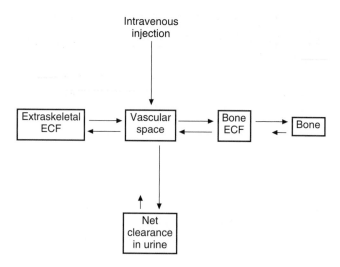

**Fig. 6-3** Technetium-99m diphosphonate distribution. Clearance from the extracellular fluid space and the vascular space is necessary for optimum visualization of the skeleton. *ECF,* Extracellular fluid.

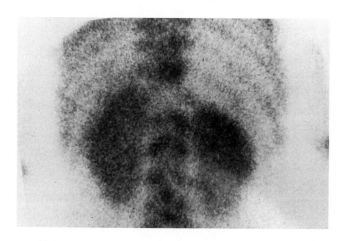

**Fig. 6-4** Complete destruction of the L1 vertebral body with corresponding photon-deficient, or cold, lesion.

nates, adsorption is is believed to occur primarily to the mineral phase of bone, with little binding to the organic phase. The uptake is significantly higher in amorphous calcium phosphate than in mature crystalline hydroxyapatite, which helps explain the avidity of the tracer for areas of increased osteogenic activity.

Another clinically important factor in regional tracer distribution is local blood flow. More radiopharmaceutical is delivered to hyperemic areas. The coupling of disease processes with both increased blood flow and increased osteogenesis for many types of lesions results in higher tracer uptake than in unaffected parts of the skeleton.

Decreased tracer localization is seen in areas of reduced or absent blood flow (bone infarction) and in areas where the skeleton has been destroyed to the point that no bone matrix elements are present for uptake to occur. This is seen in some aggressive metastases (Fig. 6-4). Cold areas are often referred to as *photon deficient.*

**Table 6-2   Technetium-99m diphosphonate: radiation absorbed dose**

| Organ | Radiation absorbed dose (rads/20 mCi) |
|---|---|
| Whole body | 0.13 |
| Skeleton | 0.70 |
| Marrow (red) | 0.56 |
| Kidneys | 0.80 |
| Bladder (2-hr void) | 2.60 |
| Ovaries (2-hr void) | 0.24 |
| Testes (2-hr void) | 0.16 |

## Dosimetry

Estimates of the radiation absorbed doses for the total body and selected organs are provided in Table 6-2. The radiation dose to the bladder wall, ovaries, and testes depends on the frequency of voiding. The estimates provided assume a 2-hour voiding cycle. Significantly higher doses can occur with infrequent voiding, and before patients are allowed to leave the imaging clinic, they are reminded to continue frequent voiding. As usual, radiopharmaceuticals should be administered to pregnant women only if clearly needed on a risk-versus-benefit basis. Tc-99m is excreted in breast milk, and formula feedings should be substituted for several days.

## TECHNIQUE

Technical details vary from department to department and include variations for special purposes that are discussed in this chapter (Box 6-1). For whole body surveys, the most common application, most departments use 20 mCi (740 MBq) of Tc-99m diphosphonate and begin imaging 2 to 3 hours after intravenous (IV) administration of the radiopharmaceutical. Dynamic imaging immediately after injection is performed to differentiate suspected osteomyelitis from cellulitis.

Imaging is accomplished with a gamma scintillation camera equipped with a low-energy, all-purpose or high-resolution collimator. For contemporary large-field-of-view cameras, either a spot view or a whole body approach may be used. Whole body imaging has the advantage of providing anatomical continuity of image data (Fig. 6-5, *A*). Spot views provide significantly higher resolution, and the highest quality bone scintigrams are obtained with high-count (1000k) regional spot views. A frequently used compromise is to obtain an initial whole body survey followed by high-resolution, high-count supplementary spot views of suspect or symptomatic

**Box 6-1   Skeletal Scintigraphy: Protocol Summary for Whole Body Survey and SPECT**

**PATIENT PREPARATION AND FOLLOW-UP**

Patient should be well hydrated
Patient should void immediately before study
Patient should void frequently after procedure (reduces radiation dose to bladder wall)
Patient should remove metal objects (jewelry, coins, keys) before imaging

**DOSAGE AND ROUTE OF ADMINISTRATION**

20 mCi (740 MBq) technetium-99m diphosphonate adult dose (standard)
Intravenous injection (site selected to avoid known or suspected pathological condition)
Adjust dosage for pediatric patients (Webster's rule; minimum 74 MBq [2mCi])

**TIME OF IMAGING**

Begin imaging 2 to 4 hr after tracer administration

**PROCEDURE**

Anterior and posterior views of the entire skeleton
Obtain a minimum of 1000k counts per view for "whole body" imaging systems
Obtain 300k to 500k counts per image if multiple spot views are used
Use the highest resolution collimator that permits imaging in a reasonable length of time
Obtain high-count (1000k) spot views or SPECT for more detail

**SPECT***

Acquisition: contoured orbit, 128 × 128 matrix, 6° intervals, 15 to 30 sec/stop
Reconstruction: filtered backprojection, Butterworth filter; cut-off 0.4, power 7

*Selection of SPECT acquisition and reconstruction parameters depends greatly on available equipment and software.

areas (Fig. 6-5). Immediately before imaging, patients are asked to empty the bladder, taking care to avoid contamination of the skin or clothing. Such areas of urinary contamination may result in misinterpretation as a soft tissue or skeletal lesion.

Special imaging techniques include dynamic scanning for the differential diagnosis of skeletal versus soft tissue disease, single-photon emission computed tomography (SPECT) for high-contrast regional imaging, and computer recording of images for quantitative analysis. Magnification imaging with a pinhole collimator or converging collimator can be helpful in children and has been used routinely in evaluation of the hip for osteonecrosis.

Skeletal SPECT is easily added as an additional part of whole body surveys for metastatic disease or more localized imaging for osteonecrosis or trauma. Some observers believe that SPECT increases study sensitivity for such conditions as spondylolysis. Without question, SPECT gives better lesion contrast for both hot and cold lesions and is superior for delineating the extent of involvement in complex structures such as the spine or facial bones. Reformatted SPECT studies using sagittal and coronal views in addition to the transaxial slices (Fig. 6-6) can

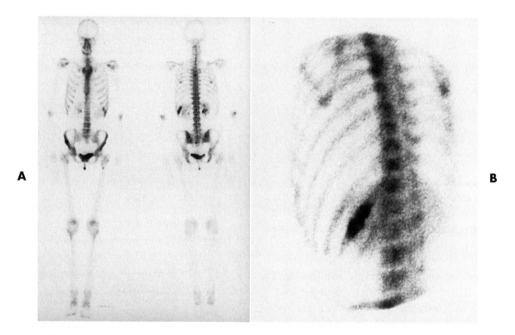

**Fig. 6-5**    **A,** Anterior and posterior whole body images of a patient with carcinoma of the breast. Whole body images have the advantage of depicting the entire skeleton in a single view. Note the abnormal uptake in one of the left lower posterior ribs. **B,** High–count density spot view of left posterior ribs from the patient in **A.** The location and appearance of the lesion are better delineated in the spot view.

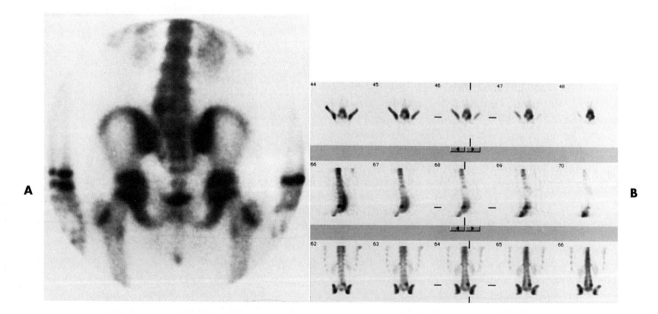

**Fig. 6-6**    **A,** Posterior skeletal scintigram of a child with back pain reveals a suspect asymmetry at the level of L5 with more uptake on the left. **B,** Corresponding SPECT study shows a focal abnormality caused by spondylolysis. SPECT provides the benefit of being able to view the lesion in three different image plans. The top row represents the transaxial planes, the middle row is sagittal views, and the bottom row is coronal views. Distinct focal uptake is demonstrated in the characteristic pars interarticularis region on each view.

also be helpful, and maximum intensity projection (MIP) images can be striking. SPECT imaging is particularly useful in correlating scintigraphic studies with other cross-sectional techniques, including CT and MRI.

A reasonable protocol for bone SPECT includes the use of a 128 × 128 matrix with contoured arc having either 60 (6° intervals) or 120 (3° intervals) stops. Imaging at each view is for 15 to 30 seconds (Box 6-1).

## APPEARANCE OF THE NORMAL SKELETAL SCINTIGRAM

The appearance of the normal skeletal scintigram changes dramatically between infancy, childhood, adolescence, and mature adulthood. In the early neonatal period skeletal tracer uptake is not as avid as it is even a few months later. For example, little activity is seen in the sutures of the skull in the first months of life, and the differentiation of increased activity in growth centers is also less in the first few months than by age 6 months. Contamination of skin and clothing is a special problem in infants because the radiopharmaceutical is excreted in the urine.

A striking feature of the growing skeleton is the marked uptake of radiopharmaceutical in growth centers (Fig. 6-7). These are hotter than surrounding bone. The observation applies to all epiphyseal and apophyseal growth centers and the sutures in the skull until their closure. The degree of uptake in the growth centers is a reflection of relative metabolic activity. The three hottest centers in order are the distal femur, proximal tibia, and proximal humerus (Fig. 6-7)—also the order of relative occurrence of osteosarcoma in children. The amount of metabolic or growth activity is paralleled by the likelihood of malignant transformation.

In adults, growth center activity normally becomes equal to activity in adjacent bone. Tracer uptake is greatest in the axial skeleton (spine and pelvis), with relatively less intense uptake in the extremities and skull. Background activity is normally seen in the soft tissues. The kidneys are routinely visualized in normal subjects and should have less intensity than the adjacent lumbar spine. If the kidneys show equal or greater intensity, a renal abnormality or concomitant drug therapy should be suspected (Box 6-2).

A number of normal variants must be recognized for correct scintigraphic interpretation. The skull frequently presents an uneven or variable activity along its margin, probably because of slight variations in calvarial thickness. Bilaterally increased radionuclide concentration in the frontal area with thinning at the midline may be due to hyperostosis frontalis interna. In slightly oblique views of the skull a flame-shaped or triangular area of

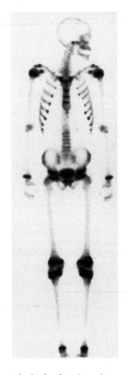

**Fig. 6-7**  Anterior whole body view in a growing adolescent. Note the increased uptake in growth centers. This study is a particularly good example of increased activity at the anterior rib ends and in the sternal ossification centers and the growth centers in the shoulders.

---

**Box 6-2  Reported Causes of Bilaterally Increased and Decreased Renal Visualization on Skeletal Scintigrams**

**INCREASED UPTAKE**

Urinary tract obstruction
Chemotherapy (doxorubicin, vincristine, cyclophosphamide)
Nephrocalcinosis
Hypercalcemia
Radiation nephritis
Acute tubular necrosis
Thalassemia

**DECREASED UPTAKE**

Renal failure
Metastatic disease—"superscan"
Metabolic bone disease—"superscan"
  Paget's disease
  Osteomalacia
  Hyperparathyroidism
Myelofibrosis—"superscan"
Nephrectomy

activity is commonly seen projecting from the base of the skull just posterior to the orbit where the sphenoid ridge meets the calvarial structures. Sutural activity is not seen discretely in adults.

The anterior aspect of the mandible may appear as a "hot spot" on lateral views of the skull. The projected bone mass of the mentum is greater in this view than the rami. The laryngotracheal cartilages are usually seen in adults, probably related to some degree of calcification. The thyroid gland also avidly accumulates unbound pertechnetate, resulting in superimposed activity in the same general region.

Some mild diffuse asymmetry in paired joints is commonly seen in adults. The phenomenon is most common in the shoulders and correlates with handedness. This normal variant appearance should be distinguished from focal asymmetry involving only part of the joint.

In high-resolution scintigrams the sternal-manubrial joint is frequently visualized as a focal hot spot. In the growing skeleton, sternal ossification centers can be confused with abnormal uptake, but these centers should not be seen in the adult.

Increased activity at the costochondral junction is abnormal in adults but is routinely seen in children and adolescents (Fig. 6-7). Increased uptake in a limited number of rib ends is usually due to trauma. Increased uptake at the costochondral junction in adults is seen in some types of metabolic bone disease.

Some asymmetry is frequently seen in the sacroiliac joints, especially in patients with scoliosis or abnormal gait. Scoliosis can also result in subtle rotation of the pelvis with apparent asymmetry of the ala iliae, especially on anterior views. Asymmetrical activity in the sacroiliac joints and pelvic structures should be interpreted with caution in patients with scoliosis.

Interpretation of uptake in the spine itself is potentially difficult in patients with marked scoliosis. The pedicles appear asymmetrical. The altered weight bearing results in remodeling and degenerative changes that can produce confusing patterns of tracer activity.

The normal spinal curvatures cause the vertebrae at different levels of the spine to be at different distances from the face of the collimator, with corresponding differences in the amount of interposed soft tissues. For example, the lower lumbar spine generally appears hotter on the anterior view than the area of the thoracolumbar junction because of the normal lumbar lordosis, which brings the spine forward, with less intervening soft tissue.

Although the marked uptake in the epiphyseal-metaphyseal area is not seen in adults, the ends of the long bones continue to demonstrate greater uptake than the diaphyses. This is due to the greater bone volume and more avid uptake of radiopharmaceutical in cancellous than compact bone.

In women, activity in the breast should reflect general soft tissue activity. Focal or asymmetrical breast activity is not normal and may indicate breast disease. After mastectomy the ribs on the operative side appear hotter because of loss of soft tissue and less attenuation.

## METASTATIC DISEASE

The most common clinical application of skeletal scintigraphy is in evaluating patients with extraskeletal primary malignancies for the presence of metastatic disease. The different kinds of information sought are summarized in Box 6-3. In many patients the presence or extent of skeletal metastasis directly influences treatment decisions and prognosis. Bone scintigraphy plays a role in treatment of bone pain and pathological fractures, which are common management problems in patients with skeletal metastatic disease.

### Pathophysiology: Basis of Scintigraphic and Radiographic Detection

Nonosseous neoplasms gain access to the skeleton by three mechanisms: (1) direct extension, (2) retrograde venous flow, and (3) via the arterial circulation after venous or lymphatic access. For epithelial tumors the initial seeding of metastatic deposits via the arterial circulation is typically in the red marrow. This helps explain the predominance of metastatic lesions in the axial skeleton. Retrograde venous flow in Batson's vertebral venous plexus is another avenue to the axial skeleton. In normal adults the red marrow is distributed to the bones of the axial skeleton, including the cranium, and the proximal portions of the femurs and humeri. Over 90% of skeletal metastatic lesions from most epithelial tumors are found in this distribution, with only a small percentage outside of red marrow–bearing areas.

As metastatic lesions grow in the marrow space, the surrounding bone remodels through osteoclastic (resorptive) and osteoblastic (depositional) activity. The relative

---

### Box 6-3   Skeletal Imaging: Applications in Patients with Extraskeletal Malignancies

Initial staging: metastatic skeletal survey
Protocol monitoring: response to chemotherapy and decision to change therapy
Radiation therapy: treatment field planning and response to radiation therapy
Detection of areas at risk for pathological fracture

degree of bone resorption and deposition elicited is highly variable among the different types of tumors and sometimes even between different locations for the same tumor. The relationship between the two remodeling processes determines whether a metastatic deposit will appear as predominantly lytic or sclerotic or will exhibit a mixed pattern radiographically.

Radionuclide bone scintigrams are sensitive for detecting the altered local metabolism in areas of skeletal remodeling associated with metastatic deposits. On the other hand, a 30% to 50% change in bone density is required before small lesions can be detected radiographically.

These observations are reflected in a characteristic sequence of image findings for skeletal scintigrams and standard radiographs. Early in the natural history of the metastatic lesion, both the skeletal scintigram and standard radiograph are normal. As the metastases grow, bone remodeling results in increased skeletal metabolism and increased tracer localization; the scintigram becomes abnormal and the radiograph remains normal. As the process continues, net calcium content and skeletal trabecular architecture change; the scintigram remains abnormal and the standard radiograph also becomes abnormal. This sequence occurs over a period of months. If healing occurs as a result of therapy, the bone scintigram may revert to normal while the radiograph typically remains abnormal, although there are occasional exceptions. If the cancerous process is indolent or diffusely lytic, the skeletal scintigram may not reveal an abnormality. This is due to a failure of the cancer to alter bone metabolism or local blood flow sufficiently to produce a focally detectable lesion. Multiple myeloma is a notorious cause of false negative skeletal scintigraphic studies on this basis.

It is important to realize that the skeletal tracers do not localize mainly in the cancerous tissue but in the remodeling, metabolically active bone surrounding or being invaded by the metastatic tissues. This is well illustrated in Fig. 6-8, which shows the growth of a metastatic lesion in the calvarium. The circular rim of increased tracer uptake is in the reactive bone surrounding the cancerous tissue. As the cancer enlarges, the rim is displaced as bone is completely destroyed. The central cancerous tissue is photon deficient without tracer uptake.

Although the bone scan is significantly more sensitive than standard radiography as a survey technique, the actual difference in sensitivity depends on the stage of disease being evaluated. In early disease the sensitivity of the bone scintigram is severalfold greater and the sensitivity is also significantly greater on a per lesion basis. However, if all patients with metastatic disease are considered, including patients with advanced disease, the relative superiority is less because both types of examina-

tion are positive in a higher percentage of cases. The accuracy of skeletal scintigraphy will never be precisely known, owing to the lack of a reference standard for comparison. The sensitivity for detecting metastatic disease is often said to be as high as 95% or above.

MRI has suggested a new approach to the early detection of skeletal metastases. The intense, uniform signal from marrow fat is altered by metastatic lesions. A number of early studies showed that lesions disrupting the marrow fat can be detected before they elicit an osteogenic response sufficient to be detected by scintigraphy. $T_2$ MRI with fat suppression (fast STIR) is now being evaluated for detection of metastases. In this technique metastases are associated with increased signal. The major problems in the use of MRI for this application are the difficulty in surveying the entire skeleton and the frequent presence of incidental benign defects or heterogeneity in marrow fat unrelated to metastatic disease, making the specificity of the observation problematic. Use of thicker sections to cover the entire skeleton results in decreased sensitivity because of partial volume effects.

## Scintigraphic Patterns in Metastatic Disease

The scintigraphic patterns encountered in skeletal metastatic disease are summarized in Box 6-4, and a decision tree or algorithm for the workup of patients with proven nonosseous primary tumors is provided in

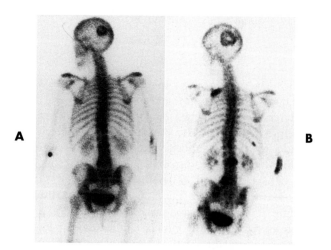

**Fig. 6-8** **A,** Initial skeletal scintigram in a patient with multiple skeletal metastases, including the skull. Note the intense uptake in the calvarial lesion with a small area of decreased uptake centrally. **B,** Several months later the metastatic disease has progressed in both the axial skeleton and the calvarium. The overall diameter of the skull lesion has increased, and the central photon-deficient area is much larger. The increased uptake is in bone at the margin of the metastatic lesion.

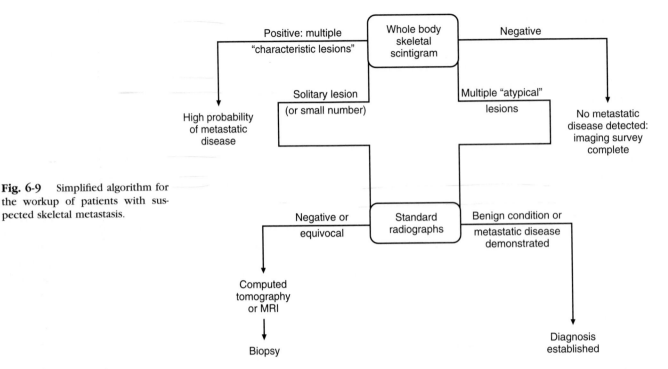

**Fig. 6-9** Simplified algorithm for the workup of patients with suspected skeletal metastasis.

## Box 6-4  Scintigraphic Patterns in Metastatic Disease

Solitary focal lesions
Multiple focal lesions
Diffuse involvement ("superscan")
Photon-deficient lesions (cold lesions)
Normal (false negative)
Flare phenomenon (follow-up studies)
Soft tissue lesions (tracer uptake in tumor)

Fig. 6-9. The point of entry in the algorithm is the whole body bone scintigram. If the examination is positive and characteristic for metastatic disease, the screening workup is complete. The classic, "typical" pattern that provides the most diagnostic certainty is the presence of multiple focal lesions distributed randomly throughout the axial skeleton (Fig. 6-10).

A number of other conditions may also result in multiple scintigraphic abnormalities (Box 6-5). A key feature in recognizing nonmetastatic causes for multifocal scan abnormalities is the pattern of distribution. For example, patients with Cushing's syndrome or osteomalacia frequently have a disproportionate number of rib lesions (Fig. 6-11) as compared with other areas. In patients with osteoporosis, dorsal kyphosis and patterns of associated fractures such as the H-type fracture of the sacrum provide clues to the correct diagnosis.

Skeletal scintigrams in older subjects almost routinely reveal evidence of osteoarthritis. This is generally recog-

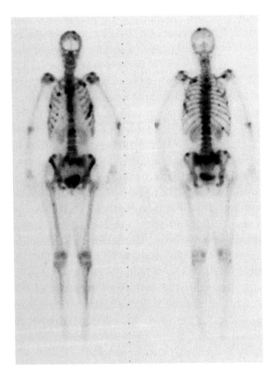

**Fig. 6-10** Anterior *(left)* and posterior *(right)* whole body scintigrams in a patient with widely distributed metastatic disease. Lesions are present in the skull, spine, ribs, pelvis, and extremities.

nized by its characteristic locations. The uptake can be quite intense and is not necessarily closely related in degree to current symptoms. Involvement of both sides of a joint is often seen and is not characteristic of metastatic disease. Medial and lateral compartment

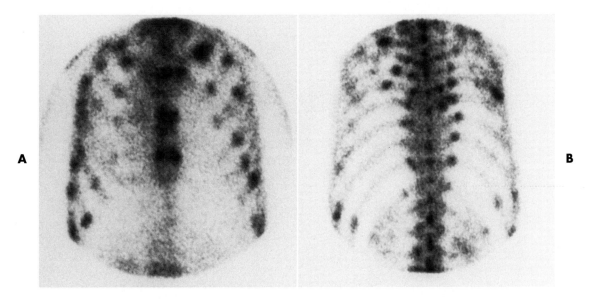

**Fig. 6-11**   **A,** Anterior and, **B,** posterior views from a skeletal scintigram of a patient with osteomalacia. The patient was referred to the nuclear medicine service to "rule out metastatic disease." The unusually large number of rib lesions alerted the nuclear medicine physician to suspect metabolic bone disease.

---

**Box 6-5   Differential Diagnosis of Multiple Focal Lesions, in Order from More Likely to Less Likely**

Metastatic disease
Arthritis
Trauma, osteoporotic insufficiency fractures
Paget's disease
Other metabolic bone disease
Osteomyelitis
Numerous other conditions (fibrous dysplasia, multiple enchondromas, infarction)

---

arthritis in the knee, changes in the hands and wrists (especially at the base of the first metacarpal), and changes in the shoulder are extremely common scintigraphic findings. Degenerative changes in the lower lumbar spine can pose a special problem because of the high incidence of both metastatic disease and degenerative disease in this location. The pattern of scintigraphic abnormality must be assessed with caution. Degenerative changes typically involve the facet joints and vertebral end-plates with hypertrophic spurring. Metastatic disease more typically involves the pedicle and body of the vertebra. The spatial resolution of conventional bone scintigrams often is not sufficient to make these distinctions. Modern SPECT imaging should be considered in difficult cases.

Trauma is a frequent cause of multiple lesions, and patients should be routinely questioned for history of trauma. In the ribs a characteristic vertical alignment of fractures occurs because of the mechanism of injury in falls or automobile accidents (Fig. 6-12). This nonrandom pattern would not be expected in metastatic disease. Displaced fractures can be recognized by their structural deformity, but otherwise a healing fracture and a metastatic lesion may appear the same scintigraphically. Persistently positive skeletal scintigrams from old trauma are a major interpretative problem. The issue is discussed in more detail later in the chapter.

Multifocal osteomyelitis can simulate metastatic disease, but it is unusual as an incidental and unsuspected problem in patients with cancer. Conversely, Paget's disease of bone is relatively common in the cancer age group, and differentiating Paget's disease from metastatic disease in specific lesions may not be possible on the bone scintigram. Paget's disease can be suspected from its characteristic patterns of involvement and the extreme intensity of tracer uptake. In particular, the involvement of a hemipelvis or a long portion of a long bone and the expansion of osseous structures point to Paget's disease. Osteoporosis circumscripta causes a characteristic rim pattern of activity in the skull but may also be difficult to distinguish from metastasis. Radiographic correlation is frequently required when the differential diagnosis rests between Paget's disease and metastatic disease.

Multiple infarctions with reactive bone causing increased tracer uptake can also mimic skeletal metastatic disease. This pattern is most commonly seen in patients with sickle cell anemia and is rarely a practical problem. It is recognized from the history and the presence of other characteristic changes on the bone scan.

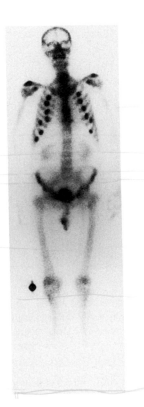

**Fig. 6-12**    Multiple rib fractures bilaterally. The pattern of vertically aligned lesions is highly characteristic for trauma and would be unusual as a pattern for metastatic disease.

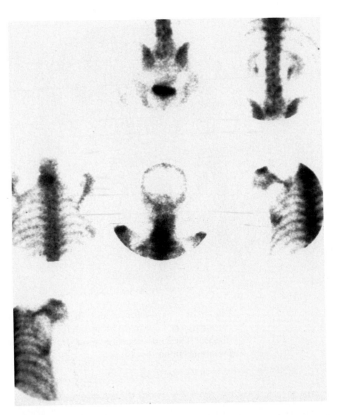

**Fig. 6-13**    Posterior spot views of a patient with suspected metastatic disease. A solitary area of abnormally increased uptake can be seen in the lower cervical spine.

**Solitary lesions**    Scans showing either solitary scintigraphic abnormalities or a small number of lesions pose special problems in interpretation and have been the subject of several major clinical studies (Figs. 6-9 and 6-13). The potential for diagnostic error results from the frequency with which incidental benign conditions involve the skeleton and are detected on bone scintigraphy. When a solitary lesion is encountered, a systematic approach, using an algorithm such as the one presented in Fig. 6-9, is important. Frequently, standard radiographs will confirm the presence of either a metastatic deposit or a benign condition, ending the diagnostic evaluation. If standard radiographs are normal or equivocal and the presence or absence of metastatic disease is important to clinical decision making, further imaging (Fig. 6-14) and if necessary biopsy should be carried out.

The most common cause of solitary benign abnormalities is degenerative arthritis, followed by healing fracture. Other benign bone lesions, including monostotic Paget's disease, enchondroma, frontal osteoma, fibrous dysplasia, and osteomyelitis, can also be the cause of solitary abnormalities.

Location and pattern are important in scintigraphy. Lesions in the anterior rib ends are rarely due to metastases. This is a location subject to trauma, and the costochondral junction can be quite positive scinti-

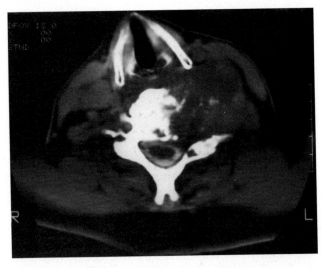

**Fig. 6-14**    Computed tomographic scan obtained at the level of scintigraphic abnormality reveals extensive destruction of the corresponding vertebral body and demonstration of a clinically palpable soft tissue mass in the neck.

graphically with no radiographic abnormality after even minor trauma. Conversely, 40% to 80% of proven solitary lesions in the spine are shown to be metastatic in origin. However, rather than attempting to assign an overall probability of malignancy or a specific probability for

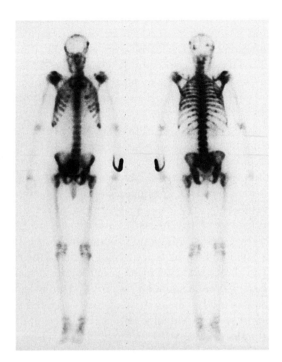

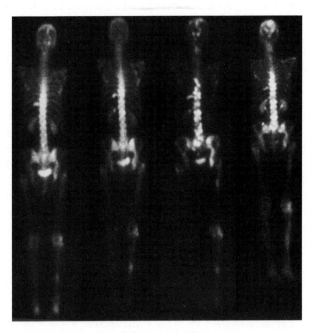

**Fig. 6-15**  "Superscan" of a patient with prostatic carcinoma. In this case the uptake is nonuniform enough that the abnormality is easily seen. The image shows an increased skeletal-to-soft tissue uptake ratio and an axial-appendicular disproportion in uptake. Visualization of the kidneys is faint, but the bladder is well visualized, indicating that failure to see the kidneys is not due to absence of tracer excretion through them. Rather, the uptake in the skeleton is so intense that the kidney activity is below the threshold for recording on the film.

**Fig. 6-16**  The flare phenomenon is demonstrated by a 10-month sequence of posterior whole body scintigrams of a patient undergoing chemotherapy for carcinoma of the breast. Note the increased intensity of uptake in the skull, spine, and pelvis, especially between the second and third images in the sequence. The scintigram appears worse, but the patient was improving clinically, with reduced bone pain and radiographic evidence of healing.

each anatomical area, it is more important simply to recognize the potential pitfall presented by the solitary lesion and have a systematic approach to it.

**Superscan**  Another scintigraphic pattern that can cause interpretative problems for the unwary is the "superscan." In some patients with breast cancer and prostatic cancer the entire axial skeleton becomes diffusely and rather uniformly involved with metastatic disease. If the involvement is uniform enough, the scan may appear deceptively normal (Fig. 6-15). A number of clues provide a tip-off, including unusually good bone-to-soft tissue background ratio, absent or faint visualization of the kidneys, and an increase in the ratio of uptake in the axial versus appendicular skeleton. One helpful rule to avoid being fooled by uniform tracer uptake is to review at least one radiograph from every patient undergoing bone scintigraphy. Virtually all patients have had chest radiographs or other studies so that sufficient correlative information is available to avoid this uncommon diagnostic pitfall.

**Flare phenomenon**  Another potentially perplexing pattern is seen in evaluating follow-up bone scans in patients undergoing cyclical chemotherapy. In some patients who have a good response to chemotheraphy, the bone scan appears to worsen paradoxically, with a "flare" of increased activity (Fig. 6-16). The hypothesis to explain the flare phenomenon is that as lesions begin to heal after therapy, an osteoblastic response occurs, resulting in increased activity on the scintigram. Some patients experience pain in these areas following the onset of chemotherapy, further confusing the issue clinically. When these lesions are followed radiographically, healing with increased sclerosis is seen over 2 to 6 months. The flare phenomenon reinforces the fact that tracer uptake is not in tumor tissue but in the surrounding bone.

**Other patterns**  Some metastatic lesions elicit a predominantly resorptive or destructive response in bone. Areas of the skeleton that are completely replaced by metastatic tumor or that are purely lytic radiographically may appear as "cold" or photon-deficient lesions on bone scan (Fig. 6-4). Therefore the focal absence of expected normal tracer uptake, as well as areas of focally increased uptake, should be sought on bone scintigrams. The photon-deficient area is often bordered by a rim of increased uptake (Fig. 6-8).

A more difficult problem is the scintigraphic detection of some lesions that are characterized by a permeative pattern radiographically. As noted in the discussion on pathophysiology, if the neoplastic process is indolent or causes no reactive bone formation, the scan may falsely appear normal. This is a particular problem with round cell tumors and multiple myeloma. If all sites of involvement are considered, the sensitivity of the bone scan in multiple myeloma is low, although studies in the literature suggest that the majority of patients have some abnormality, often related to pathological fractures. MRI is highly sensitive for detection of marrow involvement by multiple myeloma. Lesions have low signal on $T_1$ images and high signal on $T_2$ and STIR images.

## Scintigraphy in Specific Tumors

The mnemonic "Pb KTL" ("lead kettle") is useful for remembering the common nonosseous tumors that metastasize to bone: cancers of the prostate, breast, kidney, thyroid, and lung. In particular, carcinomas of the prostate, lung, and breast are among the most common causes of cancer and death from cancer.

**Carcinoma of the prostate**   Because of demographic factors and aging of the population, more cases of carcinoma of the prostate are being seen in clinical practice. Until the introduction of prostate-specific antigen (PSA), the skeletal scintigram was considered the most sensitive technique for detecting metastatic disease. Compared with scintigraphy, alkaline phosphatase testing is only half as sensitive an indicator of skeletal metastatic disease, and radiographs are normal in approximately 30% of cases with abnormal scintigrams. The likelihood of an abnormal skeletal scintigram correlates positively with clinical stage, Gleason score, and PSA level. In early stage I disease, 5% or fewer patients have abnormal scintigrams. In patients with a PSA level less than 10 ng/ml, the likelihood of bone metastases is less than 1%. Skeletal scintigrams are still indicated for symptomatic patients and to evaluate suspect areas seen radiographically.

With higher PSA levels the likelihood of detecting metastatic disease at the time of initial workup increases. Each institution should establish its own criteria for when to order baseline studies. During therapy, follow-up scintigrams are often obtained as part of chemotherapy protocols to monitor response to hormonal and drug treatment. Follow-up scintigrams are also indicated when clinical symptoms change.

Prostatic cancer and breast cancer are the two tumors most frequently associated with both the superscan and the flare phenomenon (Figs. 6-15 and 6-16). Serial imaging is useful in monitoring the response to therapy, and lesion regression can be quite dramatic. The flare phenomenon is clearly seen when the timing of the follow-up scan corresponds to osteoblastic healing. The majority of patients dying of prostate cancer have skeletal metastases. These are often dramatic and extensive. When they coalesce to involve essentially the entire axial skeleton, the superscan appearance is seen scintigraphically.

The intensity of uptake in prostatic carcinoma can be confused with Paget's disease. This is especially true when there is contiguous spread to involve a hemipelvis.

**Carcinoma of the breast**   Carcinoma of the breast has reached almost epidemic proportions in the United States. The lifetime incidence of carcinoma of the breast, which in the past was 1 in 11 or 12 women, has now increased to an estimated 1 in 9. Mammographic screening is used to make the diagnosis early, but a large number of woman still have advanced disease at diagnosis and must be evaluated for skeletal metastases.

It is now recognized that the yield for skeletal scintigraphy for stage I disease is low, probably less than 3% to 5%. Early literature on this topic had reported much higher early-stage scan positivity, but in retrospect there were many false positive interpretations because of failure to critically evaluate solitary lesions and consider benign causes of abnormal tracer uptake.

Because of the low yield in early-stage disease, the timing of skeletal scintigraphy in the management of breast cancer is controversial. In some institutions the study is performed on all patients preoperatively. Others reserve the test for patients with clinical stage II or III disease and for the routine follow-up of patients with positive nodes, who are at higher risk for skeletal metastatic disease. Conversion from scan negative to scan positive is a bad prognostic sign. A reasonable approach to patients with newly diagnosed breast cancer is to image those who have skeletal pain, those with stage II or III disease, those whose chemotherapy protocols require scintigrams, and those with a history of other malignancy.

In addition to arterial dissemination of metastases, patients with carcinoma of the breast may have local invasion of the ribs or, via the substernal nodes, of the sternum. As noted previously, both the superscan pattern and the flare phenomenon can be seen in carcinoma of the breast. Skeletal metastases are often widely disseminated. Soft tissue metastases from carcinoma of the breast may accumulate sufficient tracer to be visualized (Fig. 6-17).

After mastectomy the ipsilateral ribs appear relatively more intense than the contralateral ribs. The explanation

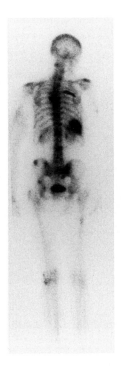

**Fig. 6-17**  Posterior whole body scintigram of a patient with widely disseminated carcinoma of the breast. The patient has multiple skeletal metastases. Uptake is intense in a soft tissue metastasis in the liver. The uptake projects just superolateral to the right kidney.

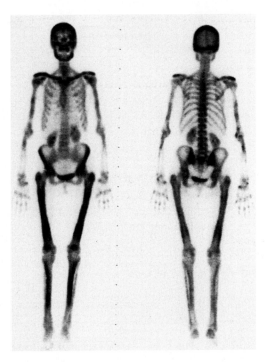

**Fig. 6-18**  Whole body anterior and posterior scintigrams of a patient with florid hypertrophic osteoarthropathy. The bones of the upper and lower extremities are diffusely involved, as are the clavicles, mandible, and skull. The patient did not have skeletal metastatic disease.

for this has been the loss of intervening soft tissue with reduced attenuation. Secondary blood flow effects may occur because of healing in the mastectomy bed. This pattern is seen less frequently with the decline in popularity of the radical mastectomy.

**Carcinoma of the lung**  Lung cancer remains the leading cause of cancer death in men and is a rapidly increasing cause of cancer death in women. Although up to 50% of patients dying of primary lung cancer have osseous metastases at autopsy, there is again incomplete agreement on when to use skeletal scintigraphy. If a curative operative attempt is anticipated, the workup should be aggressive. Skeletal scintigraphy, mediastinal and adrenal CT, and mediastinoscopy with biopsy are performed. However, if treatment is palliative with evidence of local invasion or mediastinal metastases, surveying the skeleton is less useful. With the increasing availability of F-18 fluorodeoxyglucose (FDG), many institutions are performing PET FDG studies as part of the staging evaluation.

Metastatic spread of lung cancer to bone can occur either by direct invasion or through arterial metastases. Involvement and even complete destruction of adjacent ribs are common. Although the distribution of arterially disseminated metastases is still predominantly to red marrow–bearing areas, tumor emboli may reach the distal portions of the extremities. Appendicular involvement relatively early in the course of disease is more common with aggressive lung cancers than with cancer of the breast or prostate.

Characteristic periosteal uptake is seen in patients with lung cancer and hypertrophic osteoarthropathy (Figs. 6-18 and 6-19). The scintigram typically shows parallel uptake along the medial and lateral margins of long bones, commonly restricted to the diametaphyseal area. Although the long bones of the extremities, including those in the hands and feet, are most frequently affected, the patella, scapula, skull, and clavicle can also be involved. The classic appearance is a fairly uniform "double stripe" or "parallel track" activity. It can also be patchy with skip areas.

**Other tumors of epithelial origin**  A number of other extraosseous tumors metastasize to bone. Renal cell carcinoma and thyroid carcinoma are classically included in the differential diagnosis of lesions that frequently metastasize to bone. However, these are far less common tumors than cancers of the breast, lung, and prostate. A whole body survey for metastatic disease is usually accomplished with radioiodine-131 for differentiated thyroid cancer.

GI tract and gynecological cancers do not commonly metastasize to bone early in their courses. Late-stage disease involves bone by direct extension. The success of chemotherapy, including regional chemotherapy, in controlling GI tract tumors has led to an increase in cases of skeletal involvement owing to longer survival and

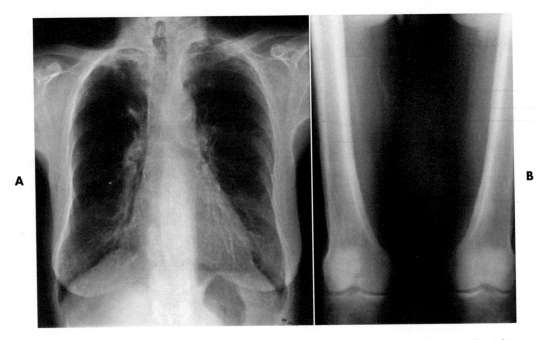

**Fig. 6-19** **A,** Radiograph of the patient in Fig. 6-18 reveals bronchogenic carcinoma in the right upper lobe just above the right hilum. **B,** Radiograph of the femurs shows characteristic periosteal new bone bilaterally on both the medial and lateral aspects of the femoral shaft.

control of the local and regional metastases that usually cause death before bone metastases are manifest.

**Neuroblastoma** Neuroblastoma has a neural crest origin and is the most common solid tumor in children that metastasizes to bone (Fig. 6-20). As with epithelial tumors in adults, radionuclide skeletal scintigraphy is far more sensitive than radiography for detecting bone involvement. On a lesion-by-lesion basis, radionuclide scintigraphy is twice as sensitive as skeletal radiography. The characteristic pattern of skeletal involvement is multifocal activity in the metaphyses. However, involvement in the skull, vertebrae, ribs, and pelvis is also common. Early, symmetrical involvement may be difficult to diagnose scintigraphically because of the normal high intensity of uptake in the ends of growing bones. MRI can be helpful in determining the extent of disease (Fig. 6-21).

A unique characteristic of neuroblastoma is the avidity of Tc-99m diphosphonate for the primary tumors. Approximately 30% to 50% of primary tumors can be demonstrated scintigraphically. Occasionally neuroblastoma is discovered in children undergoing radionuclide imaging to evaluate another condition. Particular attention should be paid to the abdomen.

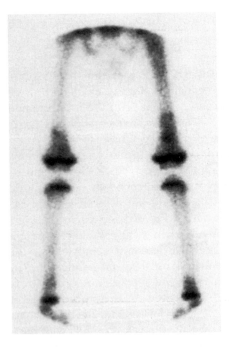

**Fig. 6-20** Lower extremity views of a child with neuroblastoma. Abnormal tracer localization is present in both femurs, more extensive on the left than the right.

## Extraskeletal Uptake in Soft Tissue Neoplasms

A number of common soft tissue neoplasms exhibit variable degrees of skeleton-seeking tracer uptake in both the primary tumor and soft tissue metastases. The

mechanism of localization is not well understood but is thought to be a combination of tumor calcification and binding to macromolecules. The degree of uptake and the consistency with which it is seen are not sufficient to use the Tc-99m-labeled bone agents as primary tumor-

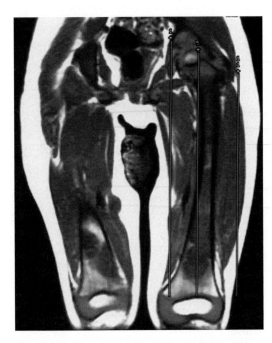

**Fig. 6-21** Magnetic resonance image corresponding to Fig. 6-20 reveals the extensive disease in the left femur and the disease in the right distal femur.

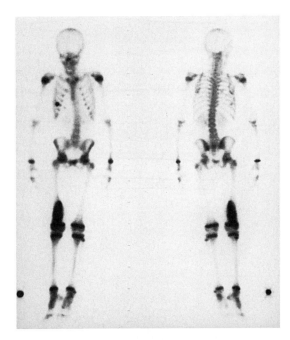

**Fig. 6-22** Anterior and posterior whole body scintigrams of a patient with osteosarcoma of the right distal femur. The degree of tracer accumulation in the lesion is striking. Note also the "watershed" phenomenon with increased tracer accumulation in all of the bones of the right lower extremity above and below the lesion. The increased blood flow induced by the osteosarcoma results in increased tracer delivery to the entire limb. This "extended" or augmented pattern of uptake adds to the difficulty in using the skeletal scintigram to determine the margins of primary bone tumors. (The focal activity over the right ribs is a marker.)

imaging agents, although this has been explored for carcinoma of the breast.

Tumors most frequently imaged, in addition to carcinoma of the breast, are carcinoma of the lung, metastatic carcinoma of the colon in the liver, melanoma, and neuroblastoma (Fig. 6-17).

## PRIMARY MALIGNANT BONE TUMORS

Uptake of bone-seeking radiopharmaceuticals in primary bone tumors is avid and frequently striking (Figs. 6-22 and 6-23). However, skeletal scintigraphy is not commonly used in the workup of patients with osteosarcoma or other primary bone neoplasms because the radionuclide technique does not answer the questions the orthopedic surgeon must address. The skeletal scintigram does not accurately portray the tumor margins in bone, nor does it allow assessment of soft tissue extent. Plain radiographs, CT, and MRI are better for making these determinations (Figs. 6-24 and 6-25). Although most primary bone tumors are monostotic, the occasional polyostotic involvement is missed without a whole body survey of some kind (Fig. 6-26).

PET imaging with FDG is being explored for primary bone tumors. FDG uptake correlates with tumor metabolism. Scans can be helpful in localizing sites for biopsy and in assessing response to preoperative radiation and chemotherapy. In institutions without access to FDG, both Tl-201 and Tc-99m MIBI have been used for

sarcoma imaging to determine whether tumors are low or high grade and to assess response to therapy. As with FDG, high-grade tumors show higher uptake. Successful radiation therapy or chemotherapy is associated with decreasing uptake.

Conventional skeletal scintigraphy may have a role if metastases are suspected. Skeletal scintigraphy is capable of demonstrating soft tissue, pulmonary, and skeletal metastatic lesions (Fig. 6-26). However, the value of scintigraphy is for surveying the entire body. If metastases are suspected in a given area, a higher resolution technique is employed. Thus pulmonary metastases are typically evaluated with CT, not scintigraphy.

The effectiveness of modern multimodality therapy for primary bone tumors has changed the pattern of metastatic disease. As patients are living longer, osseous metastases are becoming more common. Skeletal scintigraphy retains its utility for whole body survey studies for this indication.

Studies of primary tumors have led to at least one important observation about skeletal tracer uptake. Many tumors elicit marked hyperemia. The increased blood flow is not restricted to the tumor itself but affects the entire watershed distribution of regional flow, most

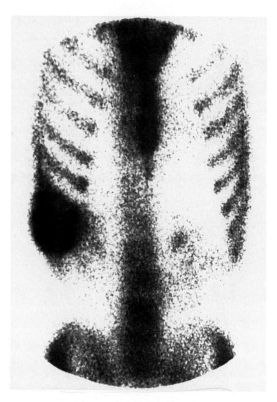

**Fig. 6-23**    Anterior spot view of a patient with a primary chondrosarcoma arising from the right anterior ribs.

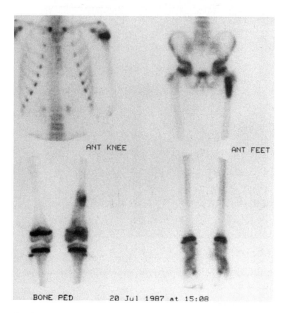

**Fig. 6-24**    Anterior spot views in a patient with osteosarcoma of the left distal femur and a metastatic lesion in the left proximal femur.

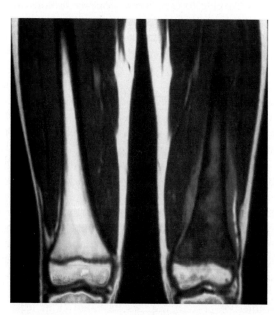

**Fig. 6-25**    Coronal view from magnetic resonance imaging (MRI) of the patient in Fig. 6-24. The MRI study provides superior anatomical information about the osseous and soft tissue extent of the tumor. However, it missed the second lesion in the proximal femur.

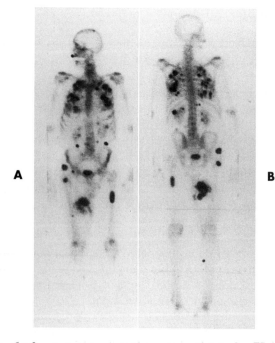

**Fig. 6-26**    **A,** Anterior and, **B,** posterior whole body scintigrams in a patient with an extraosseous osteosarcoma arising in the right medial thigh area. The lesion is widely disseminated with skeletal metastases, soft tissue metastases, and pulmonary metastases. This study is a dramatic example of the ability of skeletal scintigraphy to survey the entire body. (Courtesy of David A. Parker, M.D.)

characteristically involving an entire extremity (Fig. 6-22). Thus markedly increased tracer uptake is seen in adjacent structures. The augmented or extended uptake pattern can be seen in other hyperemia-inducing lesions, including fractures, osteomyelitis, and nerve injuries resulting in reflex sympathetic dystrophy syndrome.

## Multiple Myeloma

The primary malignant disease that most commonly involves bone is multiple myeloma. Myeloma is really a disease of the red marrow space, and the most frequently involved skeletal structures are the vertebrae, pelvis, ribs, and skull.

On skeletal radiographs the only finding in myeloma may be osteopenia. Unless an associated fracture or a focal lesion such as a plasmacytoma is present, skeletal scintigrams are often normal. As noted previously, MRI is an excellent modality for evaluating the marrow space for areas of involvement.

## BENIGN BONE TUMORS

### Osteoid Osteoma

Osteoid osteomas are often associated with excruciating bone pain that classically is greater at night. They are most common in adolescents and young adults.

Skeletal scintigraphy, now with SPECT, is highly sensitive for detecting osteoid osteomas. They can be difficult to find by standard radiography, especially in the spine. The most common location of occurrence is the femur (Figs. 6-27 and 6-28). In the spine the posterior elements are usually affected rather than the vertebral body. Some surgeons have used intraoperative scintigraphic probes to localize osteoid osteomas, which in many cases are not immediately apparent from inspecting the surface of the bone. Recently percutaneous treatment of osteoid osteomas has become possible,

using either radiofrequency-induced injury to cause the lesion to involute or image-guided curettage. CT has diminished the role of nuclear medicine in the diagnosis of osteoid osteomas.

### Other Benign Bone Tumors

Osteochondromas, chondroblastomas, and enchondromas demonstrate a spectrum of abnormalities on skeletal scintigraphy. In some cases the scintigram is normal or near normal. In other cases uptake is striking, especially for osteochondromas and chondroblastomas. Enchondromas rarely demonstrate striking uptake unless secondarily involved by fracture.

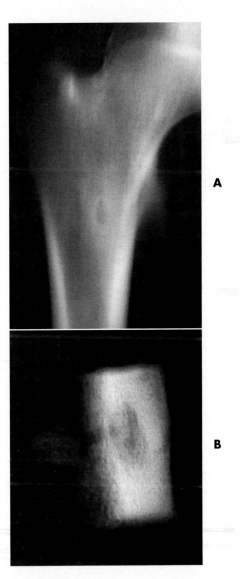

**Fig. 6-28**  **A,** Conventional tomogram of the right proximal femur reveals a characteristic radiolucent nidus surrounded by sclerotic bone. **B,** Specimen radiograph confirms the complete excision of the nidus.

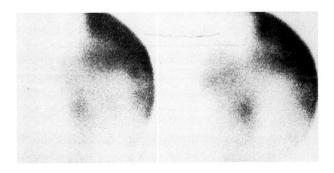

**Fig. 6-27**  Internal and external rotation pinhole spot views of the proximal femur in a patient with suspected osteoid osteoma. An area of abnormally increased uptake is demonstrated just lateral to the lesser trochanter.

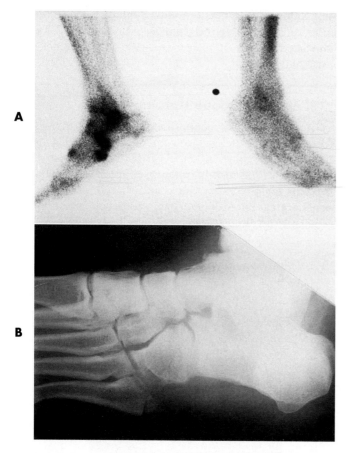

**Fig. 6-29** **A,** Skeletal scintigram of a patient who had sustained direct trauma to the right foot and ankle reveals multiple focal areas of abnormal tracer accumulation. Each of these areas was subsequently demonstrated radiographically to correspond to a fracture. **B,** Radiograph of the patient in **A,** illustrating fractures of the base of the fifth metatarsal and lateral cuneiform.

## SKELETAL TRAUMA

Skeletal trauma is common and presents both an opportunity and a problem in skeletal scintigraphy. The opportunity arises in the ability of skeletal scintigraphy to demonstrate abnormalities early after direct trauma (Figs. 6-12, 6-29, and 6-30). SPECT is also a useful adjunct early in the course of a process such as stress fracture (Fig. 6-30). The problem comes in recognizing the effects of skeletal trauma when using skeletal scintigraphy for another purpose, such as the detection of metastatic disease.

### Detection of Fractures

The time course of scintigraphic positivity after trauma is important in considering skeletal imaging to detect fractures and in understanding the problem of persistent positivity that could contribute to a false positive diagnosis of metastatic disease. According to data provided by Matin, approximately 80% of fractures can be visualized by 24 hours after trauma. The earliest scintigraphic

appearance is diffusely increased uptake, most likely the result of hyperemia at the fracture site. By 3 days, 95% of fractures are positive on scintigraphy, and in patients under the age of 65 essentially all fractures are positive by this time. Advanced age and debilitation are factors contributing to nonvisualization or delayed visualization of fractures. Maximum fracture positivity occurs 7 or more days after trauma, and delayed imaging in this time frame is recommended in difficult or equivocal cases.

The time a fracture takes to return to normal scintigraphically depends primarily on its location and the degree of damage to the skeleton. Some 60% to 80% of nondisplaced uncomplicated fractures revert to normal in 1 year and over 95% in 3 years (Table 6-3). However, many instances in which displaced fractures remained positive indefinitely have been documented, and involvement of a joint by posttraumatic arthritis causes prolonged positivity. A careful history is important. Patients undergoing metastatic skeletal survey should be routinely asked about prior trauma. In a prospective study by Kim, nearly half of patients being evaluated for skeletal metastatic disease reported previous fractures. Twenty-six percent of the fracture sites were positive at the time of scintigraphic examination, including 16 (16%) of 98 sites where the trauma had occurred more than 5 years before (Table 6-3). Structural deformity and posttraumatic arthritis were the most common reasons for prolonged positivity.

### Iatrogenic Trauma

Iatrogenic trauma to either the skeleton or soft tissues may be manifest scintigraphically. Again, the key to correct interpretation is an accurate history. Craniotomy typically leaves a rim pattern at the surgical margin that may persist for months postoperatively. Rib retraction during thoracotomy can elicit periosteal reaction and increased uptake without actual resection of bone being involved. Bone resections are recognized as photon-deficient areas, although small laminectomies are usually not appreciated scintigraphically.

The pattern in bone grafting depends on the timing postoperatively. Intercalary grafts demonstrate increased uptake at the opposed bone ends, with gradual fill-in of tracer activity as the graft is revitalized. In pedicle grafts or grafts where microvascular anastomoses are made, tracer uptake should be visualized immediately and if not seen may indicate loss of bone viability.

Areas of the skeleton receiving curative levels of ionizing radiation (typically 4000 rads or greater) characteristically demonstrate decreased uptake within 6 months to 1 year after therapy. The threshold for the effect is on the order of 2000 rads. The mechanism is probably decreased osteogenesis and decreased blood flow to postirradiated bone. The scintigraphic hallmark is a geometrical pattern of regionally decreased tracer uptake (Fig. 6-31). Some observers have reported an

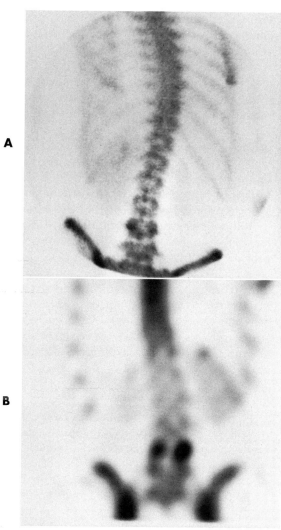

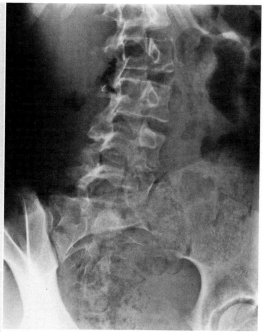

**Fig. 6-30    A,** Posterior scintigram from a child with low back pain after athletic injury. Uptake is bilaterally increased at L5. **B,** Corresponding coronal view from a SPECT study reveals a characteristic pattern for spondylolysis. **C,** Comparison radiograph reveals defect in the pars interarticularis corresponding to the area of abnormal uptake on the scintigram.

| Table 6-3 | Skeletal scintigraphy in trauma: time course from fracture to return to normal |

**Fracture type and site**

Percent of normal

**NONMANIPULATED CLOSED FRACTURES***

|  | 1 yr | 3 yr |
|---|---|---|
| Vertebra | 59 | 97 |
| Long bone | 64 | 95 |
| Rib | 79 | 100 |

**ALL FRACTURES†**

|  | <1 yr | 2-5 yr | >5 yr |
|---|---|---|---|
| All sites | 30 | 62 | 84 |

*Adapted from Matin P: The appearance of bone scans following fractures, including immediate and long term studies, *J Nucl Med* 20:1227-1231, 1979.
†Adapted from Kim HR, Thrall JH, Keyes JW Jr: Skeletal scintigraphy following incidental trauma, *Radiology* 130:447-451, 1979.

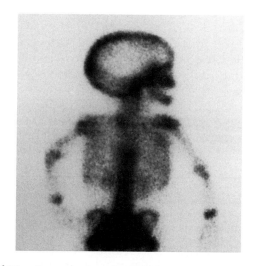

**Fig. 6-31**    Posterior view of a child after radiation therapy of the upper thoracic spine. Note the sharply marginated cut-off in the midthoracic region with greatly diminished uptake in the treated area compared with the lower thoracic spine and the lumbar spine.

actual increase in uptake immediately after therapy, but the mechanism is unknown.

## Child Abuse

The generally high sensitivity of skeletal scintigraphy would seem to make it an ideal survey test in cases of suspected child abuse. In practice, however, the sensitivity is somewhat disappointing. This probably relates to the timing of injury in relation to scintigraphy. Older fractures may have healed and not be seen scintigraphically, and skeletal scintigraphy has been reported to miss calvarial fractures in young children. In child abuse, radiographic skeletal survey is more sensitive than bone scintigraphy because of its ability to demonstrate old fractures. Scintigraphy should be reserved for cases of suspected child abuse in which radiographs are unrevealing.

## ATHLETIC INJURIES

### Stress Fractures

Normal bone is constantly remodeling. Bone resorption and deposition are balanced (Table 6-4). When the skeleton is placed under stress because of a change in activity or repetitive activity, the rate of remodeling increases. Lamellar bone is remodeled into stronger osteonal bone. If resorption and deposition remain balanced, the skeleton adapts to the new demands being made on it. However, if the rate of resorption sufficiently exceeds the rate of replacement, cortical bone is weakened and may be buttressed by periosteal and endosteal new bone. The final result of imbalance between resorption and replacement is a stress fracture (Table 6-4).

From the foregoing, it is clear that a "stress fracture" is not necessarily an all-or-none phenomenon. It is probably more useful to think of a continuum of injury from an early remodeling reaction to overt fracture. In fact, in cases diagnosed and treated early, a discrete fracture line may never develop. If skeletal scintigraphy is performed early enough and the patient's activity is changed appropriately, radiographs may never show an abnormality. If the process is allowed to continue to the point of overt fracture, healing predictably takes several months or more, compared with the several weeks required for healing of an early stress reaction.

Skeletal scintigraphy is exquisitely sensitive to the remodeling process and typically shows abnormalities 1 to 2 weeks or more before the appearance of radiographic changes in stress fractures (Table 6-4). The characteristic scintigraphic appearance is that of intense uptake at the fracture site. The configuration is oval or fusiform with the long axis of increased uptake parallel to the axis of the bone (Figs. 6-32 and 6-33).

MRI is a powerful competitor to nuclear scintigraphy for the diagnosis of stress fractures because it can provide more information and does not expose patients to ionizing radiation (Figs. 6-34 and 6-35). MRI can identify marrow edema early in the stress response, making the technique competitive in early sensitivity. MRI can also differentiate the marrow edema of the stress reaction from the presence of a true fracture. Fractures are visualized as linear abnormalities on $T_1$ scans.

## Shin Splints

The term *shin splints* is applied generically to describe stress-related leg soreness. In nuclear medicine the term is now used to describe a specific combination of clinical and scintigraphic findings. Patients complain of mild to moderate exercise-induced pain along the medial or posteromedial aspect of the tibia. This is associated with increased tracer uptake on the scintigram, typically involving greater than one third of bone length and involving the middle to distal tibia (Fig. 6-36). Most cases are bilateral although not necessarily symmetrical. The radionuclide uptake is of only mild to moderate intensity and does not have the focal aspect seen with true stress fractures. The etiology is thought to be microperiosteal tears at points of periosteal stress. The stress may be mediated by Sharpey's fibers through their connection to muscle and bone.

**Table 6-4   Sequence of findings in stress reaction**

|  | Clinical findings | X-ray | Scintigram |
|---|:---:|:---:|:---:|
| Normal (resorption = replacement) | − | − | − |
| Accelerated remodeling (resorption > replacement) | +/− | − | + |
| Fatigue (resorption >> replacement) | + | +/− | +++ |
| Exhaustion (resorption >>> replacement) | ++ | + | ++++ |
| Cortical fracture | ++++ | ++++ | ++++ |

Adapted from Roub LW et al: Bone stress: a radionuclide imaging perspective, *Radiology* 132:431-438, 1979.

The clinical significance of the shin splint pattern is quite different from that of the stress fracture pattern. Unless the tracer uptake has a focal component, the shin splint pattern does not predict further injury. Limited hyperemia on arterial phase imaging helps distinguish shin splints from stress fractures, which typically demonstrate intense hyperemia.

Unlike the situation for stress fractures, MRI does not yet have a proven role in the diagnosis of shin splints except to rule out stress fracture. Medullary and periosteal changes can be demonstrated, but useful, reproducible diagnostic criteria are not yet established.

A phenomenon perhaps related to shin splints is activity-induced enthesiopathy. The term simply refers to a disease process at the site of tendon or ligament attachment to bone. In athletes, repeated microtears with subsequent healing reaction can result in increased tracer uptake at corresponding locations. Osteitis pubis and plantar fasciitis are examples, as are Achilles tendinitis and some cases of pulled hamstring muscles. A periosteal reaction develops at the site of stress, resulting in increased skeletal tracer localization.

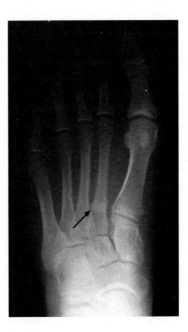

**Fig. 6-33**  A fracture with callus formation *(arrow)* is demonstrated corresponding to the base of the second metatarsal.

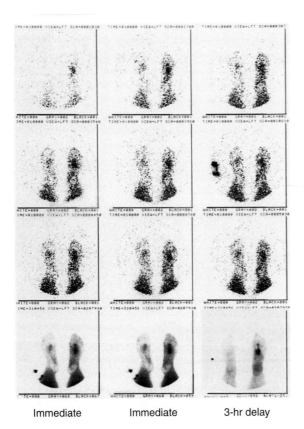

Immediate          Immediate          3-hr delay

**Fig. 6-32**  Three-phase skeletal scintigram of the feet in plantar view reveals marked early hyperemia to the left midfoot. The immediate views *(lower left and middle)* reveal increased uptake in the same area. The 3-hour delayed view shows marked focal uptake corresponding to the base and shaft of the second metatarsal, compatible with stress fracture.

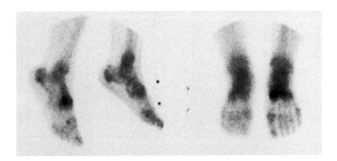

**Fig. 6-34**  Scintigrams of the feet reveal marked focal uptake at the base of the first metatarsal on the left.

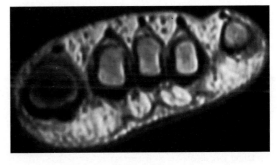

**Fig. 6-35**  Magnetic resonance image corresponding to the scintigram in Fig. 6-34 reveals abnormal signal corresponding to the area of increased tracer uptake. Note the difference in signal between the first metatarsal and the other metatarsals.

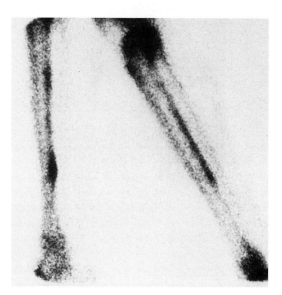

**Fig. 6-36**   Lateral views of a patient demonstrating the classic finding in shin splints of increased tracer uptake along the posterior and medial aspects of the tibia on the left. A similar pattern can be seen on the right, but with the addition of a focal area distally, which could indicate stress fracture.

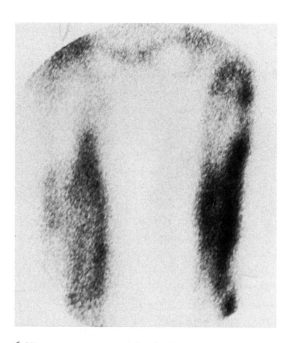

**Fig. 6-37**   Anterior view of the thighs in a patient who recently competed in a marathon. Bilateral soft tissue uptake is compatible with rhabdomyolysis.

### Rhabdomyolysis

Another athletic injury that is seen in this day of marathons and triathlons is rhabdomyolysis (Fig. 6-37). The localization of skeletal tracers in exercise-damaged skeletal muscle is probably similar to the localization in damaged myocardium. Calcium buildup in damaged tissue provides a site for radionuclide deposition.

The scintigraphic pattern reflects the muscle groups undergoing injury. In marathon runners the most striking uptake is usually in the muscles of the thigh. The time course of scintigraphic positivity appears to be similar to that for acute myocardial infarction. Matin has described a pattern of maximum positivity 24 to 48 hours following injury, with resolution by 1 week.

## BONE INFARCTION AND OSTEONECROSIS

Bone necrosis has numerous causes (Box 6-6). The appearance on skeletal scintigraphy depends greatly on the time course of the process. With acute interruption of the blood supply, newly infarcted bone appears cold or photon deficient scintigraphically. In the postinfarction or healing phase, osteogenesis and tracer uptake at the margin of the infarcted area are increased. Skeletal scintigrams can show intensely increased tracer uptake during the healing period.

---

**Box 6-6   Etiologies of Aseptic Bone Necrosis**

Trauma (accidental, iatrogenic)
Drug therapy (steroids)
Hypercoagulable states
Hemoglobinopathies (sickle cell disease and variants)
After radiation therapy (orthovoltage)
Caisson disease
Osteochondrosis (pediatric age group; Legg-Calvé-Perthes disease)
Polycythemia
Leukemia
Gaucher's disease
Alcoholism
Pancreatitis
Idiopathic

---

### Legg-Calvé-Perthes Disease

Legg-Calvé-Perthes disease most commonly affects children between the ages of 5 and 9 years, with predominance in boys (4:1 to 5:1). It is a form of osteochondrosis and results in avascular necrosis of the capital femoral epiphysis. The mechanism of injury is unknown except that the vascular supply of the femoral head is thought to be especially vulnerable in the most commonly affected age group.

The best scintigraphic technique for detecting the abnormality in the femoral head is to use some form of magnification and to image in the frogleg lateral projection. Classically, early in the course of the disease, before

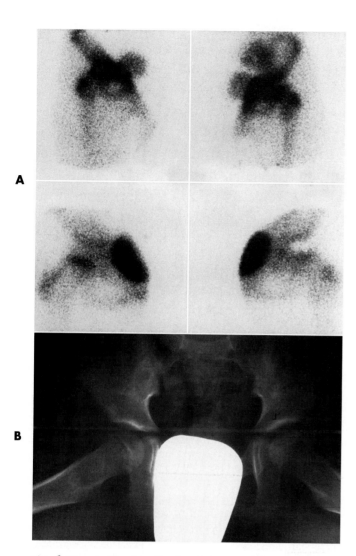

**A**

**B**

**Fig. 6-38**    **A,** The benefit of pinhole magnification is demonstrated in a comparison of the top two images, obtained with a standard parallel hole collimator, and the bottom two images of the same patient, obtained with a pinhole collimator. The characteristic lentiform area of decreased uptake is demonstrated on the left. **B,** Corresponding radiographs of the patient in **A** reveal deformity of the left femoral epiphysis with flattening, increased density, and increased distance between the epiphysis and the acetabulum.

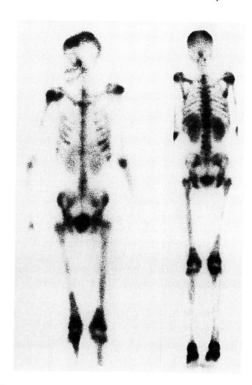

**Fig. 6-39**    Anterior and posterior whole body views of a patient with sickle cell anemia. Calvarial uptake is increased with relative thinning at the midline. There is prominent skeleton-to-soft tissue uptake. The kidneys appear large, and the spleen shows intense uptake. Uptake in the knees and ankles is greater than expected for an adult subject. The photon-deficient areas in the right femur are due to bone and bone marrow infarction.

healing has occurred, a discrete photon-deficient area can be seen in the upper outer portion of the capital femoral epiphysis with a lentiform configuration (Fig. 6-38). Areas of photon deficiency are well demonstrated by SPECT imaging.

As healing occurs, increased uptake is first seen at the margin of the photon-deficient area, and gradually the scintigram demonstrates filling in of activity. In severe cases the femoral head never reverts to normal. Increased tracer uptake is seen for a prolonged period—many months or more.

Currently MRI is the imaging modality of choice for the evaluation of Legg-Calvé-Perthes disease, as well as other causes of osteonecrosis. MRI has comparable or higher sensitivity and higher specificity than nuclear scintigraphy. MRI also provides a range of additional information, which offers the ability to evaluate articular cartilage, detect acetabular labral tears, and recognize metaphyseal cysts that are indicators of prognosis.

### Steroid-Induced Osteonecrosis

An entity that may be confusing on skeletal scintigraphy is drug-induced, especially steroid-induced, osteonecrosis. It would seem that areas of osteonecrosis would appear photon deficient on skeletal scintigraphy. However, in the vast majority of cases increased uptake is demonstrated scintigraphically. Although the pathogenesis of steroid-induced osteonecrosis is still being debated, it is a chronic process manifested by microfractures and repair. The net effect most often seen scintigraphically is increased tracer localization.

### Sickle Cell Anemia

Skeletal scintigrams in patients with sickle cell anemia have a number of characteristic features that suggest the diagnosis (Fig. 6-39). In the skull the expanded marrow space results in bilaterally increased calvarial uptake of tracer. In the extremities, patients usually have greater relative uptake compared with the axial skeleton than is seen in normal subjects. This increased uptake may be

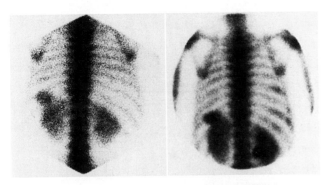

**Fig. 6-40**   Posterior views obtained at the time of onset of acute chest pain *(left)* and several days later *(right)* from a patient with sickle cell anemia. Note the uptake in the spleen on both images. Typically, once the spleen is visualized scintigraphically, it remains positive. The initial image reveals no abnormality in the ribs. The follow-up image demonstrates increased uptake, particularly in the right ribs, associated with healing of the infarctions.

related to the persistence of hematopoietic elements throughout the extremities, including the hands and feet, of patients with sickle cell anemia. As noted earlier, in normal adults the red marrow extends only to the proximal portions of the femurs and humeri. The overall skeleton-to-background ratio is usually good and is accentuated by the increased appendicular uptake.

In many patients with sickle cell anemia the kidneys appear somewhat larger than normal, which may be related to a defect in the ability to concentrate urine. Avid accumulation of skeletal tracer is sometimes seen in the spleen, presumably because of prior splenic infarction and calcification (Fig. 6-39).

Patients with sickle cell anemia are subject to infarctions in bone and bone marrow. If the involvement is primarily in the marrow space, the skeletal scintigram may be normal acutely but typically demonstrates increased uptake during the healing phase, beginning within a few days of the acute event (Fig. 6-40). MRI can demonstrate marrow infarctions immediately.

Bone marrow scans (Tc-99m sulfur colloid) are sensitive for detecting bone marrow infarction and are positive immediately after the event (Fig. 6-41). Affected areas fail to accumulate tracer and are seen as cold, or photon deficient. The problem in making the diagnosis of acute bone marrow infarction is the presence of chronic marrow defects from prior bone marrow infarctions in the majority of patients with sickle cell anemia. Thus the significance of a photon-deficient area on marrow scanning is somewhat uncertain unless a recent baseline study is available for comparison. Here again, MRI has an advantage in distinguishing acute from chronic changes.

## OSTEOMYELITIS

Acute hematogenous osteomyelitis typically begins by seeding of the infectious organism in the marrow space.

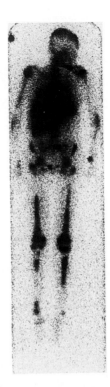

**Fig. 6-41**   Technetium-99m sulfur colloid bone marrow scan of a patient with sickle cell anemia. Note the intense uptake in the liver. The uptake in the bone marrow extends throughout the upper and lower extremities. The numerous focal defects indicate marrow infarctions. Based on one examination, new abnormalities cannot be distinguished from old ones.

Extension of the untreated process from the medullary cavity is through Volkmann canals horizontally and in the haversian canal system axially. The skeletal scintigram is almost invariably abnormal by the time clinical symptoms develop. Increased tracer uptake is the typical finding (Fig. 6-42).

In children *Staphylococcus aureus* is the most common organism and is probably responsible for 50% or more of cases. The skeletal infection is commonly associated with some other staphylococcal infection, often of the skin. Enteric bacteria and *Streptococcus* are also important pathogens.

Osteomyelitis may involve any skeletal structure. In adults the axial skeleton is affected more often than the extremities (Figs. 6-43 and 6-44). When vertebrae are involved, the organisms may be carried through the perispinous venous plexus, producing involvement at multiple levels. An exception to the axial involvement in adults is seen in diabetic patients, whose feet are commonly involved. However, the infection often begins in the soft tissues with extension to bone. Diskitis in children and adults is characterized by narrowing of the disk space and increased uptake in the adjacent vertebral bodies.

In some patients, especially children, increased pressure in the marrow space or thrombosis of blood vessels

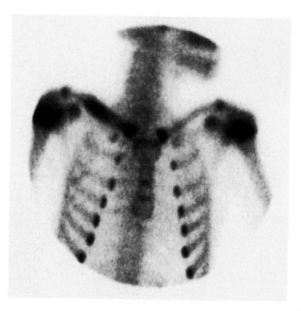

**Fig. 6-42**   Anterior scintigram in a child with osteomyelitis of the right clavicle. Uptake is markedly greater than in the left clavicle.

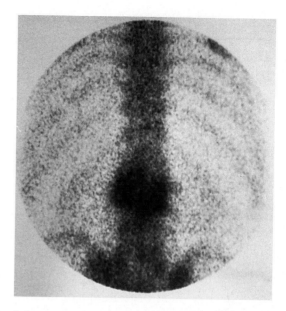

**Fig. 6-43**   Posterior spot view of an adult patient with spinal osteomyelitis. Uptake is intensely increased in the midlumbar region, involving more than one level.

results in paradoxically decreased tracer uptake and a cold or photon-deficient lesion. Organisms most commonly responsible for this pattern are coagulase-positive *Staphylococcus aureus* and *Streptococcus.*

Numerous studies in the literature document the superior sensitivity of skeletal scintigraphy compared with conventional radiography in the diagnosis of acute hematogenous osteomyelitis. False negative scintigraphic studies are unusual but have been reported in young children, especially infants under the age of 1 year. Other causes of false negative examinations are imaging very early in the course of disease and failure to recognize the significance of photon-deficient areas.

For the diagnosis of osteomyelitis, MRI is typically performed with gadolinium enhancement. Again, MRI is very sensitive but is limited as a survey technique. If clinical findings point to a specific location, MRI is useful. When polyostotic disease is suspected or clinical findings are not well localized, skeletal scintigraphy remains a useful survey technique. The characteristic appearance of osteomyelitis by gadolinium-enhanced MRI is an area of enhancement, while the centers of abscesses do not enhance. MRI is not very useful in evaluating the feet of diabetic patients, including those with Charcot's disease. The underlying changes and poor blood flow make diagnosis difficult.

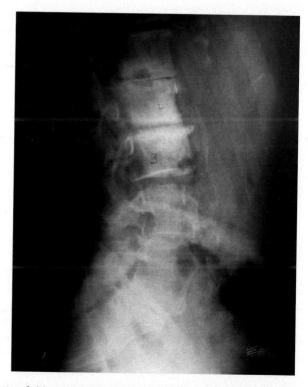

**Fig. 6-44**   Corresponding radiograph of the patient in Fig. 6-43 shows destructive and sclerotic changes involving the L2 vertebral body and adjacent portions of L1 and L3. The process has involved the intervertebral disks with loss of height in the disk space.

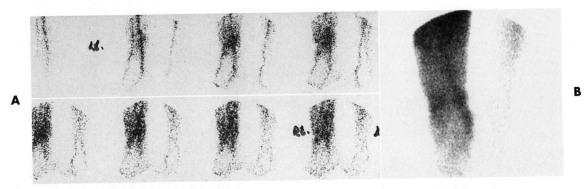

**Fig. 6-45**  **A,** Sequential images from the flow phase of a diabetic patient with cellulitis. The ankle region and the visualized portion of the leg show marked hyperemia. **B,** Follow-up blood pool images revealed diffusely increased activity in the areas corresponding to the hyperemia. No focal abnormality was demonstrated on follow-up late-phase imaging.

---

### Box 6-7   Three-Phase Skeletal Scintigraphy: Protocol Summary

**RADIOPHARMACEUTICAL DOSAGE AND ROUTE OF ADMINISTRATION**

Standard tracer and dosage are used and given as a bolus injection

**PROCEDURE**

The gamma camera is positioned before radiopharmaceutical administration immediately over the site of the suspected pathological condition

**FLOW PHASE**

Dynamic 2- to 5-sec images are obtained for 60 sec after bolus injection (30 sec in children)

**BLOOD POOL AND TISSUE PHASE**

Immediate static images for time (5 min) or counts (300k)

**SKELETAL PHASE**

Delayed 300k to 1000k images at 2 to 4 hr

---

### Box 6-8   Three-Phase Skeletal Scintigraphy: Interpretive Criteria

Osteomyelitis: *arterial* hyperemia, progressive focal skeletal uptake with relative soft tissue clearance; in children a focal cold area may be seen if osteomyelitis is associated with infarction

Cellulitis: *venous* (delayed) hyperemia, persistent soft tissue activity; no focal skeletal uptake (may have mild to moderate diffusely increased uptake)

Septic joint: periarticular increased activity on dynamic and blood pool phases that persists on delayed images; less commonly the joint structures appear cold if pressure in the joint causes decreased flow or infarction

---

### Three-Phase Scintigraphy

Dynamic, or three-phase, imaging is a special technique used in the differential diagnosis of cellulitis and osteomyelitis. This is an important differential diagnosis for diabetic patients, who have a high incidence of both problems. The distinction is clinically important because of the therapeutic implications of prolonged treatment when osteomyelitis is diagnosed.

The technique for dynamic scanning is summarized in Box 6-7, and the key diagnostic criteria are shown in Box 6-8. Cellulitis typically demonstrates delayed or venous phase hyperemia with increased uptake diffusely on the blood pool images and clearance of tracer on delayed images without focally increased uptake in bone (Fig. 6-45). The typical appearance of osteomyelities is early or arterial hyperemia with focally and possibly diffusely increased uptake of tracer on the blood pool images and progressive focal accumulation in the involved bone at delayed imaging (Fig. 6-46). Although the technique has been shown useful in distinguishing cellulitis from osteomyelitis, the pattern described for osteomyelitis is not specific. The same sequence of image findings can be seen in neuropathic joint disease; gout; fractures, including stress fracture (Fig. 6-32); and rheumatoid arthritis, among other conditions (Box 6-9). Most of these differential possibilities can be distinguished radiographically.

### Prosthesis Evaluation

Numerous attempts have been made to use skeletal scintigraphy in the evaluation of patients after total joint replacement or implantation of other metallic prostheses. The distinction between component loosening and infection is critical in guiding management.

The findings on skeletal scintigraphy are not specific enough for a reliable distinction between loosening of a prosthesis and infection (Fig. 6-47). Reactive bone around a loose prosthesis may be indistinguishable from increased tracer uptake resulting from osteomyelitis. In cases of a loose prosthesis, uptake is usually increased in the region of the greater and lesser trochanters and at the tip of the prosthesis. This is presumably due to remodeling of bone in response to movement of the prosthesis. In osteomyelitis activity is increased in the bone surrounding the prosthesis. However, a negative bone scan is useful because it helps rule out both osteomyelitis and prosthesis loosening. Some increased uptake is expected as a normal healing response for 1 year after placement of a cemented prosthesis and for 2 or 3 years after placement of a noncemented prosthesis.

The differential diagnosis between loosened prosthesis and infection is better made with tracers such as indium-111-labeled white blood cells and either contrast or radionuclide arthrography. In one approach a skeletal scintigram is first obtained with Tc-99m diphosphonate, followed by a radionuclide arthrogram using a radionuclide with higher energy than Tc-99m. Images with the two different tracers are superimposed so that skeletal anatomical landmarks can be correlated with tracer distribution on the arthrogram. If a prosthesis is firmly in place, the tracer (or radiographic contrast medium) cannot flow around it and is confined to the joint space. With prosthesis loosening, the tracer is readily detected outside the joint space. For example, with a loose femoral component, tracer may be seen all the way to the tip.

The best combination of sensitivity and specificity for detecting an infected prostheses is offered by In-111-labeled white blood cells. This tracer localizes in areas of infection and not in areas of remodeling or reactive bone. Use of In-111-labeled white blood cells has three pitfalls. First, false negative studies may occur in low-grade chronic osteomyelitis. Second, cellulitis can be difficult

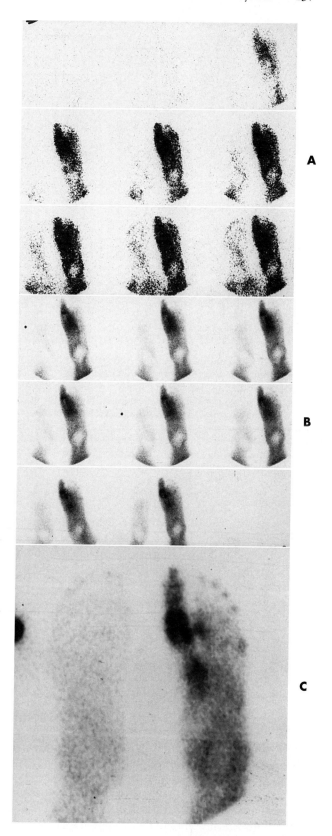

**Fig. 6-46**    **A,** Sequential dynamic images in a middle-aged man with diabetes and osteomyelitis. Note the intense arterial phase hyperemia. **B,** Blood pool images already show localization in skeletal structures. **C,** Delayed static images reveal intense focal accumulation in multiple areas of the great toe and distal first and second metatarsals.

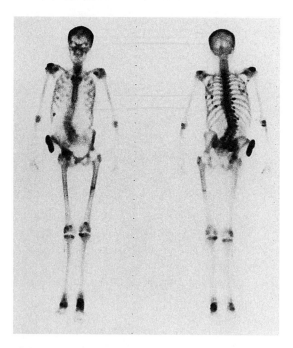

**Fig. 6-47**   Anterior and posterior whole body images in a patient with severe scoliosis and skeletal metastases from carcinoma of the breast. The patient has a left femoral prosthesis, which was subsequently shown to be loose. Uptake is increased at the tip of the prosthesis and subtly increased in the region of the trochanters, especially the greater trochanter. Uptake is intensely increased in the right femoral head because of dysplastic and degenerative arthritic changes.

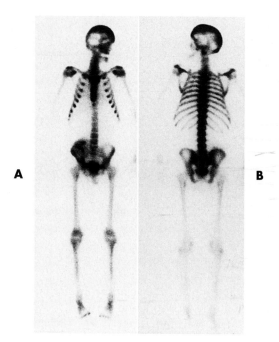

**Fig. 6-48**   **A,** Anterior and, **B,** posterior whole body images of a patient with renal osteodystrophy. The increase in skeletal–to–soft tissue uptake is striking. The patient's native kidneys had failed, and a renal transplant is in place in the right iliac fossa. The anterior rib ends are especially prominent. Otherwise, the appearance mimics that of a "superscan" seen in metastatic disease.

to distinguish from septic arthritis. Third, false positive studies can result from normal In-111 white blood cell uptake in bone marrow around a prosthesis. In some departments white blood cell and sulfur colloid marrow scanning is combined to avoid this pitfall. Infection is diagnosed only in areas of In-111 white blood cell uptake that are negative for marrow activity.

## METABOLIC BONE DISEASE

A number of metabolic conditions can result in marked abnormalities on bone scintigrams. Although these do not represent important clinical indications for bone scintigraphy, they may be encountered incidentally in other applications, most importantly during metastatic skeletal survey. Hyperthyroidism, primary hyperparathyroidism, renal osteodystrophy, osteomalacia, and hypervitaminosis D can all result in generalized increased tracer uptake throughout the skeleton that has some features in common with the superscan seen in metastatic disease (Fig. 6-48). These features are an increased skeleton–to–soft tissue ratio and faint or absent visualization of the kidneys. Increased skull activity, involve-

ment of the long bones of the extremities, and increased periarticular uptake are features that distinguish scans in these conditions from the superscan of metastatic disease.

Another striking feature occasionally seen in metabolic bone disease is "beading" of the costochondral junction akin to the rachitic rosary (Fig. 6-48). A number of other features are seen in some of the metabolic bone diseases. For example, in primary hyperparathyroidism and renal osteodystrophy, extraskeletal uptake may be seen in the lungs and stomach (Fig. 6-49). In osteomalacia, pseudofractures are commonly seen and demonstrate avid radiopharmaceutical uptake (Fig. 6-11).

### Osteoporosis

Osteoporosis is an increasingly common problem with the aging of the population. Skeletal scintigraphy does not have a role in the diagnosis of osteoporosis but is useful in surveying the entire skeleton for osteoporotic insufficiency fractures. Since these may be asymptomatic, the ability to survey the entire skeleton is advantageous. Compression fractures of the spine are common (Fig. 6-50), as are sacral insufficiency fractures. Sacral fractures are often difficult to diagnose radiographically. The most common pattern is the H or butterfly pattern,

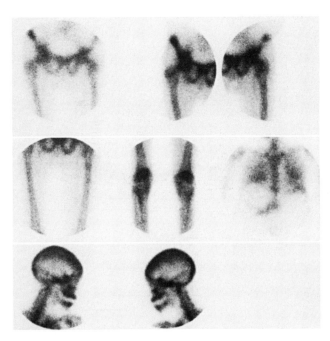

**Fig. 6-49** Multiple spot views of a patient with hyperparathyroidism. The anterior view of the lungs and upper abdomen *(middle right image)* reveals diffuse uptake in both lungs and the stomach.

with a horizontal band of increased uptake across the body of the sacrum and two vertical limbs of activity in the sacral alae (Fig. 6-51). Several pattern variations may be seen, including asymmetry of the alar activity. Less severe fractures may show only horizontal linear uptake.

### Paget's Disease

Paget's disease of bone involves the skeleton focally. The scintigraphic appearance is striking, with intensely increased tracer localization (Figs. 6-52 and 6-53). The expansion of bone demonstrated radiographically is not well assessed by scintigraphy, owing to the lower resolution of the technique, but is certainly suggested on the images. The pelvis is the most commonly involved site, followed by the spine, skull, femur, scapula, tibia, and humerus. The increased uptake is seen both in the early resorptive or lucent phase of the disease and in the proliferative or sclerotic phase. In osteoporosis circumscripta a characteristic rim of increased uptake borders the lesion.

### BONE DYSPLASIAS

Numerous bone dysplasias demonstrate increased skeletal tracer uptake (Figs. 6-54 to 6-56). Fibrous

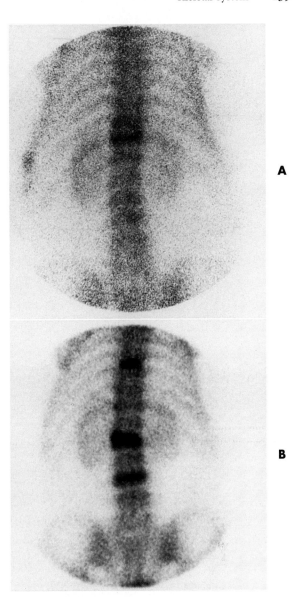

**Fig. 6-50** Surveillance images obtained several months apart. **A,** The initial study shows a single vertebral compression fracture caused by osteoporosis involving the lower thoracic spine. **B,** The subsequent study shows healing with normalization of uptake in the initial abnormality. Three new compression fractures are demonstrated in the middorsal spine and lumbar spine.

dysplasia is the most commonly encountered of these and may be monostotic or polyostotic (Fig. 6-56). The degree of increased tracer uptake is typically high, rivaling that seen in Paget's disease. Distinguishing features are the younger age of the patient and the different pattern of involvement. When Paget's disease involves a long bone, it invariably extends to at least one end of the bone. Fibrous dysplasia frequently does not involve the end of the bone. Other dysplasias associated with increased tracer uptake are listed in Box 6-10.

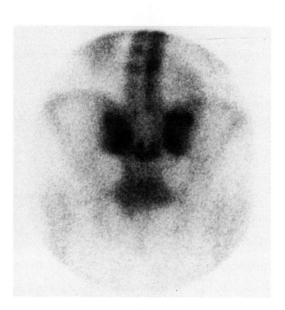

**Fig. 6-51**    Posterior spot view of a patient with osteoporosis. The patient has an H-type insufficiency fracture with a horizontal band of increased uptake across the body of the sacrum and bilaterally increased uptake in the sacral alae.

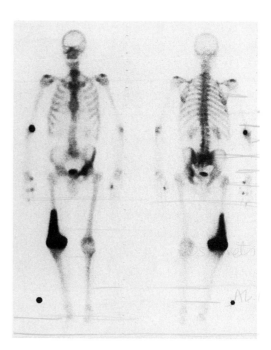

**Fig. 6-52**    Anterior and posterior whole body images of a patient with Paget's disease involving the right distal femur and the left hemipelvis. The uptake is extremely intense, with the appearance of bony expansion. The observation about expansion must be made with caution because of the extreme intensity of uptake and "blooming" of the recorded activity.

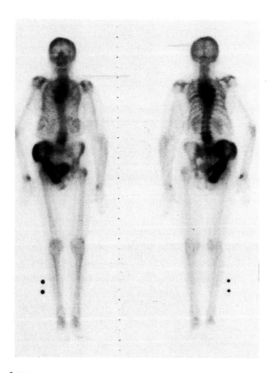

**Fig. 6-53**    Anterior and posterior whole body scintigrams of a patient with extensive Paget's disease involving the right pelvis, the lumbar spine, the thoracic spine, and a left rib.

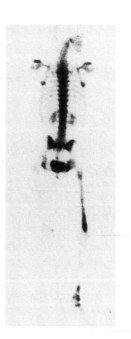

**Fig. 6-54**    Posterior whole body image from a patient with melorheostosis. Uptake is intensely increased in a somewhat patchy distribution involving the right femur.

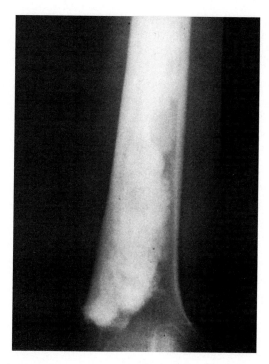

**Fig. 6-55** Spot view of the distal femur of the patient in Fig. 6-54 reveals the characteristic intensely sclerotic lesion of melorheostosis, often characterized as having the appearance of dripping candle wax.

---

**Box 6-10   Bone Dysplasias Associated with Increased Skeletal Tracer Uptake**

Fibrous dysplasia
Osteogenesis imperfecta
Osteopetrosis
Progressive diaphyseal dysplasia (Engelmann's disease)
Hereditary multiple diaphyseal sclerosis (Ribbing's disease)
Melorheostosis

---

## ARTHRITIS

Skeletal scintigraphy is a sensitive marker of both osteoarthritis (Fig. 6-57) and rheumatoid arthritis. Numerous attempts have been made over the last two decades to develop scintigraphic techniques for staging the severity of arthritis and assessing response to therapy. These have been largely unsuccessful, and skeletal scintigraphy is not commonly used to evaluate arthritis in current clinical practice. The major importance of arthritis is its ubiquitous presence in the elderly and therewith the likelihood of encountering increased

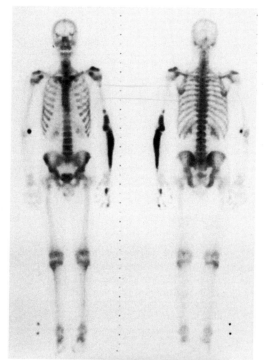

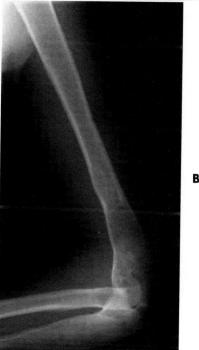

**Fig. 6-56** **A,** Whole body scintigrams of a patient with fibrous dysplasia involving the left upper extremity. Uptake is markedly increased in the distal humerus, most of the forearm, and focal areas in the hand. **B,** Corresponding radiograph of the left elbow reveals characteristic expansile lesions of fibrous dysplasia.

focal uptake in patients undergoing metastatic surveys. Arthritis in the extremities is typically not a problem. Special care must be taken in assessing the lower lumbar spine because of the common occurrence of both osteoarthritis and metastatic disease in this location.

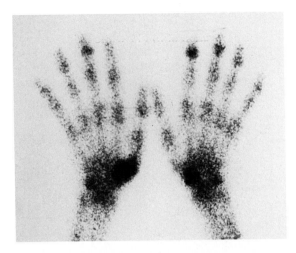

**Fig. 6-57**    Characteristic appearance of osteoarthritis in the hands and wrists. Uptake is increased in multiple distal interphalangeal joints and is particularly intense at the base of the first left metacarpal, a characteristic place for osteoarthritis.

## EXTRASKELETAL AND GENITOURINARY FINDINGS

A number of conditions causing nonosseous uptake of skeletal radiopharmaceuticals are routinely encountered in clinical practice and are discussed throughout the chapter (Box 6-11). Because of the opportunity to make an additional diagnosis, extraskeletal distribution of tracer should be inspected in every case.

Several normal or normal variant causes of extraskeletal tracer uptake are discussed earlier in the chapter in the section on the appearance of the normal scintigram. The thyroid cartilage, calcifications in blood vessels, and calcified costal cartilages can all demonstrate uptake.

The kidneys and bladder should be visible in normal subjects. Many genitourinary tract abnormalities are diagnosed incidentally by skeletal scintigraphy. Renal tumors and cysts are readily seen if large enough. Displacements of the kidney, including crossed renal ectopia and horseshoe kidney, are also readily visualized. The cause of renal enlargement or abnormally small kidneys may not be apparent on skeletal scintigraphy, but the findings should be noted for further workup. Excessive retained soft tissue background at the time of imaging may be due to poor renal function or soft tissue edema as in congestive heart failure.

Diffuse abnormal uptake in the liver is rare but can be caused by radiopharmaceutical formulation errors with colloid formation (Box 6-11). Diffuse hepatic necrosis has also been a reported cause of diffuse liver uptake. Focal liver uptake secondary to metastases is sometimes seen.

Dystrophic calcifications in the soft tissues and acute injury to myocardium and skeletal muscle can show avid

## Box 6-11    Summary of Soft Tissue Uptake on Skeletal Scintigrams

**NORMAL**

General soft tissue background
Kidneys: symmetrical, less than lumbar spine uptake
Bladder
Thyroid cartilage (common)
Costal cartilage (less common)

**ABNORMAL**

Brain: cerebrovascular accident
Lung:
    Diffuse: hyperparathyroidism, other courses of hyperalcemia
    Focal: lung cancer, other tumors    *OSA mets*
Liver:
    Diffuse: hepatic necrosis, excess colloid in radiopharmaceutical preparation, amyloidosis, *AL tox*
    Focal: metastatic tumors
Heart:
    Diffuse: amyloidosis
    Focal: myocardial infarction
Renal: diffusely increased uptake: chemotherapy, amyloidosis
Ureter: obstructive uropathy
Soft tissue:
    Diffuse: congestive heart failure, renal failure, edema, lymphedema, dermatomyositis, scleroderma
    Focal: sarcoma, metastatic tumors, dystrophic calcification, myositis ossificans, tumoral calcinosis, synovial calcinosis, dystrophic ossification
Breast:
    Diffuse: inflammation
    Focal: breast cancer (unilateral)
Stomach: intraluminal; free technetium-99m pertechnetate
Parenchyma: secondary to metastatic calcification, hyperparathyroidism
Skeletal muscle: rhabdomyolysis, myositis ossificans
Extremities: reflex sympathetic dystrophy syndrome, lymphedema
Lymph nodes: infiltrated tracer injection

**MISCELLANEOUS CONDITIONS**

Metastatic calcification: lung, stomach, kidneys, heart, liver; secondary to hypercalcemia
Free technetium-99m pertechnetate: thyroid and salivary glands (early); stomach, gastrointestinal tract

uptake. Cardiac amyloidosis can demonstrate striking uptake in the heart. Myositis ossificans avidly accumulates skeletal-seeking tracers (Fig. 6-58). The condition may develop after direct injury to muscle or as a consequence of paralysis. The maturity of the process can be assessed scintigraphically based on the relative

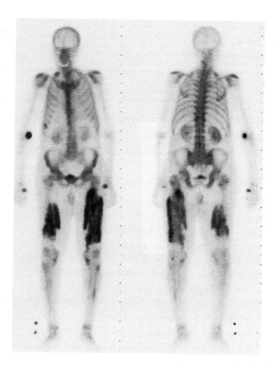

**Fig. 6-58**    Anterior and posterior whole body scintigrams of a patient with extensive myositis ossificans.

uptake of tracer in sequential studies. As the process matures, the degree of uptake diminishes. Skeletal imaging has been used to time surgical intervention, which is best performed after the lesion matures.

## BONE MARROW SCINTIGRAPHY

Bone marrow scintigraphy is not important in current practice but does have a small number of indications. The procedure is most commonly performed with Tc-99m sulfur colloid, which localizes in the reticuloendothelial elements of the red marrow.

In patients with sickle cell anemia, bone marrow imaging demonstrates the extent of marrow expansion into the extremities (Fig. 6-41). In most normal subjects the marrow is confined to the proximal thirds of the femurs and humeri. In patients with hemoglobinopathies the marrow uptake is typically seen throughout the appendages. Marrow imaging is highly sensitive for detection of bone marrow infarction and can also define the extent of involvement. The major limitation is not being able to distinguish new from chronic infarctions. Moreover, areas involved by osteomyelitis demonstrate defects on marrow imaging, so the technique is not useful in distinguishing infarction from osteomyelitis. In current practice, marrow imaging is used in some institutions in conjunction with In-111-labeled white blood cells to diagnose osteomyelitis. As noted in the discussion of prosthesis evaluation, in marrow-bearing areas the combination of In-111 white blood cell uptake and absence of Tc-99m sulfur colloid uptake is specific for osteomyelitis.

Marrow imaging has also enjoyed a vogue for the diagnosis of aseptic necrosis of the hip. Marrow elements are lost in the necrotic area. Although the technique is fairly sensitive, it has given way to MRI.

## MEASUREMENT OF BONE MINERAL

A number of methods have been developed for quantitative measurement of bone mineral mass. Until recently all of the techniques were based on the absorption of photons in bone, the differential absorption in bone tissue versus soft tissue, and calibration of absorption percentage against calcium-containing reference standards. A number of ultrasound techniques, based on the rate of sound transmission through bone, are now available.

The simplest technique is single-photon absorptiometry (SPA). In this technique a photon source, typically iodine-125, is collimated and scanned across the radius or calcaneus or both. These sites are selected for the minimal soft tissue because correction for soft tissue attenuation is not possible in the SPA technique.

Dual-photon absorptiometry (DPA) again uses a collimated photon source that is scanned over the skeletal part of interest. It is a more flexible technique because the soft tissue attenuation can be corrected based on the differential absorption of the beam at different energies. In DPA, gadolinium-153 with photon energies between 40 and 100 keV is typically used. Areas frequently studied with DPA are the lumbar spine and both the neck and intertrochanteric region of the femur. The single- and dual-photon techniques have given way to x-ray-based approaches in current practice.

Bone densitometry measurements can also be made with either dedicated x-ray densitometer devices or special quantitative computed tomography (QCT) algorithms. Single- and dual-energy techniques have been described for both x-ray and QCT. The advantage of the x-ray technique is higher photon flux compared with SPA and DPA instruments. Radiation exposure is essentially identical for dual-energy x-ray densitometry and DPA. The most versatile and widely used technique in current practice is dual energy x-ray absorptiometry (DXA). DXA is the basis for the World Health Organization (WHO) criteria for categorizing osteopenia and osteoporosis.

The main advantage of QCT is the ability to measure cortical and trabecular bone separately. Dual-energy QCT has the additional advantage over single-energy QCT of allowing correction for fat in the marrow space. Both techniques are quite flexible with respect to body part examined. QCT is an important research tool but is too expensive for population screening.

Several ultrasound devices are now approved by the U.S. Food and Drug Administration (FDA) for measurement of bone mass. Sound is transmitted faster in dense bone than in osteopenic bone, and the devices are calibrated against other methods to correlate with bone mass. Application of the technique is limited to peripheral structures such as the calcaneus. The low cost, small size, and ease of use of ultrasound devices make them attractive for population screening. However, current data indicate that spine measurements are necessary to follow the effects of therapy, since the spine is the most sensitive structure for assessing response to drug treatment.

The main application of bone mineral measurements is to establish baseline diagnostic measurements in the evaluation of patients with suspected osteopenia and osteoporosis and to follow the course of therapy. Primary osteoporosis has been divided into two subtypes. Type I or postmenopausal osteoporosis is related to decreased estrogen secretion after menopause. Type II or senile osteoporosis is presumably due to age-related impaired bone metabolism.

Risk factors for osteoporosis include female sex, Caucasian or Asian race, smoking, chronic alcohol intake, and a positive family history. Early menopause, long-term treatment with corticosteroids, and a number of nutritional disorders, including malabsorption, are also risk factors. Obesity is protective.

WHO has established a classification system for bone mass based on DXA measurements of the spine and femoral neck. A measurement in an individual is compared with the mean and standard deviation (SD) for a young control population. A reading within 1 SD is considered normal. Osteopenia is taken as 1 to 2.5 SD below the control mean, and osteoporosis is defined as 2.5 SD or greater below the control mean. When the standard deviation is reported in this way, it is referred to as the *T score*.

The use of bone mineral density has been accelerated by the availability of new drugs such as alendronate, a bisphosphonate that localizes in bone and promotes mineralization. Estrogen is also widely used in postmenopausal women but is not uniformly well tolerated, and concerns remain about its effects on other diseases such as breast cancer.

## ACKNOWLEDGMENTS

Portions of this chapter appeared in a slightly different form in Thrall JH, Ellis BI: Skeletal metastases, *Radiol Clin North Am* 25:1155-1170, 1987. Reprinted with permission.

## SUGGESTED READINGS

Brown ML: Significance of the solitary lesion in pediatric bone scanning, *J Nucl Med* 24:114-115, 1983.

Charkes ND, Young J, Sklaroff DM: The pathologic basis of the strontium bone scan, *JAMA* 206:2482, 1968.

Chilton HM, Francis MD, Thrall JH: Radiopharmaceuticals for bone and bone marrow imaging. In Swanson DP, Chilton HM, Thrall JH, editors: *Pharmaceuticals in medical imaging*, New York, 1990, Macmillan.

Collier BD, Fogelman I, Rosenthal L, editors: Skeletal nuclear medicine, St Louis, 1996, Mosby.

Corcoran RJ, Thrall JH, Kyle RW, et al: Solitary abnormalities in bone scans of patients with extraosseous malignancies, *Radiology* 121:663-667, 1976.

Fogelman I, editor: *Bone scanning in clinical practice*, London, 1987, Springer-Verlag.

Freeman LM, Blaufox MD, editors: Metabolic bone disease, *Semin Nucl Med* 27:195-305, 1997.

Freeman LM, Blaufox MD, editors: Orthopedic nuclear medicine (Part 1), *Semin Nucl Med* 27:307-389, 1997.

Freeman LM, Blaufox MD, editors: Orthopedic nuclear medicine (Part 2), *Semin Nucl Med* 28:1-131, 1998.

Kim H, Thrall JH, Keyes JW Jr: Skeletal scintigraphy following incidental trauma, *Radiology* 130:447-451, 1979.

Matin P: The appearance of bone scans following fractures including immediate and long-term studies, *J Nucl Med* 20:1227-1231, 1979.

McNeil BJ: Value of bone scanning in neoplastic disease, *Semin Nucl Med* 14:277-286, 1984.

Roub LW, Gamarman LW, Hanley EN, et al: Bone stress: a radionuclide imaging perspective, *Radiology* 132:431-438, 1979.

Saha GB: *Fundamentals of nuclear pharmacy*, New York, 1998, Springer.

Treves ST, editor: *Pediatric nuclear medicine*, New York, 1998, Springer.

# Pulmonary System

The single most important application of pulmonary scintigraphy is the evaluation of patients with suspected pulmonary embolism (PE). This frequently fatal condition continues to defy clinical diagnosis at the bedside and is all too often first diagnosed at postmortem examination. Some authorities have estimated the annual incidence of PE in the United States at over 650,000 cases per year, with over 100,000 deaths. The mortality from untreated significant PE is on the order of 30%. This mortality is reduced to 3% to 10% by treatment with anticoagulants and other therapies, including placement of a vena cava filter. The combination of nonspecificity of clinical presentation and the potentially high mortality from untreated PE has created an ongoing need for noninvasive testing. Although pulmonary angiography has been and remains the reference standard for the definitive diagnosis of PE, it is expensive, invasive, and subject to its own morbidity and mortality. The contemporary approach to the diagnosis of PE requires the judicious melding of clinical observations, application of ventilation-perfusion scintigraphy, and selective referral for pulmonary angiography. Helical computed tomography (CT) is also being critically evaluated to determine its role in the diagnosis of pulmonary embolism.

A number of less common indications for pulmonary scintigraphy merit brief discussion. These include quantitative analysis of relative lung perfusion before lobectomy or pneumonectomy, and studies in patients with adult respiratory distress syndrome.

## VENTILATION SCINTIGRAPHY

Ventilation and perfusion in the lung are coupled in many conditions and not linked directly in others. The finding of "concordant" versus "discordant" ventilation and perfusion abnormalities thus becomes pivotal in the differential diagnosis of combined ventilation-perfusion (V/Q) studies. The findings from ventilation studies lend additional specificity and significance to the patterns identified on perfusion studies.

## Radiopharmaceuticals

**Radioactive gases**    Two classes of radiopharmaceuticals are used for ventilation imaging, radioactive gases and radioaerosols. The radioactive gases include xenon-133 (Xe-133), xenon-127, and krypton-81m. The most widely used of these agents is Xe-133 (Box 7-1). Its half-life is 5.27 days, which makes it relatively easy to distribute and keep in stock in nuclear medicine pharmacies. It is available from commercial vendors in either a single-dose or a multidose vial form.

A major drawback to the use of Xe-133 is the relatively low (81-keV) energy of its principal photon. This low energy makes it difficult to perform Xe-133 ventilation studies after a perfusion study with a technetium-99m (Tc-99m) agent. There is significant Compton scatter from the 140-keV principal gamma of Tc-99m into the Xe-133 window. This "downscatter" potentially obscures abnormalities on the Xe-133 study and significantly degrades the image. Even with subtraction techniques, images are degraded. Therefore Xe-133 ventilation scintigraphy is typically performed first in combined V/Q imaging.

Xe-127 has a physical half-life of 36.4 days and three usable photons at 172 keV, 203 keV, and 375 keV, respectively. These energies are higher than that of Tc-99m, and therefore Xe-127 can be readily used following the perfusion portion of the V/Q examination. The advantage of this is the flexibility in selecting the ideal view or projection for ventilation scintigraphy, based on the results of the perfusion scintigram. Despite this theoretical advantage, Xe-127 has not become widely used because it is more expensive than Xe-133.

Krypton-81m (Kr-81m) is obtained from a rubidium-81/krypton-81m generator system. The physical half-life of the Ru-81 parent is 4.6 hours, and the generator system is good for only 1 day for all practical purposes.

The lack of general commercial availability, the high cost, and the logistical impracticality of daily generator replacement have kept Kr-81m from becoming clinically important.

Use of Kr-81m has some theoretical advantages. The generator can be continuously eluted. This feature, coupled with the short (13-second) half-life of Kr-81m, allows the operator to obtain multiple views. Also, the principal photon energy of Kr-81m is 190 keV, which readily permits ventilation studies after perfusion scintigraphy with Tc-99m-labeled agents.

Over the timeframe of ventilation scintigraphy the radioactive gases remain within the bronchoalveolar space. Sequential images during inhalation, steady-state breathing, and exhalation or washout depict the overall and regional dynamics of ventilation. It should be noted that a small amount of the radioactive gas equilibrates across the alveolar-capillary membrane with blood and is carried throughout the body in the systemic circulation. Xenon is relatively fat soluble, and a significant accumulation may be seen in the liver in patients with fatty infiltration (Fig. 7-1).

**Radioaerosols**    As an alternative to radioactive gases for ventilation studies, various radioaerosols may be used. Radioaerosols depict the distribution of ventilation during the inhalation phase. The inhaled aerosol is deposited on the lining of the bronchoalveolar spaces, so that subsequent imaging shows the regional patterns of ventilation. An advantage of the aerosol technique is the ability to image in multiple views or projections after administration of a single dose of radiotracer.

A number of radioaerosols have been tried for ventilation imaging. The current agent of choice and the only FDA-approved aerosol is Tc-99m pentetate (DTPA). Commercial nebulizers are available that provide particles of appropriate size. The ideal aerosol particle size is in the range of 0.1 to 0.5 $\mu$m. Particles smaller than this

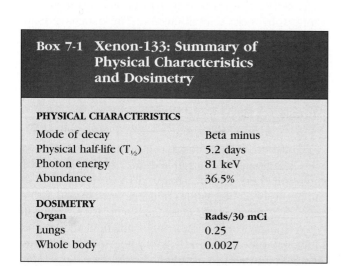

| Box 7-1 Xenon-133: Summary of Physical Characteristics and Dosimetry | |
|---|---|
| **PHYSICAL CHARACTERISTICS** | |
| Mode of decay | Beta minus |
| Physical half-life ($T_{1/2}$) | 5.2 days |
| Photon energy | 81 keV |
| Abundance | 36.5% |
| **DOSIMETRY** | |
| **Organ** | **Rads/30 mCi** |
| Lungs | 0.25 |
| Whole body | 0.0027 |

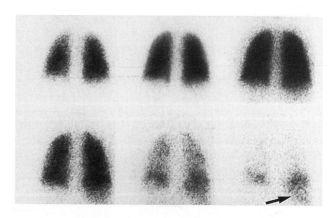

**Fig. 7-1**    Posterior view of a xenon-133 ventilation study. There is delayed washout of xenon at both lung bases, as well as significant xenon uptake in the region of the liver (*arrow on bottom right image*).

may simply be inhaled and then exhaled. Particles greater than 2 to 3 $\mu$m tend to settle out in large airways, including the trachea and bronchi. This effect may obscure the alveolar distribution in adjacent portions of the lung. In the ideal preparation the particles penetrate the lung and localize in the alveoli without significant deposition in the large airways.

Another approach with radioaerosols has used Tc-99m-labeled carbon particles. The agent has been called "Technegas" and is in a sense a "pseudogas." The particles are very small (0.005 $\mu$m) and for the most part do not settle out in the lung.

Because the radioaerosols typically use the same Tc-99m radiolabel as the pulmonary perfusion agents, the relative doses are adjusted to minimize "cross-talk," or interference between radioactivity from the two different portions of the examination.

## Technique

**Radioactive gases**  Ventilation studies with Xe-133 are ordinarily performed first during combined V/Q imaging. A large-field-of-view gamma camera with a low-energy, all-purpose collimator is used. A 20% energy window is centered at 81 keV. The usual adult dose of Xe-133 is 10 to 20 mCi (370 to 740 MBq) (Box 7-2).

A high-quality ventilation scan requires patient cooperation. The study is accomplished in three phases, the single-breath or wash-in phase, the equilibrium phase, and the washout phase. Severely tachypneic, uncooperative, or unresponsive patients may require modification of the standard protocol or an alternative approach with a radioaerosol.

The patient is placed for a posterior view. Patient orientation should be the same as subsequently used for the perfusion portion of the study. Some laboratories routinely perform both parts of the study with the patient supine. Others favor a sitting position if the patient can tolerate it. The sitting position is generally better because it permits a fuller excursion of the diaphragm and makes oblique views easier to obtain during the washout phase. Also, chest radiographs are usually obtained with the patient upright, and the best correlative information comes from comparisons in like positions.

To begin the study, the patient takes in and holds a single maximal deep inspiration. The breath is taken through a mouthpiece attached to an Xe-133 delivery apparatus. An initial image is obtained for 100,000 counts (100k).

The next phase of the study is the equilibrium phase. Typically, two images are obtained for 90 seconds each, beginning after the initial breath image is completed. During this time the patient continues to breathe a mixture of air and xenon. When Kr-81m is used, a true equilibrium is never achieved because the short (13-second) half-life does not allow complete penetration of the alveolar spaces.

In the third phase of the examination, multiple washout images are obtained. The valve on the xenon delivery apparatus is shifted from the delivery reservoir to a xenon-trapping device while the patient breathes room air. Three or four sequential 45-second washout images are obtained. As an option, additional 45-second images are obtained in both the 45° left posterior and right posterior oblique projections, followed by a final 45-second posterior view. The sitting position greatly facilitates oblique views. The patient is placed on a backless chair with a swivel seat that allows rapid positioning for the oblique images. Many patients referred for V/Q scintigraphy are uncomfortable in or unable to maintain a sitting position, and the same sequence may be obtained with the patient supine and the camera under the imaging table. The oblique views are then obtained by helping the patient roll onto a 45° bolster.

Studies with Xe-127 may be performed by use of the same protocol as with Xe-133. As discussed previously, there is flexibility in choosing the imaging view or projection and also in choosing the sequence of the ventilation and perfusion portions of the examination. The rapid clearance of xenon from the lung after the delivery apparatus is switched to room air allows

---

**Box 7-2    Protocol for Xenon-133 Ventilation Scintigraphy**

**PATIENT PREPARATION**

None

**DOSAGE AND ROUTE OF ADMINISTRATION**

Xenon-133: 10 to 20 mCi (370 to 740 MBq) adult dosage by inhalation

**PROCEDURE**

Use a wide-field-of-view camera with a parallel hole, all-purpose collimator and a 20% window centered at 81 keV

The patient is seated (if possible) with the camera positioned in the posterior view

First breath: The patient exhales fully and is asked to take a maximal inspiration and hold it long enough, if possible, to obtain 100k counts

Equilibrium: Obtain two sequential 90-sec images while the patient breathes normally

Washout: Obtain three sequential 45-sec posterior images and then left and right posterior oblique images and a final posterior image

imaging in multiple views if sufficient radioactive gas is available.

**Radioaerosols** For studies with radioaerosols the radiopharmaceutical is placed in a special nebulizer system. The patient is asked to breathe through the mouthpiece of the delivery system until sufficient radio-aerosol is delivered to the lungs. This may require several minutes. Because only 5% to 10% of the radioactivity in the nebulizer is delivered to the lung, 25 to 75 mCi of Tc-99m pentetate is placed in the nebulizer. The goal is to deliver enough radioaerosol to the lung that 150,000 to 250,000 count (150k to 250k) images may be obtained in 1 to 2 minutes.

The views obtained in radioaerosol studies should be the same as those obtained for the perfusion phase. Most nuclear medicine clinics obtain anterior, posterior, right and left lateral, and both posterior 45° oblique views. The right and left 45° anterior oblique views may also be readily obtained. The Tc-99m-DTPA aerosol remains in the lung, with a biological half-life approaching 1 hour. This is more than enough time for multiple view imaging.

## PERFUSION SCINTIGRAPHY

### Radiopharmaceuticals

The diameter of a red blood cell is approximately 7.7 μm. Larger diameter particles introduced into the bloodstream proximal to the pulmonary capillary bed lodge in the pulmonary capillaries and precapillary arterioles. If mixing has been adequate to prevent laminar flow effects, the resulting distribution of radio-activity is an accurate map of regional perfusion in the lung. Numerous particulate agents, both biodegradable and nonbiodegradable, have been studied experimentally and clinically for perfusion scintigraphy. The first studies in humans were obtained with radioiodinated (iodine-131) macroaggregated albumin.

The two agents providing the most clinical experience are Tc-99m-labeled human albumin microspheres (Tc-99m HAM) and Tc-99m-labeled macroaggregated albumin (Tc-99m MAA). Human albumin microspheres (HAM) are prepared by heating albumin in an oil emulsion and selecting particles of the appropriate size from the resulting microspheres. In suitable preparations over 95% of the microspheres are in the range of 10 to 40 μm. The ability to control the size range is a distinct advantage of HAM preparations. However, HAM preparations are not currently available commercially in the United States, and Tc-99m MAA has become the dominant agent.

In current practice MAA preparations contain particles ranging in size from a few microns to 100 μm. The majority (60% to 80%) of MAA particles in commercial preparations are in the 10- to 30-μm range.

| Table 7-1 | Dosimetry for technetium-99m macroaggregated albumin |
|---|---|

| Organ | Rad/4 mCi |
|---|---|
| Lungs | 0.880 |
| Bladder wall | 0.120 |
| Testes | 0.024 |
| Ovaries | 0.030 |
| Whole body | 0.060 |

In commercial preparations a vial that contains MAA with stannous ion is supplied. Tc-99m as sodium pertechnetate is added to the reaction vial, resulting in rapid labeling of the MAA particles.

After intravenous (IV) injection into a peripheral vein, the radiolabeled particles travel through the right atrium and right ventricle, where thorough mixing occurs. They are then filtered or trapped in the pulmonary vascular bed. In areas of absent or decreased perfusion, correspondingly fewer particles are delivered and trapped, resulting in relatively photopenic or "cold" areas.

The clearance of Tc-99m MAA from the lung is due primarily to a physical, mechanical degradation of the particles. As particles become fragmented, they may initially lodge in smaller branches of the pulmonary circulation, but eventually they gain access to the systemic circulation, where they are phagocytosed in the reticuloendothelial system and further degraded. The biological half-life of current Tc-99m MAA preparations in the lung is 2 to 3 hours. Of historical interest is the somewhat longer biological half-life of HAM (4 to 6 hours), which probably results from the spherical configuration of these particles and therefore their lower susceptibility to fragmentation. The dosimetry for Tc-99m MAA is summarized in Table 7-1.

Because any particles reaching the systemic circulation lodge in the capillary beds of critical organs of the body, right-to-left shunts are a relative contraindication to the use of Tc-99m MAA. After injection of this radiopharmaceutical into patients who have shunts, the brain, heart, kidneys, and other structures are readily visualized (Fig. 7-2). Although the process sounds alarming in theory, it is remarkably well tolerated in practice. Substantial clinical experience has been obtained in using various macroaggregates of albumin for quantitative assessment of right-to-left shunting by measuring radioactivity trapped in the lung versus the amount of activity gaining access to the systemic circulation. Also, investigators around the world have injected radiolabeled particles directly into many organs to assess relative regional blood flow, with an apparently wide margin of safety. Nonetheless, the possibility of right-to-

to ↓ central deposition —need smaller size particles, but there then don't settle peripherally but there then don't settle into periph airways ∴ can add alcohol to preparation so that parts evaporate & nebulation ∴ will ↓ absorb too & settle.

Pulmonary System  **149**

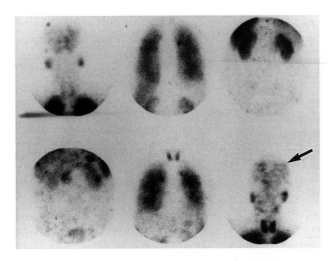

**Fig. 7-2**  Technetium-99m MAA scintigrams in a patient with right-to-left shunts in the lung. Note the uptake in the brain *(arrow, lower right image)*. Free pertechnetate would not be taken up in the cerebrum. Uptake is also marked in the salivary glands, the thyroid gland, and the kidneys and other abdominal viscera. (From Bank ER, Thrall JH, Dantzker DR: *Am J Roentgenol* 140:967-969, 1983.)

left shunting should be borne in mind when performing this study.

From time to time the question arises as to whether activity seen outside the lungs is due to right-to-left shunting or to free Tc-99m pertechnetate in the radio-pharmaceutical preparation. The distinction can be made readily by imaging the brain. Tc-99m pertechnetate and other nonparticulate potential radiocontaminants do not cross the blood-brain barrier or localize in the brain. Shunted Tc-99m MAA lodges in the cerebral circulation (Fig. 7-2).

Another important consideration is the number of radiolabeled particles constituting the diagnostic dose. If the dose of particles is too small, the distribution pattern in the capillary bed is not statistically valid. On the other hand, injecting too many particles could theoretically obstruct a hemodynamically significant portion of the pulmonary circulation. Empirically, a minimum of 60,000 particles is required to meet statistical distribution criteria in adults. In practice, an upper limit of 400,000 particles is observed. Because it is estimated that there are over 280 billion pulmonary capillaries and 300 million precapillary arterioles, administration of even 400,000 particles should result in obstruction of only a very small fraction of the cross section of the normal vascular bed. The margin of safety is quite large in normal subjects and in most patients undergoing evaluation. Caution is still advised, including the use of the minimum number of particles in patients with pulmonary hypertension who may have significantly fewer remaining pulmonary capillaries than normal. The number of particles should also be reduced for neonates

(10,000) and children under the age of 5 years (50,000 to 150,000).

Pregnancy is another situation requiring caution. When PE is a clinical consideration in pregnant patients, the minimum radiation dose is figured on a risk-versus-benefit basis. However, with perfusion imaging it is still necessary to deliver a minimum of 60,000 particles. To achieve the right balance between the amount of radioactivity and the number of particles, the amount of Tc-99m pertechnetate added to the reaction vial may have to be adjusted. Also, because the commercially available kits provide for multiple doses, the ratio of radioactivity to particles changes continuously after the initial labeling. This should be borne in mind in making dose calculations.

## Technique

The usual dose of Tc-99m MAA for pulmonary perfusion imaging is 2 to 5 mCi (Box 7-3). The dose is administered intravenously and should be given slowly over several respiratory cycles. The patient should be encouraged to breathe deeply. The injection should be made with the patient supine to foster even distribution of particles cephalocaudally in the lung. If the particles are injected with the patient sitting or standing, a basilar predominance may occur.

Once the injection is complete, imaging can begin immediately. The patient's position for imaging should

---

**Box 7-3  Protocol for Technetium-99m Macroaggregated Albumin Perfusion Scintigraphy**

**PATIENT PREPARATION AND PRECAUTIONS**

Right-to-left shunts are a relative contraindication
Pregnant women: Adjust dosage and observe requirement for a minimum of 60,000 particles
Pulmonary hypertension or pneumonectomy: Reduce number of particles to 60,000

**DOSAGE AND ROUTE OF ADMINISTRATION**

Tc-99m MAA: 4 mCi (148 MBq) adult dosage
Intravenous administration over several respiratory cycles with the patient supine

**PROCEDURE**

Use a wide-field-of-view gamma camera with a low-energy high-resolution or all-purpose collimator and a 20% window centered at 140 keV
Obtain anterior, posterior, right lateral, left lateral and right and left lateral posterior oblique images (anterior oblique images optional)
Obtain 500k to 750k counts/image

be the same as that selected for the ventilation portion of the study. A large-field-of-view gamma scintillation camera equipped with an all-purpose or high-resolution collimator is used. A 20% window is centered at 140 keV. Images are obtained in the anterior, posterior, right and left lateral, and both 45° posterior oblique views. The 45° anterior oblique images are also commonly obtained. A minimum of 500,000 counts per image is recommended.

Some laboratories image the more normal lung in the lateral view for 500,000 counts and the contralateral, more abnormal lung for the same time as was required for the initial lateral view. The rationale is to recognize and prevent misleading patterns that would result from shine-through of activity from right to left or vice versa. For example, the right lateral view in a patient without a right lung can appear surprisingly normal because of shine-through from the left! The combined count- and time-based approach alerts the observer to the true differences in right lung versus left lung activity.

Care is taken during the venipuncture not to draw blood into the syringe. Occasionally a small clot forms in the syringe when this happens. Adherence of Tc-99m MAA particles to the clot results in a spurious hot spot in the lung because of reinjection of the small clot. Also, the syringe should be agitated just before injection to avoid sedimentation or settling out and aggregation of particles. The particles should be injected through a 23-gauge or larger needle to prevent fragmentation during dose administration.

## APPEARANCE OF NORMAL SCINTIGRAMS

### Appearance of the Normal Ventilation Scintigram

In normal subjects the initial breath or wash-in image reveals homogeneous distribution of radioactive xenon. In subjects taking an effective deep breath the distribution is fairly complete. In the equilibrium phase the appearance is again homogeneous, with the full outline of the lungs demonstrated. The spine attenuates activity in the midline and appears as a linear photopenic area separating the left and right lungs. In some thin subjects a relative photopenia is also seen on the left side, corresponding to the projected area of the heart (Fig. 7-3, *A*).

During the washout phase a progressive and uniform decrease occurs in activity from the lungs. The half-time of washout should be 2 minutes or less, and the last washout image should have faint or no discernible activity. In an otherwise normal subject washout may

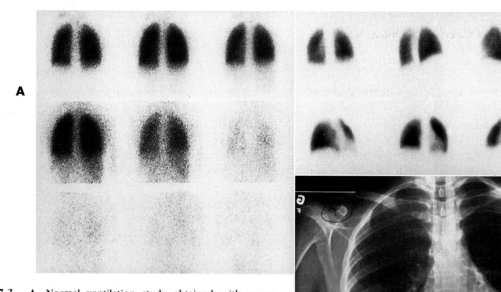

**Fig. 7-3** **A,** Normal ventilation study obtained with xenon-133. The initial breath *(left)* and equilibrium images are in the upper row followed by the sequential washout images in the middle and lower rows. Xenon is uniformly distributed with no evidence of air trapping. Minimal activity is seen in the region of the liver. **B,** The corresponding technetium-99m MAA study also demonstrates homogeneous distribution of tracer activity throughout the lungs. The defect resulting from the cardiac structures is clearly visualized. No focal abnormalities are demonstrated. **C,** Corresponding chest radiograph reveals fully expanded lungs with no cardiovascular or pulmonary abnormalities.

appear delayed as a result of the subject's inability to breathe comfortably through the mouthpiece of the delivery apparatus. The left and right posterior oblique images should not reveal any focal accumulations at the time they are obtained.

In some subjects discernible activity accumulates in the right upper quadrant of the abdomen in the area of the liver. Significant accumulation is usually due to fatty infiltration of the liver (Fig. 7-1). Distribution of radio-aerosols is similar to that in initial breath xenon studies. In radioaerosol studies activity may be seen in the larger airways and activity from swallowed radiopharmaceutical is sometimes seen in the stomach (Fig. 7-4).

## Appearance of the Normal Perfusion Scintigram

The scintigram in healthy subjects should show homogeneous, uniform distribution of tracer throughout the lungs (Fig. 7-3, *B*). The hilar structures are frequently perceived as photopenic areas corresponding to the large airway and vascular structures in the hilum. The area of the heart is obviously photopenic on the anterior view and is seen as variable degrees of apparent regionally decreased activity on other views, depending on the habitus of the patient. Again, in thin subjects a cardiac "defect" may be seen on the posterior view and an area of decreased activity corresponding to the heart is frequently seen on the left lateral view.

The spine and sternum effectively attenuate activity in the midline, resulting in a separation of the left and right lungs.

The pulmonary outline on the perfusion images commonly appears slightly smaller than on the ventila-

tion images. This is due to the lower spatial resolution on the ventilation study (lower photon energy and fewer counts).

The location of the diaphragms, the size of the heart, and the size of hilar defects should correspond to the location and appearance of these structures as seen on chest radiographs (Fig. 7-3, *C*). Comparison with the chest radiographic findings is most useful when the radiograph has been obtained with the subject in the same position as for the perfusion and ventilation images. This is another reason for performing all three examinations with the subject upright if possible. The upright position usually results in better excursion of the diaphragm and fuller expansion of the lungs than the supine position.

The perfusion images should be scrutinized for extrapulmonary activity that may indicate either a right-to-left shunt or a radiopharmaceutical contaminant in the preparation. Uptake in the thyroid and stomach typically indicates free pertechnetate, uptake in the liver indicates colloidal impurities, and uptake in the brain indicates right-to-left shunting as described in the discussion of radiopharmaceuticals.

## PULMONARY EMBOLISM

By far the most important indication for V/Q imaging is suspected PE. This condition in many respects is a medical orphan. PE is not the province of any medical specialty, and patients to be evaluated for the disorder come from every service in the hospital. The majority of physicians initially encountering patients with PE do not have special expertise in its diagnosis or management. In many institutions the radiologist serves as the de facto expert because all patients undergoing diagnostic evaluation go through the nuclear medicine or angiography laboratory for study. Thus the radiologist has an opportunity to become a key person in the diagnosis and management of patients with PE. The importance of establishing a correct specific diagnosis of PE is motivated by the high death rate among untreated patients but also by a high complication rate in patients undergoing anticoagulant therapy. For example, in the Prospective Investigation of Pulmonary Embolism Diagnosis (PIOPED) study, 8% of patients experienced a major bleeding complication as defined by a drop in hemoglobin level of 2 g or more or by the development of a cerebral hemorrhage or hemarthrosis.

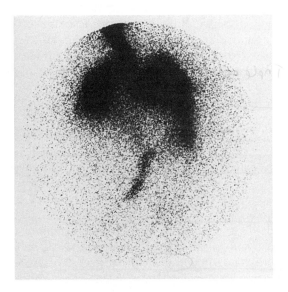

**Fig. 7-4**    Technetium-99m DTPA aerosol study reveals intense uptake in the trachea and midabdominal activity as a result of swallowed radiopharmaceutical in the stomach.

### Predisposing Factors

A number of associated clinical conditions are thought to predispose to PE. These include recent surgery (within 3 months), immobilization, thrombophlebitis, and underlying malignancy or some other cause of a hypercoagulable state. In women pregnancy and estrogen use have been considered risk factors. The majority of pulmonary emboli arise from venous thromboses in the lower extremities and pelvis. The predisposing factors mentioned here are all associated with an increased likelihood for the development of thrombophlebitis and deep vein thrombosis.

## Clinical Presentation

The signs and symptoms of PE vary widely among patients and are generally nonspecific. Overall, the clinical presentation depends on the size and number of emboli and therefore the percentage of the pulmonary circulation that has been occluded. The signs and symptoms also depend on whether associated pulmonary infarction is causing pleuritic chest pain and hemorrhage with associated hemoptysis.

The majority of patients have tachypnea, dyspnea, chest pain, and cough. Patients are frequently apprehensive and may have a sense of impending doom. Tachycardia is commonly present. Less common findings are hemoptysis, wheezing, and such severe symptoms as marked hypotension and syncope. In massive PE the first presentation may be fatal with cor pulmonale and circulatory collapse.

The classic presenting triad of dyspnea, pleuritic chest pain, and hemoptysis is infrequently encountered in contemporary practice. This may be due to earlier presentation of patients today than when this triad was first described, since infarction-related hemoptysis may not develop for a day or more after the event.

## Radiographic Findings

Radiographic findings are nonspecific and depend on whether the pulmonary emboli are associated with infarction. PE without infarction is more common than with infarction but can still be massive and fatal. PE without infarction may not have associated chest radiographic findings. When abnormalities are seen, they may include an increase in the size of the central pulmonary arteries because of the presence of a large embolus. Local oligemia may be observed in the area distal to an occluding PE. Oligemia may involve an entire lung if the clot is proximal and is referred to as Westermark's sign. A small pleural effusion may be present. In severe cases acute cor pulmonale may be seen with cardiac enlargement and prominence of the superior vena cava and azygos vein.

In patients with related pulmonary infarction all of the aforementioned chest radiographic findings may be present. In addition, typical findings include an elevated hemidiaphragm on the involved side, small pleural effusions, atelectasis with linear opacities, and parenchymal opacity corresponding to the infarct per se. The last

finding may not be apparent if the patient is studied immediately after the onset of symptoms. Large pleural effusions are not characteristic of PE.

The parenchymal opacities associated with pulmonary infarctions can vary in appearance depending on the location of the involved tissue. A characteristic pleura-based, wedge-shaped density (Hampton's hump) can be seen with a rounded or hump-shaped surface toward the hilum. However, not all lobules are pleura based and infarction can be associated with a wide variety of opacity shapes. All of the above features can also be seen on CT scans.

## Laboratory Findings

The majority of patients with PE have abnormalities in serum enzymes, and classically the oxygen pressure ($Po_2$) is low. The patients tend to hyperventilate, which is associated with a respiratory alkalosis. The majority of patients also have electrocardiographic abnormalities, but these are transient and may not be detected. Use of laboratory indicators of clot formation to help rule out PE has attracted recent attention, but these are not well enough established to rely on clinically, although determination of D-dimer is promising.

## Diagnosis

Over the years a number of diagnostic schemes have used information from chest radiographs and ventilation-perfusion studies to arrive at probability estimates for PE. If PE were the only condition affecting pulmonary perfusion, the diagnosis would be straightforward. However, innumerable pulmonary and cardiac conditions may distort pulmonary perfusion. The chest radiograph and ventilation studies are used to help identify the possible presence of these nonembolic causes of perfusion abnormality. As a corollary observation, the more extensive the preexisting pulmonary morbidity, the greater the difficulty of ruling in or ruling out superimposed PE.

## Terminology

A special set of terms has been developed for use in the diagnostic schemes employed in the interpretation of V/Q scans. The diagnostic schemes require correct application of the concepts embodied in this terminology.

The first concept is that of the matched versus mismatched perfusion defect (Box 7-4). A perfusion defect is said to be *matched* if there is a corresponding ventilation abnormality. The ventilation abnormality may be the absence of ventilation in the corresponding area, as might be seen in pleural effusion or secondary to tumor, or may reflect altered ventilatory dynamics, as

## Box 7-4  Ventilation-Perfusion "Match-Mismatch" Concept

V/Q match: Both scintigrams are abnormal in the same area; defects of equal size

V/Q mismatch: *Abnormal* perfusion in an area of *normal* ventilation or much larger perfusion abnormality than ventilation defect

## Box 7-5  Terminology for Ventilation-Perfusion Scintigraphy

| | |
|---|---|
| **SEGMENTAL DEFECT** | Caused by occlusion of a branch of the pulmonary artery; characteristically wedge shaped and pleural based; conforms to segmental anatomy of the lung |
| Large segmental defect | >75% of a lung segment |
| Moderate segmental defect | 25%-75% of a lung segment |
| Small segmental defect | <25% of a lung segment |
| **NONSEGMENTAL DEFECT** | Does *not* conform to segmental anatomy or does not appear wedge shaped or neither conforms to segmental anatomy nor appears wedge shaped |

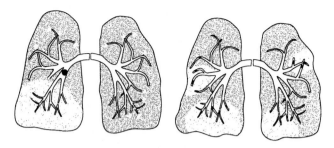

**Fig. 7-5**  Branching pattern of the pulmonary arteries. Emboli may be due to larger, more proximal clots as illustrated in the diagram on the left or to showers of smaller clots lodging more distally. In either case the resulting defects should be pleura based and correspond to the segmental anatomy of the lung.

## Box 7-6  Causes of Nonsegmental Defects

Pacemaker artifact
Tumors
Pleural effusion
Trauma
Hemorrhage
Bullae
Cardiomegaly
Mediastinal and hilar adenopathy
Atelectasis
Pneumonia
Aortic ectasia or aneurysm

might be seen in chronic airway disease with both delayed wash-in and delayed washout.

A *V/Q mismatch* refers to an area of abnormal perfusion that demonstrates normal ventilation. The concept also applies to a comparison of the perfusion scintigram with the chest radiograph. In most diagnostic schemes a perfusion defect that is substantially larger than a corresponding radiographic or ventilatory abnormality is considered to be mismatched.

The distinction of whether a given perfusion defect is matched or mismatched is fundamental. Typically, matched defects are due to nonembolic causes. Acute PE classically results in V/Q mismatch. That is, there is a perfusion defect because the embolus blocks blood flow, but ventilation remains normal because the airway has no corresponding blockage.

The next important concept embodied in the diagnostic terminology is the difference between a *segmental* and a *nonsegmental defect* (Box 7-5). Perfusion defects caused by blockage of the pulmonary arterial tree should reflect the branching or arborization of the pulmonary circulation in its classic segmental pattern (Fig. 7-5). Thus a classic *segmental defect* corresponds to one or more bronchopulmonary segments, is wedge shaped, and is pleura based. The term *nonsegmental defect* is reserved for abnormalities that do not correspond to the pulmonary segments, are not pleura based, and do not have the classic wedge shape. Causes of nonsegmental defects are summarized in Box 7-6. Many of the conditions resulting in nonsegmental defects are apparent radiographically, such as pleural effusion and tumors.

Assessment of the size of a given defect and determination of the number of defects present in each category are important for the correct application of the clinical diagnostic schemes. By convention a defect is considered *large* if it equals more than 75% of the size of a lung segment, *moderate* if it is between 25% and 75% of the size of a lung segment, and *small* if it is less than 25% of the size of a lung segment. Having a diagram of the segmental anatomy of the lungs available for reference is useful when interpreting V/Q studies (Fig. 7-6).

The complexity of interpretation of combined ventilation and perfusion studies has led to the use of probability categories rather than the simple assignment of positive or negative. If no abnormalities are demon-

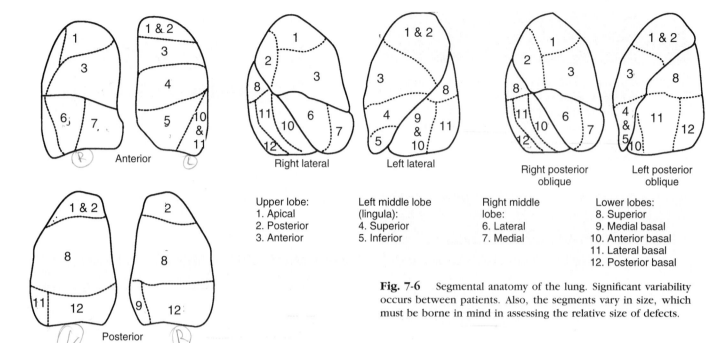

Upper lobe:
1. Apical
2. Posterior
3. Anterior

Left middle lobe (lingula):
4. Superior
5. Inferior

Right middle lobe:
6. Lateral
7. Medial

Lower lobes:
8. Superior
9. Medial basal
10. Anterior basal
11. Lateral basal
12. Posterior basal

**Fig. 7-6**  Segmental anatomy of the lung. Significant variability occurs between patients. Also, the segments vary in size, which must be borne in mind in assessing the relative size of defects.

### Box 7-7  Modified PIOPED Criteria for Combined Study Interpretation

**HIGH PROBABILITY (>80%)**

*Two or more large mismatched segmental defects* without radiographic abnormality (or a perfusion defect that is substantially larger than the radiographic abnormality)

Any combination of mismatched defects equivalent to the above (two moderate defects = one large defect)

**INTERMEDIATE PROBABILITY (INDETERMINATE) (20%-80%)**

One moderate mismatched segmental defect with normal radiograph

One large or two moderate mismatched segmental defects with normal radiograph

Three moderate mismatched segmental defects with normal radiograph

One large and one moderate mismatched segmental defect with normal radiograph

Mismatched ventilation, perfusion, and radiographic defects

Difficult to categorize as high or low probability

Not meeting the stated criteria for high or low

**LOW PROBABILITY (<20%)**

Nonsegmental perfusion defects (e.g., small pleural effusion with blunting of costophrenic angle, cardiomegaly, elevated diaphragm or enlargement of the aorta, hila, or mediastinum, stripe sign)

Any perfusion defect with a substantially larger radiographic abnormality

Matched ventilation and perfusion defects with normal chest radiograph

Small subsegmental perfusion defects

**NORMAL**

No perfusion defects

*PIOPED*, Prospective Investigation of Pulmonary Embolism Diagnosis.

strated, the combined study is considered normal. Depending on the number, size, and combined patterns of demonstrated abnormalities, abnormal studies are classified in the different diagnostic schemes as *low* probability, *intermediate* probability (also referred to as *indeterminate*), or *high* probability.

### Diagnostic Criteria

Numerous diagnostic schemes using the terminology and probability categories previously described have been proposed over the years. The criteria summarized in Box 7-7 are modified from those used in the multiinstitutional PIOPED study of the accuracy of V/Q scintigraphy sponsored by the National Institutes of Health. The original PIOPED criteria were derived from the literature and drew heavily on the work of Dan Biello. The scheme represented in Box 7-7 differs from the original PIOPED criteria based on a performance analysis of the original criteria. For example, in the original criteria a single moderate mismatched V/Q defect with a correspondingly normal radiograph was considered low probability, but it is included as intermediate probability in the criteria presented in Box 7-7, based on the

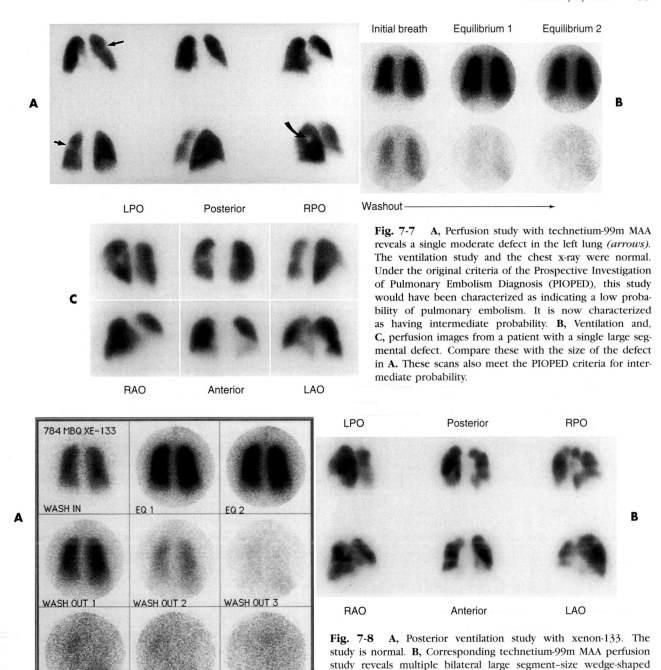

LPO    Posterior    RPO

Washout ⟶

RAO    Anterior    LAO

**Fig. 7-7** **A,** Perfusion study with technetium-99m MAA reveals a single moderate defect in the left lung *(arrows).* The ventilation study and the chest x-ray were normal. Under the original criteria of the Prospective Investigation of Pulmonary Embolism Diagnosis (PIOPED), this study would have been characterized as indicating a low probability of pulmonary embolism. It is now characterized as having intermediate probability. **B,** Ventilation and, **C,** perfusion images from a patient with a single large segmental defect. Compare these with the size of the defect in **A.** These scans also meet the PIOPED criteria for intermediate probability.

784 MBQ XE-133   WASH IN   EQ 1   EQ 2   WASH OUT 1   WASH OUT 2   WASH OUT 3   POST TRAP   RPO TRAP   LPO TRAP

LPO    Posterior    RPO

RAO    Anterior    LAO

**Fig. 7-8** **A,** Posterior ventilation study with xenon-133. The study is normal. **B,** Corresponding technetium-99m MAA perfusion study reveals multiple bilateral large segment–size wedge-shaped pleura-based defects. This pattern fits the high-probability diagnostic category.

PIOPED experience (Fig. 7-7). An important note is that the number of combinations of diagnostic findings in the intermediate (indeterminate) category exceeds any practical ability to enumerate them individually. The criteria account for this by specifying that if an abnormal study does not meet the criteria for high or low probability, it should be considered indeterminate. It cannot be emphasized enough that the specific criteria in different published diagnostic schemes are highly variable, particularly in separating low- from intermediate-probability studies.

The scintigraphic hallmark of PE is a perfusion defect corresponding to a bronchopulmonary segment that exhibits normal ventilation, with no abnormality on chest radiograph (or a radiographic abnormality that is *much* smaller than the perfusion defect). When two or more such large-segment defects or their equivalent are seen, the likelihood of PE is over 80% (Figs. 7-8 and 7-9).

At the other end of the spectrum, when the perfusion study is completely and unequivocally normal, without a segmental or other defect, the likelihood of PE is less than 5% and the likelihood of significant morbidity or mortality from PE is probably less than 1% (Fig. 7-3).

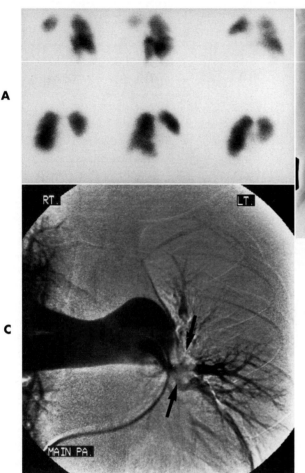

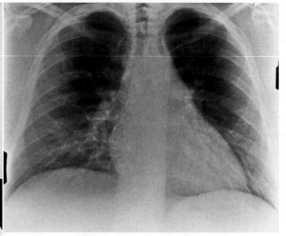

**Fig. 7-9   A,** High-probability study. Technetium-99m perfusion study reveals absence of activity in the entire left lower lobe and left middle lobe. The study also shows a moderate-size segmental defect at the right base and a small defect in the region of the right middle lobe. The xenon-133 ventilation scan was normal. **B,** Corresponding chest radiograph does not show focal abnormalities. No secondary signs of embolism, such as pleural effusion, oligemia, or apparent hilar enlargement, can be seen. **C,** Pulmonary arteriogram with an injection in the main pulmonary artery reveals extensive clot in the left-sided circulation *(arrows)*. Some contrast is seen distal to the clots, which do not completely occlude the involved arteries in this case.

In the experience of most investigators studying PE, if a patient has a limited number of matched abnormalities in ventilation and perfusion but the radiograph of the respective area is normal, the probability of PE is still low, on the order of 5% to 15% or 5% to 20% (Fig. 7-10).

## Practical Approach to Interpreting the Ventilation-Perfusion Scintigram

The complexity of interpreting V/Q studies, including integration of information from the chest radiograph, warrants a rigorous systematic approach. This is not a study that can or should be interpreted hastily. The following approach is used successfully in a number of institutions.

First, the chest radiograph is reviewed and all abnormalities are recorded. Ideally the radiograph is obtained at the same time as the V/Q study and with the patient in the same position. The most common chest radiographic abnormalities in patients with PE are pleural effusion, an elevated hemidiaphragm, and atelectasis. Oligemia (Westermark's sign) and opacities associated with pulmonary infarction are less common; enlargement of the pulmo-

nary artery is also less common. Although large pleural effusions are rarely caused by PE, they can obscure significant portions of the pulmonary parenchyma, and large effusions often render V/Q scintigraphy indeterminate. Other common findings resulting from intercurrent disease in patients referred for suspected PE are cardiomegaly, pulmonary parenchymal opacities, hilar enlargement, and signs of airway disease. Occasionally a pneumothorax is seen and may account for the patient's clinical signs and symptoms.

After review of the chest radiograph all segmental or subsegmental perfusion defects are identified on the perfusion scan and recorded by location. The ventilation scan is then reviewed in the area of each perfusion defect. The number and location of V/Q mismatches are recorded, and each in turn is compared with the corresponding area on the chest radiograph. If the perfusion defect has no radiographic explanation and the ventilation scan is normal, the mismatched areas are candidates for sites of PE. Some authorities assign high probability in the face of one or more large segment-sized mismatches. The PIOPED criteria (Box 7-7) require two segment-sized defects or their aggregate equivalent for a classification of high probability. The larger the

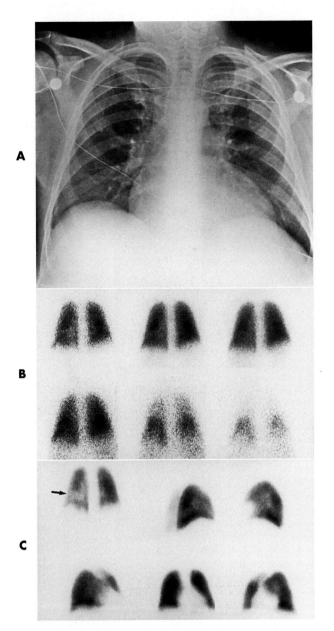

**Fig. 7-10** **A,** Chest radiograph reveals some cardiomegaly and blunting of the right costophrenic angle. The lungs are clear, without focal opacities. **B,** Ventilation study with xenon-133 reveals good distribution on the initial breath image and equilibrium images *(top row)*. The washout images show significant delay in clearance from the lung bases bilaterally. **C,** Corresponding technetium-99m MAA perfusion study reveals a large area of relatively decreased perfusion in the left lower lobe *(arrow)* and a smaller area at the right base in the general region of the ventilation abnormalities. The combination of matched ventilation-perfusion defect with no corresponding radiographic abnormality indicates a low probability of pulmonary embolism.

number of mismatched segments, the higher the likelihood of PE.

If no moderate or large segmental mismatches are demonstrated, attention is turned to seeing whether the study can be categorized as low probability or less. Areas

of V/Q match and no corresponding radiographic abnormality have empirically been associated with a low probability of PE (Box 7-7). The presence of any number of small subsegmental perfusion defects with a correspondingly normal chest radiograph also falls in the low-probability category. Finally, any perfusion defect with a substantially larger chest radiographic abnormality and nonsegmental perfusion defects resulting from an identifiable cause such as enlargement of the heart, aorta, or hila fall in the low-probability category.

If the study cannot be categorized as high probability, low probability, or normal, it is by definition indeterminate, and the various radiographic, perfusion, and ventilation abnormalities are described for documentation in the report. It should be emphasized again that the threshold for reaching the intermediate or indeterminate category is now taken as a single moderate segmental mismatch. Also falling into the intermediate category are the presence of two or three moderate segmental mismatches or one moderate and one large segmental mismatch. Once the aggregate number and size of defects reach two large segment size defects or greater, the threshold for high probability is reached.

Approaching the diagnosis by adhering to institutionally agreed-on diagnostic criteria keeps the observer from pingponging back and forth between abnormalities. It also makes the results of the V/Q study more reliable and more meaningful to the clinician receiving the report than would a less organized or even a gestalt approach.

## Accuracy of Ventilation-Perfusion Scintigraphy

In the PIOPED trial the specificity of a V/Q study with a high probability was 97%. However, only 41% of patients shown by angiography to have PE had a high-probability pattern scintigraphically. In a way this is a disappointingly low sensitivity, but it must be remembered that V/Q scintigraphy is not a test of PE per se but a test of lung function. By setting the threshold for a high-probability interpretation at the level of two or more large-segment mismatches, the specificity is kept high at the expense of sensitivity. If the criteria were relaxed—for example, to require only one large mismatch or one large and one moderate mismatch for assignment of high probability for PE—the sensitivity for detecting PE would go up, but at the expense of specificity (Figs. 7-11 and 7-12). The high specificity allows us to recommend that in the appropriate clinical setting a high-probability interpretation provides sufficient diagnostic certainty for a clinician to begin anticoagulation without resorting to pulmonary angiography. Patients with significant risk factors for anticoagulation may still require angiography.

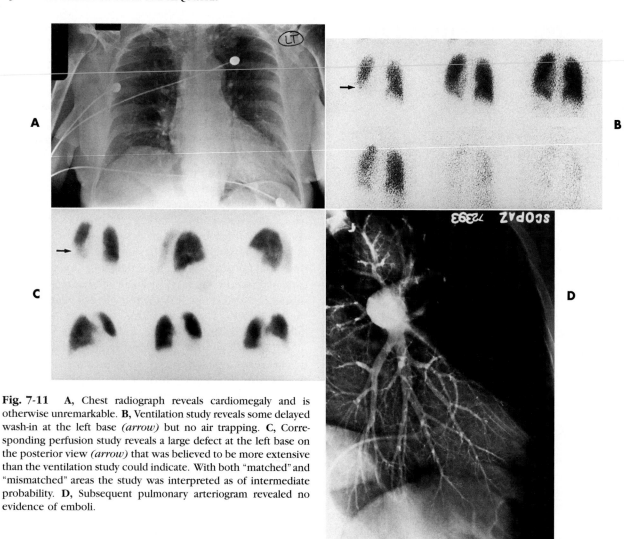

**Fig. 7-11    A,** Chest radiograph reveals cardiomegaly and is otherwise unremarkable. **B,** Ventilation study reveals some delayed wash-in at the left base *(arrow)* but no air trapping. **C,** Corresponding perfusion study reveals a large defect at the left base on the posterior view *(arrow)* that was believed to be more extensive than the ventilation study could indicate. With both "matched" and "mismatched" areas the study was interpreted as of intermediate probability. **D,** Subsequent pulmonary arteriogram revealed no evidence of emboli.

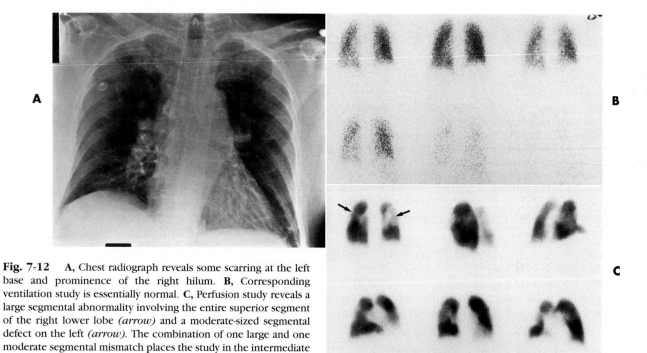

**Fig. 7-12    A,** Chest radiograph reveals some scarring at the left base and prominence of the right hilum. **B,** Corresponding ventilation study is essentially normal. **C,** Perfusion study reveals a large segmental abnormality involving the entire superior segment of the right lower lobe *(arrow)* and a moderate-sized segmental defect on the left *(arrow)*. The combination of one large and one moderate segmental mismatch places the study in the intermediate probability category.

In the PIOPED series the percentage of patients with angiographically demonstrated thromboemboli and intermediate-probability study interpretations was 33%. When both clinical outcome and angiographic findings were used, the occurrence of PE in the low-probability and the normal or near-normal interpretive categories was 12% and 4%, respectively.

A unique feature of the PIOPED study was a complete clinical evaluation of the patients before they underwent scintigraphy or angiography. Each patient was assigned a "clinical science" probability of having PE. When the clinical probabilities were compared with the scan-based probabilities, the results were striking. Of patients with a high-probability scintigraphic interpretation and a high clinical probability of having PE, 96% were shown to have PE by angiography. On the other hand, when the clinical probability was low and the scintigraphic interpretation was normal or near-normal, only one (<2%) of 61 patients was found to have PE by angiography. These remarkable observations illustrate the importance of interpreting test results in the clinical context.

Another important observation from the PIOPED study is the low likelihood of an adverse clinical outcome in patients with low-probability and normal scintigraphic patterns. In the study 150 patients who had either a low-probability or normal/near-normal scan but who did not undergo angiography were followed up for at least 1 year. No patient had an adverse event or readmission to the hospital for suspected PE. Some may well have had small pulmonary emboli, but none received anticoagulant therapy and the clinical course was unremarkable. This finding supports several other studies that suggest a benign clinical course in low-probability cases.

### Differential Diagnosis

Differential possibilities for V/Q mismatch are listed in Box 7-8. These are potential causes of false positive interpretations. One of the most vexing is chronic PE with incomplete resolution of clot and incomplete restoration of pulmonary perfusion. If an old examina-

tion or baseline study is available for comparison, it should be consulted to avoid this pitfall. In one large study assessing the sensitivity and specificity of V/Q scintigraphy, in which observers were blinded to prior history and prior test results, chronic PE was the most common cause of false positive interpretations. Unfortunately, in clinical practice many patients coming for evaluation have not undergone prior scintigraphic studies. A clinical history can prevent this kind of misinterpretation.

Data on the time course of the resolution of PE are disappointingly scarce in the literature, probably because most studies have been retrospective. Sequential follow-up V/Q scans are generally not obtained on a routine basis. Factors favoring early, complete resolution are small size of the emboli, no preexisting or intercurrent comorbidity, and younger patient age. Small emboli in otherwise healthy young subjects may resolve in 24 hours. Large emboli in older patients with underlying lung disease may never resolve completely (Fig. 7-13). An important point is that the pattern of perfusion defects may change even without recurrent emboli. As large proximal clots break up, either spontaneously or because of therapy, they may relodge more peripherally.

The large vascular structures of the lung, especially the pulmonary veins, are relatively compressible compared with the larger bronchi. Hilar tumors, either primary or metastatic to the lung, may obstruct these

---

**Box 7-8    Conditions Associated with Ventilation-Perfusion Mismatch**

Acute pulmonary embolism
Chronic pulmonary embolism
Other causes of embolism (drug abuse, iatrogenic)
Bronchogenic carcinoma (other tumors)
Mediastinal or hilar adenopathy with obstruction of pulmonary artery or veins
Hypoplasia or aplasia of pulmonary artery
Swyer-James syndrome (some cases)
Post radiation therapy
Vasculitis

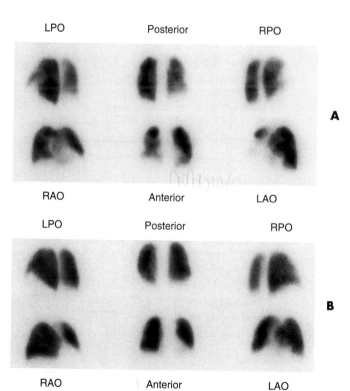

**Fig. 7-13    A,** Perfusion scintigram reveals multiple segmental defects in a patient with angiographically proven pulmonary emboli. **B,** Follow-up study 4 months later shows significant but not complete resolution.

vessels, decreasing regional perfusion. This pattern can mimic PE unless a mass is discernible on the chest radiograph.

Common conditions resulting in matched V/Q abnormalities are summarized in Box 7-9 (Fig. 7-14). In patients with asthma, bronchoconstriction causes a reflex decrease in perfusion. The classic pattern on V/Q scintigraphy is multiple matched ventilation and perfusion defects. Patients with congestive heart failure have variable degrees of perfusion abnormality that are due to pulmonary congestion and pleural fluid. In areas of blebs and bullae, destruction of the lung parenchyma results in absence of perfusion. During the wash-in phase of the ventilation study the corresponding areas demonstrate decreased tracer distribution. During equilibration the radioactive xenon can gain access to the bullae, with evidence of trapping and delayed clearance on the washout phase of the ventilation study. Obviously, on ventilation studies performed with radioaerosols, bullae are seen as cold areas. Chronic bronchitis and bronchiectasis cause actual destruction of the

---

**Box 7-9  Conditions Typically Associated with V/Q Matched Abnormalities**

Chronic obstructive pulmonary disease
Bronchitis and bronchiectasis
Blebs and bullae
Congestive heart failure
Pulmonary edema
Pleural effusion
Asthma
Pulmonary trauma, hematoma
Inhalation injury
Mucus plugs
Bronchogenic carcinoma (other tumors)

---

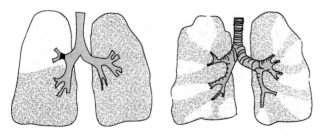

**Fig. 7-14**  Ventilation abnormalities may be due to obstructions in larger airways as might be caused by bronchogenic carcinoma or by mucus plugs. Constriction of smaller bronchi in asthma can also cause ventilation abnormalities *(right diagram)*.

bronchial walls, with decreased perfusion in the affected area. Correspondingly, ventilation is decreased with delayed wash-in and air trapping occurs with delayed clearance.

## Special Signs

A number of special signs can aid in the interpretation of V/Q studies. The *stripe sign* refers to a margin of radioactivity between a perfusion defect and the pleural surface of the lung. Because the pulmonary circulation branches progressively toward the pleural surface, most pulmonary emboli result in pleura-based and wedge-shaped defects. The presence of interposed activity (the stripe) suggests a parenchymal abnormality such as pulmonary hemorrhage or other fluid accumulation rather than PE.

The *swinging heart* sign refers to unusually large cardiac defects seen on lateral views when the patient has been imaged lying down and turned to the right and left sides for the lateral views. The heart has a certain mobility in the chest and may displace or compress lung tissue, resulting in this somewhat confusing appearance.

Fluid in the pleural space can be difficult to recognize if patients are imaged in the supine position. Fluid in a layer between the lung and the gamma camera increases attenuation of activity. If the fluid is unilateral, a uniform difference in intensity between the two lungs is seen (Fig. 7-15). Unless the cause is recognized, this can be quite confusing because the asymmetry is seen only on the dependent view. Similarly, if the patient is imaged in the upright position, a subpulmonic collection of fluid may be missed if radiographic/scintigraphic correlation is not carried out carefully. Fluid in the interlobar fissures causes curvilinear perfusion defects (*fissure sign*) that may or may not have corresponding radiographic findings (Fig. 7-16).

Patients with pacemakers have easily recognizable imaging defects. The pacemakers have clear borders and do not correspond in shape or location to pulmonary segments, nor are they seen as defects on orthogonal views (Fig. 7-15). Smaller defects may be seen if electrocardiographic monitoring leads are left on the patient.

## Computed Tomography in the Diagnosis of Pulmonary Embolism

With the availability of electron beam and helical CT, a number of investigators have explored the use of these modalities in the diagnosis of PE. Early reports in highly selected patient populations were optimistic. Although it is too early to come to a definitive conclusion about the role of CT, a number of observations can be made. First, clots can be directly visualized as negative filling defects on contrast-enhanced CT scans (Figs. 7-17 and 7-18). Second, the ability to see clots is better in the larger, more central vessels. Visualization of subsegmental vessels is a problem. Third, the specificity of CT scanning when interpreted by an experienced practitioner is very high, in the same range (>95%) as the high-probability category for V/Q scintigraphy. Thus the direct identification of a clot by CT scanning and the finding of a high-probability V/Q scan are both associated with a high positive predictive value for the presence of PE.

Questions that remain to be answered about the CT approach are the optimal selection of technical param-

eters such as collimation, pitch, and reconstruction interval and the optimal parameters for the use of contrast material, including volume, concentration, and timing. The work to date is likely to be repeated with multislice CT scanners.

Unless and until additional research demonstrates improved sensitivity for the CT technique, V/Q scintigraphy will remain the preferred approach. V/Q scintigraphy uses less toxic radiopharmaceuticals than radiographic contrast media, and the negative predictive value of normal V/Q scans is superior to that of a negative CT scan. Nonetheless, institutions that have CT scanners but do not have access to V/Q imaging may well adopt the CT approach.

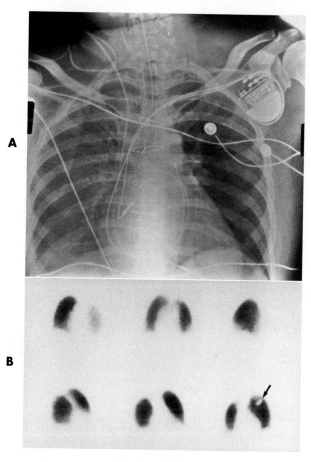

**Fig. 7-15**    **A,** Chest radiograph reveals the uniformly greater density in the right lung compared with the left lung, which is caused by layering out of fluid posteriorly when the patient is supine. The patient has a pacemaker in the left axilla. **B,** Corresponding technetium-99m MAA perfusion study reveals uniformly decreased activity in the right lung as seen on the posterior view. Apparent activity is equal in both lungs on all other views, tipping off the observer to the explanation for the discrepancy in the posterior view. The pacemaker causes a well-defined defect *(arrow).*

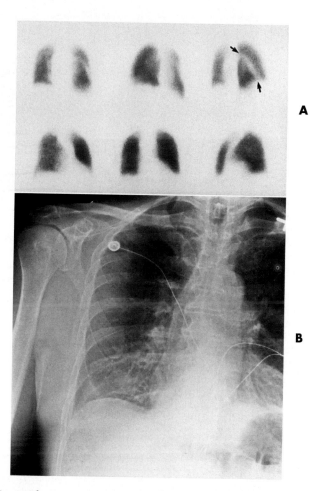

**Fig. 7-16**    **A,** Technetium-99m MAA perfusion scan reveals a curvilinear defect in the area of the major fissure of the right lung ("fissure sign") *(arrows).* The study is otherwise unremarkable. **B,** Corresponding chest radiograph reveals blunting of the right costophrenic angle but provides no indication of the extensive fluid accumulation in the fissure.

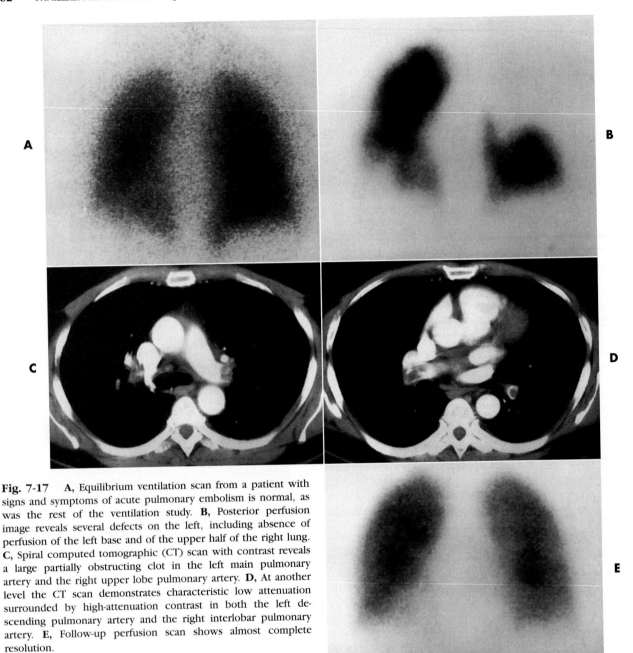

**Fig. 7-17** **A,** Equilibrium ventilation scan from a patient with signs and symptoms of acute pulmonary embolism is normal, as was the rest of the ventilation study. **B,** Posterior perfusion image reveals several defects on the left, including absence of perfusion of the left base and of the upper half of the right lung. **C,** Spiral computed tomographic (CT) scan with contrast reveals a large partially obstructing clot in the left main pulmonary artery and the right upper lobe pulmonary artery. **D,** At another level the CT scan demonstrates characteristic low attenuation surrounded by high-attenuation contrast in both the left descending pulmonary artery and the right interlobar pulmonary artery. **E,** Follow-up perfusion scan shows almost complete resolution.

## OTHER APPLICATIONS OF VENTILATION-PERFUSION SCINTIGRAPHY

A number of other clinical applications have been suggested for V/Q scintigraphy. None of these has approached the importance of evaluating patients with suspected PE. In some institutions patients undergoing lung resection are studied with quantitative V/Q imaging. The percentage of overall ventilation and perfusion of each lung can be determined. For example, if a patient has an apparently operable lung carcinoma on one side but poor overall lung function, an estimate of the remaining postoperative lung function can be critical in making the decision to operate. In patients undergoing unilateral lung transplantation, quantitative imaging is useful for monitoring the function of the transplanted lung (Figs. 7-19 and 7-20).

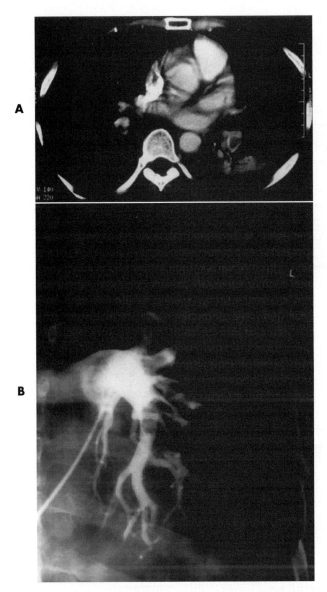

**Fig. 7-18**    **A,** Helical computed tomography demonstrates characteristic low attenuation in the lumen of the left descending pulmonary artery with surrounding contrast media. This pattern is characteristic of pulmonary embolism. **B,** Corresponding pulmonary angiogram confirms the presence of multiple clots in the pulmonary circulation.

## DETECTION OF VENOUS THROMBOSIS

Although the major thrust of this chapter is the diagnosis of PE, the search for the origin of emboli is also a clinical objective. The development of new techniques for detecting venous thrombi has produced substantial advancements over the past decade. The traditional radiographic test is contrast venography. This procedure is somewhat cumbersome to perform, and in patients

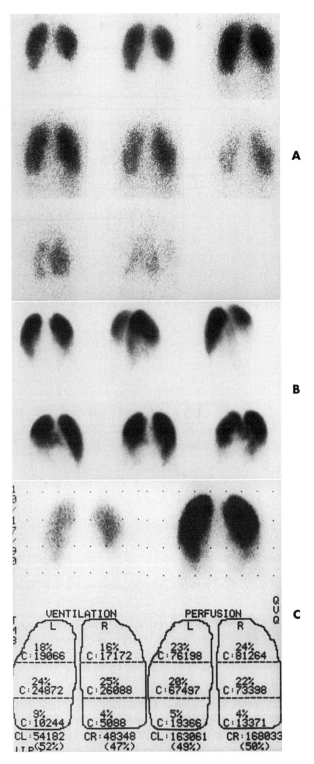

**Fig. 7-19**    **A,** Xenon-133 ventilation study in a patient with alpha-1-antitrypsin disorder. Extensive ventilation abnormality is visible at the lung bases bilaterally with delayed wash-in and air trapping. **B,** Corresponding technetium-99m perfusion study reveals fairly symmetrical perfusion deficits at both lung bases. **C,** Preoperative quantitative analysis of right and left lung ventilation and perfusion reveals essentially symmetrical function.

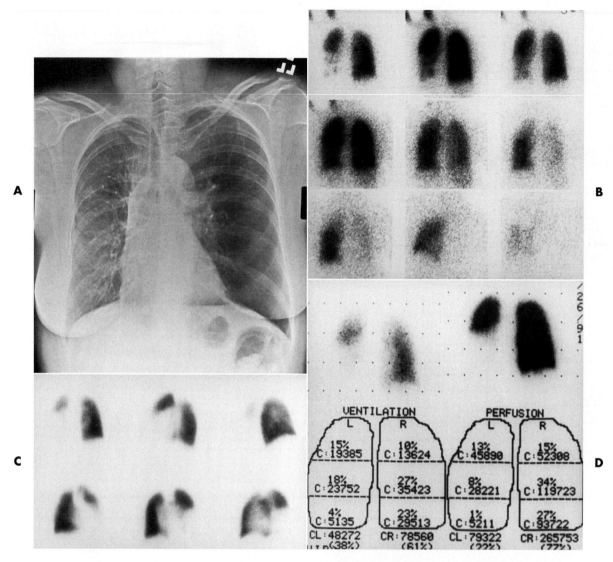

**Fig. 7-20** **A,** Patient with the alpha-1-antitrypsin deficiency underwent right lung transplantation. Postoperative chest radiograph reveals hyperlucency of the left lung compared with the transplanted right lung. **B,** Postoperative ventilation study reveals continued ventilation abnormality in the native left lung and normal ventilatory dynamics in the transplanted right lung. **C,** Corresponding perfusion study reveals essentially normal homogeneous perfusion on the right with marked abnormality on the left. **D,** Postoperative quantitative analysis of ventilation and perfusion confirms the improved function on the right. The right lung accounts for 61% of the ventilation and 77% of the perfusion.

with significant venous compromise it may actually result in phlebitis because of stasis of contrast media. Also, contrast venography does not permit the diagnosis of pelvic venous thrombosis.

Some nuclear medicine clinics take advantage of the dosage administration process for pulmonary perfusion scanning to perform a combined radionuclide venogram and perfusion study. The radiopharmaceutical is administered through a vein in the foot and forced into the deep system through application of a tourniquet above the ankle. Interpretation below the knee is difficult because of the number of deep veins and the

inability to resolve them as individual structures scintigraphically. However, above the knee, radionuclide venography is very sensitive in demonstrating venous thrombosis. In addition to venous obstruction (Fig. 7-21), the key diagnostic findings are the presence of collaterals and focal accumulations of Tc-99m MAA at the trailing end of thrombi (Fig. 7-22). The radionuclide technique also has some utility in the iliac external and inferior vena caval systems. The dilutional effects that hamper contrast venography are not a problem in the same way. Abnormalities in the external iliac veins and vena cava can be demonstrated. The technique obvi-

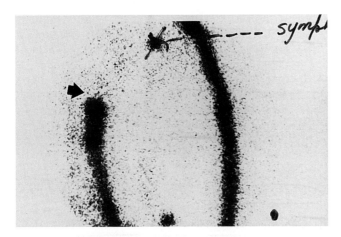

**Fig. 7-21** Radionuclide venogram demonstrates venous obstruction on the right caused by thrombus *(arrow)*.

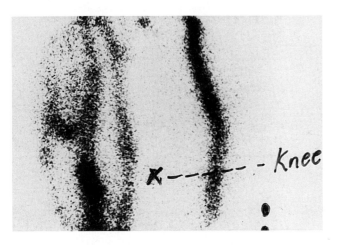

**Fig. 7-22** Radionuclide venogram demonstrates extensive collateralization, indicating obstruction of the deep venous system.

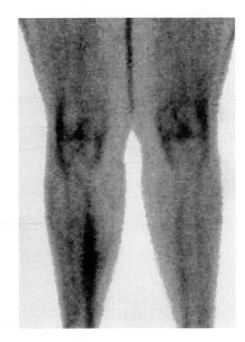

**Fig. 7-23** Acute thrombophlebitis detected by technetium-99m apcitide. Uptake is increased in the area of the right calf.

ously does not provide information about the internal iliac veins.

A number of new radionuclide techniques have been described. Antifibrin monoclonal antibodies labeled with a variety of radionuclides, including Tc-99m, have shown some promise. The advantage of the antifibrin technique is the ability to identify thrombi owing to direct uptake of the radiopharmaceutical. Although early experience suggests that sensitivity is greater in the thigh, the technique is also applicable below the knee. Further advances in "hot spot" radionuclide imaging techniques for detection of thrombi are likely to be made.

Various radiolabeled peptides are being tested. One of these, Tc-99m apcitide, has recently undergone clinical trials with moderately encouraging results. It has been approved by the FDA and is commercially available. The agent is a synthetic peptide that binds to glycoprotein IIb/IIIa on the surface of activated platelets. Areas

of acute thrombophlebitis accumulate the tracer (Fig. 7-23). An advantage over Doppler ultrasound is the ability to visualize disease below the knee. The efficacy of Tc-99m apcitide is apparently not adversely affected by anticoagulation.

Doppler imaging in conjunction with various compression techniques continues to be used to assess the integrity of the venous system. Thrombosed veins are not compressible and exhibit altered flow patterns. The technique is best applied above the knee because of difficulty in identifying the venous structures in the calf.

## ADULT RESPIRATORY DISTRESS SYNDROME

The rate of clearance of aerosolized Tc-99m-DTPA is significantly affected by the presence of pulmonary disease. The clearance half-time is approximately 80 minutes in healthy subjects. In patients with adult respiratory distress syndrome the clearance is faster, probably because of more rapid diffusion of Tc-99m-DTPA across the airspace epithelium to the pulmonary circulation. Other conditions associated with more rapid clearance are cigarette smoking, alveolitis, and hyaline membrane disease in infants. A clear-cut clinical utility has not been established for the application of the technique, although possibly serial studies could be used to guide therapy and assess its efficacy.

## SUGGESTED READINGS

Alavi A, Palevsky HI, editors: Nuclear medicine's role in thromboembolic disease, *Semin Nucl Med* xxi:273-346, 1991.

Alderson PO, Martin EC: Pulmonary embolism: diagnosis with multiple imaging modalities, *Radiology* 164:297-312, 1987.

Alderson PO, Rujanavech N, Secker-Walker RH, et al: The role of 133Xe ventilation studies in the scintigraphic detection of pulmonary embolism, *Radiology* 120:633-640, 1976.

Bedont RA, Datz FL: Lung scan perfusion defects limited to matching pleural effusions: low probability of pulmonary embolism, *AJR* 145:1155-1160, 1985.

Biello DR, Mattar AG, McKnight RC, et al: Ventilation-perfusion studies in suspected pulmonary embolism, *AJR* 133:1033-1037, 1979.

Biello DR, Mattar AG, Osei-Wusu A, et al: Interpretation of indeterminate lung scintigrams, *Radiology* 133:189-194, 1979.

Carson JL, Kelley MA, Duff AH, et al: The clinical course of pulmonary embolism: one year follow-up of PIOPED patients, *N Engl J Med* 326:1240-1245, 1992.

Carter WD, Brady TM, Keyes JW, et al: Relative accuracy of two diagnostic schemes for detection of pulmonary embolism by ventilation-perfusion scintigraphy, *Radiology* 145:447-451, 1982.

Drucker EA, Rivity SM, Shepard J, et al: Acute pulmonary embolism: assessment of helical CT for diagnosis, *Radiology* 209:235-241, 1998.

Freitas JE, Sarosi MG, Nagle CC, et al: Modified PIOPED criteria used in clinical practice, *J Nucl Med* 37:1573-1578, 1995.

Gottschalk A, Juni JE, Sostman HD, et al: Ventilation-perfusion scintigraphy in the PIOPED study. I. Data collection and tabulation, *J Nucl Med* 34:1109-1118, 1993.

Gottschalk A, Sostman HD, Coleman RE, et al: Ventilation-perfusion scintigraphy in the PIOPED study. II. Evaluation of the scintigraphic criteria and interpretations, *J Nucl Med* 34:1119-1126, 1993.

Jacobson AF, Patel N, Lewis DH: Clinical outcome of patients with intermediate probability lung scans during six-month follow-up, *J Nucl Med* 38:1593-1596, 1997.

Lee ME, Biello DR, Kumar B, et al: "Low probability" ventilation-perfusion scintigrams: clinical outcomes in 99 patients, *Radiology* 156:497-500, 1985.

Magnussen JS, Chicco P, Palmer AW, et al: Optimization of the scintigraphic segmental anatomy of the lungs, *J Nucl Med* 38:1987-1991, 1997.

PIOPED Investigators: Value of the ventilation/perfusion scan in acute pulmonary embolism: results of the prospective investigation of pulmonary embolism diagnosis (PIOPED), *JAMA* 263:2753-2759, 1990.

Remy-Jordin M, Remy J, Deschildre F, et al: Diagnosis of pulmonary embolism with spiral CT: comparison with pulmonary angiography and scintigraphy, *Radiology* 200:699-706, 1996.

Sostman HD, Coleman RE, DeLong DM, et al: Evaluation of revised criteria for ventilation-perfusion scintigraphy in patients with suspected pulmonary embolism, *Radiology* 193:103-107, 1994.

Sostman HD, Gottschalk A: A prospective validation of the stripe sign in ventilation-perfusion scintigraphy, *Radiology* 184:455-459, 1982.

Tourassi GD, Folyd CE, Coleman RE: Improved noninvasive diagnosis of embolism with optimally selected clinical and chest radiographic findings, *Acad Radiol* 3:1012-1018, 1996.

Trujillo NP, Pratt JP, Tahisani S, et al: DTPA aerosol in ventilation/perfusion scintigraphy for diagnosing pulmonary embolism, *J Nucl Med* 38:1781-1783, 1997.

# CHAPTER 8

# Infection and Inflammation

*Leukopenic pts (<3000) → Ga*
*Abdominal ⎤*
*Osteomyelitis ⎦ In¹¹¹ better*
*Diskitis Ga*
*FUO — ??In¹¹¹ better.*
*IBD —⎤ Tc HMPAO WBCS.*
*Paeds ⎦*

*Urgent results → Tc HMPAO WBCs*

Nuclear medicine imaging has played a role in the diagnosis and localization of infection since the early 1970s, when gallium-67 (Ga-67) citrate was first noted to have an infection-seeking property in addition to its already appreciated tumor avidity. In the mid-1980s, in vitro labeling of leukocytes with indium-111 (In-111) oxine was FDA approved for imaging of infection. Although In-111 oxine–labeled leukocytes are widely and successfully used for localizing infectious and other inflammatory processes, the method has disadvantages, including a lengthy preparation time and routine imaging 24 hours after injection. In addition, it has relatively high dosimetry, which dictates a low administered dose, long imaging times, and suboptimal imaging characteristics. Furthermore, transmission of bloodborne infections to personnel and patients is a serious potential problem.

The more recent availability of a technetium-99m (Tc-99m)-labeled white blood cell radiopharmaceutical (Tc-99m hexamethylpropylene amine oxime [HMPAO] leukocytes) has resulted in better images and lower radiation dose to the patient, but the problem of handling blood products remains. A number of new radiopharmaceuticals with various mechanisms of uptake, such as nonspecific immune globulin, monocolonal antibodies, and chemotactic peptides, are under investigation,

## Box 8-1    Status of U.S. Food and Drug Administration Approval for Infection-Imaging Radiopharmaceuticals

**APPROVED**

Gallium-67 citrate
Indium-111 oxine-labeled leukocytes
Technetium-99m HMPAO–labeled leukocytes

**INVESTIGATIONAL**

Radiolabeled:
  Nonspecific immunoglobulins
  Monoclonal antigranulocyte antibodies
  Albumin nanocolloid
  Chemotactic peptides
  Cytokines and chemokines (interleukins)
  Liposomes

**Table 8-1    Physical characteristics of gallium-67 and indium-111**

| Radionuclide | Half-life (hr) | Photopeak (keV) | Relative abundance of photons per 100 disintegrations (%) |
|---|---|---|---|
| Gallium-67 | 78 | 91-93 | 41 |
| | | 185 | 23 |
| | | 300 | 18 |
| | | 394 | 4 |
| Indium-111 | 67 | 173 | 89 |
| | | 247 | 94 |

and some of these are expected to become available in the near future (Box 8-1). Most of these latter methods do not require cell labeling and thus avoid its problems.

## PATHOPHYSIOLOGY OF INFLAMMATION AND INFECTION

Inflammation is a response of tissues to injury that brings cells of the immune system and other specialized serum proteins and chemical mediators to the site of damage. Infection implies the presence of microorganisms, although there can be inflammation without infection. The inflammatory reaction is triggered by products of tissue injury. In addition to infection, tissue injury can result from trauma, foreign particles, ischemia, and neoplasm. Infection can be present without inflammation, as occurs in severely immunosuppressed patients.

The classic signs of inflammation are redness, swelling, heat, and pain. The inflammatory response results in regionally increased blood flow, increased permeability of the venules in the affected region, and emigration of leukocytes out of the blood vessels into the tissues (chemotaxis). The plasma carries to the site of inflammation leukocytes and a variety of proteins, such as opsonins, complement factors, and antibodies, as well as chemical mediators, such as histamine, serotonin, and bradykinin, that modulate the inflammatory response.

Early identification and localization of infection are important for the appropriate and timely selection of therapy. Traditional radiological imaging methods, such as computed tomography (CT), magnetic resonance imaging (MRI), and ultrasonography, can be used to diagnose infection and inflammatory processes by detecting the resulting anatomical changes. However,

these techniques may be unsuccessful in locating the site of infection. In the early phase of infectious and inflammatory processes, anatomical change may be insufficient. In addition, diagnostic changes can be difficult to differentiate from successfully treated processes or postoperative changes. Furthermore, these methodologies usually image a body region, not the whole body.

In many cases radionuclide imaging methods can be used to diagnose and pinpoint the site of infection. Since scintigraphic methods are physiologically based, infection and inflammation can be diagnosed in their earliest stages and the results are not affected by prior therapy or surgery. Radionuclide studies also permit whole body imaging.

## GALLIUM-67 CITRATE

Ga-67 was developed as a bone-seeking radiopharmaceutical but found use clinically as a tumor-imaging agent. Its infection-seeking property was subsequently noted in the early 1970s, and Ga-67 became the mainstay of infection scintigraphy for over a decade. It still has important clinical utility in specific clinical situations.

### Chemistry and Physics

Gallium is a group III element in the Periodic Table with biological behavior similar to iron. The radionuclide Ga-67 is cyclotron produced. It decays by electron capture, emits a spectrum of gamma rays (93, 185, 300, 394 keV), and has a physical half-life of 78 hours (Table 8-1).

### Pharmacokinetics and Normal Distribution

Ga-67 citrate acts like a ferric ion analog and circulates in blood bound to transferrin. It is transported to cellular receptors and incorporated intracellularly. Within 24

low specific activity — more atoms to make up same amount of activity

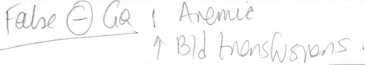

*False ⊖ Ga ↑ Anemia*
*↑ Bld transfusions.*

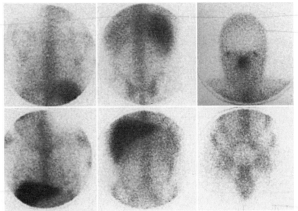

**Fig. 8-1**   Normal gallium-67 distribution at 48 hours. Greatest uptake is in the liver. Bone and marrow uptake are also prominent. Lesser uptake is seen in the spleen and scrotum. Lacrimal gland and nasopharygeal uptake is present. *Left column,* Posterior *(above)* and anterior chest *(below). Middle column,* Posterior *(above)* and anterior abdomen *(below). Right column,* Anterior head *(above)* and pelvis *(below).*

---

**Box 8-2   Mechanisms of Localization of Infection-Seeking Radiopharmaceuticals**

| RADIOPHARMACEUTICAL | MECHANISM |
| --- | --- |
| Gallium-67 citrate | Vascular permeability, binding to lactoferrin *transferrin* |
| Leukocytes | Diapedesis and chemotaxis |
| Nonspecific IgG antibodies | Increased vascularity, nonimmunological |
| Monoclonal antigranulocyte antibodies | Antibody-antigen binding to activated leukocytes |
| Chemotactic peptides | Binding to activated leukocytes |
| Nanocolloids | Increased vascular permeability |
| Liposomes | Increased vascular permeability |

---

hours of administration, 15% to 25% of the injected dose is excreted via the kidneys. Subsequently the colon is the major route of excretion. Total body clearance is slow, with a biological half-life of 25 days. Ga-67 uptake is highest in the liver, but normal uptake also takes place in the salivary glands, spleen, bone, marrow, and lacrimal glands (Fig. 8-1). Lacrimal gland uptake is due to the binding of Ga-67 to lactoferrin. Ga-67 is excreted in breast milk.

In vivo, Ga-67 distribution can be altered by whole body irradiation, an excess of carrier gallium or ferric ion (as with multiple transfusions), or gadolinium exposure (e.g., after an MRI study). The mechanism for the latter two is saturation of the protein-binding sites.

---

## Mechanism of Uptake

After transport to the site of inflammation or infection by transferrin, localization depends on various factors. An *adequate blood supply* is a primary requisite for localization. The Ga-67–transferrin complex is delivered to an inflammatory site as a result of increased blood flow and *increased vascular permeability* of the capillaries (Box 8-2).

Although *bacterial uptake* and *binding to leukocytes* occur, these do not seem to be the major mechanisms of localization. The neutrophil plays an important indirect role. After migration to a site of infection, neutrophils degranulate and deposit large amounts of lactoferrin. Physiologically lactoferrin traps free ferric ions, which inhibit bacterial growth. Ga-67 localizes at the site of inflammation by binding to lactoferrin, since Ga-67 has a higher affinity for lactoferrin than for the transporting protein, transferrin.

## Imaging Characteristics

Ga-67 is not an optimal imaging agent. It emits four photopeaks ranging from 100 to 400 keV (Table 8-1). The lower energy photons result in a high percentage of scatter relative to usable photons. The higher energy photons are difficult to collimate and not efficiently detected by present-day thin gamma camera crystals. For maximal sensitivity the three lower photopeaks (93, 185, and 300 keV) should be acquired.

## Methodology

For imaging of infection the usual administered adult dose of Ga-67 is 5 mCi (pediatric dose 40 mCi/kg). Image acquisition is typically performed at 48 hours (Box 8-3). This allows time for background clearance that results in an improved target-to-background ratio. However, imaging at 6 to 24 hours is sometimes useful. In patients with suspected intraabdominal abscess, early diagnosis may allow prompt intervention.

Early imaging at 24 hours can sometimes help differentiate infection from physiological bowel clearance. Abdominal activity not seen at 24 hours but seen at 48 hours probably represents normal bowel clearance and not a site of acute infection. Further delayed imaging, laxatives, and enemas may be needed to confirm this.

Opinion differs regarding the routine preimaging use of laxatives and enemas to facilitate normal bowel clearance. Vigorous bowel cleansing is not always effective and can produce mucosal irritation and inflammation, which may result in increased Ga-67 uptake.

*In pts c̄ Iron overload — decreased uptake*
*∴ see ↑ renal excretion, ↓ bone.*

## Normal Distribution

Table 8-2 compares the normal distribution of the various infection-imaging radiopharmaceuticals. The organ with the greatest Ga-67 uptake is the liver. Lesser uptake is seen in the spleen. Uptake in bone and bone marrow can be seen prominently throughout the axial and proximal appendicular skeleton (Fig. 8-1). Other normal sites of variable uptake and distribution are the nasopharynx and the lacrimal and salivary glands. The kidneys and bladder are seen during the first 24 hours after tracer injection owing to normal renal clearance. By 48 to 72 hours the kidneys are only faintly visualized except in patients with renal failure.

After 24 hours, biological clearance is mainly through the large bowel. Diffuse lung uptake is often seen at 24 hours but clears by 48 hours. Breast uptake is variable, depending to some extent on the phase of the woman's hormonal cycle. Uptake may be quite prominent post partum (Fig. 8-2). Thymus uptake is sometimes noted in children, most commonly after chemotherapy (Fig. 8-3). Other areas of low-grade normal uptake are the scrotum, testes, and female perineum.

Postoperative sites may have Ga-67 uptake for 2 to 3 weeks. Uptake may occur in sterile abscesses associated with frequent intramuscular injections (for example, insulin injections in diabetics, depot injections of iron). Increased salivary gland uptake may be seen after local external beam irradiation or chemotherapy.

---

### Box 8-3    Gallium-67 Citrate Imaging: Protocol Summary

**PATIENT PREPARATION**

No recent barium contrast studies

**RADIOPHARMACEUTICAL**

Gallium-67 citrate, 5 mCi (185 MBq) injected intravenously *kids 40 mci/kg*

**INSTRUMENTATION**

Camera: Large-field-of-view gamma camera
Photopeak: 20% window over 93-, 185-, and 300-keV
  photopeaks
Collimator: Medium (or high) energy

**IMAGING PROCEDURE**

24-hr images (optional): Site of suspected infection if
  early intervention considered; abdominal images
  may be helpful for interpreting activity seen at 48
  hours
48-hr images: Whole body imaging, including head and
  extremities, unless the site of suspected infection is
  limited to one site, e.g., hip prosthesis
Delayed 72- to 96-hr images of abdomen as indicated
  to differentiate intraabdominal infection from normal
  bowel clearance; laxatives or enemas as needed
SPECT of the abdomen, pelvis, or chest as indicated

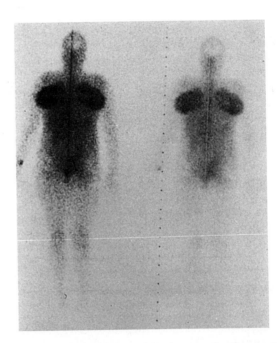

**Fig. 8-2**    Postpartum gallium-67 uptake in the breast. Breast uptake is normal but can vary from patient to patient and is often quite intense post partum. Two intensity settings are shown.

---

### Table 8-2    Normal distribution of radiopharmaceuticals used for infection

| Radiopharmaceutical | Liver | Spleen | Marrow | Bone | Gastrointestinal | Genitourinary | Lung |
|---|---|---|---|---|---|---|---|
| Gallium-67 | *** | * | * | * | *** | *Female peri (contam) transitory* | |
| Indium-111 leukocytes | ** | *** | ** | | | | * |
| Technetium-99m HMPAO leukocytes | ** | *** | ** | | ** | ** | * |
| Antigranulocyte antibodies | ** | * | *** | | ** | | |
| Nonspecific immunoglobulin G antibodies | *** | ** | ** | | * | * | * |

## Dosimetry

The target organ for Ga-67 is the large intestine (0.90 rad/mCi or 4.5 rads/5 mCi). The marrow receives 2.9 rads and the liver 2.3 rads. The whole body absorbed dose is 0.26 rad/mCi (Table 8-3).

## Clinical Applications

In addition to acute localized infections such as abscess, Ga-67 can detect infection without well-formed borders or pus, such as cellulitis, peritonitis, and other inflammatory and granulomatous processes. Leukocytic infiltration is not necessary for Ga-67 to detect foci of infection, making it valuable for studying leukopenic patients. Although radiolabeled leukocytes have replaced Ga-67 for many of its earlier indications, Ga-67 still plays an important role in the detection of a variety of pulmonary interstitial and granulomatous diseases.

**Pulmonary infection and inflammatory disease** Ga-67 citrate accumulates in virtually all pulmonary infections, inflammatory sites, and interstitial and granulomatous diseases (Box 8-4), including pneumonia, lung abscesses, tuberculosis, pneumoconioses, idiopathic pulmonary fibrosis, sarcoidosis (Fig. 8-4), *Pneumocystis carinii* infection (Fig. 8-5), adult respiratory distress syndrome, and cytomegalovirus (CMV) infec-

tion, as well as in therapeutic drug–induced pulmonary reactions (Box 8-5).

*Sarcoidosis*  Sarcoidosis is a chronic granulomatous disease of unknown etiology. Pulmonary manifestations usually predominate, but the disease may involve any organ of the body.

PATHOGENESIS  Sarcoidosis is a multisystem disease characterized by an accumulation of T-lymphocytes, mononuclear phagocytes, and noncaseating epithelioid granulomas. Intrathoracic manifestations consist of hilar or mediastinal adenopathy, endobronchial granuloma formation, interstitial or alveolar pulmonary infiltrates, or pulmonary fibrosis.

An increase in both the relative and absolute numbers of T-lymphocytes, monocytes, and macrophages in the lung can be demonstrated with bronchoalveolar lavage. The lung function abnormalities are typical of interstitial lung disease. The alveolitis is seen on the chest radiograph as an infiltrative process.

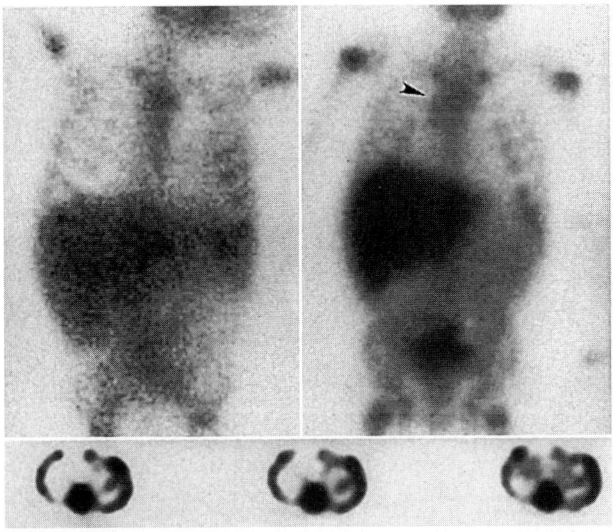

**Fig. 8-3**  Gallium-67 uptake in thymus and heart. A 20-month-old child received azothioprine and steroids for treatment of idiopathic myocarditis. **A,** *Left,* Pretherapy planar image of the chest showed no abnormal uptake. *Right,* Posttherapy planar image shows prominent uptake by the thymus *(arrowhead).* **B,** In contrast to the planar study, the pretherapy SPECT study showed myocardial uptake (best seen on middle image). Three sequential transverse slices through the myocardium are shown.

**Table 8-3**  Radiation dosimetry for gallium-67 citrate, indium-111 oxine leukocytes, and technetium-99m HMPAO leukocytes

| Organ | Ga-67 (5 mCi) | In-111 oxine WBCs (500 µCi) | Tc-99m HMPAO WBCs (10 mCi) |
|---|---|---|---|
|  | Rads | | |
| Bladder wall |  |  | 2.8 |
| Large intestine | 4.5 |  | 3.6 |
| Liver | 2.3 | 2.66 | 1.5 |
| Bone marrow | 2.9 | 1.99 | 1.6 |
| Spleen | 2.7 | 20.00 | 2.2 |
| Ovaries | 1.4 | 0.20 | 0.3 |
| Testes | 1.2 | 0.014 | 1.9 |
| Total body | 1.3 | 0.37 | 0.3 |

*WBCs,* White blood cells.

**Box 8-4  Interstitial and Granulomatous Pulmonary Diseases Associated with Gallium-67 Uptake**

Tuberculosis +MAI
Histoplasmosis
Sarcoidosis
Idiopathic pulmonary fibrosis (all causes)
*Pneumocystis carinii*
Cytomegalovirus
Pneumoconioses (asbestosis, silicosis)
Hypersensitivity pneumonitis
Lymphoma

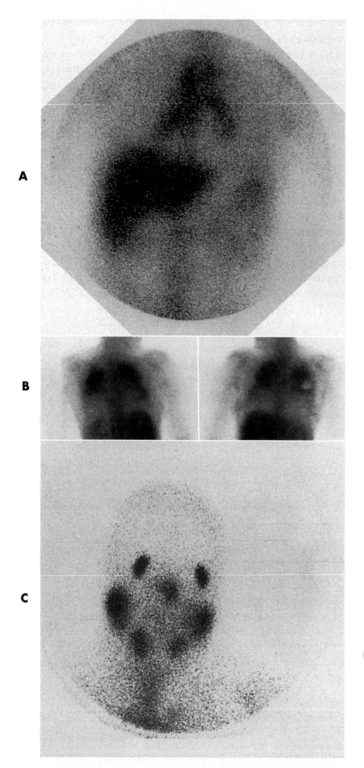

**Fig. 8-4** **A,** Lambda sign. Paratracheal and hilar nodal uptake with early active sarcoidosis. **B,** Diffuse pulmonary gallium-67 uptake. Different patient with active sarcoidosis diffusely involving predominantly the upper lobes. The cold defect is due to a pacemaker. **C,** Panda sign in sarcoidosis. Prominent Ga-67 uptake is seen in the parotid, salivary, and lacrimal glands in a patient with sarcoidosis.

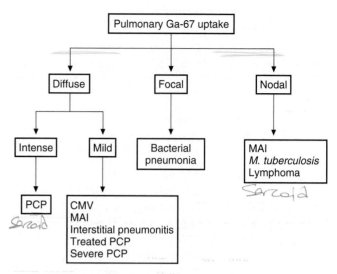

**Fig. 8-5** Diagnostic decision tree pattern of pulmonary gallium-67 uptake in immunosuppressed patients. *Ga,* Gallium; *MAI, Mycobacterium avium-intracellulare; PCP, Pneumocystis carinii* pneumonia; *CMV,* cytomegalovirus.

---

**Box 8-5    Therapeutic Agents Associated with Gallium-67 Lung Uptake**

Cytoxan                Amiodarone
Busulfan               Nitrofurantoin
Bleomycin

---

CLINICAL MANIFESTATIONS  The lung is almost always involved in sarcoidosis, and the initial presentation is usually pulmonary. However, as many as 20% of patients are asymptomatic and have only an abnormal chest radiograph at initial examination. One third of patients present with complaints of dysnea and dry cough. Systemic symptoms such as weight loss, fatigue, weakness, malaise, and fever are common (40%). Extrathoracic disease is less common but can involve any organ, most commonly the liver and spleen, but also the skin, eyes, heart, central nervous system, bones, and muscle.

The clinical course is variable. Spontaneous resolution occurs in about one third of patients. Another 30% to 40% have a smoldering or progressively worsening course, 20% have permanent loss of lung function, and 5% to 10% die of respiratory failure.

Chest radiographic findings can be categorized into four types (Box 8-6): no abnormality (type 0), bilateral hilar adenopathy (type I), bilateral adenopathy with diffuse parenchymal abnormalities (type II), and diffuse parenchymal changes without hilar adenopathy

## Box 8-6 Classification of Chest Radiographic Findings in Sarcoidosis

| TYPE | RADIOGRAPHIC FINDINGS |
|------|----------------------|
| ∅ I | Hilar and/or mediastinal node enlargement with normal lung parenchma |
| II | Hilar and/or mediastinal node enlargement and diffuse interstitial pulmonary disease |
| III | Diffuse pulmonary disease without node involvement |
| IV | Pulmonary fibrosis |

(type III). Although patients with type I radiographs tend to have a reversible form of the disease and those with types II and III usually have chronic progressive disease, these patterns do not necessarily represent consecutive stages of sarcoidosis.

DIAGNOSIS AND ASSESSMENT OF DISEASE ACTIVITY  The diagnosis of sarcoidosis is based on a combination of clinical, radiographic, and histological findings. The chest radiograph cannot be the sole criterion for diagnosis, since the typical bilateral hilar adenopathy may be seen with other diseases. Biopsy evidence of a mononuclear cell granulomatous inflammatory process is mandatory for a definitive diagnosis. Since the lung is so frequently involved, it is the most common biopsy site, usually via fiberoptic bronchoscopy. However, biopsy may be performed on any involved organ.

Various other diagnostic tests and methods have been used clinically to diagnose sarcoidosis. The *Kveim-Siltzbach test* requires intradermal injection of human sarcoid tissue. A nodule develops at the injection site in 4 to 6 weeks in patients with sarcoidosis. Biopsy reveals noncaseating granulomas in 70% to 80% of patients. *Serum markers,* such as angiotensin-converting enzyme (ACE), have been used to diagnose sarcoidosis. However, ACE measurement is negative in two thirds of patients with sarcoidosis and false positive results are common. *Bronchoalveolar lavage* with examination for inflammatory cells is an accurate method of making the diagnosis. The finding of an increased percentage of T-lymphocytes has been used as an indication for therapy.

Glucocorticoids effectively suppress the activated T-cells at the disease site and the clinical manifestations of the disease. To decide if therapy is indicated, however, clinicians need to determine disease activity because glucocorticoids are associated with significant long-term complications. The chest radiograph is not a sensitive indicator of disease activity. The serum ACE level is not generally believed to be specific enough, but it is easy to obtain and relatively inexpensive. Brochoalveolar lavage and Ga-67 scans are commonly used as indicators of disease activity.

GALLIUM-67 SCINTIGRAPHY  Although Ga-67 has been used in the diagnosis of sarcoidosis, its primary usefulness is for the evaluation of disease activity and guidance in therapeutic decisions. Ga-67 can distinguish active granuloma formation and alveolitis from inactive disease and fibrotic changes. Increased Ga-67 uptake in the lungs is more than 90% sensitive for clinically active sarcoidosis. Scans are typically negative in inactive cases. In addition, Ga-67 can localize nonpulmonary sites of disease involvement.

Some controversy exists as to whether increased pulmonary Ga-67 uptake correlates with the degree of inflammation, serum ACE levels, or the percentage of T-lymphocytes obtained from bronchoalveolar lavage. Proponents believe that Ga-67 uptake does indeed correlate with disease activity and is more sensitive than serum ACE levels for following disease activity. Studies have shown a correlation between the degree of uptake on serial Ga-67 scans and response to therapy with corticosteroids, both early in treatment and after 1 year of therapy.

Ga-67 is more sensitive than a chest radiograph for detecting early disease. Pulmonary uptake on scintigraphy can be seen before characteristic abnormalities are present on radiographs. Up to one third of patients have normal radiographs at this stage of disease. Patients with a normal Ga-67 scan nearly always have a negative biopsy. In addition, patients with a history of sarcoidosis and an abnormal chest radiograph, but inactive disease, have a negative Ga-67 study. In these cases the abnormal radiograph represents past, not present, disease.

Characteristic patterns of Ga-67 uptake are seen in sarcoidosis. Typical early disease shows only bilateral hilar Ga-67 uptake. Bilateral hilar with paratracheal uptake has been called the "lambda sign" (Fig. 8-4, *A*). When present, pulmonary uptake is characteristically intense and symmetrical (Fig. 8-4, *B*) and may or may not be associated with hilar and mediastinal involvement.

In contrast, patients with malignant lymphoma typically have asymmetrical hilar or mediastinal uptake, often involving the anterior and paratracheal nodes. Although paraaortic, mesenteric, and retroperitoneal lymph node involvement may be seen in sarcoidosis, it is much more common in lymphoma.

Prominent uptake in the nasopharyngeal region and the parotid, salivary, and lacrimal glands has been referred to as the "panda sign" (Fig. 8-4, *C*). The combination of ocular involvement (iritis or iridocyclitis) with accompanying lacrimal gland inflammation and bilateral salivary gland involvement is known clinically as uveoparotid fever (Mikulicz's syndrome).

The degree of pulmonary uptake can be judged subjectively relative to uptake in the liver, bone marrow, and soft tissue. Uptake in the lung greater than in the liver is highly positive for sarcoidosis, whereas lung uptake less than soft tissue uptake is regarded as negative. Numerous semiquantitative indexes of Ga-67 uptake have been proposed. Although more objective quantification may be desirable, the problem with these methods is that uptake by normal overlying soft tissue, bone, and bone marrow limits the accuracy and clinical utility of Ga-67.

Low-grade pulmonary uptake can sometimes be hard to ascertain because of the normal distribution in overlying soft tissue, sternum, breasts, ribs, scapulae, and spine. Since the heart may obscure much of the left lung field in the anterior view, the posterior view is usually preferable for estimating uptake. Oblique views or single-photon emission computed tomography (SPECT) can be useful for discerning mediastinal and hilar uptake or confirming pulmonary uptake when there is prominent overlying activity.

*Idiopathic interstitial pulmonary fibrosis*  The etiology of idiopathic interstitial pulmonary fibrosis is unknown. Typically the disease follows a pathological progression through stages of alveolitis, with derangement of the alveolar-capillary units, ultimately leading to end-stage fibrotic disease. Ga-67 has been used to monitor the course of disease and response to therapy. The amount of Ga-67 uptake correlates with the degree of cellular infiltration, but, unlike the situation with sarcoidosis, it does not predict the results of steroid treatment.

*Adverse pulmonary drug reactions*  Ga-67 uptake can be an early indicator of drug-induced lung injury before the chest radiograph is abnormal. Therapeutic drugs known to cause lung injury and to result in Ga-67 uptake include cytoxan, nitrofurantoin, bleomycin, and amiodarone (Box 8-5). Lung uptake may also be seen after lymphangiography caused by a chemical-induced alveolitis.

**Infection in immunosuppressed patients**  The clinical presentation, physical findings, and radiological abnormalities in immunosuppressed patients are often obscured by an impaired inflammatory response as a result of the underlying disease or therapy. Furthermore, many of the organisms causing infection, such as *Pneumocystitis carinii, Cryptococcus,* and CMV, produce a minimal inflammatory response even in healthy hosts.

Immunosuppression is seen most commonly in patients with AIDS and those receiving drugs for cancer chemotherapy or organ transplantation. The diagnostic sensitivity of ultrasonography, CT, and MRI depends on the presence of normal anatomical markers, which can be disrupted by previous surgical procedures or disease. Monitoring the effects of therapy is complicated by the slowness of response, the lack of microbiological methods for assessing response, and the need for extended courses of therapy for some opportunistic infections.

*Pulmonary infections*  Ga-67 citrate can be helpful in the differential diagnosis of pulmonary disorders in immunosuppressed patients. It is useful to classify the patterns of pulmonary uptake on Ga-67 scans as diffuse parenchymal, focal parenchymal, lymph node, or normal (Fig. 8-5).

DIFFUSE PULMONARY UPTAKE  *Pneumocystis carinii* pneumonia (PCP) is often the first pulmonary manifestation of AIDS. The chest x-ray findings are usually abnormal, with bilateral diffuse infiltrates originating from the hilum and extending peripherally. However, the radiograph may show a lobar or nodular infiltrate or even be normal.

Ga-67 scans show abnormalities in approximately 90% of cases. Pulmonary Ga-67 uptake is often positive before the chest radiograph becomes abnormal. With severe pulmonary involvement that can be visualized on the chest radiograph, the lung uptake of Ga-67 may actually decrease, reflecting a deficient immune response. This has been associated with a poor prognosis.

The characteristic Ga-67 pattern of PCP infection is that of *diffuse* bilateral pulmonary uptake, either uniform or nonuniform, without nodal or parotid uptake (Fig. 8-6). However, increased Ga-67 uptake in an

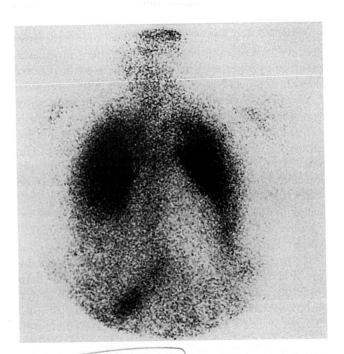

**Fig. 8-6**  *Pneumocysitis carinii.* Diffuse intense homogeneous or heterogeneous uptake is typical of this infection. The characteristic pattern is different from that of most other common pulmonary infections in AIDS patients.

immunocompromised patient may have other causes, including CMV, bacterial pneumonitis, lymphocytic interstitial pneumonitis, or the effects of various drug therapies. As the intensity of Ga-67 uptake increases, the diagnosis of PCP becomes increasingly likely. In the proper clinical setting, with pulmonary uptake greater than liver uptake and a normal chest radiograph, the predictive value for PCP approaches 95%.

Ga-67 uptake at initial presentation of PCP is typically higher than that seen after the treatment of recurrences. Prophylactic aerosolized pentamidine therapy can result in an atypical and heterogeneous pattern of uptake. Reports suggest that Ga-67 may also have value for monitoring the response to therapy.

With CMV infection, diffuse Ga-67 lung uptake is usually low grade, with perihilar prominence. This finding may be accompanied by ocular uptake caused by retinitis, adrenal and renal uptake, and often persistent colon uptake associated with diarrheal symptoms.

Although the radiographic appearance in lymphoid interstitial pneumonia may be normal or similar to that seen in PCP, viral infections, or miliary tuberculosis, Ga-67 has a characteristic pattern of low-grade diffuse pulmonary uptake, without nodal uptake, and symmetrically increased parotid uptake.

FOCAL PULMONARY UPTAKE  Focal pulmonary uptake is a less common pattern that is typically seen with bacterial pneumonia. Corresponding infiltrates can usually be seen on chest radiographs. Intense Ga-67 uptake in a lobar configuration in the absence of nodal and parotid uptake suggests bacterial pneumonia. When multiple sites of focal accumulation are present, bacterial causes are less common and aggressive infections caused by *Actinomyces, Nocardia,* and *Aspergillus* should be considered. These latter infections are frequently accompanied by local bone invasion.

NODAL UPTAKE  Nodal uptake may be seen with *Mycobacterium avium-intracellulare* (MAI) infection, tuberculosis, lymphoma, and occasionally PCP, although the last-named usually has increased pulmonary uptake as well. Other causes of increased nodal uptake are lymphadenitis, cryptococcal infection, and herpes simplex.

Infection with MAI causes widespread disease in 25% to 50% of AIDS patients and requires more aggressive therapy than that used for tuberculosis. Delay in diagnosis, often because of initial treatment for PCP, contributes to a high morbidity. Patchy lung uptake with hilar and nonhilar nodal (axillary and inguinal) Ga-67 uptake suggests MAI infection.

NEGATIVE GALLIUM-67 UPTAKE  The absence of Ga-67 uptake in conjunction with a negative chest radiograph excludes pulmonary infection with a high degree of certainty. When the chest x-ray findings are positive,

particularly in a patient with deteriorating respiratory status, Kaposi's sarcoma must be seriously considered.

*Malignancy*  AIDS-related lymphoma is less common than mycobacterial infection and can be differentiated on Ga-67 scintigraphy by its characteristic bulky nodal pattern of uptake. Kaposi's sarcoma is Ga-67 negative, but positive on thallium-201 imaging.

*Gastrointestinal infections*  Intraabdominal infections are common in immunocompromised patients. However, radionuclide imaging has not played a major role in their evaluation, probably because the patterns of accumulation are nonspecific and many of the infection-seeking radiopharmaceuticals are normally cleared through the bowel.

Oral and esophageal candidiasis are common fungal infections in immunosuppressed patients. The diagnosis is usually based on an upper gastrointestinal series or endoscopy but can be made with Ga-67 scintigraphy. Debilitating diarrhea is commonly caused by the protozoon *Cryptosporidium*. Proximal small bowel Ga-67 uptake has been reported with cryptosporidial infection.

As a general rule, In-111-labeled leukocytes are superior to Ga-67 for diagnosing intestinal infection because of the latter's normal intestinal clearance. When stool cultures are negative for *Salmonella* or *Shigella,* diffuse colonic uptake that does not change with time is probably due to CMV infection or antibiotic-induced colitis. The additional findings of eye, adrenal, esophageal, and low-grade pulmonary uptake are most suggestive of CMV. Multifocal activity (paratracheal and bowel) is indicative of mycobacterial infection.

**Abdominal and pelvic infections**  Radionuclide whole body scintigraphy is particularly useful when the site of infection cannot be localized. With localizing symptoms, ultrasonography is usually the imaging modality of choice for examining the right upper quadrant, pelvis, and kidney region, and CT can be used to examine the remainder of the abdomen.

When the source of the infection remains uncertain, scintigraphy can be helpful. Although Ga-67 scintigraphy has been used to diagnose intraabdominal infection, In-111 leukocyte scintigraphy is usually preferable because the radiopharmaceutical is not cleared through the intestines or kidneys and the study can be completed within 24 hours. Scintigraphy can be used to determine if a fluid collection identified by ultrasonography or CT represents a site of infection or rather a sterile fluid collection. Intrahepatic abscesses may be diagnosed with Ga-67 scintigraphy, although normal hepatic uptake may complicate interpretation. A concomitant Tc-99m sulfur colloid study serving as a template for normal liver can aid in making the diagnosis (Fig. 8-7). Ga-67 scans can be used to confirm the diagnosis of active retroperitoneal fibrosis.

**Genitourinary infections**   Because 10% to 25% of the injected Ga-67 citrate dose is excreted via the kidneys during the first 24 hours, the diagnosis of renal inflammatory disease must be made from images obtained 48 to 72 hours after tracer injection. Renal

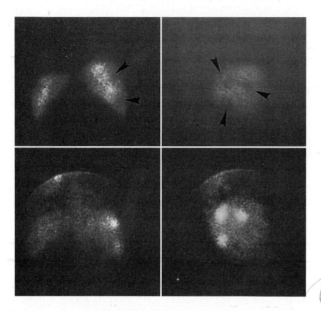

**Fig. 8-7**   Multiple liver abscesses. The diagnosis was made with gallium-67 in conjunction with a technetium-99m sulfur colloid scan of the liver and spleen. Posterior *(left)* and right lateral *(right)* views are displayed. *Top,* Tc-99m sulfur colloid study. *Bottom,* Comparable Ga-67 study. Note increased focal uptake on the Ga-67 scan corresponding to the focal photopenic defects seen on the Tc-99m sulfur colloid study *(arrowheads).*

parenchymal infection such as pyelonephritis or diffuse interstitial nephritis (Fig. 8-8), lobar nephronia (focal interstitial nephritis), and perirenal infections (Fig. 8-9) can be diagnosed with Ga-67 scintigraphy. Interpretive caution is indicated when patients have renal or hepatic failure or iron overload, in which renal uptake is increased.

**Bone infections**   Since Ga-67 is normally taken up by bone, increased abnormal uptake will be seen whenever bone remodeling occurs, as in patients with underlying bone disease, previous surgery, fractures, and prosthetic devices. For greater specificity in the diagnosis of osteomyelitis, the combination of a bone scan and a Ga-67 scan has been recommended.

The combination of Ga-67 and bone scan is interpreted as positive for osteomyelitis if the Ga-67 uptake is incongruent with the bone scan; that is, either there is greater uptake on the Ga-67 study than on the bone scan, or the uptake occurs in a different distribution on the two studies. Low-grade uptake (less than bone) on the Ga-67 scan or congruent uptake (Fig. 8-10) is interpreted as a negative study. However, intense congruent uptake is considered equivocal and infection cannot be excluded.

In general, In-111 oxine leukocytes are more accurate than Ga-67 for diagnosing osteomyelitis. However, Ga-67 scintigraphy is useful for diagnosing disk space infections, which often have a soft tissue component (Fig. 8-11).

*Pseudomonas* necrotizing external otitis is a life-threatening infection seen in diabetic patients. It has a poor prognosis. Increased uptake of Ga-67 can differentiate this disease from other, less serious causes of

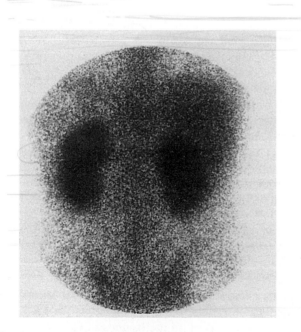

**Fig. 8-8**   Interstitial nephritis. Bilateral intense renal gallium-67 uptake is seen at 48 hours (posterior view). Normal uptake is seen in the liver, bone, and bone marrow.

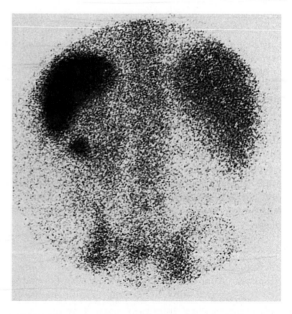

**Fig. 8-9**   Perirenal abscess. In this patient fever and pain developed after renal stone removal and nephrostomy. Focal increased gallium-67 uptake is seen just inferior to the spleen and adjacent to the left kidney, consistent with an abscess.

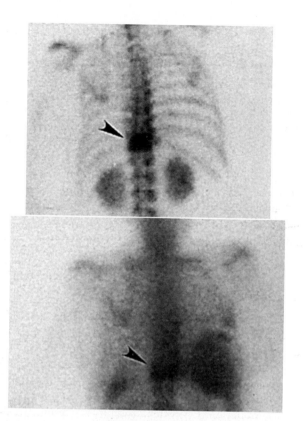

therapy-resistant external otitis. The increased uptake is seen in the temporal bone on both Tc-99m bone scans and Ga-67 scans. The bone scan can be used to establish the initial diagnosis, whereas the Ga-67 scan is particularly useful for evaluating the effectiveness of therapy.

**Fever of unknown origin**    Fever of unknown origin is rigidly defined by clinicians as a fever of at least 38.3° C that occurs on more than three occasions, remains without a diagnosed cause for at least 3 weeks, and results in at least 7 days of hospitalization.

For patients who have not had recent surgery, Ga-67 is a sensitive test for uncovering the source of the fever. In addition to localizing acute infection, Ga-67 can detect chronic and indolent infections, granulomatous infections, and even tumor sources of fever. However, postoperative patients with fever are usually better served with In-111-labeled leukocytes, since the fever is most commonly due to an acute infection and In-111 leukocytes do not have the bowel clearance problem of Ga-67 to confound intraabdominal interpretation.

## RADIOLABELED LEUKOCYTES

Scintigraphy of radiolabeled leukocytes is a physiologically appealing method for detecting infection. In 1976 McAfee and Thakur demonstrated that In-111 oxine could be used to label mixed leukocytes in vitro. Over the years many studies have proved the clinical utility of In-111 oxine–labeled leukocytes for detecting the site of infection and inflammation.

**Fig. 8-10**    Evaluation for osteomyelitis: combined gallium-67 and bone scan. Fever after laminectomy raised the question of infection. Vertebral Ga-67 uptake *(bottom)* was judged to be less than that seen on the technetium-99m medronate (MDP) bone scan *(top)*, and the study was interpreted as negative for vertebral osteomyelitis or soft tissue infection. The low-grade Ga-67 uptake was the result of reactive healing bone.

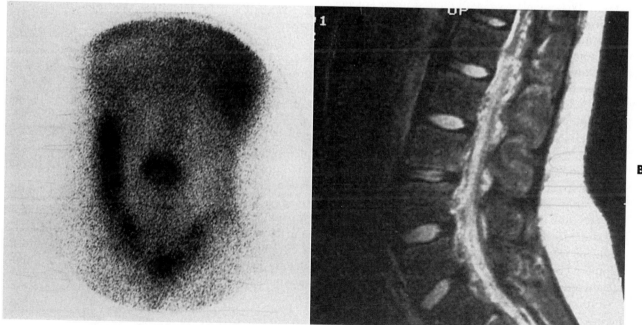

**Fig. 8-11**    Disk space infection. **A,** Prominent focal gallium-67 uptake seen at L3-4 (posterior view). **B,** Magnetic resonance imaging showed only a narrowed interspace with evidence of degenerative disk disease.

More recently it was demonstrated that the Tc-99m-labeled cerebral perfusion agent HMPAO could bind to leukocytes. This radiopharmaceutical has some advantages over In-111 oxine and has found clinical applicability and wide acceptance. Both agents are now in clinical use.

Both methods of labeling leukocytes have the disadvantage of requiring cell labeling, which is time consuming and technically demanding and exposes personnel to bloodborne diseases. Nonspecific radiolabeled gamma globulin, monoclonal antibodies against white blood cells, chemotactic peptides, and other creative methodologies are under investigation.

## Leukocyte Physiology

Leukocytes are the major cellular components of inflammatory and immune responses. They protect against infection and neoplasia and assist in the repair of damaged tissue. The nucleated precursor cells differentiate into mature cells within the bone marrow. The normal blood leukocyte count of 4.5 to $11.0 \times 10^6$ cells/mm$^3$ includes the granulocyte series of neutrophils (55% to 65%), eosinophils (3%), and basophils (0.5%), as well as lymphocytes (25% to 35%) and monocytes (3% to 7%). Leukocytes spend a small part (6 to 7 hours) of their short life span in the peripheral blood, using it mainly for transportation to sites of need.

Neutrophils exist in two compartments: 2% to 3% are in a circulating pool and the remainder are in a "marginated" pool adherent to vascular endothelial cells in tissues. Normally about 90% of the neutrophil pool resides in the bone marrow, with the rest in the spleen, liver, lung, and to a lesser extent the gastrointestinal tract and oropharynx. These marginated cells can be marshalled into the circulating pool by exercise, epinephrine, or exposure to bacterial endotoxin.

In response to an acute inflammatory stimulus, neutrophils migrate toward an attractant (chemotaxis) and enter tissues by crawling (diapedesis) between postcapillary endothelial cells. They increase their adhesiveness, aggregate, adhere to endothelial surfaces, phagocytose the infectious agent or foreign body, and enzymatically destroy it within cytoplasmic vacuoles. Both adherence and migration of neutrophils are inhibited by exposure to corticosteroids or ethanol. Neutrophils survive in tissues for only 2 to 3 days.

Eosinophils mediate allergic reactions and help protect against parasitic infestations.

Lymphocytes play an important part in immune reactions. Although their nonimmunological role in inflammation is less well understood, they arrive at inflammatory sites during the chronic phases of many inflammatory responses.

The T-lymphocytes are responsible primarily for cell-mediated immune responses. These cells originate from the marrow and are processed into mature T-lymphocytes in the thymus. They represent 50% to 80% of peripheral lymphocytes and concentrate in the marrow, spleen, tonsils, intestines, thymus, and lymph nodes. They recirculate and have a life span of 100 to 200 days. B-lymphocytes are involved primarily in antibody synthesis, do not usually recirculate, and have a short turnover in the lymph nodes and spleen.

Monocytes act as tissue scavengers, phagocytosing damaged cells and bacteria and detoxifying chemicals and toxins. At sites of inflammation they transform into tissue macrophages. They also have immunological functions.

## Indium-111 Oxine–Labeled Leukocytes

For over two decades In-111 oxine–labeled leukocytes have been used to image infection and inflammation. The scintigraphic images reflect the distribution of white blood cells in the body. Since an abscess or other localized infection consists primarily of leukocytes, the radiopharmaceutical localizes at the site of infection.

**Chemistry and physics**  Indium is a group III element in the Periodic Table. The radionuclide In-111 is cyclotron produced. It decays by electron capture, emitting two gamma photons of 173 and 247 keV (Table 8-1). It has a physical half-life of 67 hours (2.8 days), which allows imaging at 24 hours. Oxine (8-hydroxyquinolone) is a lipid-soluble complex that chelates metal ions such as In-111.

**Mechanism of uptake**  Because of its lipid solubility the In-111 oxine complex readily diffuses through cell membranes. Intracellularly the complex dissociates. The In-111 binds to nuclear and cytoplasmic proteins, while the oxine diffuses back out of the cell. In-111 oxine labels blood cells indiscriminately, whether granulocytes, lymphocytes, monocytes, platelets, or erythrocytes. However, during the labeling process most of the erythrocytes and platelets are removed. Pure granulocyte preparations have been used, but they require more complex separation methods and have not shown a clear clinical advantage.

Alternatives to oxine have been proposed. Tropolone, unlike oxine, has the advantage that it can be labeled with In-111 in plasma. Imaging is possible at 4 hours. However, studies have not shown improved accuracy with tropolone-labeled leukocytes. Mercaptopyridine-*N*-oxide (MERC), another chelating agent proposed as an alternative to oxine, has potential advantages. It can also label cells efficiently in plasma, is less cytotoxic than oxine, and results in less uptake in muscle, liver, and spleen. However, neither tropolone nor In-111 MERC is approved for clinical use.

*kidneys vs TC*

**Pharmacokinetics and normal distribution** After infusion the radiolabeled leukocytes are distributed to the blood pool, lungs, liver, and spleen. Early lung uptake occurs because of cellular activation as a result of in vitro cell manipulation. By 4 hours lung activity and blood pool activity have decreased considerably. At 24 hours blood pool activity is not normally seen. Its persistence indicates a high percentage of erythrocyte or platelet labeling.

On images obtained at 18 to 24 hours after tracer injection the most intense uptake is seen in the spleen, followed by the liver and then the bone marrow (Fig. 8-12). Each receives about one third of the total activity. Table 8-2 compares the normal distribution of radiolabeled white blood cells with other infection-seeking scintigraphic agents.

**Dosimetry** The spleen receives the highest radiation-absorbed dose with In-111 oxine–labeled white blood cells, approximately 15 to 20 rads (Table 8-3). This is of particular concern for pediatric patients.

**Methodology** To be labeled efficiently, leukocytes must be removed from plasma because In-111 has a higher affinity for serum transferrin than for oxine. The cell labeling process takes roughly 2 hours. Careful handling is necessary to avoid damaging the cells. Red blood cells and platelets must be removed, since they are

many times more numerous than white blood cells. Hydroxyethyl starch (Hetastarch), a settling agent, hastens erythrocyte clumping. A technique that simultaneously combines red blood cell sedimentation with centrifugation (Box 8-7) to reduce platelets and proteins results in a high yield of leukocytes.

Proper labeling does not adversely affect normal physiological function, and the tag usually remains stable in vivo for over 24 hours. Labeling efficiencies of 75% to 95% are obtainable.

*Neutropenic patients* An In-111 oxine leukocyte study may be suboptimal because of the patient's low granulocyte count. Although a leukocyte count above 5000/mm$^3$ is preferred, diagnostic scintigraphy can often be performed on patients with lower cell counts (3000/mm$^3$). Cross-matched donor leukocytes have

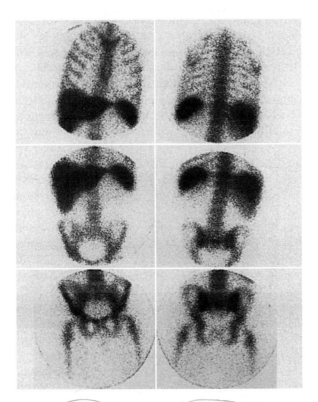

**Fig. 8-12** Normal distribution of indium-111 oxine leukocytes at 24 hours. The greatest uptake is seen in the spleen, followed by the liver, then the bone marrow. No intestinal or renal activity is seen.

---

### Box 8-7    Labeling Autologous Leukocytes with Indium-111 Oxine

**PREPARATION**

Patient's peripheral leukocyte count should be greater than 4000 cells/ mm$^3$.

**PROCEDURE**

1. Collect autologous blood:
   Draw 30 to 50 ml into an ACD anticoagulated syringe using a 19-gauge needle.
2. Isolate leukocytes:
   Separate red blood cells (RBCs) by gravity sedimentation and 6% Hetastarch, a settling agent.
   Centrifuge the leukocyte-rich plasma (LRP) at 300 to 350 *g* for 5 min to remove platelets and proteins. A white blood cell (WBC) button forms at the bottom of the tube.
   Draw off and save the leukocyte-poor plasma (LPP) for later washing and resuspending.
3. Label leukocytes:
   Suspend WBCs (LRP) in saline (includes granulocytes, lymphocytes, monocytes, and some RBCs).
   Incubate with In-111 oxine for 30 min at room temperature and gently agitate.
   Remove unbound In-111 by centrifugation. Save wash for later calculation of labeling efficiency.
4. Prepare injectate:
   Resuspend 500 μCi In-111 leukocytes in saved plasma (LPP).
   Inject via peripheral vein within 2 to 4 hr.
5. Perform quality control:
   Microscopic examination of cells.
   Calculate labeling efficiency: Assay the cells and wash in dose calibrator. ($E = C/[C + W] \times 100\%$, where $C$ is the activity associated with the cells, $W$ is the activity associated with the wash, and $E$ is the labeling efficiency.)

been used successfully for patients with severe leukopenia. An alternative method that does not require cell labeling or heterologous cells would be preferable, such as the use of nonspecific immunoglobulins, radiolabeled antibodies, or infection-seeking peptides. This would be particularly advantageous for imaging of HIV-positive patients, whose blood products expose medical personnel to some risk. It is hoped that such an agent will be clinically available in the near future.

*Quality control* Viability studies of labeled leukocytes are complex and time consuming and therefore are not routinely performed in clinical settings. With cell damage, increased lung retention is seen. With excessive erythrocyte and platelet labeling, blood pool clearance is slower.

Routine quality control should include a microscopic examination to look for structural integrity, erythrocyte contamination, and the presence of clumping. Labeling efficiency should be calculated (Box 8-7).

The ultimate test of viability of leukocytes is their in vivo function as manifested by a normal distribution within the body and their ability to detect infection. If the infused white blood cells become nonviable, as might result from an interval greater than 4 hours between labeling and reinfusion, a change in the normal distribution can be seen; for example, the normal high spleen to liver ratio will not be present.

**Imaging protocol** In-111 oxine leukocyte images are routinely acquired 18 to 24 hours after radiopharmaceutical injection (Box 8-8). This allows sufficient time for leukocyte localization and blood pool clearance. Further delayed images do not usually give additional information.

Earlier imaging (at 4 hours) is somewhat less sensitive for detecting infection but may occasionally be useful for rapid diagnosis of an abscess that requires prompt intervention. However, 4-hour imaging is mandatory for the localization of inflammatory bowel disease because inflamed mucosal cells slough, become intraluminal, and move distally by 24 hours. Twenty-four-hour images may result in misleading and erroneous information.

*Dual-isotope studies* In some cases diagnostic accuracy is improved by performing an ancillary study, such as an In-111 leukocyte plus a Tc-99m bone marrow study to diagnose osteomyelitis. Dual-isotope studies require special attention to the imaging characteristics of the radionuclides, such as their photopeaks, half-lives, and relative administered doses, and to the camera's capability for simultaneous multichannel acquisition.

The problem of downscatter or even upscatter must be considered. One approach is to perform Tc-99m scanning first. With a 6-hour half-life, less than 6% of Tc-99m activity will remain at 24 hours and less than 1% at 24 hours. For an In-111 leukocyte study the blood required for cell labeling can be drawn immediately before injection of the Tc-99m tracer, and the In-111-

---

**Box 8-8  Indium-111 Oxine Leukocyte Scintigraphy: Protocol Summary**

**RADIOPHARMACEUTICAL**

In-111 oxine in vitro labeled leukocytes, 500 μCi (18.5 MBq)

**INSTRUMENTATION**

Camera: Large field of view
Windows: 20% centered over 173 and 247 keV photopeaks
Collimator: Medium energy

**PATIENT PREPARATION**

Draw 50 ml of blood to radiolabel cells in vitro

**PROCEDURE**

Inject in vitro labeled cells intravenously, preferably by direct venipuncture through a 19-gauge needle. Contact with dextrose in water solutions may cause cell damage.
Imaging at 4 hr may be helpful to diagnose an acute abscess and is critical in localizing inflammatory bowel disease.
Perform routine whole body imaging at 24 hr.
Acquire anterior abdomen for 500k counts, then other images for equal time. Include anterior and posterior views of the chest, abdomen, and pelvis, and spot images of specific areas of interest (e.g., feet) for a minimum of 200k counts or 20 min.
Perform SPECT in selected cases.

---

labeled cells can be reinjected after imaging for the bone scan. The In-111 imaging is then performed at 18 to 24 hours. However, with a 3-hour delay between injection and bone scan imaging, the problem of cell viability must be considered.

An alternative approach is to perform both studies simultaneously, using a dual-isotope acquisition technique. This approach ensures identically positioned images for comparison. When this method is used, only the upper 247-keV photopeak of In-111 should be employed because of overlap of the 140-keV Tc-99m and the 173-keV In-111 windows. Downscatter (i.e., In-111 in the Tc-99m window) is a theoretical problem. However, the activity ratio of In-111 (500 μCi) to Tc-99m (20 mCi) is quite low, minimizing this potential problem.

**Image interpretation**

*Abnormal uptake* Activity outside the expected normal distribution of In-111 oxine leukocytes is evidence for infection or inflammation (Figs. 8-13 to 8-18). Focal uptake equal to or greater than that in the liver or spleen is typical for an abscess; activity equal to that of

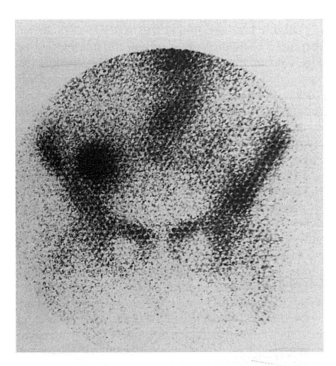

**Fig. 8-13**   Intraabdominal abscess. Anterior view of pelvis. Focal indium-111 leukocyte uptake seen in the right lower quadrant represents a perforated appendix with abscess formation.

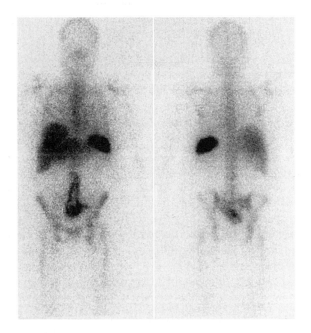

**Fig. 8-14**   Postoperative abscess. Dehiscence of the incision site because of abscess inferior and deep to incision. Whole body indium-111 oxine leukocyte scan.

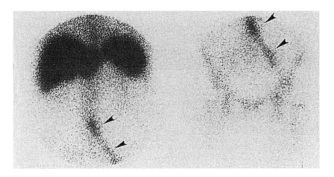

**Fig. 8-15**   Infected aortofemoral graft. *Left,* Anterior abdomen. *Right,* Pelvis. Indium-111 leukocyte uptake confirms the clinical suspicion that the surgical graft is infected *(arrowheads).*

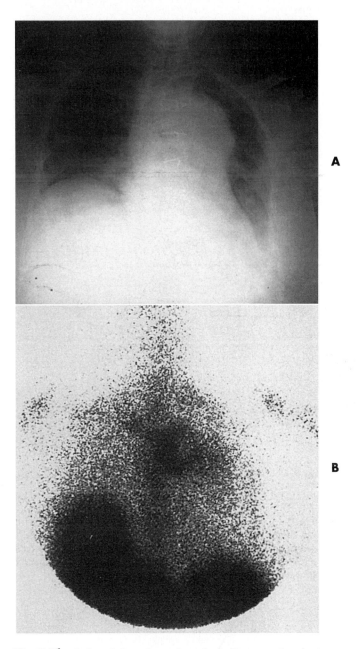

**Fig. 8-16**   Infected thoracic aortic graft. **A,** Postoperative chest radiograph. **B,** Indium-111 leukocytes localize in the region of the aortic knob.

the liver generally signifies a clinically important inflammatory site; and activity less than that of the bone marrow usually suggests a low-level inflammatory response.

*Accuracy*   Generally the accuracy of In-111 leukocyte scintigraphy for diagnosing infection is quite good.

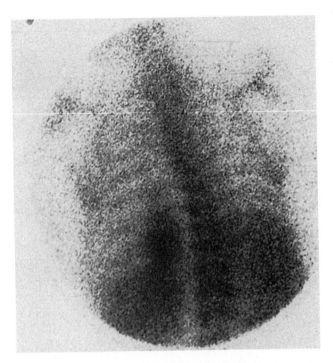

**Fig. 8-17** Pneumonia. Posterior chest. Focal indium-111 leuko-cyte uptake in the left lower lobe. The purpose of the study was to locate the source of postoperative fever. Pneumonia was not suspected on the basis of clinical findings. The last chest radiograph had been 10 days earlier. A subsequent radiograph confirmed the diagnosis.

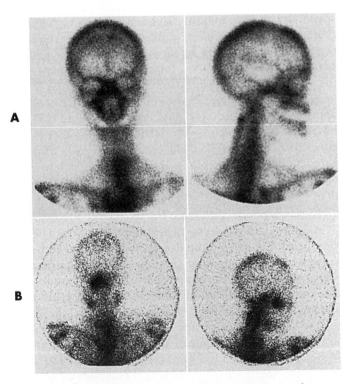

**Fig. 8-18** Osteomyelitis of the right maxillary sinus. History of bilateral sinus surgery. **A,** Bone scan shows fairly symmetrical ethmoid and maxillary sinus uptake. **B,** Indium-111 oxine leuko-cyte study shows uptake just right of midline in a pattern different from the bone scan, consistent with focal maxillary infection, abscess, or osteomyelitis. Osteomyelitis was confirmed at surgery.

---

**Box 8-9  Causes of False Negative and False Positive In-111 Leukocyte Studies**

**FALSE NEGATIVE**

Encapsulated, nonpyogenic abscess
Vertebral osteomyelitis
Chronic low-grade infection
Parasitic, mycobacterial, or fungal infections
Intrahepatic or perihepatic or splenic infection
Hyperglycemia
Steroids

**FALSE POSITIVE**

Gastrointestinal bleeding
Pseudoaneurysm
Healing fracture
Soft tissue tumor
Swallowed leukocytes; oropharyngeal, esophageal, or lung disease
Surgical wounds, stomas, or catheter sites
Hematomas
Tumors
Accessory spleens

---

One investigation reported a high false negative rate for chronic infection. However, a subsequent larger series found no significant difference in sensitivity for detection of acute or chronic infections. Although chronic inflammations consist largely of monocytes, macrophages, lymphocytes, and plasma cells, they also have significant neutrophilic infiltration and at times frank pus. In addition, the In-111 mixed cell population contains many radiolabeled lymphocytes.

Tuberculosis and fungal infections are detected by In-111 leukocytes, but with a decreased sensitivity. Ga-67 is preferable for these cases. Although conflicting data exist regarding the sensitivity of In-111 leukocyte scintigraphy for detecting infection in patients who are receiving antibiotics, it is probably not a significant factor. Questions have been raised about the sensitivity of In-111 leukocyte scintigraphy when the patient is undergoing therapy that alters leukocyte function, such as hyperglycemia, steroid therapy, chemotherapy, hemodialysis, and hyperalimentation. Data are sparse.

*Interpretive pitfalls* The practitioner should keep in mind interpretive pitfalls and potential false positive findings (Box 8-9).

Leukocytes may accumulate at sites of inflammation without clinical infection, such as at placement sites of intravenous catheters; nasogastric, endogastric, and drainage tubes; tracheostomies; colostomies; and ileostomies. Unless very intense, this uptake should be considered normal.

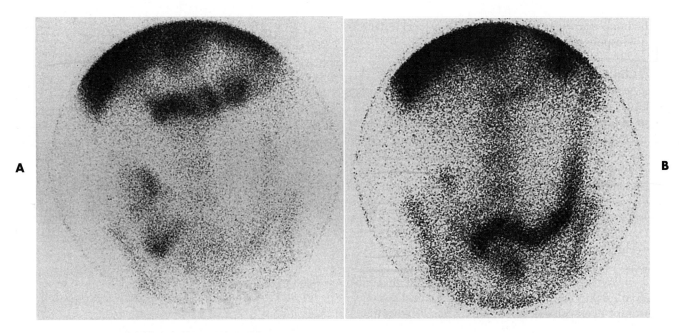

**Fig. 8-19**    False positive indium-111 leukocyte study. The intraluminal activity was due to gastrointestinal bleeding. Images obtained at, **A,** 4 hours and, **B,** 24 hours. Note movement of tracer through the bowel. No intraabdominal infection was diagnosed. The acute bleeding resolved without specific therapy.

Uninfected postsurgical wounds commonly show faint uptake for up to 10 days. If uptake is intense, persists, or extends beyond the surgical wound site, infection should be suspected. Low-grade uptake is often noted at sites of bone fracture.

Intraluminal intestinal activity may be the result of swallowed or shedding cells that occur with herpes esophagitis, pharyngitis, sinusitis, and pneumonia (Fig. 8-19). False positive studies of the abdomen may also be due to gastrointestinal bleeding, noninfected hematomas, and accessory spleens (Fig. 8-20). Rarely, tumors have increased uptake.

**Dosimetry**  The target organ for In-111 oxine–labeled leukocytes is the spleen, which in an adult receives a radiation dose of 15 to 20 rads. Children receive a somewhat higher splenic dose because of the smaller volume of distribution. However, the whole body absorbed dose is only 0.37 rad (Table 8-3).

**Disadvantages**  In-111 is cyclotron produced and must be ordered the day before the study. A total of 50 to 75 ml of blood must be drawn for labeling. Radiolabeling must be performed in a well-equipped laboratory with a laminar flow hood. Considerable expertise is needed to radiolabel the cells. The in vitro labeling procedure requires a minimum of 2 hours.

Lacking facilities and personnel for radiolabeling, most hospitals send the patient's blood to an outside commercial radiopharmacy. The additional time required for transportation can mean that leukocytes are not reinfused for 3 to 4 hours or longer after the blood is drawn. The longer the interval between withdrawal and

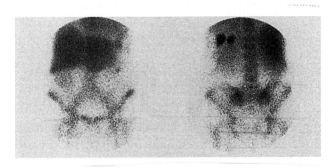

**Fig. 8-20**    Potential false positive indium-111 leukocyte scan caused by accessory spleens. This 78-year-old woman with bacterial endocartititis had previously undergone splenectomy. The In-111 leukocyte study was ordered to localize any extracardiac infection. A technetium-99m sulfur colloid study confirmed that the focal uptake in the left upper quadrant represented accessory spleens (see Fig. 10-48, *B*).

reinfusion, the higher the liklihood that the cells will lose viability.

The 18- to 24-hour delay between reinjection of the cells and imaging is suboptimal from the standpoint of clinical decision making. Another disadvantage is the relatively high radiation dose to the spleen (15 to 20 rads). This is particularly an issue for pediatric patients. Dosimetry limits the administered dose to 500 μCi in adults. Imaging time is thus long and the images are suboptimal.

Handling of blood products is a serious potential problem for the technician and technologist. A potentially catastrophic problem is accidental reinfusion of cells into the wrong patient, which unfortunately has been reported.

## TECHNETIUM-99M HMPAO–LABELED LEUKOCYTES

Leukocytes labeled with Tc-99m have theoretical advantages over In-111-labeled leukocytes. Tc-99m, being generator produced on site, could be immediately available for radiolabeling. The radiation dose to the patient would be significantly lower, permitting a higher administered activity. The higher photon yield of Tc-99m and its more optimal photopeak would result in superior image resolution that might translate into improved infection detectability and accuracy.

### Mechanism of Uptake

Tc-99m HMPAO is a radiopharmaceutical approved for cerebral perfusion imaging (see Chapter 12). It is lipophilic and readily crosses cell membranes. This property allows it to cross the blood-brain barrier and be taken up by cortical brain tissue. Intracellularly it changes into a hydrophilic complex and becomes trapped, bound to the mitochondria and the nucleus. It was appreciated that these properties could be used to radiolabel leukocytes.

### Radiolabeling

Unlike In-111 oxine, Tc-99m HMPAO leukocyte labeling can be performed in plasma. HMPAO preferentially labels granulocytes, a potential advantage for imaging acute purulent processes. The radiolabeling process does not adversely affect leukocyte function. The U.S. Food and Drug Administration (FDA) views Tc-99m HMPAO–labeled leukocytes as an alternative use of an approved radiopharmaceutical.

### Pharmacokinetics and Normal Distribution

Tc-99m HMPAO–labeled leukocytes are distributed in the body similarly to In-111 oxine leukocytes, with localization in the spleen, kidney, and bone marrow (Fig. 8-21). The biological half-life in blood is somewhat shorter than that of In-111 oxine leukocytes (4 versus 6 hours) because of slow elution of the Tc-99m HMPAO from circulating labeled cells. Early lung uptake similar to that seen with In-111 oxine occurs but decreases significantly by 4 hours.

Unlike In-111 oxine–labeled leukocytes, Tc-99m HMPAO–labeled leukocytes are cleared by the hepatobiliary and renal systems because of excretion of a secondary hydrophilic complex, which is similarly seen

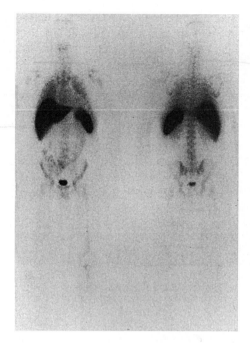

**Fig. 8-21** Normal technetium-99m HMPAO leukocyte distribution. The distribution is similar to that of indium-111 oxine leukocytes (Fig. 8-12), with highest uptake in the spleen, followed by the marrow and spleen. Image quality is superior for the Tc-99m-labeled agent. Some bowel and urinary clearance is seen on this image obtained 4 hours after injection. Low-grade normal pulmonary uptake is also seen. The study was performed because of suspected infection of a left knee prosthesis. It was reported as negative.

with Tc-99m HMPAO cerebral perfusion imaging. The kidneys and bladder may be seen as early as 1 hour after injection. The gallbladder is visualized in 4% of patients at 1 hour and in about 10% by 24 hours. Biliary clearance and bowel activity are routinely seen by 3 to 4 hours and increase with time.

### Dosimetry

With Tc-99m HMPAO leukocytes the colon is the organ receiving the highest radiation dose, 3.6 rads, followed by the bladder with 2.8 rads and the spleen with 2.2 rads (Table 8-3). This is in marked contrast to In-111 oxine–labeled white blood cells, which have a splenic radiation dose of more than 15 to 20 rads.

### Methodology

Box 8-10 describes a typical protocol. Early imaging at approximately 1 to 2 hours, before normal bowel and renal clearance of the radiopharmaceutical, is mandatory for diagnosis of intraabdominal infection or inflammatory bowel disease. For imaging of the distal extremies, such

---

**Box 8-10    Technetium-99m HMPAO Leukocyte Scintigraphy: Protocol Summary**

**RADIOPHARMACEUTICAL**

Tc-99m hexamethylpropylene amine (HMPAO) in vitro labeled leukocytes, 10 mCi (370 MBq)

**INSTRUMENTATION**

Camera: Large field of view; two-headed camera preferable for whole body imaging
Windows: 15%, centered over 140-keV photopeaks
Collimator: Low energy, high resolution

**PATIENT PREPARATION**

Draw 50 ml of blood to radiolabel cells in vitro

**PROCEDURE**

Radiolabel the patient's leukocytes in vitro with Tc-99m HMPAO.
Reinject labeled cells intravenously, preferably by direct venipuncture through 19-gauge needle. Contact with dextrose in water solutions may cause cell damage.
Imaging by 2 hr is mandatory to diagnose intraabdominal infection or localize inflammatory bowel disease. Imaging at 4 hr or later may be advantageous for peripheral skeletal imaging, e.g., osteomyelitis of feet.
Whole body imaging: Two-headed camera with whole body acqusition for 30 min; 10-min spot images for regions of special interest
SPECT in selected cases

---

**Table 8-4    Advantages and disadvantages of indium-111 oxine versus technetium-99m HMPAO–labeled leukocytes**

|  | In-111 oxine | Tc-99m HMPAO |
|---|---|---|
| Radionuclide immediately available | No | Yes |
| Stable radiolabel, no elution from cells | Yes | No |
| Allows labeling in plasma | No | Yes |
| Dosimetry | Poor | Good |
| Early routine imaging | No | Yes |
| Long half-life allows for delayed imaging | Yes | No |
| Imaging time | Long | Short |
| Permits dual isotope imaging | Yes | No |
| Bowel and renal clearance | No | Yes |
| Image resolution | Good | Fair |

---

**Box 8-11    Optimal Imaging Time for Infection-Seeking Radiopharmaceuticals**

| RADIOPHARMACEUTICAL | TIME (HR) |
|---|---|
| Gallium-67 | 48 |
| Indium-111 leukocytes | 24 |
| Nonspecific IgG antibodies | 10-24 |
| Antigranulocyte monoclonal antibodies | 1-6 |
| Technetium-99m HMPAO leukocytes | 1-4 |
| Chemotactic peptides | 1-4 |
| Technetium-99m nanocolloids | 1 |
| Fluorine-18 fluorodeoxyglucose | 1 |

---

as for the diagnosis of osteomyelitis, delayed imaging at 4 to 6 hours may be preferable because this allows more time for soft tissue clearance.

## Clinical Applications of Radiolabeled Leukocytes

The choice of which agent to use, Tc-99m HMPAO or In-111 oxine leukocytes, is determined by several factors. Both radiopharmaceuticals have distinct advantages and disadvantages (Table 8-4).

In some cases the specific clinical indication dictates the choice. For example, Tc-99m HMPAO leukocytes are believed to be superior for the diagnosis and localization of inflammatory bowel disease, and In-111 oxine leukocytes are preferable for other intraabdominal infections. However, for many other clinical situations the results to date have not proved to be significantly different. The decision is based on other factors (Box 8-10). Tc-99m HMPAO is preferable for pediatric patients because of the

lower radiation dose. If the results are needed urgently because of impending surgical intervention, Tc-99m HMPAO can be imaged the same day and might be preferable (Box 8-11). However, for most cases the decision is based on the physician's preference and experience.

**Pediatric patients**   The use of In-111 leukocytes poses problems for pediatric patients. Labeling requires a large volume of blood (20 to 50 ml). The child receives a relatively high radiation dose to the spleen. The low weight-adjusted administered dose results in a poor count rate, long imaging times, and poor resolution. Thus In-111-labeled leukocytes are not commonly used for children. Of the two approved radiopharmaceuticals, Tc-99m HMPAO–labeled leukocytes are preferred for use in children.

### Osteomyelitis

*Pathogenesis*   Bone infection is usually bacterial in origin. Microorganisms reach bone by three mechanisms: hematogenous spread, extension from a contiguous site of infection, and direct introduction of organisms into bone by trauma and surgery.

Acute hematogenous osteomyelitis involves bone with red marrow. In children the long bones are most commonly affected because of the relatively slow blood flow in metaphyseal sinusoidal veins and the paucity of phagocytes. Infection is often secondary to staphylococcal skin infection. In adults acute osteomyelitis rarely involves the long bones because adipose tissue has replaced red marrow. Instead, it most commonly occurs in vertebral bodies, where the marrow is cellular and has an abundant vascular supply. The initiating event is usually septicemia, often secondary to a urinary tract infection, bacterial endocarditis, or intravenous drug abuse. Infection usually begins in the vertebral body near the anterior longitudinal ligament and spreads to adjacent vertebrae by direct extension through the disk space or via communicating venous channels. Because the disk in an adult does not have a vascular supply, disk space infection caused by hematogenous infection is always due to osteomyelitis in an adjacent vertebra.

Extension from a contiguous site of infection is a common cause for osteomyelitis. Osteomyelitis may be secondary to soft tissue infection after trauma, radiation therapy, burns, or pressure sores. In patients with vascular insufficiency, organisms can enter the soft tissues through a cutaneous ulcer, often in the foot, and cause cellulitis and then osteomyelitis.

Direct introduction of organisms into bone may occur during open fractures, open surgical reduction of closed fractures, or penetrating trauma by foreign bodies such as bullets. Osteomyelitis may also arise from perioperative contamination of bone during surgery for nontraumatic orthopedic disorders, as in laminectomy, diskectomy, or placement of a joint prosthesis. The causative organism is often normal flora, such as *Staphylococcus epidermidis*.

*Pathology*   Pathological findings during the acute phase of osteomyelitis include neutrophilic inflammation, edema, and vascular congestion. Because of the bone's rigidity, intramedullary pressure increases, compromising the blood supply and causing ischemia and vascular thrombosis. After several days the suppurative and ischemic injury may cause bone to fragment into devitalized segments called sequestra. Inflammation spreads via haversian and Volkmann's canals to reach the periosteum, where abscesses form. This can lead to soft tissue abscesses or sinus tracts.

With persistent infection, chronic inflammatory cells (lymphocytes, histiocytes, and plasma cells) join the neutrophils. Fibroblastic proliferation and new bone formation occur. Periosteal osteogenesis may surround the inflammation to form a bony envelope, or involucrum. Occasionally a dense fibrous capsule confines the

infection to a localized area of suppuration (Brodie's abscess).

Hematogenous osteomyelitis acquired in childhood or adulthood may be manifested as intermittent or persistent drainage from sinus tracts communicating with the involved bone, usually the femur, tibia, or humerus, or as a soft tissue infection overlying it. Signs of infection may recur after years of quiescence.

*Clinical diagnosis*   Biopsy with culture is the most definitive basis for the diagnosis, but this is invasive and often contraindicated. Noninfected bone may become contaminated if there is an overlying soft tissue infection, and there is risk of pathological fractures in the small bones of the hands and feet. Noninvasive methods are preferred.

*Conventional imaging*   Plain radiography should be performed whenever osteomyelitis is suspected. However, the characteristic changes of permeative radiolucencies, destructive changes, and periosteal new bone formation may take 10 to 14 days to develop.

Although not used for diagnosis, CT can be helpful in defining the cortical extent of bone infection and can guide biopsy in suspected vertebral osteomyelitis. However, for the most part MRI has replaced CT because it can image the marrow, as well as demonstrate the extent of cortical infection. MRI has a reported sensitivity for osteomyelitis of 95% and a specificity of 88%. Typical findings include low signal intensity on $T_1$-weighted images and high signal intensity on $T_2$-weighted images. However, any disease that replaces bone marrow and causes increased tissue water, such as healing fractures, tumors, and Charcot joints, may not be distinguishable. Artifacts caused by joint implants can degrade images sufficiently to make diagnosis impossible.

*Scintigraphy*   The best method for diagnosis of osteomyelitis depends on the clinical situation as discussed in the following sections (Box 8-12).

---

**Box 8-12   Scintigraphic Diagnosis of Osteomyelitis in Different Clinical Situations**

Normal x-ray: three-phase bone scan

Neonates: three-phase bone scan; if negative, Tc-99m HMPAO

Suspected osteomyelitis in non-marrow-containing skeleton (distal extremities): bone scan + leukocyte study

Suspected osteomyelitis in bone marrow-containing skeleton (hips and knees): marrow scan + leukocyte study

Suspected vertebral osteomyelitis: gallium-67

BONE SCAN    In patients who do not have an associated underlying condition, the three-phase bone scan is the radionuclide procedure of choice for making the diagnosis of osteomyelitis. Its overall accuracy approaches 95%. However, the specificity is considerably poorer in patients with underlying conditions such as prior bone disease, fractures, orthopedic implants, and neuropathic joints (Table 8-5).

GALLIUM-67 CITRATE    Since Ga-67 is taken up by normal bone, uptake will be increased in regions that have increased bone turnover, similar to the uptake seen with the bone scan. As mentioned in more detail in the discussion of Ga-67, for better specificity the Ga-67 images should be interpreted in conjunction with a bone scan. A positive study is defined as one in which Ga-67 uptake is incongruent with the bone scan. However, the accuracy of the combined two studies is inferior to that of labeled leukocytes (Table 8-5).

RADIOLABELED LEUKOCYTES    For confirmation or exclusion of the diagnosis of osteomyelitis in patients with underlying bone disease, prostheses, and other confounding conditions, radiolabeled leukocytes, labeled with either In-111 oxine or Tc-99m HMPAO, have proved helpful. Some investigations have found an accuracy of over 90%, although others have not found the accuracy to be as high.

A problem in correct interpretation of radioloabeled leukocyte studies is the underlying assumption that the marrow distribution is normal and that identification of an area of abnormal uptake is consistent with infection. However, marrow distribution may not be normal for various reasons. For example, marrow distribution is frequently altered in the presence of previous disease, orthopedic hardware, infarction, or tumor. In these cases it may be difficult to ascertain whether focal uptake represents infection or atypical distribution of normal marrow.

One approach to improving the diagnostic accuracy of radiolabeled leukocytes in the preceding situations has been to interpret the study in conjunction with a bone scan. However, this has not improved the overall accuracy, probably because the two radiopharmaceuticals represent very different physiological processes, one that of cortical bone uptake and the other bone marrow uptake.

A more successful and rational approach is to use a bone marrow study as a template for the patient's marrow distribution. Tc-99m sulfur colloid marrow scintigraphy is the most commonly used technique. The distribution of the two radiopharmaceuticals, Tc-99m sulfur colloid and radiolabeled leukocytes, should be similar unless localized infection is present.

Osteomyelitis is usually seen on marrow imaging as a photopenic defect at the involved site because the marrow is displaced by the infection. This spatial incongruity, with accumulation of In-111 leukocytes where there is no marrow uptake, is diagnostic of infection. The accuracy for the combined study approaches 95%.

INFECTED JOINT PROSTHESES    The infection rate after primary hip or knee replacement is only 1% and after revision surgery is less than 3%. However, when infection occurs, this complication can be quite serious. Prosthetic joint infection may be difficult to diagnose because the symptoms and signs of infection are frequently indolent. Joint aspiration has a low sensitivity for the diagnosis of infection (12% to 66%). Radiography also has poor sensitivity, and bone scans have poor specificity.

Infection scintigraphy can be helpful in evaluating the complications of hip prosthesis, but accurate interpretation of scintigraphic uptake patterns requires a familiarity with the type of implant, its age, and the varying patterns seen after implantation of various joints.

Characteristic bone scan findings have been described for both loosening and infection of hip prostheses. In patients with a cemented total hip prosthesis studied more than 12 months after insertion, focal uptake at the tip of the femoral component is characteristic of loosening, and diffuse uptake around the femoral component is associated with infection. However, these patterns are not highly accurate. Furthermore, the cementless or porous coated prosthesis depends on bony ingrowth for stabilization. Thus ongoing new bone formation is part of the fixation process, and this results in periprosthetic uptake on bone scintigraphy in a variable pattern for a prolonged period, making interpretation more difficult.

Bone scintigraphy is a particular problem when patients have knee prostheses. More than half of all femoral components and three fourths of all tibial components show periprosthetic uptake more than 12 months after placement. Thus, for patients with cement-

**Table 8-5    Diagnosis of osteomyelitis: summed results from a literature review**

| Type of study | Sensitivity (%) | Specificity (%) |
|---|---|---|
| Three-phase bone scan (normal x-ray) | 94 | 95 |
| Three-phase bone scan (underlying bone disease) | 95 | 33 |
| Gallium-67 | 81 | 69 |
| Indium-111 leukocytes | 88 | 85 |
| Technetium-99m HMPAO | 87 | 81 |
| Leukocytes (vertebral) | 40 | 90 |
| Leukocytes + bone marrow | 95 | 90 |
| Antigranulocyte (LeukoScan) | 92 | 88 |
| Magnetic resonance imaging | 95 | 87 |

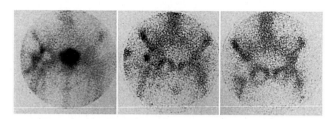

**Fig. 8-22** Infected hip prosthesis. *Left,* Technetium-99m medronate (MDP) bone scan shows increased uptake in the region of the right hip prosthesis laterally, consistent with heterotopic calcification. *Middle,* Indium-111 leukocyte study shows focal intense uptake just lateral to the femoral head and more diffuse uptake within the joint space consistent with infection. *Right,* Tc-99m sulfur colloid marrow study shows a normal bone marrow distribution with cold head of the femur consistent with prosthesis. The mismatch of the bone marrow and In-111 leukocyte study indicates an infected prosthesis.

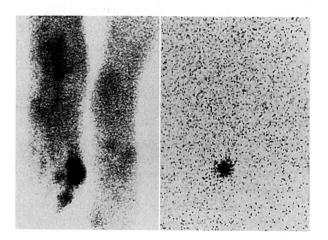

**Fig. 8-23** Diabetic foot, osteomyelitis. A diabetic patient with peripheral vascular disease, cellulitis, and infection in the region of the first metatarsal. *Left,* The 2-hour delayed bone scan shows markedly increased uptake in the distal first metatarsal. The first two phases of the study were also positive. *Right,* Indium-111 oxine leukocyte study was performed to confirm the diagnosis. Intense uptake is seen in the same distal metatarsal. No uptake is noted in other areas of the foot that were hot on the bone scan (i.e., the distal phalanx of the first toe and the second distal metatarsal). This is due to the lack of infection in these areas and lack of red marrow in the foot.

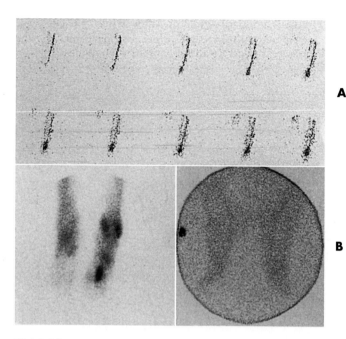

**Fig. 8-24** Positive three-phase bone scan and negative indium-111 leukocyte study for osteomyelitis. **A,** Radionuclide angiogram shows increased flow in the region of the distal left midfoot. **B,** *Left,* A 3-hour delayed image shows increased uptake by the third metatarsal. Ankle uptake is also noted. *Right,* The In-111-leukocyte study is negative for infection. Radiograph showed a metatarsal fracture.

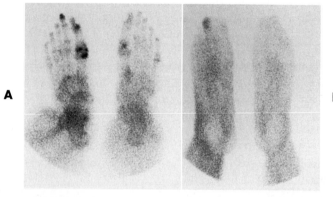

**Fig. 8-25** Osteomyelitis confirmed with technetium-99m HMPAO leukocytes. A diabetic patient with purulent drainage of the distal second digit of the right foot. **A,** Bone scan shows increased uptake on the distal second digit of the right. The first two phases were also positive. **B,** Tc-99m HMPAO leukocyte study was positive as well, consistent with osteomyelitis.

less hip replacement or total knee replacement, bone scintigraphy is most useful when the scan is normal or when serial studies over time are available for comparison.

Ga-67 scintigraphy in conjunction with bone scintigraphy is only moderately accurate (approximately 80%) in the diagnosis of infected joint prostheses. The accuracy of the combination of bone imaging with leukocyte scintigraphy approaches 85%.

If leukocytes are used alone, false positive interpretations may result. Insertion of the shaft of a hip prosthesis invariably results in marrow displacement. The best results for the diagnosis of infected hip prostheses are obtained when the combination of In-111 oxine leuko-

cytes and Tc-99m sulfur colloid marrow scintigraphy is used (Fig. 8-22). The accuracy is reported to be greater than 90%.

DIABETIC FOOT  Over 90% of foot ulcers in diabetic patients serve as a portal of entry for infection. The use of In-111-labeled leukocyte scintigraphy has proved accurate in confirming or excluding the diagnosis of osteomyelitis (Figs. 8-23 to 8-25). One problem in evaluating the diabetic foot is that leukocytes also

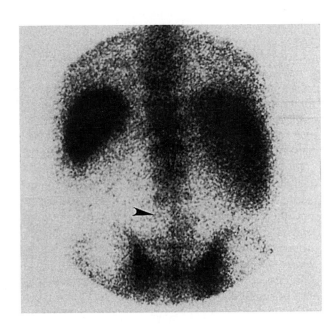

**Fig. 8-26**    Vertebral osteomyelitis. A cold defect at L5 was seen with indium-111 leukocyte scintigraphy. Biopsy was necessary to make the diagnosis of osteomyelitis.

accumulate in neuropathic joints and fractures. Although this uptake is generally of low intensity, it can pose a diagnostic dilemma. The improved resolution of Tc-99m HMPAO white blood cells may be an advantage in trying to diagnose osteomyelitis in the small bones of the feet. Marrow scintigraphy is less useful for evaluation of the feet because of the lack of red marrow in the distal extremities.

In-111 scintigraphy can be useful for monitoring response to therapy. Scintigraphic findings of infection should revert to normal after 2 to 8 weeks of appropriate antibiotic therapy.

Vᴇʀᴛᴇʙʀᴀʟ Oꜱᴛᴇᴏᴍʏᴇʟɪᴛɪꜱ    Vertebral osteomyelitis is a special case in regard to scintigraphy. Poor sensitivity for radiolabeled leukocytes has been repeatedly reported, with false negative results occurring in 10% to 40% of patients who have osteomyelitis of the central skeleton. The labeled leukocyte study commonly shows a photopenic or cold defect at the site (Fig. 8-26). Thus infection cannot be differentiated from metastasis, fracture, Paget's disease, surgical defects, or irradiation. The reason for this is uncertain, although it may be related to associated infarction. Therefore, although Ga-67 is often used in the diagnosis of vertebral osteomyelitis, its specificity is poor.

**Intraabdominal infection**    Because of the morbidity and mortality associated with intraabdominal infection, prompt diagnosis is critical. Ga-67 is not optimal because of its considerable normal bowel clearance and 48-hour optimal imaging time. In-111-labeled leukocytes have a distinct advantage in imaging of the abdomen (Fig. 8-3). The radiopharmaceutical is not cleared through the bowel. Combined data from three large

series showed an overall sensitivity of approximately 90% for In-111 oxine leukocytes in detecting intraabdominal infection.

Early imaging (at 4 hours) with In-111 leukocytes has been shown to be less sensitive for the detection of infection and is not recommended as a routine. However, imaging at 1 to 4 hours may expedite the diagnosis in acutely ill patients with suspected acute appendicitis, diverticulitis, and ischemic bowel disease. These diseases are associated with increased blood flow and marked leukocyte infiltration, making for rapid intensive leukocyte uptake.

Tc-99m HMPAO label has potential advantages because of its superior image quality and preferential labeling of granulocytes, resulting in rapid uptake in lesions. On first consideration it might not be considered an optimal radiotracer because of its intraabdominal clearance. However, if imaging is done early, before bowel clearance, its accuracy is good. A large study found that the sensitivity for detecting abdominal infection and inflammatory disease was 88% at 30 minutes and 95% at 2 hours. Initial imaging must be done by 1 to 2 hours. Delayed imaging is occasionally helpful to confirm that the early detected abnormal activity is a fixed pattern. A shifting pattern of activity over time implies intraluminal transit of labeled leukocytes, for example, as seen with inflammatory or ischemic bowel disease, fistula, or abscess in communication with bowel, or some other false positive cause (Box 8-9).

Abnormal leukocyte uptake has been described in a variety of noninfectious inflammatory diseases, including severe pancreatitis, polyarteritis nodosa, rheumatoid vasculitis, and acute cholecystitis. For the routine diagnosis of acute cholecystitis, the Tc-99m hepatoiminodiacetic acid (HIDA) study is preferable because cell labeling is unnecessary and the HIDA study has a high accuracy. However, in selected cases In-111 leukocytes may prove useful, such as in the clinical situation in which a false positive HIDA is possible (prolonged fasting, hyperalimentation, severe concurrent illness) or in the case of a suspected false negative HIDA study (acute acalculous cholecystitis).

**Inflammatory bowel disease**    Ulcerative colitis and Crohn's disease (granulomatous or regional enteritis) are characterized by intestinal inflammation. Although barium enema examination and colonoscopy are routinely used to make these diagnoses, the procedures are often contraindicated in severely ill patients. Studies have shown good correlation between the site and amount of In-111 leukocyte uptake compared with the endoscopic and radiological localization.

Imaging should be performed at 4 hours rather than the usual 24 hours because shedding of leukocytes into the bowel lumen from the inflammatory sites and subsequent peristalsis may result in incorrect assignment of disease to sites distal to the true lesion. The In-111 leukocyte study is useful not only in acute fulminant enteritis or colitis, but also for evaluating areas hard to see with endoscopy and for monitoring the effectiveness of therapy. Inactive colitis is not detected by scintigraphy.

In-111-labeled leukocytes can differentiate reactivation of inflammatory bowel disease from abscess formation resulting from bowel perforation. The latter is a serious clinical problem, requiring very different therapy (surgical rather than medical). In-111 leukocyte uptake in an abscess is usually focal, whereas uptake in inflamed bowel typically follows the contour of the intestinal wall (Fig. 8-27). Leukocyte uptake may also be seen in ischemic colitis (common in elderly patients), pseudomembranous colitis (antibiotic related), and bowel infarction.

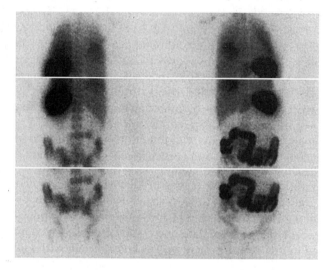

**Fig. 8-27**    Cytomegalovirus infection detected with technetium-99m HMPAO leukocytes. HIV-positive patient with fever and diarrhea. *Left column,* Posterior views. *Right column,* Anterior views of chest *(upper),* abdomen *(middle),* and pelvis *(lower).* Imaging was performed at 90 minutes, before bowel clearance would normally be seen. Tc-99m HMPAO uptake is seen in the right lung base and the bowel. A pneumonic infiltrate was found on chest radiograph. Cytomegalovirus was confirmed as the cause of the colitis.

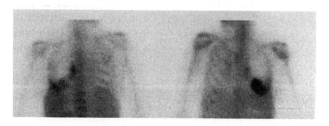

**Fig. 8-28**    Postoperative empyema diagnosed with technetium-99m HMPAO leukocytes. The infection occurred after thoracotomy for lung cancer. *Left,* Posterior view. *Right,* Anterior view.

Tc-99m HMPAO–labeled leukocytes are now generally preferred to In-111-labeled leukocytes because of their superiority for the localization of disease to specific bowel segments and particularly for their ability to identify small bowel disease. Although In-111 leukocytes give reliable images of the colon, they are more likely to miss small bowel disease. Accurate results with T-99m HMPAO leukocytes can be obtained as early as 1 hour after injection.

Crohn's disease and ulcerative colitis can usually be distinguished from each other by the distribution of disease activity. Rectal sparing, small bowel involvement, and skip areas suggest Crohn's disease, whereas continuous colonic involvement from the rectum without small bowel involvement suggests ulcerative colitis.

**Renal disease**    In-111-labeled leukocytes can detect and localize genitourinary infection. The radiolabeled cells accumulate at sites of acute pyelonephritis, focal nephritis (lobar nephronia), and renal or perirenal abscess. However, In-111-labeled leukocytes have limited utility for evaluation of renal transplants. Almost all transplant recipients exhibit uptake, regardless of the presence or absence of clinically significant disease or rejection.

**Cardiovascular disease**    In-111-labeled leukocytes are not useful in making the diagnosis of subacute bacterial endocarditis. The vegetative lesions often contain high concentrations of bacteria, platelets, and fibrin adherent to damaged valvular endothelium but relatively few leukocytes. Uptake can be seen in acute myocardial infarction and cardiac transplant rejection, but the study is not generally used for making these diagnoses.

Radiolabeled leukocytes can be used to diagnose surgical prosthetic graft infection (Fig. 8-15). Infection of arterial prosthetic grafts, such as femoropopliteal and aortofemoral grafts, is associated with significant morbidity (amputation) and mortality. Ultrasound, CT, and MRI are often unable to distinguish infection from aseptic fluid collections around the graft. Prompt diagnosis of graft infection is critical but often delayed because of the indolent and insidious course of such infections.

**Pulmonary infection**    Pulmonary uptake of In-111 leukocytes should be interpreted cautiously. Low-grade diffuse uptake has been associated with a variety of noninfectious causes, including atelectasis, congestive heart failure, and adult respiratory distress syndrome, and therefore should not be considered diagnostic of infection.

Focal intense uptake is likely to be due to infection (Fig. 8-17). Tuberculosis and chronic granulomatous diseases do not usually take up In-111-labeled leukocytes. Ga-67 is the preferred agent for the scintigraphic evaluation of most pulmonary diseases.

## PROMISING INFECTION-SEEKING RADIOPHARMACEUTICALS

Alternative infection-seeking radiopharmaceuticals have been under investigation with the hope that they might overcome some of the disadvantages of the present approved radiopharmaceuticals. A major advantage of most discussed in this section is that they do not require cell labeling and therefore transmission of bloodborne diseases is not a concern. Some of the interesting and promising new approaches are briefly described.

### Radiolabeled Lymphocytes

Lymphocytes are potentially useful for diagnosing chronic and more indolent inflammatory processes such as rejection of kidney and heart transplants. Only preliminary studies have been reported. Unlike neutrophils, lymphocytes are quite radiosensitive. Concerns have been expressed about the radiation effect on function and, more important, the potential for oncogenesis because of the lymphocytes' long life span.

### Nonspecific Immunoglobulin G Antibodies

The utility of radiolabeled human immunoglobulin (HIG) for imaging of infection was fortuitously discovered during investigations of monoclonal antibodies. Surprisingly, the nonspecific polyclonal immunoglobulins were found to be equally effective. The mechanism is not well understood. Accumulation is probably not due to an immunological mechanism, but rather to the increased vascular permeability associated with inflammatory processes. Radiolabeled HIG has a number of advantages. It comes in kit form, can be labeled with Tc-99m or In-111, and does not require complicated and time-consuming in vitro cell labeling or the handling of blood products. The normal distribution of In-111-labeled HIG includes the liver, spleen, and bone marrow (Table 8-4). The gastrointestinal and genitourinary systems show varying degrees of uptake. Preliminary results have been good, with accuracy greater than 90%. Uptake has been seen with a wide variety of infectious agents, including *Mycoplasma, Pneumocystis, Candida, Histoplasma,* and tuberculosis. Chronicity of infection, antibiotics, antiinflammatory drugs, and corticosteroids do not seem to affect the sensitivity.

### Monoclonal Antibodies

Radiolabeled monoclonal antibodies directed against specific leukocyte cell-surface antigens have been investigated. One agent, LeukoScan (Immunomedics, Morris Plains, N.J.), is in phase III clinical investigations and may soon be approved for clinical use. It is a Tc-99m-labeled antigranulocyte (IgG1) antibody Fab' fragment. Fab' fragments result in less immunoreactivity (human antimurine antibody [HAMA] response) than whole antibodies and have a better target-to-background ratio owing to rapid renal clearance. Clinical trials, particularly for musculoskeletal infection, have found the accuracy of LeukoScan imaging to be equal or superior to that of In-111 leukocyte imaging. Imaging can be performed within 1 to 6 hours after injection.

### Chemotactic Peptides

Produced by bacteria, chemotactic peptides bind to receptors on the cell membrane of polymorphonuclear leukocytes, stimulating the cells to undergo chemotaxis. Analogs of these peptides have been synthesized and radiolabeled. Localization at sites of infection is rapid owing to the small size of these compounds; they easily pass through vascular walls and quickly enter an abscess. The highest target-to-background ratio occurs at 1 hour. Animal studies have been promising, and human studies are pending.

### Radiolabeled Colloids

Tc-99m nanocolloid, most commonly used for bone marrow imaging and lymphoscintigraphy, has also been investigated for imaging of infection and is used for this purpose in Europe. These human serum albumin colloids are less than 50 nm in diameter and are preferentially taken up by the reticuloendothelial system of the marrow and to a lesser extent by the liver and spleen. They leave the circulation and localize in the extracellular space at sites of infection, probably because of increased vascular permeability. This radiopharmaceutical has shown utility in the early diagnosis (within 60 minutes) of bone and joint infections. However, the radiotracer has poor sensitivity for infections outside the musculoskeletal system.

### Fluorine-18 Fluorodeoxyglucose

Fluorine-18 fluorodeoxyglucose (F-18 FDG) is used primarily in positron emission tomography for tumor imaging. However, it has been noted that uptake of F-18 FDG is often increased in active infection. Clinical trials to define its clinical utility are under way.

### Other Agents

Other single-photon radiopharmaceuticals with various physiological mechanisms are under investigation. Among these are radiolabeled liposomes, cytokines, and chemokines, such as interleukins.

## SUGGESTED READINGS

Coleman RE, Datz FL: Detection of inflammatory disease using radiolabeled cells. In Sandler M, Coleman RE, Wackers FJTh, et al, editors: *Diagnostic nuclear medicine,* ed 3, Baltimore, 1996, Williams & Wilkins.

Datz FL, Taylor AT Jr: Cell labeling: techniques and clinical utility. In *Freeman and Johnson's clinical radionuclide imaging,* ed 3, Update, 1986, Grune & Stratton.

Hakki S, Harwood SJ, Morrissey MA, et al: Comparative study of monoclonal antibody in diagnosing orthopedic infection, *Clin Orthop Rel Res* 335:275-285, 1997.

Kipper SL: Radiolabeled leukocyte imaging of the abdomen. In Freeman LM, editor: *Nuclear medicine annual 1995,* New York, 1995, Raven Press.

McAfee JG, Samin A: In-111 labeled leukocytes: a review of problems in image interpretation, *Radiology* 155:221-229, 1985.

Merkel KD, Brown ML, Dewanjee MK, Fitzgerald RH Jr: Comparison of indium-labeled-leukocyte imaging with sequential technetium-gallium scanning in the diagnosis of low-grade musculoskeletal sepsis, *J Bone Joint Surg* 67A: 465-476, 1985.

Oyen WJG, Boerman OC, van der Laken CJ, et al: The uptake mechanism of inflammation- and infection-localizing agents, *Eur J Nucl Med* 23:459-465, 1996.

Palermo F, Boccaletto F, Paolin A, et al: Comparison of technetium-99m-MDP, techetium-99m WBC and technetium-99m-HIG in musculoskeletal inflammation, *J Nucl Med* 39:516-521, 1998.

Palestro CJ, Torres MA: Radionuclide imaging in orthopedic infections, *Semin Nucl Med* 27:334-345, 1997.

Peters AM: Imaging inflammation and infection Tc-99m HMPAO labeled leukocytes. In Henkin RE, Boles MA, Dillehay GL, editor: *Nuclear medicine,* St Louis, 1996, Mosby.

Rubin RH, Fishchman AJ: Radionuclide imaging of infection in the immunocompromised host, *Clin Infect Dis* 22:414-422, 1996.

Schauwecker DS: The scintigraphic diagnosis of osteomyelitis, *AJR* 158:9-18, 1992.

Oncology has always represented a substantial portion of nuclear medicine practice, but in recent years tumor imaging has become a major area of growth. Use of gallium-67 (Ga-67) studies has had a resurgence. Technetium-99m (Tc-99m) sestamibi, originally a cardiac agent, has become an important tumor-imaging agent and is approved by the U.S. Food and Drug Administration (FDA) for evaluation of breast masses. New monoclonal antibodies have been approved by the FDA for the imaging of patients with colon, prostate, and lung cancer, and others are expected to become available in the near future for both imaging and therapy. A new generation of peptide-based imaging agents is emerging. The first one is a somatostatin receptor imaging agent that has been approved for localization of neuroendocrine tumors. Fluorine-18 fluorodeoxyglucose (F-18 FDG) oncological imaging has come of clinical age with use of positron emission tomography (PET) and single-photon emission computed tomography (SPECT). Clinical interest has also been renewed in lymphoscintigraphy for the preoperative evaluation of melanoma and breast cancer patients.

Numerous radionuclide imaging studies that detect primary and metastatic tumors are described in other chapters. Most are organ specific, not tumor specific (Box 9-1); among these are Tc-99m medronate (MDP) bone scans, iodine-123 (I-123) and Tc-99m pertechnetate thyroid scans, Tc-99m sulfur colloid liver-spleen scans, and Tc-99m diethylenetriamine pentaacetic acid (DTPA) and glucoheptonate brain scans. Although these studies can detect malignant tumors, the hot spot (increased uptake) or cold spot (decreased uptake) abnormalities are nonspecific and may also have benign or nontumor etiologies. A few radionuclide studies discussed in other chapters are tumor type specific, such as I-131 whole body scans for thyroid cancer, Tc-99m hepato-iminodiacetic acid (HIDA) scans for benign and malignant hepatocyte tumors, and adrenal tumor imaging with I-131 meta-iodo-benzyl-guanidine (MIBG) and I-131-6-beta-iodomethyl-19-norcholesterol (I-131 NP-59).

This chapter focuses on radiopharmaceuticals not discussed elsewhere in the text, both nonspecific tumor-imaging radionuclides, such as Ga-67, thallium-201 (Tl-201), Tc-99m sestamibi (MIBI), Tc-99m tetrofosmin, and F-18 FDG, and newer tumor-specific radiopharmaceuticals, such as monoclonal antibodies and peptides. Important new developments in the use of lymphoscintigraphy for sentinel node detection in melanoma and breast cancer are reviewed.

## GALLIUM-67 TUMOR IMAGING

Although initially investigated as a bone-imaging agent, Ga-67 citrate was first used clinically in 1969 for tumor detection in patients with Hodgkin's disease. Its uptake in many other tumors was subsequently appreciated. Ga-67 was found to have a high sensitivity for detection of Hodgkin's disease, non-Hodgkin's lymphoma, metastatic melanoma, and hepatocellular carcinoma. Although GA-67 is taken up by numerous other tumors, such as those of the lung, head and neck, and soft tissue, its clinical role in these diseases has been less certain. In recent years pretherapy staging and posttherapy evaluation of patients with Hodgkin's disease and non-Hodgkin's lymphoma have become the most common clinical indications for Ga-67 tumor scintigraphy.

### Chemistry and Physics

Gallium is a group III element in the Periodic Table with biological behavior similar to that of iron. The radionuclide Ga-67 is cyclotron produced. It decays by electron capture and emits a spectrum of gamma rays ranging from 91 to 394 keV (approximately 100, 200, 300, and 400 keV) (Table 9-1). The lower three photopeaks are used for imaging because of their higher abundance. Physical half-life is 78 hours.

Ga-67 does not have optimal physical characteristics for scintigraphic imaging. Neither the low- nor the high-

| Table 9-1 | Physical characteristics of tumor-imaging radionuclides | | | | | |
|-----------|-------------------------|------------------------|--------------------------------|-----|------------------|-----------------------|

| Radionuclide | Chemical or Pharmaceutical | Physical half-life (hr) | Principal mode of isotopic decay | Photopeaks keV | Photopeaks Percent abundance | Usual administered dose (mCi) |
|--------------|----------------------------|-------------------------|----------------------------------|------|--------------------|--------------------------------|
| Gallium-67 | citrate | 78 | Electron capture | 93 | 41 | 10 |
| | | | | 185 | 23 | |
| | | | | 300 | 18 | |
| | | | | 394 | 4 | |
| Thallium-201 | chloride | 73 | Electron capture | 69-83 | 94 | 3 |
| Technetium-99m | sestamibi tetrofosmin CEA-SCAN | 6 | Isomeric transition | 140 | 88 | 25 |
| Fluorine-18 | fluorodeoxyglucose | 2 | Positron (beta +) (97%) Electron capture (3%) | 511 | 194 | 10 |
| Indium-111 | OncoScint ProstaScint | 67 | Electron capture | 173 247 | 90 94 | 5 |

energy photons are well suited for present-day gamma camera crystals. The high-energy photons penetrate the collimator septa and result in unavoidable scatter.

## Pharmacokinetics and Normal Distribution

Ga-67 citrate acts like a ferric ion analog in the blood and circulates bound to transferrin. The radiopharmaceutical is transported to cellular receptors and incorporated intracellularly. The kidney excretes 15% to 25% of the administered dose within the first 24 hours. From that point on, however, the colon is the major route of excretion. Total body clearance is slow, with a biological half-life of 25 days. Two days after injection about 75% of the administered dose remains in the body. Ga-67 uptake is highest in the liver and occurs to a lesser extent in the salivary glands, spleen, bone marrow, and lacrimal glands. Uptake in the lacrimal glands is due to lactoferrin binding. Ga-67 is also excreted in breast milk.

Alterations in biodistribution and uptake can result from a number of factors, including prior administration of the magnetic resonance imaging (MRI) contrast agent gadolinium, radiation therapy, chemotherapy, and iron saturation. Since iron competes with gallium for binding to serum transferrin, iron overload syndromes (e.g., repeated transfusions) saturate the receptors and cause decreased hepatic and marrow uptake and increased renal uptake.

The pharmacokinetics and distribution of Ga-67 citrate are not optimal from an imaging standpoint. It has slow background clearance, so that good imaging is not possible until 48 or 72 hours after injection. The considerable normal uptake by the liver, bone, and bone marrow makes tumor detection difficult in or adjacent to these organs. Slow large bowel clearance is a problem in abdominal imaging and often necessitates delayed imaging at 4 to 7 days. Nevertheless, the tumor avidity of Ga-67 makes it a clinically useful radiopharmaceutical.

## Mechanism of Tumor Localization

The mechanism by which Ga-67 is taken up by tumors is complex. Multiple mechanisms have been described, and their relative importance is uncertain and may vary by tumor type. An adequate blood supply is essential for delivery of Ga-67 to the tumor site. The increased vascular permeability of the tumor probably plays a role in cell entry.

Specific tumor-associated transferrin receptors are known to bind Ga-67 to the tumor cell surface. Ga-67 is then transported intracellularly and binds to cytoplasmic proteins, such as ferritin and lactoferrin, which are often found in high concentration in tumors, and also to macromolecules within organelles. Ga-67 is taken up only by actively growing and viable tumors, not by tumor necrosis or fibrosis. The degree of uptake is directly related to tumor metabolism.

## Dosimetry

With a typical administered Ga-67 dose of 10 mCi in an adult, the large intestine receives the highest radiation, about 9 rads, the spleen and bone marrow receive 5 to 6 rads, and the liver receives 4.6 rads (Table 9-2).

## Methodology

Advancements in instrumentation and methodology have resulted in markedly better image quality and tumor detectability than in the early years of

**Table 9-2    Radiation absorbed dose for Ga-67, Tl-201, Tc-99m-MIBI, Tc-99m tetrofosmin, and F-18 FDG**

| Organ | Ga-67 (rads/10 mCi) | Tl-201 (rads/3 mCi) | Tc-99m MIBI (rads/30 mCi) | Tc-99m tetrofosmin (rads/30 mCi) | F-18 FDG (rads/10 mCi) |
|---|---|---|---|---|---|
| Kidney | 4.1 | **3.6** | 2.0 | 1.4 | 0.8 |
| Thyroid | | 1.5 | 0.7 | 0.6 | |
| Heart wall | | 1.5 | 0.5 | 0.5 | 1.5 |
| Liver | 4.6 | 1.8 | 0.6 | 0.5 | 0.7 |
| Spleen | 5.3 | | | | 1.9 |
| Bone marrow | **5.8** | | | | |
| Bone | 4.4 | | | | |
| Gallbladder | | | 2.0 | **5.4** | |
| Testes | 2.4 | 1.6 | 0.3 | 0.4 | |
| Ovaries | 2.8 | 1.5 | 1.5 | 1.1 | 0.6 |
| Brain | | | | | 0.7 |
| Urinary bladder | | | 2.0 | 2.2 | **4.1** |
| Large intestine | 9.0 | 1.2 | **5.4** | 3.4 | |
| Breasts | | | 0.2 | 0.4 | |
| Total body | 2.6 | 0.7 | 0.5 | 0.6 | 0.4 |

Target organ in boldface type.

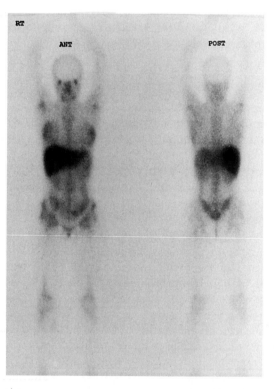

**Fig. 9-1**    Normal gallium-67 distribution. Whole body scan of a 50-year-old woman, obtained 72 hours after injection. Highest uptake is seen in the liver, followed by the bone and marrow. Prominent uptake is seen in the left side of the colon and the sigmoid. Note normal lacrimal uptake, nasopharyngeal activity, and breast and soft tissue distribution in this thin patient.

Ga-67 imaging (Figs. 9-1 to 9-5). Some of these advances include improved gamma camera resolution, multi-headed detectors, fast dedicated computers, quality SPECT instrumentation and software, and multichannel acquisition.

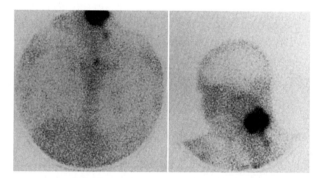

**Fig. 9-2**    Hodgkin's disease. This 25-year-old man had a mass in the left side of the neck. *Right,* Left lateral view. Large region of increased gallium-67 uptake in left side of the neck and small nodal focus just inferior to it. *Left,* Anterior view. Small focus can be seen inferior to mass on left side of neck. There is also focal uptake in the mediastinum (proven with SPECT).

Although in the past 3 to 5 mCi of Ga-67 was used for both tumor and infection imaging, 8 to 10 mCi is now routine for tumor imaging. The resulting higher count rate makes possible high-quality planar and SPECT imaging and increased tumor detectability. Delayed imaging gives time for bowel and background clearance, resulting in an improved target-to-background ratio and better abdominal imaging, as well as high-quality SPECT at delayed imaging times. The higher dose is acceptable because of the clear-cut benefit versus the very low risk in these cancer patients. Use of multiple photopeaks, usually three (93, 185, and 300 keV) (Table 9-1), is recommended to maximize the count rate.

Bowel cleansing before imaging has been advocated to minimize the problem of slow bowel clearance and the need for delayed imaging. However, this is controversial.

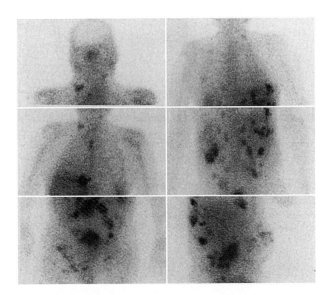

**Fig. 9-3**   Non-Hodgkin's lymphoma. A 67-year-old man with multiple sites of gallium-67 uptake by tumor both above and below the diaphragm. *Left,* Anterior spot views of the head, chest, and abdomen and pelvis *(top to bottom). Right,* Posterior views of the chest and abdomen and right lateral view of the abdomen and pelvis *(top to bottom).*

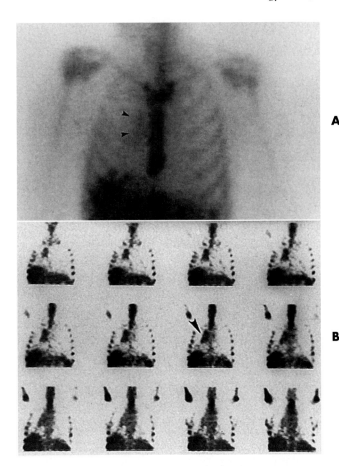

**Fig. 9-4**   Gallium-67 chest SPECT. A 35-year-old man with Hodgkin's disease. **A,** Anterior planar chest image shows low-intensity uptake in the right hilum *(arrowheads).* **B,** SPECT shows definite hilar uptake *(arrowhead)* on sequential coronal chest sections owing to the improved contrast resolution of SPECT.

Although the exact protocol varies by laboratory, planar and SPECT images are typically obtained at 48 to 72 hours. Planar images can be obtained as long as 7 to 10 days after injection, and good SPECT images at 5 to 6 days. Box 9-2 describes a typical Ga-67 tumor imaging protocol.

Because chemotherapy and radiation therapy before Ga-67 imaging can result in altered biodistribution, Ga-67 injection should follow chemotherapy by at least 3 weeks, although some data suggest that 1 week may be sufficient. When the Ga-67 study is urgently needed, such as when chemotherapy is given in 2-week cycles and reevaluation is required before the next cycle, Ga-67 should be injected at least 1 week after prior treatment and 48 hours before the next therapy.

### Image Interpretation

**Normal gallium-67 distribution**   The liver has the highest uptake of Ga-67, followed by bone and marrow and then the spleen (Fig. 9-1). The kidneys are seen on early imaging at 6 to 24 hours but appear only faintly by 48 to 72 hours. Uptake is variable in the salivary and lacrimal glands and nasal mucosa. Female breast uptake varies with the hormonal status and may be particularly prominent post partum (Fig. 9-1; see Fig. 8-2). Soft tissue background activity can be high. This depends to a large extent on body habitus and decreases with delayed imaging. Increased salivary gland uptake is noted after head and neck irradiation and can persist for years.

Large bowel clearance is variable and can pose interpretive problems in differentiating tumor from normal transit of radiopharmaceutical. Laxatives and enemas may speed clearance, but delayed imaging is often necessary to differentiate intraabdominal tumor from normal intestinal activity clearance. Tumor uptake remains fixed, while normal Ga-67 clearance takes place in the large bowel.

Faint symmetrical hilar uptake may be seen normally and is common after chemotherapy. More prominent hilar node uptake sometimes poses an interpretive problem owing to concomitant inflammatory disease. Asymmetrical and intense nodal uptake is abnormal. CT can be helpful in problem cases. If Ga-67 uptake occurs before treatment and CT does not show abnormality, the uptake probably has no clinical significance. However, when a corresponding CT abnormality is seen, persistent or new Ga-67 may cause a problem on a posttreatment scan. Tl-201 can help differentiate benign nodal uptake from tumor, since Tl-201, a tumor-avid agent, is not usually taken up in inflammation.

Faint or absent liver uptake can result from competition from extensive tumor metastases or occasionally from nonmalignant causes of hepatic insufficiency. Chemotherapeutic agents, such as vincristine administered

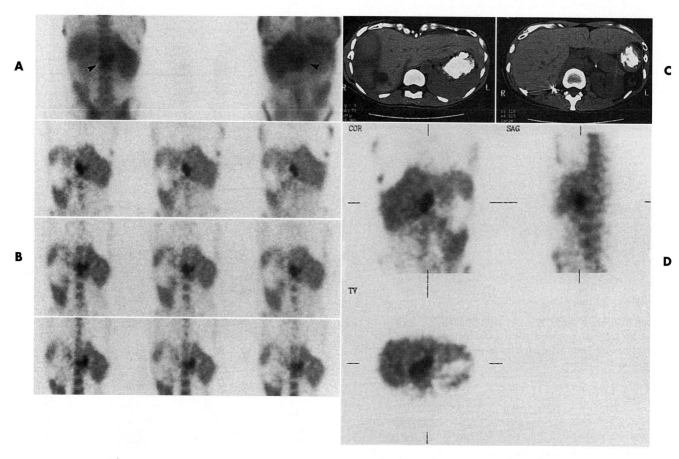

**Fig. 9-5** Gallium-67 abdominal SPECT. A 26-year-old woman with non-Hodgkin's lymphoma. **A,** The anterior *(right)* and posterior *(left)* planar images suggest uptake in the spine or prevertebral region *(arrowheads).* **B,** High-contrast SPECT sequential coronal views clearly confirm prevertebral periaortic node involvement. Also seen is a subcapsular defect in the right lobe of the liver caused by hematoma as a complication of liver biopsy. **C,** Computed tomography. *Left,* Superior cut shows the large hematoma. *Right,* The tumor mass is anterior to the spine in a lower cut. **D,** Three-view SPECT display shows the tumor to be anterior to the spine, perhaps best seen in the sagittal view.

within 24 hours of Ga-67 injection, can depress liver uptake. Iron overload syndromes may also decrease liver uptake and increase renal clearance. Renal uptake is increased with interstitial nephritis because of chemotherapy or nephrotoxic antibiotics. Renal failure results in prolonged background clearance.

Several potential interpretive problems should be kept in mind. Ga-67 is taken up at sites of infection or inflammatory disease (see Chapter 8) and increased bone turnover. Bone marrow biopsy can result in focal uptake. Postoperative surgical wounds have increased uptake for 2 to 3 weeks. Soft tissue uptake can be seen at therapeutic injection sites. Contrast lymphangiography can result in a chemical pneumonitis with prominent pulmonary uptake, so Ga-67 imaging should be performed first. Axillary node uptake may be missed if imaging is not performed with the arms elevated (Fig. 9-6). Breast uptake is sometimes confused with intratho-

racic disease on planar imaging. Oblique, lateral views or SPECT can clarify this question.

## Tumor Detectability

Tumor detectability with Ga-67 depends on multiple factors. One of these is tumor histology, since uptake varies by tumor type (Table 9-3). Within a tumor type, high-grade tumors are more likely to take up Ga-67 than low-grade tumors. Lesion size is another important factor. Tumors less than 2 cm in diameter are not reliably detected with conventional planar imaging, those 2 to 5 cm in diameter can usually be seen, and occasional tumor masses greater than 5 cm may be poorly visualized because of tumor necrosis. SPECT allows detection of smaller lesions (1 to 1.5 cm) because of its better contrast resolution. Detectability also depends on anatomical location of the tumor. Superficial lesions are

## Box 9-2    Gallium-67 Citrate Tumor Imaging: Protocol Summary

**PATIENT PREPARATION**

Optional bowel preparation

**RADIOPHARMACEUTICAL DOSE**

Adult dose 10 mCi
Pediatric dose 75 to 100 mCi/kg (minimum 500 mCi)

**INSTRUMENTATION**

Camera: Large field of view; dual-headed camera preferable
Collimator: Medium-energy parallel hole
Photopeaks: 20% windows around 93, 184, and 296 keV
Computer acquisition matrix: 128 × 128 byte mode

**PROCEDURE**

Whole body images initially at 48 to 72 hr and at 5 to 10 days as needed
SPECT of chest, abdomen, or both at 48 to 72 hr and delayed SPECT as needed up to 5 to 6 days
1. Inject Ga-67 intravenously.
2. Planar imaging: For dual-headed camera, simultaneous anterior and posterior whole body scanning mode requires 30-40 min. For single-headed camera, obtain 500k spot images of anterior chest and equal time for posterior chest, anterior and posterior abdomen, pelvis, and anterior head. Regions of special interest require 1000k. Image axillae with arms elevated.
3. SPECT:

| Camera: | Single-headed | Dual-headed |
|---|---|---|
| Collimator: | Medium energy | Two medium energy |
| Rotation: | 360° | 360° |
| Patient: | Supine | Supine |
| Computer acquisition parameters: | | |
| | 64 × 64 matrix | 128 × 128 matrix |
| | 128 images/ 360° arc | 120 images/360°, 60 stops/head |
| | 20 sec/image | 40 sec/stop at 48 hr |
| Processing: | Filtered back-projection | Filtered back-projection |
| | Attenuation correction: | Attenuation correction: |
| | Chest: no | Chest: no |
| | Abdomen: yes | Abdomen: yes |

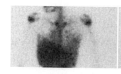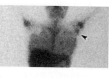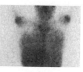

**Fig. 9-6**    Axillary node uptake of gallium-67. Initial study *(left and middle)*. Left axillary Ga-67 uptake *(arrowhead)* is seen only with the arms elevated. A follow-up study 3 months later *(right)* shows resolution of the nodal involvement.

## Table 9-3    Sensitivity of gallium-67 for tumor detection

| Tumor | Sensitivity (%) | Clinical utility |
|---|---|---|
| Hodgkin's disease | >90 | +++ |
| Non-Hodgkin's lymphoma | 85 | +++ |
| Hepatocellular carcinoma | 90 | +++ |
| Soft tissue sarcomas | 93 | +++ |
| Melanoma | 82 | ++ |
| Lung cancer | 85 | ++ |
| Head and neck tumors | 75 | ++ |
| Abdominal and pelvic tumors | 55 | + |

disease than does planar imaging (Fig. 9-5). SPECT is mandatory for state-of-the-art Ga-67 imaging.

Detection of tumor in the liver and spleen is complicated by the normal uptake of Ga-67 in these organs. One method of improving tumor detectability is to first obtain a Tc-99m sulfur colloid study. Cold regions (photopenic defects) on the Tc-99m sulfur colloid study that "fill in" (uptake equal to or greater than adjacent liver) on Ga-67 imaging are abnormal and positive for tumor (or infection). This observation is useful for diagnosing hepatocellular carcinoma in a cirrhotic liver (Fig. 9-7).

Bowel preparation with laxatives and enemas is ordered routinely in some laboratories to clear intestinal activity before imaging, although others have not found this helpful. Alternatively, bowel preparation can be ordered as needed to clear problematic intraabdominal activity. Excessive enema use may induce mucosal inflammation and Ga-67 uptake.

more easily detected than more central ones. SPECT can help here as well.

Detection of tumors involving the mediastinum requires oblique views or preferably SPECT. Otherwise, normal overlying soft tissue, sternum, and spine uptake may hinder detection (Fig. 9-4). Similarly, abdominal SPECT better detects and localizes paraaortic nodal

## Clinical Applications

**Hodgkin's disease and non-Hodgkin's lymphoma**
Aggressive combination chemotherapy, with or without radiation therapy, can produce cure and long-term complete remission in a large percentage of patients with Hodgkin's disease, as well as many with high- and intermediate-grade non-Hodgkin's lymphoma. However, response varies widely among patients. Prognosis for

both diseases depends on the stage of disease and tumor histology.

Hodgkin's disease and non-Hodgkin's lymphoma differ clinically and pathologically (Table 9-4). Hodgkin's disease is usually seen initially as localized disease in the neck or supraclavicular area and spreads in an orderly

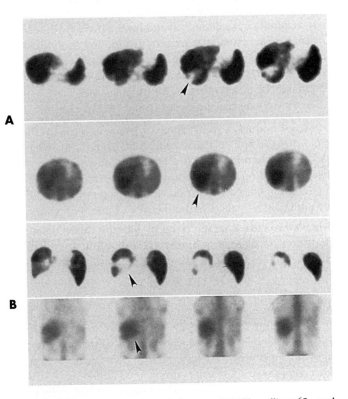

**Fig. 9-7**   Hepatocellular carcinoma: SPECT gallium-65 and technetium-99m sulfur colloid. **A,** Transaxial and, **B,** coronal SPECT slices. SPECT was performed with an aging single-headed rotating gamma camera. The Tc-99m sulfur colloid liver spleen slices *(top)* show a large defect *(arrowheads)* in the posterior aspect of the right lobe. In comparable sections the Ga-67 study *(bottom)* shows increased uptake *(arrowheads)* in the same area, consistent with the suspected tumor.

manner to contiguous lymph nodes. It is associated with a high cure rate. Non-Hodgkin's lymphoma is characterized by various histological patterns (Box 9-3), multicentric disease, a highly variable clinical course that may be indolent or rapidly lethal, and a high incidence of extranodal tumor involvement. Although mediastinal masses are common with Hodgkin's disease, 80% of patients with non-Hodgkin's lymphoma have abdominal presentations involving mesenteric and retroperitoneal nodes. Treatment and prognosis depend on the stage of disease and the histological subtype.

Classification schemes for malignant lymphomas have changed over the years. Although older schemes were based on morphological features of the lymphoma, more recent schemes emphasize its B-cell or T-cell origin (Box 9-3 and Table 9-5). Approximately 90%

---

**Box 9-3   Revised European-American Lymphoma (REAL) Classification**

**B-CELL NEOPLASMS**

Precursor B-cell neoplasm: B-cell lymphoblastic lymphoma
Peripheral B-cell neoplasms
   Chronic lymphoma or leukemia
   Mantle cell lymphoma
   Follicular lymphoma
   Marginal cell lymphoma
   Hairy cell leukemia
   Plasma cell myeloma
   Diffuse large B-cell lymphoma
   Burkitt's lymphoma

**T-CELL AND NATURAL KILLER CELL NEOPLASMS**

Precursor T-cell neoplasm: T-cell lymphoblastic leukemia/lymphoma
Peripheral T-cell and natural killer-cell neoplasms
   Chronic lymphoma or leukemia
   Large lymphocyte leukemia
   Mycosis fungoides
   Peripheral T-cell lymphomas
   Angiocentric lymphoma
   Intestinal T-cell lymphoma

---

**Table 9-4   Hodgkin's disease versus non-Hodgkin's lymphoma**

|  | Hodgkin's disease | Non-Hodgkin's lymphoma |
|---|---|---|
| Cellular derivation | Unresolved Reed-Sternberg | 90% B-cell 10% T-cell |
| Site of disease |  |  |
| Localized | Common | Uncommon |
| Nodal spread | Contiguous | Discontiguous |
| Extranodal | Uncommon | Common |
| Mediastinal | Common | Uncommon |
| Abdominal | Uncommon | Common |
| Bone marrow | Uncommon | Common |
| Systemic symptoms | Uncommon | Common |
| Curability | >75% | <25% |

---

**Table 9-5   Rye classification of Hodgkin's disease**

| Histological subgroup | Incidence (%) | Prognosis |
|---|---|---|
| Lymphocyte predominant | 2-10 | Excellent |
| Nodular sclerosis | 40-80 | Very good |
| Mixed cellularity | 20-40 | Good |
| Lymphocyte depleted | 2-15 | Poor |

of malignant lymphomas are of B-cell and 10% are of T-cell origin.

Ga-67 has been used for staging, detecting relapse or residual disease, and monitoring the response to radiation or chemotherapy (Figs. 9-8 and 9-9). Thus it permits decisions regarding the need for further therapy, second-line chemotherapy, or high-dose chemotherapy and bone marrow transplantation.

*Accuracy* Much of the data from the older medical literature underestimates present-day accuracy of Ga-67 for tumor imaging. Many of these studies were performed with low doses (3 to 5 mCi), older camera technology, and outdated methodologies. Despite these limitations, past investigations noted a high sensitivity for Ga-67 in Hodgkin's disease (>90%), although a somewhat lower sensitivity in non-Hodgkin's lymphoma (70% to 85%). Most intermediate- and high-grade non-Hodgkin's lymphomas are Ga-67 positive, whereas only half of low-grade tumors are Ga-67 positive. More recent studies using SPECT have found higher accuracy for Ga-67 in these diseases than is reported in the older literature.

*Tumor staging* Appropriate treatment planning requires a determination of the extent of disease. Various clinical staging classifications have been used (Box 9-4). No consensus has been reached on the use of staging

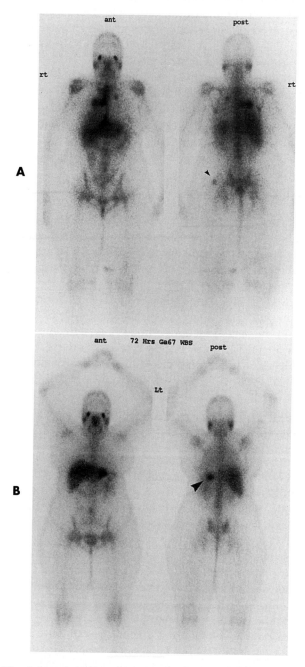

**Fig. 9-8** Hodgkin's disease: response to chemotherapy. A 30-year-old woman with nodular sclerosing Hodgkin's disease. **A,** Whole body gallium-67 scan shows multiple sites of tumor in the right perihilar and peritracheal regions, anterior mediastinum, and right and left lungs. Note uptake in the left buttock at the site of injection *(small arrowhead)*. **B,** Follow-up scan after a course of chemotherapy shows resolution of Ga-67 uptake in the chest. New uptake in the stomach is secondary to gastritis, best seen in posterior view *(large arrowhead)*. Gastric localization was confirmed by SPECT.

| **Box 9-4   Ann Arbor Staging System for Hodgkin's Disease** | |
|---|---|
| Stage I | Involvement of single lymph node region or single extralymphatic site |
| Stage II | Involvement of two or more lymph node regions on the same side of diaphragm; can also include localized involvement of extralymphatic site |
| Stage III | Involvement of lymph node regions or extra-lymphatic sites on both sides of diaphragm |
| Stage IV | Disseminated involvement of one or more extralymphatic organs with or without lymph node involvement |

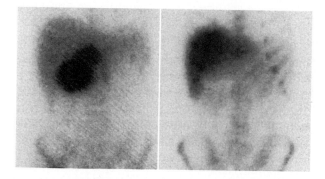

**Fig. 9-9** Non-Hodgkin's lymphoma: response to therapy. Resolution of gallium-67 uptake after appropriate therapy in a patient with non-Hodgkin's lymphoma. *Left,* A large portal hepatic mass is seen before therapy. *Right,* After therapy a residual mass was seen on computed tomography. No Ga-67 uptake is detected, although a photopenic mass effect appears to be present just below the liver because of residual nonviable tumor.

laparotomy and splenectomy for patients with Hodgkin's disease. CT is generally considered the primary imaging method for staging. However, Ga-67 can be used. The advantages of Ga-67 are that it is noninvasive and provides whole body screening. One study of 170 patients reported a sensitivity of 93% for Hodgkin's disease and 89% for non-Hodgkin's lymphoma with high specificity. Ga-67 scans were thought to complement CT and alter staging.

The primary role of Ga-67 at most centers lies in its usefulness in evaluating the effectiveness of therapy. However, a pretherapy scan is important to ensure that the tumor is gallium avid. Ga-67 can detect both nodal and visceral tumor involvement in Hodgkin's disease and in high- and intermediate-grade non-Hodgkin's lymphomas. Some disagreement exists about its sensitivity in low-grade disease. However, it is a highly sensitive method for detecting mediastinal disease, intraabdominal and paraaortic nodal involvement, and superficial regional lymph nodes.

*Response to therapy*   It is critical to identify patients who have had an incomplete or slow response to first-line chemotherapy. Induction of dose-intensive salvage therapy before the development of extensive disease may benefit patients who have had only a partial response to chemotherapy. Ga-67 can stratify low- and high-risk disease patients early in the course of treatment. High-risk patients with aggressive disease may benefit from new treatment approaches, such as second-line and very high dose chemotherapy with bone marrow transplantation. Recent studies have suggested that Ga-67 scintigraphy performed during chemotherapy, even after a single therapy cycle, can predict therapeutic outcome. This information permits a change to other treatment before the number of resistant cells grows to a bulk that will not be affected by chemotherapy.

Patients with bulky disease often have a residual mass seen radiographically. Residual radiographic abnormalities are seen in 64% to 83% of patients with mediastinal disease and 30% to 50% of patients with abdominal masses. However, radiographs or CT cannot reliably distinguish between complete and partial remissions. The residual mass may be the result of ineffectively treated tumor or of necrosis and fibrosis. Needle aspiration and biopsy are invasive and subject to sampling errors.

Ga-67 can resolve the dilemma of a residual post-therapy mass by virtue of being an indicator of tumor viability. The reported sensitivity and specificity for detecting mediastinal tumors are high for Hodgkin's disease (95% and 90%, respectively) and for non-Hodgkin's lymphoma (92% and 99%, respectively). The amount of Ga-67 uptake directly correlates with the amount of viable tumor.

SPECT can often demonstrate disease when planar images are normal or equivocal. SPECT can separate superimposed normal Ga-67 activity (e.g., uptake by soft tissue, sternum, liver, or bone) from an underlying pathological condition, which is often a problem with planar imaging alone (Figs. 9-4 and 9-5). The sensitivity of SPECT for tumor detection is 85% to 96% compared with planar imaging's sensitivity of 69%. False positive studies are uncommon in patients with known biopsy-proven disease. However, uptake at sites of infection, inflammation, or increased bone turnover can complicate interpretation in some patients.

**Malignant melanoma**   Most malignant melanomas and metastases are gallium avid. Ga-67 has been used to detect metastases and determine response to therapy for patients with metastatic melanoma receiving chemotherapy or immunotherapy. The overall sensitivity and specificity for detecting metastatic melanoma are reported to be 82% and 99%, respectively.

**Hepatocellular carcinoma**   Although hepatocellular carcinoma is most often seen initially as a single mass lesion in an otherwise normal liver, the tumor is frequently multifocal in patients with cirrhosis. Because most hepatomas are gallium avid, Ga-67 has been used to differentiate hepatoma from regenerating hepatic nodules ("pseudotumors") seen on CT in patients with cirrhosis (Fig. 9-7). Approximately 90% of hepatomas are gallium avid, with 63% concentrating more Ga-67 activity than the liver, 25% having uptake equal to surrounding liver, and 12% showing less uptake. Of course, other hepatic lesions such as abscess or metastatic disease may also take up Ga-67. However, biopsy will probably still be required.

**Lung cancer**   Overall sensitivity of Ga-67 for lung cancer has been reported to be 85% to 90%. However, on the important issue of the use of Ga-67 to stage patients and determine operability, the general consensus is that its accuracy is suboptimal. In contrast, F-18 FDG PET imaging has proved accurate and cost effective for staging lung cancer (see discussion under "Fluorine-18 Fluorodeoxyglucose").

Ga-67 has been used to determine the local extent of disease and the presence or absence of distant metastases for patients with pleura-based mesotheliomas. Ga-67 imaging is more accurate than chest radiography for differentiating malignant mesothelioma from benign pleural thickening.

**Head and neck tumors**   Varying results have been reported for Ga-67 in head and neck tumors. Sensitivity for tumor detection has ranged from 56% to 86%. CT and MRI are the primary imaging modalities. Ga-67 is usually reserved for detection of recurrent tumor after therapy when normal anatomical landmarks have been disrupted. The prognosis is poor for patients with recurrent tumor detected by Ga-67 compared with patients whose residual mass is gallium negative and therefore represents effectively treated tumor.

**Abdominal and pelvic tumors** Sensitivity of Ga-67 for pelvic and abdominal tumors is generally poor: esophageal cancer 41%, gastric tumors 47%, colon cancer 25%, pancreatic tumors 15%, and similar results for gynecological tumors. However, Ga-67 has been used successfully to detect metastases from draining nodes in testicular cancer. Uptake depends to some extent on histological type: 74% sensitivity for metastatic embryonal cell carcinoma, 57% for metastatic seminoma, and 25% for testicular teratomas.

**Soft tissue sarcomas** Most soft tissue sarcomas are gallium avid. Ga-67 has a 93% overall sensitivity for disease detection with good sensitivity for primary lesions, local recurrences, and metastatic disease. Liposarcoma, usually a low-grade tumor, has a high false negative rate. A Ga-67-positive site that becomes negative after therapy is indicative of a favorable clinical response.

## THALLIUM-201, TECHNETIUM-99m SESTAMIBI, TECHNETIUM-99m TETROFOSMIN TUMOR IMAGING

Radiopharmaceuticals initially approved as myocardial perfusion–imaging agents have recently been found to have tumor-imaging capabilities. Tl-201, used since the late 1970s for cardiac imaging, was the first cardiac agent demonstrated to have tumor avidity. Subsequently, Tc-99m sestamibi was noted to have similar tumor uptake and for many uses became the preferred agent owing to its better imaging characteristics. The newest cardiac agent, Tc-99m tetrofosmin, has qualities similar to Tc-99m MIBI, although a smaller amount of data has been published.

### Radiopharmaceuticals

#### Thallium-201 chloride

*Chemistry and physics* Tl-201 chloride (Tl-201) is a metallic element in group IIIA of the Periodic Table. It decays by electron capture, emitting a cluster of x-rays ranging from 69 to 83 keV (94% abundant) and two gamma rays, 167 keV (10% abundant) and 135 keV (3% abundant) (Table 9-1). Physical half-life is 73 hours.

*Pharmacokinetics and normal distribution* After intravenous injection Tl-201 is distributed throughout the body in proportion to regional blood flow. The heart receives 3% to 5% of the administered dose, the liver 15%, and the kidneys 3.5%, with lesser amounts to the spleen, skeletal muscles, and brain (Fig. 9-10). Cardiac uptake is maximal at 10 minutes and is probably similar for most tumors. Biological clearance is primarily via the kidneys and to a much lesser extent through the intestines. Total body clearance is slow, with a 40-hour biological half-life.

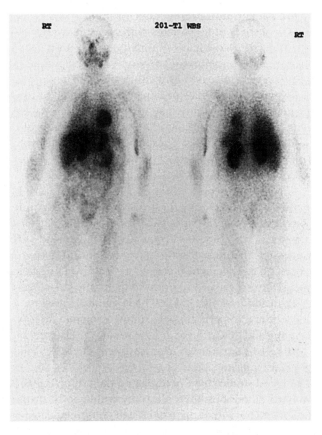

**Fig. 9-10** Normal resting thallium-201 distribution. Imaging started 15 minutes after injection. Uptake is prominent in the kidneys, heart, liver, and to a lesser extent the bowel. Normally the thyroid would be prominently seen. This patient has undergone total thyroidectomy for thyroid cancer. Adherence of Tl-201 to the arm vein on the side of the intravenous injection is common.

| Box 9-5 Factors Determining Tumor Cell Uptake of Thallium-201 and Technetium-99m Sestamibi | |
|---|---|
| **THALLIUM-201** | **Tc-99m SESTAMIBI** |
| Blood flow | Blood flow |
| Tumor viability | Tumor viability |
| Tumor type | Tumor type |
| Sodium-potassium ATPase system | Lipophilic cation |
| Cotransport system | Large negative transmembrane potential |
| Calcium ion channel system | |

*Mechanism of tumor uptake* Multiple mechanisms are involved in the uptake of Tl-201 by tumors (Box 9-5). Blood flow is critical for delivery of the radiotracer. Thallium was first used as a perfusion agent. In the myocardium uptake is directly related to blood flow. Biologically, Tl-201 is handled similarly to potassium.

Tl-201 entry into tumor cells is dependent on the cell membrane adenosine triphosphatase (ATPase) system, which actively extrudes sodium from the cell in exchange for potassium and thallium. Thus a high intracellular/extracellular gradient is maintained. This transport system is inhibited by ouabain. A second cotransport system is inhibited by furosemide. Tl-201 is accumulated by viable tumor tissue, minimally by connective tissue, and not at all by necrotic tissue. It resides in free form in cytosol, and only a small amount localizes in the nuclear, mitochondrial, or microsomal cell fractions.

### Technetium-99m sestamibi

*Chemistry and physics* Tc-99m sestamibi (Tc-99m MIBI) is a lipophilic cationic complex (methoxy-isobutyl-isonitrile) (Cardiolite, marketed as Miraluma for breast tumor imaging, DuPont Pharmaceuticals) empirically designed for myocardial perfusion imaging and approved by the FDA in 1990. The Tc-99m radiolabel, with its single 140-keV photopeak, is ideal for gamma camera imaging.

*Pharmacokinetics and normal distribution* Compared with Tl-201, Tc-99m MIBI has less cardiac uptake (2%) and remains fixed in the heart. MIBI clears rapidly from the blood and localizes in skeletal muscle, liver, and kidneys (Fig. 9-11). Initial hepatic uptake is considerable, and then the agent is cleared into the biliary system and bowel. Intestinal and urinary clearance makes subdiaphragmatic tumor imaging more difficult.

*Mechanism of tumor uptake* The cellular uptake of Tc-99m MIBI is related to its lipophilicity and charge. MIBI probably diffuses passively into the cell, where a

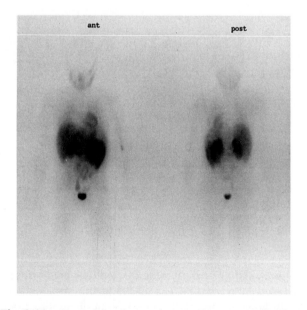

**Fig. 9-11** Normal resting technetium-99m sestamibi distribution. Imaging at 60 minutes after injection. There is prominent uptake by heart and liver. Hepatobiliary clearance and gallbladder filling are seen, as is intestinal and urinary clearance.

strong electrostatic attraction occurs between the positive charge of the lipophilic Tc-99m MIBI molecule and the negatively charged mitochondria. Approximately 90% of Tc-99m MIBI is concentrated within the mitochondria.

The retention of Tc-99m MIBI in tumor cells is also related to its rate of transport out of the cell. A cellular membrane glycoprotein, P-glycoprotein (Pgp), is responsible for pumping cationic and lipophilic substances out of the cell. This enhanced excretion mechanism is thought to be responsible for multidrug resistance (MDR). Malignant cells have increased expression of the MDR-1 gene, which encodes for Pgp. Thus increased amounts of the chemotherapeutic drugs are transported out of the tumor cells. MIBI is treated as a substrate similar to chemotherapeutic agents. With high levels of Pgp, more MIBI is transported out of the tumor cells. It has been postulated that Tc-99m sestamibi imaging might be used as an MDR indicator and thus predict chemotherapy efficacy.

### Technetium-99m tetrofosmin

*Chemistry and physics* Tc-99m tetrofosmin (Myoview, Amersham) is a lipophilic cationic diphosphine (trans-dioxo-bis) complex. When Tc-99m pertechnetate is added to tetrofosmin in the presence of stannous reductant, a lipophilic, cationic Tc-99m tetrofosmin complex is formed.

*Pharmacokinetics and normal distribution* Myocardial uptake of Tc-99m tetrofosmin is rapid. Only 1.2% of the dose localizes in the heart. Like sestamibi it is not cleared from the myocardium, but it is cleared more rapidly from the lung, blood, and liver. Approximately 66% of the injected dose is excreted within 48 hours, 40% in the urine and 26% in the feces. Clearance from the liver is faster than that of sestamibi, which may be advantageous for detection of tumors in the inferior quadrant of the right breast.

*Mechanism of tumor uptake* The mechanisms of tetrofosmin uptake and sestamibi uptake are probably similar. Both are lipophilic cationic complexes, and the uptake of both correlates with perfusion, high intracellular levels of mitochondria, and cell viability. Accumulation and retention in the mitochondria are mediated by the negative potential of the mitochondrial membrane. Tetrofosmin is also a substrate for Pgp. The Na,K-ATPase pump is only partially involved in the cellular uptake of tetrofosmin.

### Dosimetry

Tl-201 results in a somewhat higher radiation dose to the patient than that of the Tc-99m-labeled agents (Table 9-2). The kidney is the target organ for Tl-201, receiving 3.6 rads per 3 mCi, while the testicle receives about 1.6 rads. With a 30-mCi administered dose of the technetium agents (Tc-99m sestamibi and Tc-99m tetrofosmin), the organs receiving the largest radiation dose are the large bowel (5.4 and 3.4 rads, respectively) and gallbladder (2 and 5.4 rads, respectively). The kidney receives the next highest dose (2 and 1.4 rads, respectively).

## Methodology

The study methodology depends to a large extent on the clinical indication. This determines whether whole body imaging or regional imaging is required and whether planar imaging or SPECT is indicated. The optimal time to begin tumor imaging with these agents is approximately 5 to 30 minutes after injection. Specific protocols are discussed under "Clinical Applications."

The technetium-labeled agents have better imaging characteristics than Tl-201. Thallium is suboptimal because of its low-energy (69- to 83-keV) mercury x-ray emission and low allowable administered dose (3 mCi), which limits photon yield. Because of the better dosimetry of the Tc-99m-labeled agents, higher doses (25 to 30 mCi) are administered. Thus imaging time can be shorter and the images better.

## Clinical Applications

Tl-201, Tc-99m sestamibi, and Tc-99m tetrofosmin are taken up in a large number of benign and malignant tumors. Clinical utility has been demonstrated in the tumors discussed in the ensuing sections. The use of technetium-labeled agents for localization of parathyroid adenomas is reviewed in Chapter 14.

**Brain tumors** The first radiopharmaceutical used for brain tumor imaging was F-18 FDG, which was used in PET imaging. The positron radiopharmaceutical can be used to judge tumor grade based on the degree of uptake and, perhaps more important, can be used to evaluate the effectiveness of therapy by differentiating persistent or recurrent tumor from radiation necrosis. SPECT with Tl-201 provides similar information.

The uptake of Tl-201 in gliomas correlates with tumor grade: the greater the uptake, the higher the tumor grade (see Fig. 12-25). CT and MRI often cannot differentiate postoperative or postradiation changes from residual viable tumor. Tl-201 can be used to determine therapeutic effectiveness because it is taken up only by viable tumor. In HIV-positive patients, Tl-201 has been used to characterize intracerebral masses, for example, to differentiate malignant lymphoma from infectious etiologies such as toxoplasmosis. Tl-201 uptake is strongly consistent with tumor. Tc-99m MIBI can be used similarly but has the potential disadvantage for imaging of being taken up by the choroid plexus.

**Breast cancer** Mammography is the accepted first-line imaging method for breast cancer detection. Al-

though quite sensitive overall (85% to 90%), its positive predictive value for malignancy is low (20% to 30%) and thus many women undergo unnecessary surgical biopsies. Mammography also has a poor negative predictive value in women who have dense breasts, implants, or severe dysplastic disease or who have undergone breast surgery or radiotherapy. The false negative rate in this group of patients approaches 30%.

Ultrasonography can differentiate cyst from solid tumor, but it is otherwise nonspecific. MRI is very sensitive for tumor detection and can add diagnostic information in some cases, but its specificity is not high. A noninvasive imaging test with high positive and negative predictive values could obviate the need for surgical biopsy in many women.

Tl-201 is taken up by adenocarcinoma of the breast. In a study of 45 patients with breast lesions greater than 1.5 cm, Tl-201 had a sensitivity of 97% for detecting breast cancer. In that study fibrocystic disease showed no Tl-201 uptake. The smallest detectable primary lesion was approximately 1 cm in diameter. Most of these patients had palpable lesions.

Because of the better imaging characteristics of Tc-99m MIBI, studies of its utility for breast imaging were undertaken. Over 20 studies have been reported. In 1997, Tc-99m MIBI became the first radiopharmaceutical to be approved by the FDA for breast imaging.

In a large multicenter trial of 673 patients from 30 institutions, an overall sensitivity of 85% and specificity of 81% were reported for diagnosis of breast cancer in patients who had a palpable breast mass or a mammographically detected lesion. Sensitivity was better for palpable masses (sensitivity 95%, specificity 74%) than for nonpalpable lesions (sensitivity 72%, specificity 86%). Sensitivity was also lower for lesions less than 1 cm in diameter. Fibroadenomas are the most common cause for false positive studies. The positive and negative predictive values for axillary node metastatic involvement are approximately 83% and 82%, respectively.

*Methodology* A typical imaging protocol is described in Box 9-6. Tc-99m MIBI scintimammography is best performed with the patient lying on a specially designed imaging table with cutouts that allow one breast to hang dependent with the patient in the prone position. Thus lateral images of each breast can be obtained without background activity from the chest wall and heart. Supine images are obtained for two-dimensional tumor localization. A narrow Tc-99m photopeak window of 10% is recommended to minimize table scatter, which can complicate image interpretation. SPECT has not proven advantageous.

*Image interpretation* Breast tumor scintigraphy should be interpreted in conjunction with the physical examination, mammography, and ultrasonography if available. An abnormal study consistent with malignancy

## Box 9-6   Scintimammography: Protocol Summary

**PATIENT PREPARATION**

None

**DOSE**

Tc-99m sestamibi 25 mCi

**INSTRUMENTATION**

Camera: Large field of view with low-energy all-purpose collimator; 10% photopeak over 140 keV.

**IMAGING PROTOCOL**

Position patient prone on table with cutouts so that breasts hang dependent.

Inject Tc-99m sestamibi intravenously.

Begin imaging 5 min after injection. Ten minutes per image. Marker images may be shorter.

| | |
|---|---|
| Prone | Lateral of breast with palpable nodule or mammographically detected mass |
| | Repeat lateral image with radioactive marker over palpable nodule |
| | Lateral of opposite breast |
| Supine | Chest, including axilla |
| | Chest with marker over palpable nodule |
| Optional | Posterior oblique image if lesion close to chest wall |

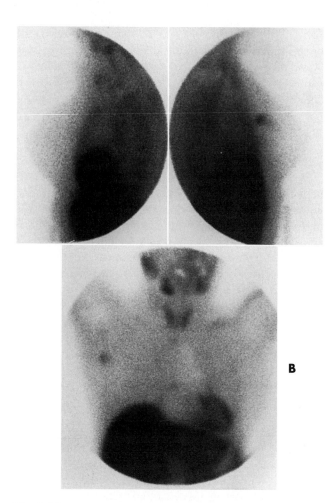

**Fig. 9-12**   Scintimammography. Large palpable breast mass imaged with technetium-99m sestamibi. **A,** Laterals of right and left breast. Intense focal uptake in right breast near axilla consistent with malignancy. **B,** Anterior view helps with localization. Uptake seen in upper outer quadrant.

will show focal increased uptake in the region of the palpable or mammographically detected mass (Fig. 9-12). Diffuse uptake is nonspecific and usually does not indicate malignancy.

*Clinical role*   The ultimate clinical role for Tc-99m MIBI breast imaging is uncertain. Some are concerned that the sensitivity and negative predictive value of this technique are not high enough and that many patients and surgeons will not accept a false negative rate of 15% in deciding whether biopsy is indicated. New dedicated breast-imaging devices with better camera sensitivity and image resolution are being developed and may answer these concerns.

The present technique is clearly useful for certain subgroups of patients, such as selected patients with nondiagnostic mammograms, those with dense breasts or architectural distortion (e.g., from surgery and breast implants), and those with fibrocystic disease who are at increased risk for malignancy.

**Bone and soft tissue tumors**   Tl-201 can successfully differentiate malignant from benign bone lesions. A high correlation has been found between Tl-201 uptake and response to chemotherapy (Fig. 9-13). The lack of Tl-201 uptake is associated with tumor necrosis. Tl-201 is superior to both Tc-99m MDP and Ga-67 for imaging of bone and soft tissue tumors. This is not surprising because uptake of the latter two radiopharmaceuticals is determined by factors other than tumor response to therapy, such as bone repair. Tumor response to therapy results in decreased Tl-201 uptake. Tc-99m sestamibi has performed similarly.

**Thyroid cancer**   Although I-131 scintigraphy is successfully used for evaluating patients with differentiated thyroid cancer, it has disadvantages. The patient must discontinue thyroid hormone replacement therapy for 4 to 6 weeks before the study to ensure hypothyroidism and an elevated thyroid-stimulating hormone level. In addition, the 364-keV gamma emissions of I-131 are not optimal for imaging. Diagnostic images require a relatively high administered dose of I-131 (2 to 5 mCi) and long imaging times. The false negative rate is 10%.

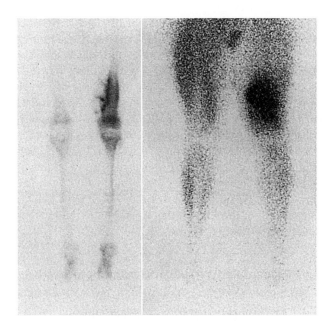

**Fig. 9-13**    Thallium-201 uptake in osteosarcoma. *Left,* Tc-99m HDP bone scan shows uptake in the distal left femur extending into soft tissue medially in a young patient with an osteosarcoma. *Right,* Tl-201 study shows a pattern of uptake similar to that with Tc-99m HDP, but Tl-201 more clearly shows soft tissue involvement superomedially. Thallium study demonstrates viable tumor.

Several studies have investigated the use of Tl-201 for thyroid cancer imaging. A major advantage is that the patient can continue taking thyroid hormone therapy. Tl-201 can effectively localize thyroid cancer. The downside is that Tl-201 is not specific for thyroid cancer and does not predict the potential therapeutic effectiveness of I-131. In clinical practice the clearest role for Tl-201 is for localization of tumor when the I-131 whole body scan is negative but the patient's serum thyroglobulin level is elevated. Some thyroid tumors then respond to high-dose radioactive iodine I-131 therapy, as evidenced by a fall in the serum thyroglobulin level. An I-131 scan 5 to 7 days after therapy may then show tumor uptake even though it was not seen on the routine 2- to 5-mCi I-131 diagnostic scan.

**Kaposi's sarcoma**    Tl-201 is useful in the differential diagnosis of chest disease in AIDS patients. Kaposi's sarcoma is Ga-67 negative but Tl-201 positive. Most infectious pulmonary diseases are gallium avid (e.g., *Pneumocystis,* atypical and typical *Mycobacterium*). Tl-201 scintigraphy is usually negative in infectious and inflammatory disease.

**Other tumors**    A variety of other tumors, such as lung cancer, lymphoma, and head and neck tumors, have been imaged with the thallium and technetium radiopharmaceuticals. However, the clinical role of these agents is uncertain and requires further investigation.

## FLUORINE-18 FLUORODEOXYGLUCOSE TUMOR IMAGING

For many years F-18 FDG tumor imaging with PET has been hailed as an exciting new tumor-imaging modality. Studies demonstrated F-18 FDG uptake in a wide variety of tumors. However, PET was generally considered an expensive research tool with an uncertain clinical role.

F-18 FDG imaging has had a slow acceptance for several reasons. First, in the past, imaging with F-18 FDG required an expensive PET camera, a cyclotron to produce positron radiopharmaceuticals, and many support personnel, including chemists, physicists, engineers, and computer specialists. Thus F-18 FDG imaging was expensive and for the most part limited to large academic medical centers. Second, the FDA hindered the development of F-18 FDG with an overly aggressive attempt to regulate it. Third, F-18 FDG PET imaging was commonly not reimbursed by insurance companies or Medicare. Thus, as of 1998 only about 50 clinical and 25 research centers in the United States were performing PET.

Now a dramatic change is occurring. F-18 FDG imaging is becoming a reality for a rapidly increasing number of U.S. hospitals. The reasons are many. A growing body of scientific evidence presented in peer-reviewed publications supports F-18 FDG PET as an accurate, clinically useful, and cost-effective clinical tumor-imaging modality. The cost of PET has decreased significantly. Self-contained cyclotrons are now available that can be housed in a nuclear medicine department and do not require large support staff. More important, cyclotrons on site are no longer necessary for clinical F-18 FDG PET imaging. Regional commercial radiopharmacies are providing local delivery of F-18 FDG in a manner similar to other single-photon radiopharmaceuticals.

The PET camera is now only moderately more expensive than the multiheaded SPECT gamma cameras used routinely in most nuclear medicine clinics. Furthermore, FDG can now be imaged with a dual-headed SPECT gamma camera using either 511-keV high-energy collimators or, preferably, specially adapted coincidence imaging detectors. These systems have become commercially available. Thus FDG imaging can be performed at any nuclear medicine laboratory, using the same camera, with some modifications, that performs bone and Ga-67 scans. This has fueled the regional distribution of F-18 FDG.

In the past, regulatory issues also hindered the growth of PET, but more recently the FDA has been restrained by the U.S. Congress and by the courts from interfering with the production and clinical use of F-18 FDG. Reimbursement by insurers has improved dramatically. Recognizing the proven cost-effectiveness of PET, most insurance companies now pay for clinically indicated PET studies. Medicare is now routinely reimbursing for lung cancer staging and evaluation of single pulmonary nodules, colorectal cancer, malignant melanoma, and malignant lymphoma. Clinical F-18 FDG tumor imaging has arrived.

## Physical Properties

The radionuclide F-18 is cyclotron produced and has a physical half-life of 109 minutes. It decays by positron (beta plus) particle emission (positive electron) (antimatter) (Table 9-1). The distanced traveled by positron particles in matter is short (2 to 8 mm). Once the positron has lost its kinetic energy, it interacts with an electron. Both particles are annihilated, and two 511-keV gamma photons are emitted $(E = mc^2)$ at 180° angles.

## Mechanism of Uptake

FDG is a glucose analog and is used as a tracer of glucose metabolism. It enters cells by the same transport mechanism as glucose. Intracellularly it is phosphorylated by hexokinase to FDG-6-phosphate. Unlike glucose-6-phosphatase, FDG-6-phosphate cannot progress into further glucose enzymatic pathways (Fig. 9-14) but rather is trapped intracellularly in proportion to the glycolytic rate of the cell. A characteristic of malignant cells is enhanced glucose metabolism.

Because the brain cortex uses primarily glucose as its substrate, FDG accumulation is high. The myocardium uses various substrates depending on availability and

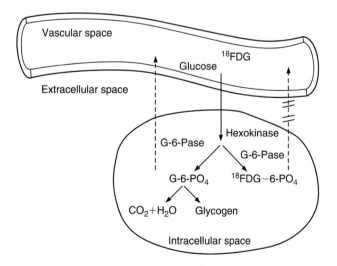

**Fig. 9-14**   Mechanism of fluorine-18 fluorodeoxyglucose uptake. F-18 FDG is a glucose analog. Like glucose, it is transported into the cell and phosphorylated by hexokinase. However, unlike glucose, it cannot be acted on by glucose-6-phosphatase or progress through further enzymatic pathways. It cannot cross cell membranes and becomes trapped intracellularly. The degree of uptake is determined by cellular metabolism.

hormonal and metabolic status. In the fasting state the myocardium uses primarily free fatty acids, but postprandially or after a glucose load, glucose utilization and FDG uptake are increased. Therefore for cardiac studies an intravenous glucose load is administered to promote cardiac uptake of FDG. However, for tumor imaging the fasting state is mandatory. Elevated levels of glucose in the blood compete with FDG uptake and will result in decreased tumor uptake.

## Normal Distribution and Pharmacokinetics

F-18 FDG uptake in the brain and heart is high. Liver uptake is considerably less. Unlike glucose, FDG is excreted via the kidneys. Some gastrointestinal clearance occurs. In the resting state accumulation of FDG in muscles is low, but muscular exertion increases the accumulation of FDG. The tumor-to-background ratio increases with time because of background clearance.

### Dosimetry

The effective radiation absorbed dose to the patient from F-18 FDG is detailed in Table 9-2. The bladder receives the highest dose, 4 rads/10 mCi.

### Methodology

The patient must fast for at least 4 hours before the procedure to maximize tumor uptake. Serum glucose is usually measured in diabetic patients. The usual injected dose of F-18 FDG is 10 mCi (370 MBq). Good hydration helps to prevent F-18 FDG accumulation in urinary tract structures, which could affect interpretation, and also minimizes the radiation dose to the patient. Imaging starts 30 to 90 minutes after injection.

With PET, limited-field tomography and whole body imaging can be performed. Limited-field PET, such as imaging of the chest or abdomen, is most commonly used to delineate metabolic activity when imaging by another modality produced an indeterminate result. Transmission images using a radioactive or x-ray source are necessary to correct for attenuation as well as for quantification. Whole body imaging is usually performed for tumor screening and clinical follow-up. With the proper software, attenuation correction can also be performed with whole body imaging. Reconstruction and processing methods are system dependent.

Quantification is not routinely performed in the clinical setting. It typically requires dynamic acquisition, arterial blood sampling, and computer modeling and processing. Semiquantification, such as the commonly used standardized uptake value (SUV), is more easily determined for clinical purposes but still is done only in selected cases, such as to differentiate tumor uptake from lesser degrees of uptake seen in inflammatory states and to quantify treatment response over time.

The SUV normalizes the amount of FDG accumulation in a region of interest (ROI) to the injected dose and patient's body weight. An ROI is flagged on the abnormality on an attenuation-corrected image, and the mean activity (mCi/ml) is measured. Both quantitative and semiquantitative methods require a calibration factor to translate scanner counts into well-counter counts, similar to the method for thyroid uptake calculation. The decay-corrected activities are then used to compute the SUV by the following formula:

$$SUV = \frac{\text{Mean ROI activity (mCi/ml)}}{\text{Injected dose (mCi)/Body weight (g)}}$$

## Image Interpretation

Normal physiological uptake is seen in the brain, myocardium, liver, spleen, stomach, intestines, and kidneys. Thymus uptake is sometimes seen, especially in younger patients. Uptake in the paraspinal, neck, and other skeletal muscles may occur because of muscular exertion. Images without attenuation correction have the appearance of prominent peripheral skin activity.

Healing surgical wounds may show increased FDG uptake for up to 6 months after surgery. Increased uptake is also seen in lactating breasts. Uptake may be noted in granulomatous tissue, infections, and other inflammatory-type reactions.

Chemotherapy and radiation therapy may decrease tumor uptake of FDG. Increased uptake in the pulmonary parenchyma can be seen in radiation pneumonitis, in therapy with such agents as bleomycin, and in the pleura after radiation therapy.

## Clinical Applications

A growing body of evidence supports the use of F-18 FDG in differentiating malignant from benign disease, staging and grading malignant disease, differentiating recurrent disease from therapy-induced changes, and monitoring response to therapy.

**Lung cancer** Lung cancer is the leading cause of cancer death in the United States for men and women. The 5-year survival of patients with lung cancer is approximately 14% and has remained unchanged over several decades. The clinical features, staging, and prognosis of small cell lung cancer and non–small cell lung cancer (NSCLC) are different, and these cancers are approached clinically as distinct malignancies. Small cell lung cancer accounts for 20% to 30% of lung cancer. It has usually spread systemically by the time of diagnosis. Surgery rarely results in cure, and treatment is almost always chemotherapy.

Both small cell lung cancer and squamous cell carcinoma are strongly associated with smoking. Squamous cell carcinoma accounts for 30% of all lung cancers. It arises from the proximal segmental bronchi.

Adenocarcinoma is not related to smoking. It is increasing in incidence and now accounts for 40% of lung cancers. These tumors are peripheral in origin and arise from alveolar surface epithelium of bronchial mucosal glands. Large cell carcinoma is the least common type of NSCLC and accounts for 15% of all lung cancers.

*Solitary pulmonary nodule* Lung cancer commonly is discovered as a focal lung abnormality on a chest radiograph, often as part of a routine physical examination or preoperative evaluation. Over 130,000 new solitary pulmonary nodules are diagnosed each year in the United States. Further evaluation with chest CT or serial radiographs is often performed. In the vast majority of cases benign focal lung lesions cannot be clearly differentiated from malignant ones by chest radiography, CT, or MRI.

An examination of tissue, obtained by bronchoscopic, percutaneous, or open lung biopsy, is necessary to make the diagnosis. In patients 35 years of age and older, about one third of single pulmonary nodules are carcinoma. For smokers the incidence is approximately 50%. In regions with endemic fungal disease, such as histoplasmosis or coccidioidomycosis, a young patient may be followed with serial chest radiographs after detection because of the high incidence of benign disease. A nodule that does not change in size for 2 or more years is considered benign. However, a tissue sample is still required in the majority of cases.

Numerous studies have shown the utility of imaging for characterizing solitary pulmonary nodules as benign or malignant when they were indeterminate on chest radiography or CT (Fig. 9-15). Data from almost 900 patients in over 20 centers have shown a high accuracy

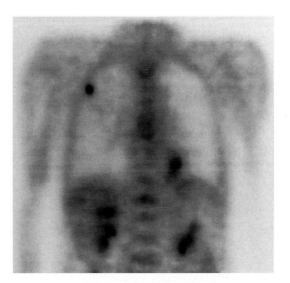

**Fig. 9-15** Solitary pulmonary nodule. This 65-year-old man was found to have a pulmonary nodule of indeterminate etiology on chest radiograph. Fluorine-18 fluorodeoxyglucose positron emission tomography findings are positive and consistent with malignancy in the right upper lobe. Focal uptake left of midline above the diaphragm is the heart.

## Box 9-7    TNM Staging of Non–Small Cell Lung Cancer

**PRIMARY TUMOR (T)**

Tx   Positive malignant cells; no lesion seen
T0   No evidence of primary tumor
TIS  Carcinoma in situ
T1   <3 cm in greatest dimension
T2   >3 cm in greatest dimension; distal atelectasis
T3   Extension into chest wall, diaphragm, mediastinal pleura, or pericardium; <2 cm from carina or total atelectasis
T4   Invasion of mediastinal organs; malignant pleural effusion

**NODAL INVOLVEMENT (N)**

N0   No involvement
N1   Ipsilateral bronchopulmonary or hilar
N2   Ipsilateral mediastinal or subcarinal; ipsilateral supraclavicular
N3   Contralateral mediastinal, hilar, or supraclavicular

**DISTANT METASTATIC INVOLVEMENT (M)**

M0   None
M1   Present

**Table 9-6    TNM stage grouping**

| Stage 0    | TIS      | N0       | M0 |
|------------|----------|----------|----|
| Stage I    | T1, T2   | N0       | M0 |
| Stage II   | T1,T2    | N1       | M0 |
| Stage IIIa | T3       | N0,N1    | M0 |
|            | T1-3     | N2       | M0 |
| Stage IIIb | Any T4   | Any N3   | M0 |
| Stage IV   | Any T    | Any N    | M1 |

of FDG PET. Sensitivity and specificity have been reported to be approximately 96% and 88%, respectively. An SUV of approximately 2.5 has been found to indicate malignancy, although the exact number varies by technique and institution. The positive predictive value of FDG far exceeds that of CT. The specificity is somewhat lower in areas with a high incidence of endemic tuberculosis or fungal disease. Studies have shown that the use of FDG PET can significantly reduce the expense associated with extended workup and thoracotomy for patients with pulmonary nodules of uncertain etiology.

*Staging of bronchogenic carcinoma* Accurate tumor staging is essential for the management of patients with NSCLC. The primary tumor in lung parenchyma or the bronchial wall ultimately invades lymphatic and vascular structures. The metastatic spread of lung cancer follows these lymphatic channels to involve bronchopulmonary (N1), mediastinal (N2-3), and supraclavicular (N3) lymph nodes (Box 9-7).

Staging of lung cancer by anatomical extent of the primary lung tumor (T), regional lymph nodes (N), and metastases (M) is used in the management of lung cancer. The staging of lung cancer (Table 9-6) includes clinical, surgical, and pathological assessment. However, clinical staging frequently understates the stage compared with final staging based on surgery and pathology. The 5-year survival is highly correlated with the stage of disease.

NSCLC is usually treated by resection of the primary lesion with lobectomy. Determining the presence of hilar or mediastinal involvement is critical for determining operability, prognosis, and appropriate therapy. In the absence of hilar or mediastinal node disease, survival approaches 50% at 5 years. With hilar or mediastinal involvement the disease-free survival rate is less than 10% at 5 years; thoracotomy does not improve survival and is not indicated.

CT has been the primary imaging modality for staging lung cancer. Its high spatial resolution makes it a sensitive screening modality. However, normal-sized nodes may harbor tumor and benign inflammatory nodes may be enlarged. A multiinstitutional study of NSCLC found that CT was only 52% sensitive and 69% specific for malignancy. MRI was 48% sensitive and 64% specific. Although mediastinoscopy establishes the diagnosis, it carries surgical risk and is subject to sampling error. Preoperatively, approximately 20% to 30% of lung tumors are considered resectable on the basis of conventional imaging procedures. Up to 20% of these tumors are found to be unresectable at surgery.

Although CT and MR diagnosis depends on morphological criteria, F-18 FDG provides information on the metabolic characteristics of the tissue. Numerous studies have demonstrated that FDG PET is more accurate and cost effective than CT for staging of patients with NSCLC (Table 9-7). Although PET can better determine the extent of mediastinal involvement than CT (Fig. 9-16), PET may not detect bronchial wall, pleural, and vascular invasion, so that anatomical imaging is necessary and complementary.

F-18 FDG PET provides additional information not easily obtained with other imaging techniques. Whole body PET imaging can identify unsuspected distant metastatic disease. Abnormalities thought to be metastases on CT scans may be found to be benign with PET scanning. NSCLC frequently metastasizes to the adrenal glands over the course of the disease, with an incidence as high as 60%. However, adrenal masses noted on CT at the time of initial presentation are often benign. In a study of 33 adrenal masses detected by CT, F-18 FDG PET had a 92% sensitivity and 100% specificity for malignancy.

FDG PET also has an important role in evaluating tumor response to therapy. Often, even with effective ther-

**Table 9-7    Staging of lung cancer: fluorine-18 fluorodeoxyglucose positron emission tomography (PET) versus computed tomography (CT)**

| Study | Year | No. of patients | PET Sensitivity (%) | PET Specificity (%) | CT Sensitivity (%) | CT Specificity (%) |
|---|---|---|---|---|---|---|
| Wahl | 1994 | 19 | 82 | 81 | 64 | 44 |
| Buchpiguel | 1994 | 26 | 93 | 84 | 93 | 42 |
| Patz | 1994 | 21 | 100 | 74 | 85 | 54 |
| Bury | 1995 | 20 | 90 | 80 | 63 | 66 |
| Valk | 1996 | 76 | 83 | 94 | 63 | 73 |

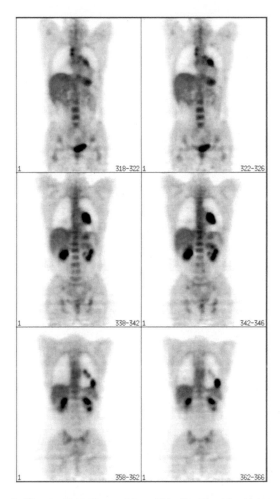

**Fig. 9-16** Lung cancer staging. This 57-year-old male smoker has a 2.8-cm mass in the left lower lobe and a 3-cm mass in the left hilum seen on CT. The staging fluorine-18 fluorodeoxyglucose PET scan shows not only these two lesions but abnormal uptake in the mediastinum and right paratracheal region consistent with tumor adenopathy. The PET scan has changed the patient's lung cancer staging from operable to nonoperable.

apy, a residual pulmonary mass remains. CT or MR usually cannot differentiate residual viable tumor from an effectively treated fibrotic or necrotic mass. Even a negative tissue biopsy is not definitive because of the possible errors of tissue sampling. FDG PET can make this deter-

mination with high accuracy. During the same scanning procedure, FDG PET can detect distant metastases.

**Colorectal cancer**    Colon cancer is the third most common malignancy in men and women and the second most common cause of cancer death in the United States. At the time of diagnosis 35% of patients have localized disease, 40% have regional lymph node metastases, and 25% have distant metastases. The 5-year survival rate decreases from 90% for patients without metastases to 60% for those with regional lymph node metastases and only 6% for those with distant metastases.

Metastatic tumor resection for cure is indicated for patients with hepatic, pulmonary, or pelvic metastases, if the tumor is thought to be localized and resectable. Accurate noninvasive detection of operable disease plays an important role in the selection of patients who might benefit from surgery. Surgical treatment of recurrences can lead to a cure in up to 25% of patients. Other distant metastases are a contraindication to resection.

Serum carcinoembryonic antigen (CEA) levels are used clinically to monitor patients for recurrence. The sensitivity of serum CEA for detecting recurrent tumor is 60% and the specificity is 85%. Serum CEA does not provide information about tumor location. CT sensitivity for detecting metastatic liver tumors is only approximately 70%, and it underestimates the number of lobes involved in a third of patients. CT portography is more sensitive (80% to 90%) but has a high false positive rate. When preoperative conventional imaging evaluation indicates localized hepatic recurrence, 25% to 50% of patients are found to have nonresectable tumor at surgery. A more accurate means is needed for diagnosis and staging of recurrent colorectal cancer.

Numerous studies have demonstrated that FDG PET has an important role in the localization of recurrent colorectal cancer. It has proved to be more sensitive and specific than CT. Its sensitivity for detecting metastatic colorectal cancer in the liver is greater than 90% (Table 9-8). FDG PET also allows simultaneous evaluation of the entire body for extrahepatic tumor (Figs. 9-17 and 9-18).

**Table 9-8    Detection of colorectal cancer metastases: positron emission tomography (PET) versus computed tomography (CT)**

| Study | Year | No. of patients | PET Sensitivity (%) | PET Specificity (%) | CT Sensitivity (%) | CT Specificity (%) |
|---|---|---|---|---|---|---|
| Gupta | 1991 | 24 | 100 | 85 | 70 | 43 |
| Gupta | 1993 | 16 | 90 | 66 | 60 | 100 |
| Falk | 1994 | 16 | 87 | 67 | 67 | 100 |
| Vitola | 1996 | 24 | 90 | 100 | 86 | 58 |
| Delbeke | 1997 | 61 | 93 | 89 | 79 | 58 |

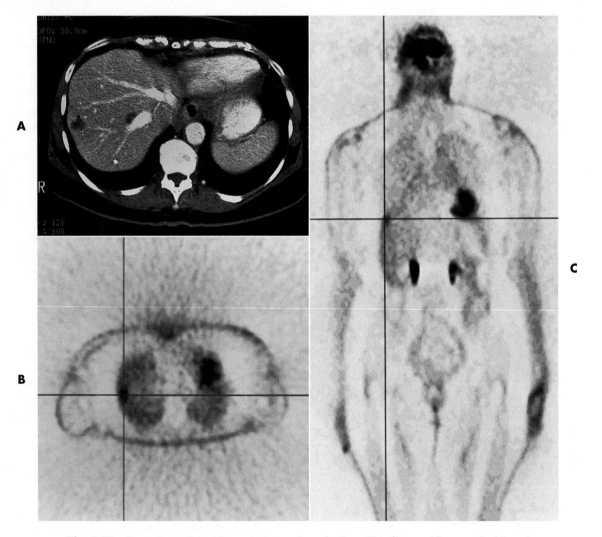

**Fig. 9-17**    Recurrent colorectal cancer metastatic to the liver. This 45-year-old woman had bowel resection 1 year ago. **A,** Computed tomography now shows a single 1.5-cm lesion in the right lobe of the liver. **B,** Fluorine-18 fluorodeoxyglucose uptake on transaxial positron emission tomography section confirms that this was a malignant lesion. **C,** No other liver lesions are noted. No metastatic lesions outside the liver were seen on the whole body scan. Therefore the patient is a candidate for surgical resection of this solitary hepatic metastasis.

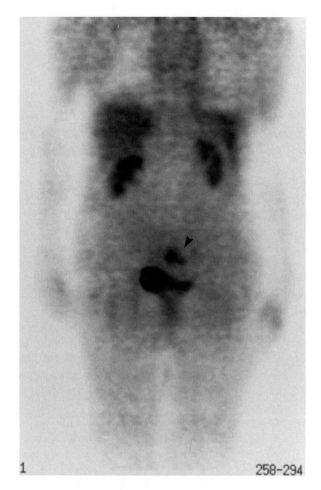

**Fig. 9-18** Recurrent colorectal carcinoma. A 63-year-old woman had primary resection of a colorectal cancer in the rectosigmoid area. Six months later the serum carcinoembryonic antigen level began to rise. Fluorine-18 fluorodeoxyglucose positron emission tomography is consistent with recurrent tumor at the site of the previous resection.

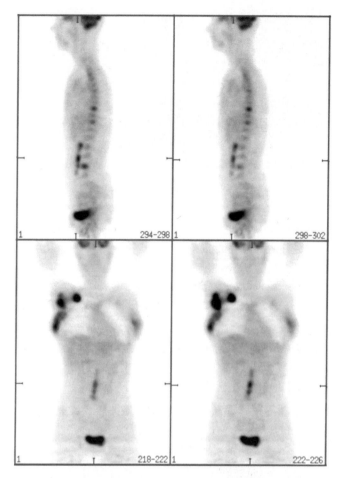

**Fig. 9-19** Malignant lymphoma. This 39-year-old woman presented with non-Hodgkin's lymphoma in the right breast and axilla. She was referred for pretherapy staging. The fluorine-18 fluorodeoxyglucose PET scan shows intense uptake not only in the known lesions, but also in retroperitoneal nodes and two thoracic and one lumbar vertebral bodies.

In one study of 378 patients, FDG PET detected unsuspected metastases in 27% of patients and had a clinical impact in 37%. The most common result of FDG PET in patients with colorectal cancer is that those who would not benefit can avoid surgery. In addition, the reduction in health care cost could have a large economic impact. Another clinical indication for FDG imaging is to localize tumor in patients with a rising serum CEA level but negative conventional imaging. FDG PET has also been used to monitor the success of therapy.

**Lymphoma** F-18 FDG has been used in Hodgkin's disease and non-Hodgkin's lymphoma for staging and monitoring of response to therapy. CT and F-18 FDG PET are comparable in their ability to localize disease in untreated lymphoma. CT is unable to distinguish between active or recurrent disease and residual scar tissue after therapy. F-18 FDG PET can accurately determine the effectiveness of therapy and determine whether a residual mass after therapy is viable tumor or is fibrosis and necrotic tissue.

**Malignant melanoma** The presence of lymph node metastases is a crucial prognostic indicator in malignant melanoma. However, accurate staging is difficult. For high-risk melanoma, F-18 FDG PET can be useful for detecting subclinical lymph nodes noninvasively and visceral metastases. PET has been found superior to other staging methods at primary diagnosis and during follow-up.

**Breast cancer** A limited number of studies have shown that FDG PET can detect primary breast cancer, as well as its regional and distant metastases. The accuracy of FDG PET seems to be similar to that of Tc-99m MIBI. Whole body F-18 FDG PET may play a role when tumor recurrence or metastases from breast cancer are suspected but other conventional diagnostic

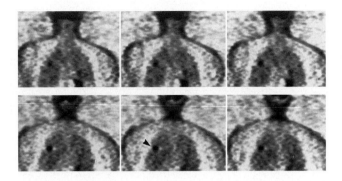

**Fig. 9-20**   SPECT fluorine-18 fluorodeoxyglucose imaging of single pulmonary nodule. A 65-year-old male smoker with a 3-cm lung nodule detected on routine chest x-ray examination. The fluorine-18 fluorodeoxyglucose SPECT study is consistent with malignancy *(arrowhead).*

tests are negative. It may also have utility in restaging and monitoring of patients receiving chemotherapy or radiation therapy. Further investigation is indicated.

**Brain tumors**   The glucose metabolic rate has been linearly correlated with histological grade in astrocytomas, permitting noninvasive tumor grading and providing prognostic information. PET F-18 FDG studies have been used to detect tumor recurrences and differentiate postoperative and postradiation changes from tumor recurrence (Fig. 12-24).

**Miscellaneous malignancies**   F-18 FDG PET shows promise as an important clinical imaging tool for a variety of other malignant tumors, including malignant lymphoma (see Fig. 12-24), melanoma, head and neck cancer, thyroid cancer, hepatocellular carcinoma, ovarian carcinoma, pancreatic cancer, and musculoskeletal tumors.

Preliminary data suggest that F-18 FDG SPECT with specially adapted coincidence detectors can locate malignant tumors (Fig. 9-20), although it is less sensitive than PET for small lesions.

Although most oncological studies to date have used F-18 FDG, future investigation will include other radiolabeled compounds, such as those that measure blood flow, oxygen metabolism, amino acid incorporation (protein synthesis), and cell division rates by analysis of carbon-11 thymidine incorporation.

## MONOCLONAL ANTIBODIES

Monoclonal antibody imaging has the potential for targeting specific tumor types. In recent years important clinical advances have been made in the development of antibodies for diagnosis and therapy. Four radiolabeled monoclonal antibodies have been approved by the FDA for imaging cancer of the colon, ovary, prostate, and lung. Other antibodies are under investigation and await the results of further clinical trials and approval. In addition to these important advances in tumor imaging, radioactive monoclonal antibodies will soon be available for radiation therapy for B-cell lymphoma.

### Mechanism of Uptake

Antibodies are proteins produced in the bone marrow, lymph nodes, and spleen by plasma cells in response to exposure to foreign antigens. Each plasma cell produces a specific antibody against a single antigenic determinant. However, animals immunized with an antigen produce and secrete into their blood a mixture of antibodies from many plasma cells, each against different antigenic determinants. Medically useful antibodies (e.g., gamma globulin) have been produced in rabbits or other animals for human use, but these polyclonal antibodies bind to multiple different antigenic sites and are thus nonspecific.

Kohler and Milstein won the Nobel Prize in 1975 for describing a methodology that could produce unlimited quantities of a single monoclonal antibody (MoAb) that bound to only one antigenic site. The technique involved fusing mouse myeloma cells with lymphocytes from the spleen of mice immunized with a particular antigen (Fig. 9-21). These "hybridoma" cells retain both the specific antibody production capacity of the lymphocytes and the immortality of the myeloma cancer cells. Immunoassays screen the hybrid cells to identify specific cell lines that produce a MoAb with desired features, such as high affinity to and specificity for the antigen of interest. The individual hybridoma cells can be maintained in culture to produce large quantities of the monoclonal antibody.

Unique cell surface antigens are expressed in many disease states, so that antibody targeting is possible. Many tumors have antigens (e.g., CEA) preferentially expressed on their surfaces. Other tumors have an increased number of expressed antigens, while some antigens are expressed similarly on normal tissues and on tumors. In the latter case antibodies have clinical utility when the native cells are surgically absent, so that only malignant cells will be detected; ProstaScint, the prostate monoclonal antibody, is an example of this approach.

Antibodies consist of two identical heavy (H) and light (L) chains linked by a disulfide bridge (Fig. 9-22). Each chain is made up of a *variable* region (Fab'), responsible for specific antigenic binding to cell surfaces, and a *constant* region (Fc), responsible for effector functions such as complement fixation and antibody-dependent cell cytotoxicity. Antibody fragments have some biological properties more desirable than those of the intact molecule, such as less antigenicity and advantages for imaging. The more rapid blood clearance results in less background activity and an improved target-to-background ratio.

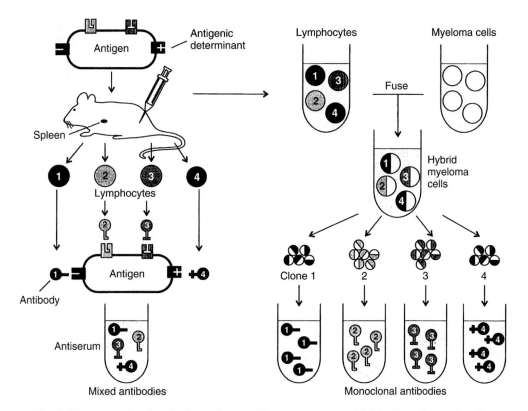

**Fig. 9-21**   Monoclonal antibody production. The process starts with injection of an antigen into a mouse, causing proliferation of B-lymphocytes that can make antibody to the antigen. The mouse spleen is removed, and the B-cells are harvested. Many of the B-cells are capable of making antibody to the specific antigen. If they were cultured at this point *(left)*, they would make a mix of antibodies and would soon die off. If instead the B-cells are mixed with mouse myeloma cells in polyethylene glycol, some of the normal B-cells will fuse with the myeloma cells, producing a population of hybridomas that can be cultured indefinitely. When this population is selectively cloned for those that make the desired antibody, a pure culture of target antibody-producing cells can be grown in great quantities. Its product is the desired monoclonal antibody.

Chemists have attached various radionuclides, such as I-131, I-123, In-111, and Tc-99m, to MoAbs. Each has distinct advantages and disadvantages (Table 9-9). Radiolabeling must be done without changing the antibody's immunoreactivity or biological properties so that the resulting radiopharmaceutical can be used successfully for immunoscintigraphy.

Early antibody imaging studies used polyclonal antibodies, often labeled with I-131. Although they showed promising results in a variety of tumors, I-131 had imaging and dosimetric disadvantages for diagnostic studies. Subsequently, MoAbs were labeled with radionuclides, such as In-111, that had shorter half-lives and better imaging characteristics. The 2.8-day half-life of In-111 allowed time for the slow radiopharmaceutical accumulation and background clearance of whole antibodies. The best target-to-background ratio for imaging occurred 48 to 72 hours after injection. With the development of antibody fragments and their more rapid background renal clearance, high target-to-background

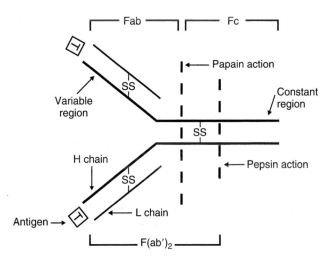

**Fig. 9-22**   IgG antibody. The molecule can be digested enzymatically by papain, resulting in three parts, two Fab′ fragments and one Fc fragment, or by pepsin to produce F(ab′)$_2$ fragments and subfragments of Fc. Fab′ may be produced by splitting the disulfide bond of F(ab′)$_2$.

| Radionuclide | Energy (keV) | Half-Life | Advantages | Disadvantages |
|---|---|---|---|---|
| Technetium-99m | 140 | 6 hr | Pure gamma<br>Inexpensive<br>High photon flux | Complex chemistry<br>Short half-life<br>High counts in kidney, bladder |
| Indium-111 | 173, 247 | 2.8 days | Gamma emitter | Affinity for liver and RES<br>Delayed imaging possible |
| Iodine-123 | 159 | 2.8 days | Gamma emitter<br>Ease of labeling | Dehalogenates<br>Cyclotron produced<br>Expensive due to short half-life |
| Iodine-131 | 364 | 8 days | Ease of labeling | Dehalogenates<br>Low count rate<br>Poor image quality<br>High radiation dose |

**Table 9-9   Radionuclides used for immunoscintigraphy: advantages and disadvantages**

ratio could be obtained on the day of injection. Thus labeling with Tc-99m became possible with the advantage of its optimal imaging characteristics.

## Human Antimouse Antibody

Monoclonal antibodies for clinical use are animal byproducts, produced by the immunization of mice. The immune system recognizes these mouse proteins as foreign and mounts an immunological response against them. This human antimouse antibody (HAMA) response may be mild with fever and hives, severe with shortness of breath and hypotension, or even fatal as a result of anaphylaxis. Some antibodies are more immunogenic than others. Antibodies can be delivered as whole and intact or as fragments. Active regions can be used, and portions of the antibody that contribute to the HAMA response can be deleted. However, the potential for serious reactions is a serious clinical concern.

## Clinical Applications

The FDA has approved four radiolabeled monoclonal antibodies for oncological diagnostic imaging: OncoScint for colorectal and ovarian cancer, CEA-SCAN for colorectal cancer, ProstaScint for prostate cancer, and Verluma for small cell carcinoma of the lung.

**Colorectal cancer** Colorectal cancer is the third most common malignancy in the United States. Five-year survival is 85% with localized disease, 50% with regional spread, and less than 7% with distant metastases. The first recurrence occurs at a single site in 75% of cases. These sites include the liver (33%), local or regional sites (21%), intraabdominal sites (18%), and retroperitoneal lymph nodes (10%).

CEA arises from ectodermally derived epithelium of the digestive system, expressed only during embryological development. CEA is expressed by colorectal cancer and other solid tumors. Over 95% of colorectal cancers express CEA at the cell surface. It is shed into the bloodstream and is detectable in 65% of patients with colorectal carcinoma. The serum CEA level has been used as a tumor marker to assess the adequacy of surgical resection and the effectiveness of chemotherapy and to detect early recurrence. However, one third of patients with recurrence do not have elevated serum CEA levels. Most recurrences and metastases occur in the abdomen and pelvis. Colonoscopy and barium studies produce a low yield in determining sites other than local recurrence because they detect only intraluminal disease. CT and MRI have limited sensitivity for evaluating the extrahepatic abdomen, assessing tumors in normal-sized lymph nodes, and distinguishing postoperative and postradiation changes from tumor.

*Radiopharmaceuticals*

OncoScint CR/OV (Colorectal/Ovarian) OncoScint (Cytogen Corp., Princeton, N.J.) was the first monoclonal antibody approved as a tumor-imaging agent by the FDA (1994). It is a B72.3 murine IgG monoclonal antibody directed against a high-molecular-weight tumor-associated glycoprotein (TAG-72), which is expressed by the majority of colorectal and ovarian carcinomas.

In vitro, OncoScint is reactive with 83% of colorectal cancers, 97% of epithelial ovarian carcinomas, and the majority of breast, non–small cell lung, pancreatic, gastric, and esophageal cancers. It is generally not immunoreactive with normal adult tissues.

The antibody is linked to In-111 by conjugation to the Fc portion, which preserves the immunoreactivity of the antibody (Fig. 9-23). OncoScint is approved for

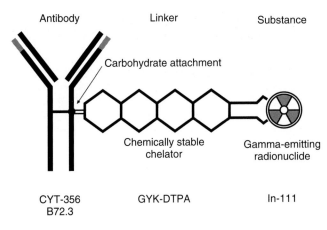

Antibody          Linker          Substance

Carbohydrate attachment

Chemically stable          Gamma-emitting
chelator                    radionuclide

CYT-356          GYK-DTPA          In-111
B72.3

**Fig. 9-23** Indium-111 OncoScint CR/OV and In-111 ProstaScint formulation. The site of attachment of the linker does not interfere with the effector or binding functions of the antibody. (Courtesy Cytogen Corp., Princeton, N.J.)

**Table 9-10  Comparison of OncoScint CR/OV and CEA-SCAN**

| | OncoScint CR/OV | CEA-SCAN |
|---|---|---|
| Radionuclide | In-111 | Tc-99m |
| Monoclonal antibody type | B72.3 | IMMU-4 reactive with CEA |
| | Whole antibody | Fab' fragment |
| HAMA | 40% | <1% |
| Liver metabolism and uptake | High | Low |
| Renal metabolism and uptake | Low | High |
| Plasma half-life | Slow (50 hr) | Rapid (Initial $T_{1/2}$ 1 hr, final $T_{1/2}$ 13 hr) |
| Urinary excretion | 10% at 72 hr | 28% at 24 hr |

**Table 9-11  Imaging sensitivity of OncoScint and CEA-SCAN versus computed tomography by anatomical site**

| | Sensitivity for colorectal tumor localization (%) | | | |
| Anatomical site | In-111 OncoScint | CT | Tc-99m CEA-SCAN | CT |
|---|---|---|---|---|
| Pelvis | 74 | 57 | 69 | 39 |
| Abdomen (extrahepatic) | 66 | 34 | 55 | 32 |
| Liver | 41 | 84 | 63 | 64 |

localization and determination of the extent of extrahepatic metastatic tumor in patients with known colorectal or ovarian cancer.

CEA-SCAN (Tc-99m CEA)   CEA SCAN (Immunomedics, Morris Plains, N.J.) was approved in 1996 for imaging of colorectal cancer. It is a Tc-99m-labeled Fab' fragment of the CEA antibody IMMU-4. Removal of the Fc group of IgG, the most immunogenic part of the molecule, eliminates much of the immunogenicity ordinarily observed with mouse-derived antibody products.

PHARMACOKINETICS   The pharmacokinetics of OncoScint and Tc-99m CEA SCAN are very different, largely because the former radiopharmaceutical is a whole antibody and the latter is an antibody fragment. Table 9-10 compares the pharmacokinetics of OncoScint and CEA-SCAN.

An advantage of the Tc-99m-labeled Fab' fragment is its rapid renal clearance from the blood, allowing for same day high tumor-to-background ratio imaging. At 1, 5, and 24 hours after infusion, 63%, 23%, and 7%, respectively, of the injected dose is present in the circulation. Over 24 hours, 28% of the dose is excreted in the urine. Liver metabolism is low compared with that for the whole antibody.

INDICATIONS   The FDA approved CEA-SCAN for detection of the presence, location, and extent of recurrent, metastatic, and occult colorectal carcinoma involving the liver, extrahepatic abdomen, and pelvis in patients with histologically confirmed colorectal carcinoma. Its major role to date has been in the evaluation of recurrent disease. The two most common clinical indications are a patient with a rising serum CEA level but negative conventional imaging and a patient with known potentially resectable disease who requires preoperative evaluation to exclude the presence of unresectable disease. The CEA-SCAN can assure the surgeon that the patient

has no other metastatic disease that would contraindicate surgical treatment.

The role of OncoScint or Tc-99m CEA in primary disease is not well established. Possible applications might be the detection of synchronous lesions, preoperative determination of the extent of regional disease, or search for occult metastases. Although these indications are included under FDA approval, further clinical investigation is needed to confirm their utility.

ACCURACY   In a multicenter trial 192 patients with colorectal carcinoma were imaged with OncoScint CR/OV and CT. The overall sensitivity was 69%, specificity 76%, positive predictive value 97%, and negative predictive value 19%. Scans detected occult disease in 10% and changed patient management in 25%. Although CT was more sensitive than antibody imaging of the liver, OncoScint was superior for the pelvis and extrahepatic abdomen (Table 9-11). The combined sensitivity of CT and OncoScint immunoscintigraphy (88%) was higher than the sensitivity of either study alone.

In a multicenter trial of 210 patients with advanced recurrent or metastatic colorectal carcinomas, the sensitivity of Tc-99m CEA for detection of metastatic colon cancer in the abdomen, liver, and pelvis was 55%, 63%, and 56%, compared with 32%, 64%, and 48% for CT (Table 9-11). Tc-99m CEA was superior to CT in the extrahepatic abdomen and pelvis. The accuracy of CT and CEA-SCAN was similar in the liver. The combination of Tc-99m CEA and CT increased the overall sensitivity from 66% to 78% while only slightly decreasing specificity (from 89% to 83%).

Tc-99m CEA is superior to OncoScint in several respects. First, it has better imaging characteristics because of the Tc-99m radiolabel. Second, the more rapid clearance of the Tc-99m CEA antibody fragments results in a higher target-to-background ratio at an earlier imaging time (day 1 versus day 2 or 3). Because of the absence of high liver uptake with CEA-SCAN, it is also superior to In-111 OncoScint in detecting liver metastases. While liver metastases are often photopenic with OncoScint, they are usually hot or target lesions with Tc-99m CEA. Finally, CEA-SCAN has a much lower incidence of HAMA response, less than 1% versus 40% for OncoScint.

METHODOLOGY   Imaging protocols for Tc-99m CEA-SCAN and In-111 OncoScint are described in Box 9-8.

DOSIMETRY   The estimated radiation absorbed patient doses for OncoScint CR/OV and CEA-SCAN are detailed in Table 9-12. The highest radiation dose from In-111 OncoScint occurs in the spleen (16 rads) and red marrow (12 rads). For Tc-99m CEA the highest dose is in the kidney (11 rads), followed by the urinary bladder and spleen (both 1.8 rads).

ADVERSE EFFECTS   The incidence of side effects with OncoScint is less than 4%. Most are not serious and are readily reversible, generally without intervention. Adverse effects with Tc-99m CEA have also been uncommon and self-limiting.

The incidence of elevated HAMA with CEA-SCAN is less than 1%, compared with a 40% incidence with OncoScint, although HAMA levels generally decrease with time and half of cases become seronegative. This has implications for using OncoScint in a serial manner to evaluate the effectiveness of therapy or as a prelude to therapy with an MoAb. At present only single administrations have been approved. HAMA can interfere with murine-based immunoassays of CEA and CA-125, producing falsely high values. Alternative assay methods that are not adversely affected are available. HAMA can alter the biodistribution and pharmacokinetics of MoAbs and may interfere with the quality or sensitivity of the imaging study.

IMAGE INTERPRETATION: NORMAL DISTRIBUTION   In-111 OncoScint images show prominent blood pool in the heart and major vessels, as well as uptake in the bone marrow, liver, spleen, and bowel and faint activity in the kidneys

---

## Box 9-8   Technetium-99m CEA-SCAN and Indium-111 OncoScint Imaging: Protocol Summary

**PREPARATION**

None.
Optional: Insert Foley catheter before SPECT pelvic imaging.

|  | Tc-99m CEA-SCAN | In-111 OncoScint |
|---|---|---|
| **RADIOPHARMACEUTICAL** | | |
| Dose: | 30 mCi intravenously | 5 mCi intravenously |
| **INSTRUMENTATION** | | |
| Camera: | Large-field-of-view gamma camera Dual-headed camera preferable | Large-field-of-view gamma camera Dual-headed camera preferable |
| Collimator: | Low-energy, high-resolution | Medium-energy collimator |
| Photopeaks: | 15% symmetric window around 140 keV | 20% window around 173, 247 keV |
| Computer: | 128 × 128 word matrix size | 128 × 128 word matrix |
| **IMAGING PROCEDURE** | | |
| Image: | Commence imaging 2 hr after injection | Imaging at 48-72 hr and 72-120 hr |
| Planar images: | 10 min/view spot images chest to pelvis | Planar: 1000k or 10 min/view |
| SPECT: | Abdomen and pelvis With two-headed camera: 60 stops/head, 40 sec each Optional 24-hr planar imaging (20 min/view) or SPECT (50% increased acquisition time) | Abdomen and pelvis Two-headed camera: SPECT imaging protocol similar to Ga-67 |

---

and bladder. Greatest uptake on the Tc-99m CEA-SCAN is seen in the kidney and spleen, followed by the liver (Fig. 9-24). Bladder activity can result in artifact. Urinary catheterization may be necessary. The greater the delay after injection, the greater the nonspecific bowel activity. Colostomy sites can accumulate radiotracer, and uptake may be seen at surgical incision sites.

**Table 9-12    Dosimetry: monoclonal antibody radiopharmaceuticals**

| Organ | OncoScint (rads/5 mCi) | CEA-SCAN (rads/30 mCi) | ProstaScint (rads/5 mCi) | Verluma (rads/30 mCi) | OctreoScan (rads/6 mCi) |
|---|---|---|---|---|---|
| Gallbladder wall | | | 7.3 | **5.6** | |
| Large intestine | 3.1 | | 7.6 | 2.7 | 1.6 |
| Kidney | 9.7 | **11.1** | 12.4 | 3.9 | 10.8 |
| Urinary bladder | 2.8 | 1.8 | 2.2 | | 6.1 |
| Liver | 15.0 | 1.1 | **18.5** | 1.3 | 2.4 |
| Lungs | 4.9 | | 5.6 | 0.7 | |
| Adrenal glands | 4.5 | | 5.3 | | 1.5 |
| Ovaries | 2.9 | 0.5 | 0.9 | | |
| Heart wall | 3.2 | | 7.8 | | |
| Spleen | **16.0** | 1.8 | 16.3 | 0.6 | **14.8** |
| Thyroid | 1.5 | | 1.4 | 0.9 | 1.5 |
| Testes | 1.4 | 0.5 | 5.6 | 0.5 | 0.6 |
| Red marrow | 12.0 | | 4.3 | 0.5 | 0.7 |
| Total body | 2.7 | 0.5 | 2.7 | 0.5 | 2.6 |

Target organ (highest radiation absorbed dose) appears in boldface type.

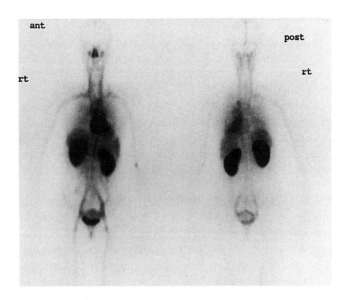

**Fig. 9-24**    Technetium-99m CEA-SCAN normal distribution. The kidneys have the greatest uptake of the radiopharmaceutical. Renal clearance into the bladder is seen. Cardiac and vascular blood pool is prominent. Lesser distribution is seen in the liver and spleen. The focal uptake above the bladder is the uterine blood pool.

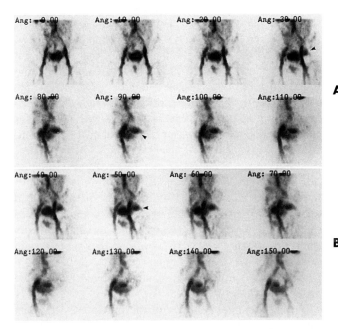

**Fig. 9-25**    Technetium-99m CEA, local recurrence of colorectal cancer. Patient had rising serum CEA level several months after primary resection of tumor in the rectosigmoid area. This reconstructed volume display of sequential projection angles [Ang: = degrees] shows tumor recurrence in the rectal area *(arrowheads)*.

IMAGE INTERPRETATION: ABNORMAL UPTAKE    Uptake is more likely to represent tumor if located in an expected lymph node distribution or an organ under investigation (Fig. 9-25). Distant metastases can also be detected (Fig. 9-26). With Tc-99m CEA, only hot or rimmed lesions should be considered positive for tumor involving the liver. Large lesions with considerable necrosis may appear cold.

Gamma detector probes are increasingly used for intraoperative localization of metastases seen on the CEA-SCAN. The intraoperative probes are also some-times used to detect liver metastases too small for scan detection.

**Ovarian cancer**    Ovarian cancer is the fourth most frequent cause of cancer deaths in women. The overall 5-year survival rate is 39%. Ovarian cancer is difficult to diagnose and stage with current imaging methods because it frequently metastasizes as small (<2 cm) peritoneal implants not detectable on CT. CT also cannot

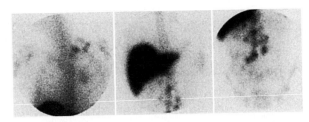

**Fig. 9-26** Distant recurrent colorectal cancer with indium-111 OncoScint. Tumor uptake is seen in the left supraclavicular nodes and left hilum *(left)*, in the periaortic nodes, and more diffusely throughout the abdomen *(middle and right)*. Retrosternal uptake was detected with SPECT.

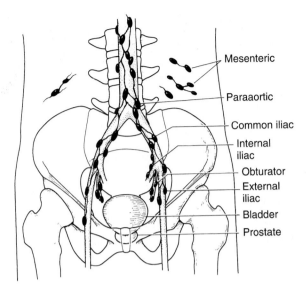

**Fig. 9-27** Pelvic and abdominal lymph node anatomy. A knowledge of this anatomy is critical for proper interpretation of indium-111 ProstaScint studies.

detect tumor in normal-sized lymph nodes, demonstrate diffuse miliary disease, or distinguish adhesions or scar from tumor. Serum CA-125 assay, a tumor marker, has a high false negative rate and does not predict the location or extent of disease. Exploratory laparotomy is the best approach to surgical staging. However, it does not detect extraabdominal tumors, is expensive, has a 20% complication rate, and gives false negative results in 20% to 50% of patients based on the results of second-look surgery.

*OncoScint CR/OV* Studies suggest that OncoScint can locate and define the extent of extrahepatic ovarian cancer, detect occult disease, including miliary spread, and potentially direct the surgical approach for ovarian cancer. In a multicenter trial of patients with primary or recurrent disease, OncoScint had a sensitivity of 60% to 70% and a specificity of 55% to 60%. The positive predictive value was 83%, and the scan was able to detect occult disease in 35%, including some with normal CA-125 levels. The antibody scan changed patient management in 25% of cases. It was superior to CT for patients with recurrent disease and carcinomatosis (60% versus 30%). However, it has not gained widespread use for this approved indication. Tc-99m CEA-SCAN has not been used or approved for ovarian cancer.

**Prostate cancer** Cancer of the prostate is the most frequently diagnosed malignant tumor in men in the United States and the second leading cause of cancer death. Its incidence is increasing. The 5-year survival is approximately 50%. Although many patients have symptoms for which they seek medical evaluation, the diagnosis is often suspected on the basis of screening prostate-specific antigen (PSA) levels drawn on men older than 50 years. Ultrasound-guided needle biopsy is used to obtain tissue from suspect nodules.

Staging of prostate cancer is based on the combination of physical examination, histopathological Gleason's score, and serum PSA. Bone scans are indicated for patients with serum PSA greater than 10 to 20 ng/ml or with a high Gleason's score. Lymph node involvement is the most common pattern of metastatic spread, usually occurring in a stepwise fashion from periprostatic or

obturator nodes, to internal and external iliac nodes, and then to common iliac and periaortic nodes (Fig. 9-27). Frequent sites of distant metastases are the skeleton, liver, and lungs.

Initial therapy involves either surgery or radiation therapy. Radical prostatectomy, the best chance for cure, is not undertaken when there is evidence of nodal involvement or distant spread. Thus definition of the status of pelvic lymph nodes draining the prostate gland is critical to staging and management. CT and MRI have limited value owing to their low sensitivity for detecting nodal involvement. Even with favorable indicators of intracapsular disease before surgery, patients are frequently found to have extracapsular disease at surgery. The rate of local recurrence after surgery is 15% to 20%.

Lymphadenectomy, the most accurate technique for detecting nodal involvement, may fail and lead to surgery for patients with occult disseminated disease. Patients with high PSA levels and a high Gleason's score are usually treated with local radiation therapy, since they are at risk for local recurrence. Radiation therapy can be performed as the initial treatment or following radical prostatectomy.

If after initial treatment the PSA fails to fall to undetectable levels or subsequently rises, residual or recurrent cancer is likely. Radiation therapy of the prostate fossa or the pelvis is often given even in the absence of positive biopsy or positive imaging results. If disease is localized to the prostate fossa or pelvis, radiation therapy offers the potential for effective treatment. However, if recurrence involves periaortic lymph nodes or other distant sites, radiation therapy exposes the patient to significant morbidity with no potential for cure owing to the presence of tumor outside the radiation therapy field. In this situation In-111 Prosta-Scint can play an important role.

*Indium-111 ProstaScint* In-111 ProstaScint (Capro-mab Pendetide, Cytogen Corp., Princeton, N.J.) is a conjugate of the monoclonal antibody 7E11-C5.3 (CYT-356), a linker-chelator (GYK-DTA), and In-111 (Fig. 9-23). CYT-356 is an intact murine immunoglobulin reactive with prostate-specific membrane antigen (PMSA), a glycoprotein expressed by more than 95% of prostate adenocarcinomas. ProstaScint was approved in 1996 as an imaging agent for the detection of soft tissue metastases for patients with prostate cancer who were at high risk for metastatic disease.

PHARMACOKINETICS AND NORMAL DISTRIBUTION   In-111 ProstaScint follows a monoexponential clearance pattern with a biological half-life of 72 hours. Ten percent is excreted in the urine within 72 hours, and a smaller amount is excreted through the bowel. Normal distribution includes the liver, spleen, bone marrow, and blood pool structures. Clearance occurs into the bowel and bladder.

ACCURACY   In a multicenter trial, 152 patients with a tissue diagnosis of prostate cancer scheduled for pelvic lymphadenectomy had ProstaScint scans. Other standard noninvasive imaging, including bone scans, CT, and MRI, was negative or equivocal. The patients were considered at high risk for the presence of lymph node metastases based on PSA or Gleason's score. The imaging results were correlated with histological analysis of pelvic lymph nodes. ProstaScint correctly identified lymph node metastases in 40 of 64 patients (sensitivity 62%), compared with a sensitivity of 4% for CT and 15% for MRI. Of 88 patients without pelvic nodal metastases, 63 were correctly identified as normal (specificity 72%) (Table 9-13). The specificity of ProstaScint may actually be higher than these results suggest, since 15 patients with a false positive study had biochemical evidence of disease after radical prostatectomy, suggesting that disease was missed.

Results were similar in a multicenter series of 183 patients in whom residual or recurrent prostate cancer after radical prostatectomy was strongly suspected based on rising PSA levels but bone scans and standard imaging methods gave negative results. Although the accuracy of ProstaScint scanning is only fair, it far surpasses all other available imaging modalities.

Minor adverse events have been reported in 4% of patients. Most common have been liver enzyme elevations, hypotension, and hypertension, each occurring in 1% of patients or less. Elevated HAMA titers have been observed in 8%. A similar incidence (4%) of adverse events was seen in patients undergoing repeated injections.

INDICATIONS   In-111 ProstaScint is indicated for patients who have biopsy-proven prostate cancer that is thought to be clinically localized after standard diagnostic evalu-

### Table 9-13   Comparison of ProstaScint with pelvic lymph node dissection

|  | ProstaScint scan positive | ProstaScint scan negative |  |
|---|---|---|---|
| Biopsy positive | 40 | 24 | Sensitivity 62% |
| Biopsy negative | 24 | 63 | Specificity 72% |

### Box 9-9   Indium-111 ProstaScint Imaging: Protocol Summary

**RADIOPHARMACEUTICAL**

Dose: 5 mCi In-111 ProstaScint intravenously.

**INSTRUMENTATION**

Camera: Large-field-of-view SPECT gamma camera; dual-headed camera preferable
Collimator: Medium-energy collimator
Photopeaks: 20% window around 173, 247 keV
Computer: 128 (128 matrix size)

**IMAGING PROCEDURE**

Image:
30 min after radiopharmaceutical injection: planar and SPECT "blood pool" imaging of abdomen and pelvis
3 to 5 days: repeat planar and SPECT images of abdomen and pelvis (SPECT technique: two-headed camera: 60 stops/head, 40 sec each)
**or**
at 3 to 5 days radiolabel the patient's RBCs with Tc-99m and acquire *dual-isotope* SPECT of abdomen and pelvis
Occasionally, repeat delayed imaging required to permit time for blood pool, bladder, or bowel clearance

ation but who are at high risk for pelvic lymph node metastases. It is most commonly used in postprostatectomy patients when occult metastatic disease is suspected because of a rising PSA level but the standard workup is negative or equivocal. Radiation therapy is indicated if disease is localized to the prostate bed and pelvic lymph nodes, but not if the scan shows activity in periaortic lymph nodes or other distant sites. In the latter case hormonal manipulations, systemic chemotherapy, or orchiectomy would be more appropriate treatment options.

METHODOLOGY   An imaging protocol for In-111 ProstaScint is described in Box 9-9. SPECT of the abdomen and pelvis is mandatory. Blood pool images are necessary for correct interpretation. They may be acquired either by imaging on day 1 at 30 minutes after In-111 ProstaScint injection or, alternatively, by radiolabeling the patient's red blood cells and acquiring dual-isotope Tc-99m RBC and In-111 ProstaScint planar and SPECT images at 3 to 5 days. We perform the study on both day 3 and day 5. The day 3 images often have problematic bowel activity, and the day 5 images sometimes have a low count rate and are suboptimal. Review of the two study days together gives us the most confidence in interpretation.

DOSIMETRY    The highest In-111 ProstaScint radiation dose is received by the liver (18.5 rads per 5 mCi administered dose), followed by the spleen (16.3 rads) and kidneys (12.4 rads) (Table 9-12).

INTERPRETATION    There is a steep learning curve for interpretation of In-111 ProstaScint SPECT studies. The FDA approved this radiopharmaceutical for clinical use and interpretation only by physicians who have undergone specific training in the acquisition and interpretation of these studies. There are several reasons for the concern about interpretive difficulty. In the pelvic SPECT there is a paucity of normal anatomical landmarks. The individual cross-sectional images have low counts and poor resolution. Bowel and bladder clearance can complicate interpretation.

The dual-isotope acquisition method allows single-day imaging and perfect image registration of the two studies. For correct interpretation the physician must be familiar with pelvic lymph node anatomy and common patterns of tumor spread (Fig. 9-27). The 3- and 5-day images must be carefully correlated with the blood pool images, since right-to-left vascular asymmetries may otherwise be misinterpreted as nodal disease on the In-111 ProstaScint images. An abnormal scan shows increased uptake in the prostate fossa, at pelvic, abdominal, or chest lymph node sites, or less commonly in bony structures. Pelvic lymph node metastases are best seen on the SPECT studies and rarely seen on planar studies (Fig. 9-28). However, both planar and SPECT

images may show periaortic lymph or thoracic lymph node metastases (Fig. 9-29). ProstaScint is considerably less sensitive (50%) than bone scans for detecting bone metastases.

**Lung carcinoma**    Lung cancer can be divided into two distinct diseases based on tumor biology and chemotherapy responsiveness: small cell carcinoma of the lung (SCLC) and non–small cell lung cancer (NSCLC). SCLC accounts for 25% of all new lung cancers in the United States. Survival is poor, 18% at 5 years with limited disease and only 2% with distant metastases. Two thirds of patients with SCLC have metastatic spread at the time of diagnosis. Thus only one third would be expected to respond to local therapy. Staging determines the extent of disease at the time of presentation and guides therapy. Patients with limited disease are treated with local radiation therapy and systemic chemotherapy, whereas patients with extensive disease receive palliative treatment with chemotherapy alone.

NSCLC is primarily a surgical disease; resection is the treatment for choice for localized disease. Accurate staging is essential to determine whether the patient is potentially curable. The standard diagnostic imaging staging method is CT. Mediastinoscopy with lymph node biopsy is indicated to evaluate enlarged or equivocal lymph nodes. The patient is considered a candidate for primary tumor resection if no evidence of tumor spread to extrathoracic sites, the contralateral chest, or the mediastinum is found. CT relies on lymph node size to detect metastatic disease. However, normal-sized nodes may contain microscopic tumor. Because of this, CT lacks sensitivity and may underestimate the extent of lung cancer. Thus patients may undergo unnecessary

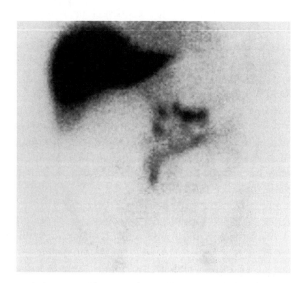

**Fig. 9-29**    Indium-111 ProstaScint shows paraaortic and mesenteric lymph nodes. This planar abdominal image showed no change in distribution between days 3 and 6, excluding bowel activity as the cause for this activity.

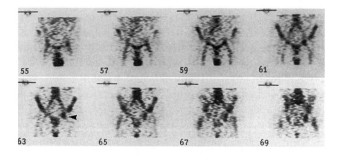

**Fig. 9-28**    Indium-111 ProstaScint detects metastases to regional nodes. Sequential coronal images show prominent uptake in external iliac nodes (*arrowhead*).

surgery. In addition, enlarged nodes may be due to reactive hyperplasia or infection, resulting in false positive findings. Although mediastinoscopy may improve accuracy, it is invasive and expensive.

*Verluma*  Verluma (Tc-99m Nofetumomab, DuPont Pharmaceuticals, Billerica, Mass.) is a Tc-99m-labeled Fab' fragment of a murine IgG2b monoclonal antibody NR-LU-10 directed against a 40-kilodalton glycoprotein expressed on a variety of carcinomas, including SCLC, NSCLC, and cancers of the breast, ovary, colorectum, and prostate. Tc-99m Verluma was approved by the FDA in 1996 as a diagnostic imaging agent for staging of patients with newly diagnosed SCLC.

PHARMACOKINETICS  Renal clearance is the main route of excretion, with 64% of the injected dose excreted within the first 22 hours. The secondary route of elimination is hepatobiliary, with clearance into the gallbladder and intestines. HAMA develops in only 6% of patients.

ACCURACY  Tc-99m Verluma was compared with conventional diagnostic methods in a multicenter trial of 96 patients with SCLC, of whom 42% had limited and 58% had extensive disease as evaluated with standard imaging modalities. Tc-99m Verluma correctly staged 82% of patients. The positive predictive value for demonstrating extensive disease was 94%. Sensitivity for tumor detection was 77%, compared with 88% for a battery of standard diagnostic tests. Tc-99m Verluma had the highest accuracy for clinical staging of any single diagnostic test.

Although approved for SCLC, Tc-99m Verluma is taken up by other tumors. In addition to NSCLC, uptake has been reported in gastrointestinal, breast, ovarian, pancreatic, renal, and cervical cancers. The ultimate role of Tc-99m Verluma in these cancers is uncertain and will require further investigation.

METHODOLOGY  Imaging is performed about 18 hours after injection of the radiopharmaceutical (30 mCi) (Box 9-10). SPECT of the chest is routine.

DOSIMETRY  The target organ receiving the highest radiation dose is the gallbladder with 5.6 rads/30mCi, followed by the large bowel with 2.7 rads (Table 9-12).

## Future of Monoclonal Antibody Imaging

In the first edition of this book in 1995, only one oncological monoclonal antibody had been approved for clinical diagnostic imaging. Now four are available. There is every reason to expect that other antibodies will be approved and available in the near future.

Radiolabeled monoclonal antibodies for B-cell lymphoma offer considerable therapeutic promise. About 80% of non-Hodgkin's lymphomas are of B-cell origin. Several companies are developing and investigating similar therapeutic antibodies. Studies report a 75% response rate, with 50% having a complete response, in patients with low- and intermediate-grade tumors previously unresponsive to standard chemotherapy. This would be a major therapeutic advance.

## PEPTIDE RECEPTOR IMAGING

Tumor cells, despite their seemingly uncontrolled metabolism and growth, are in fact modulated by various endogenously produced peptides, including numerous hormones and growth factors that interact with receptors on the tumor surface. Among these peptides are somatostatin, vasoactive intestinal peptide, tumor necrosis factor, and angiogenesis factor. Much work is being done to radiolabel these peptides for tumor imaging and ultimately for radiation therapy.

Somatostatin is a peptide hormone produced in the hypothalamus, pituitary gland, brainstem, gastrointestinal tract, and pancreas. It acts as a neurotransmitter that inhibits peptide formation and secretion by neuroendocrine cells. Outside the central nervous system its hormonal activities include inhibition of the release of growth hormone, insulin, glucagon, gastrin, serotonin, and calcitonin. It also has an antiproliferative effect on tumors and plays a role in the modulation of immunological activity.

Somatostatin receptors have been identified on many different cells and tumors of neuroendocrine origin (Fig. 9-30). Neuroendocrine cells are derived from the neural crest and have in common their ability to synthesize amines from precursors and produce peptides that act as hormones and neurotransmitters. Tumors with somatostatin receptors fall into three categories: (1) neuroendo-

---

**Box 9-10   Technetium-99m Verluma Imaging: Protocol Summary**

**RADIOPHARMACEUTICAL**

Dose: Indium-111 Technetium-99m Verluma, 30 mCi intravenously

**INSTRUMENTATION**

Camera: large-field-of-view SPECT gamma camera; dual-headed camera preferable
Collimator: low-energy high-resolution collimator
Photopeaks: 15% window around 140 keV
Computer: 128 × 128 matrix size

**IMAGING PROCEDURE**

Whole body planar imaging the morning (about 18 hr) after injection
SPECT imaging of chest after whole body scan

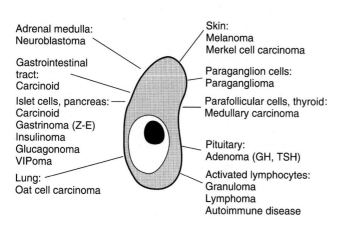

**Fig. 9-30**   Neuroendocrine cells and tumors originating from each cell type.

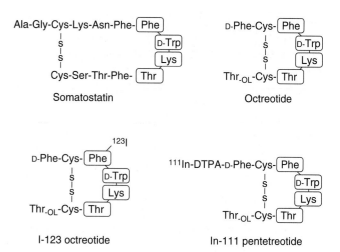

**Fig. 9-31**   Comparison of somatostatin analog octreotide, iodine-123 octreotide, and indium-111 pentetreotide (Octreo-Scan).

crine tumors or APUDomas (amine precursor uptake decarboxylation), such as pituitary adenomas, gastric endocrine-producing tumors (carcinoid, gastrinoma, insulinoma), pheochromocytomas, and medullary thyroid cancer, and small cell lung cancers; (2) central nervous system tumors (astrocytomas, meningiomas, and neuroblastomas); and (3) other tumors, including lymphoma and breast, lung, and renal cell cancer.

A somatostatin analog, octreotide (Sandostatin, Novartis, Basel, Switzerland) is an FDA-approved therapeutic agent used to treat symptoms of metastatic carcinoid and vasoactive intestinal peptide tumors and to suppress growth hormone in acromegaly. Octreotide was initially radiolabeled with I-123, but an In-111-radiolabeled analog has been found superior (Fig. 9-31). A Tc-99m-labeled analog is also under investigation.

---

### Indium-111 OctreoScan

In-111 pentetreotide (OctreoScan, Mallinckrodt, St. Louis, Mo.) has been approved by the FDA for imaging of neurorendocrine tumors. A variety of receptor-positive tumors have been imaged with this agent. It has successfully detected most APUDomas, including pituitary tumors, pancreatic islet cell tumors, carcinoids, medullary thyroid carcinoma, paragangliomas, pheochromocytomas, and neuroblastomas. Other tumors with somatostatin receptors that have been imaged include meningioma, astrocytroma, malignant thymoma, breast cancer, SCLC, and lymphoma.

**Pharmacokinetics and normal distribution**   In-111 OctreoScan is rapidly cleared by the kidneys. Only 2% undergoes hepatobiliary excretion. At 4 hours after injection 10% of the dose is still in circulation, at 24 hours less than 1%. This rapid clearance enhances the target-to-background ratio. Normal uptake occurs in the

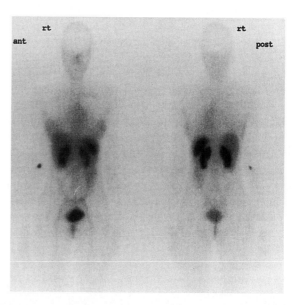

**Fig. 9-32**   Normal distribution of indium-111 OctreoScan. Anterior *(left)* and posterior *(right)* views. Imaging at 24 hours. Note intensive uptake and retention in kidneys and spleen and lesser uptake in liver. Heart and vascular blood pool seen, as well as urinary and bowel clearance.

thyroid gland, liver, gallbladder, spleen, kidneys, and bladder. The kidneys retain considerable radiotracer and appear quite intense even on delayed imaging (Fig. 9-32).

**Accuracy**   The accuracy of In-111 OctreoScan for diagnosis of various neuroendocrine tumors is noted in Table 9-14. Many of these tumors are small and can easily be missed on conventional imaging. The ability to perform whole body imaging is particularly advantageous.

For most neuroendocrine tumors, such as gastrinoma and carcinoid, the sensitivity is very high. Two excep-

| Table 9-14 | Accuracy of indium-111 OctreoScan in multicenter trial | |
| --- | --- | --- |

| Tumor type | No. consistent/total patients* | Percent |
| --- | --- | --- |
| Carcinoid | 190/237 | 80 |
| Insulinoma | 8/11 | 31 |
| Gastrinoma | 40/42 | 95 |
| Glucagonoma | 8/11 | 73 |
| Small cell carcinoma of lung | 2/2 | 100 |
| Pheochromocytoma | 9/9 | 100 |
| Paraganglioma | 6/7 | 86 |
| Medullary thyroid carcinoma | 12/22 | 54 |
| Vipoma | 6/7 | 86 |
| Pituitary adenoma | 24/30 | 80 |

*Other methods included biopsy, computed tomography, ultrasonography, magnetic resonance imaging, angiography.

tions are insulinoma and medullary carcinoma of the thyroid, with only 50% sensitivity. The sensitivity for pheochromocytoma and neuroblastoma is high (approximately 90%), similar to that obtained with I-131 MIBG imaging (see Chapter 14). However, for adults MIGB scanning is generally agreed to be preferable, even though the image quality is poorer and the radiation dose is higher than with OctreoScan. The advantage of I-131 MIBG is the higher target-to-background ratio and better specificity. An important disadvantage of OctreoScan is its persistent high kidney activity, which makes interpretation of the adjacent adrenal gland more difficult. The reported sensitivity for other tumors, such as lymphoma and lung and breast cancer, is about 70% each; however, clinical utility has not been established.

**Methodology**  Box 9-11 describes a typical imaging protocol for In-111 OctreoScan. Sandostatin therapy is generally discontinued 3 to 7 days before the study, although there are case reports of better visualization of metastases while patients were taking the drug. Early imaging at 4 hours is advantageous since bowel activity is absent at this early time, although the background activity is still high. Because of continuing background clearance the tumor to nontumor ratio increases over 24 hours, improving tumor detectability.

**Dosimetry**  The estimated radiation-absorbed dose to the patient from OctreoScan is shown in Table 9-12. The spleen is the target organ, receiving the highest absorbed dose of 14.7 rads per 6 mCi administered dose, followed by the kidneys, which receive 10.8 rads.

**Image interpretation**  Many neuroendocrine tumors can be diagnosed with planar imaging (Fig. 9-33). However, SPECT can be helpful, particularly in the abdomen. The target-to-background ratio is usually quite

| Box 9-11 | Indium-111 OctreoScan: Protocol Summary |
| --- | --- |

**RADIOPHARMACEUTICAL**

Dose: 6 mCi In-111 OctreoScan intravenously

**PREPARATION**

Bowel preparation with laxative and enema; hydration
Discontinue octreotide therapy 3 to 7 days before injection

**INSTRUMENTATION**

Camera: Large-field-of-view SPECT gamma camera
        Dual-headed camera preferable
Collimator: Low-energy high-resolution collimator
Photopeaks: 20% window around 173 and 245 keV
Computer: 128 × 128 word mode matrix size

**IMAGING PROCEDURE**

4 hr: Planar images of abdomen and pelvis, 500,000 counts or 15 min; SPECT of abdomen
24 hr: Planar whole body imaging, 300,000 counts or 15 min; SPECT of abdomen and other regions as clinically indicated

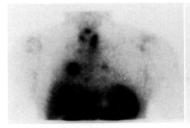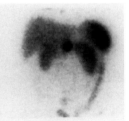

**Fig. 9-33**  Metastatic carcinoid tumor. Anterior planar views of chest *(left)* and abdomen *(right)*. Extensive metastatic disease in a 38-year-old woman with a 10-year history of carcinoid. Multiple sites of thoracic, mediastinal, and paratracheal uptake, as well as uptake in the midabdomen, representing paraaortic adenopathy. The patient also had multiple other sites not shown here, including many soft tissue metastases.

high. The region between the kidneys can be difficult to scan because of the high renal uptake.

## NeoTect

NeoTect (Tc-99m Depreotide, Diatide, Inc., Londonderry, N.H.) is a synthetic peptide with high-affinity binding to somatostatin receptors. Although developed to diagnose neuroectodermal tumors, it has proved inferior to octreotide (see next section). Pulmonary malignancies has been shown to have somatostatin receptors. NeoTect has recently been approved by the

FDA for imaging of lung masses seen on x-ray or CT. The clinical indication is similar to that of F-18 FDG: to confirm pulmonary malignancy of a lung mass and for clinical staging.

**Accuracy** In one study NeoTect had an overall sensitivity of 70% and specificity of 86% for predicting histological findings. It was able to improve the predictive value of malignancy from 85% with CT to 97% with NeoTect.

**Dosimetry** Because NeoTect is a Tc-99m radiolabeled radiopharmaceutical, the radiation absorbed dose is low. The kidneys are the target organs with 0.33 rad/mCi (15 to 20 mCi administered dose).

## Future of Peptide Scintigraphy

In-111 octreotide is only the first of many radiolabeled peptides that will likely find their way into the future practice of nuclear medicine. A new Tc-99m-labeled somatostatin receptor imaging agent is discussed above. Peptides have several potential advantages over monoclonal antibodies. They are simpler and less expensive to produce. They have low antigenicity (no HAMA) and no risk of biological contamination. The potential for peptide imaging and therapeutic agents seems considerable.

## LYMPHOSCINTIGRAPHY

### Melanoma

Radionuclide lymphoscintigraphy has been used for many years to define the lymphatic drainage of melanoma. In the past, some surgeons believed that aggressive routine resection of the draining lymphatic bed

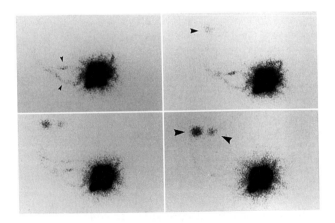

**Fig. 9-34** Melanoma lymphoscintigraphy. Filtered technetium-99m sulfur colloid injected intracutaneously around melanoma lesion. Note early lymphatic drainage *(small arrowheads, upper left)* at 10 minutes, first appearance of sentinel node *(medium arrowhead, upper right)* at 20 minutes, and visualization of two nodes at 40 minutes *(lower left)* and 1 hour *(large arrowheads, lower right)*.

could improve survival. Lymphoscintigraphy was particularly helpful for patients with neck and central torso lesions, since the lymphatic drainage pattern is unpredictable. However, recent studies have shown that routine nodal dissection does not improve survival, except in a subgroup of patients with intermediate-thickness melanoma (1 to 4 mm) who are 60 years of age or less. The finding of cancer-positive nodes can help identify high-risk patients who might be candidates for interferon adjuvant therapy.

Recent studies have shown that sentinel lymph node biopsy is an accurate alternative to routine nodal dissection. Many now consider it to be the standard of care. Studies have shown an orderly progression of lymph node tumor spread. The "sentinel" lymph node is defined as the first node of a regional lymphatic basin draining the primary tumor. Lymphoscintigraphy is used to identify the sentinel node, on which biopsy is subsequently performed (Fig. 9-34). Patients with negative sentinel nodes do not require further surgery and are at low risk, whereas those with positive sentinel nodes require nodal dissection and may be candidates for adjuvant therapy. Vital blue dye has been used to detect the sentinel node intraoperatively but has limitations because of its rapid transit. If surgery is not prompt, the dye may move beyond the sentinel node to other nodes. The newest development in the nuclear technique is use of an intraoperative gamma probe detector that provides accurate localization of the node at the time of surgery.

### Breast Cancer

The surgical management of breast cancer has evolved over recent years from radical surgical procedures toward lesser surgical procedures. This has brought the value of axillary lymph node dissection into close scrutiny. With the success of sentinel node identification for melanoma, surgeons have become interested in this approach to determine whether a patient with newly diagnosed breast cancer has regional tumor spread to axillary nodes. Involvement of the regional nodal basin is the single most important independent variable in predicting prognosis.

Controversy exists over the role of axillary dissection in the management of operable breast cancer. Advocates of axillary dissection contend that it has benefit, since it provides regional control of axillary disease, but critics say than overall survival depends primarily on the development of distant metastases and is not influenced by axillary dissection. They contend that adjuvant chemotherapy with or without nodal irradiation is preferable to axillary dissection. Axillary lymph node dissection is associated with considerable morbidity, including wound infection, seroma, paresthesia, and chronic limb edema.

Recent experience has shown that the intraoperative gamma probe has a greater than 90% accuracy for detecting sentinel lymph nodes. Studies of this technique in patients with small invasive primary breast cancer (<1 cm, T1 or T2 lesions) have shown that less than 30% have metastatic disease in axillary nodes and that only those patients require axillary node dissection. The false negative rate of the technique is low.

## Radiopharmaceuticals

Over the years a number of radiopharmaceuticals have been used for lymphoscintigraphy, including Tc-99m sulfur colloid, Tc-99m human serum albumin (HSA), Tc-99m nanocolloid, and Tc-99m antimony sulfur colloid. Although Tc-99m antimony sulfur colloid was used extensively in the past, it is no longer available. Tc-99m HSA is not particulate and shows poor retention within the lymph nodes. Tc-99m nanocolloid is used in Europe but is not available in the United States.

Colloidal clearance rate depends greatly on particle size. A large portion of unmodified larger Tc-99m sulfur colloid particles is retained at the injection site. Therefore the Tc-99m sulfur colloid is first filtered using a 0.22-μm filter to ensure a more uniform smaller colloidal particle that is more conducive to lymphatic drainage.

## Methodology

*Melanoma* The methodology of scanning in cases of melanoma varies. Some surgeons order lymphoscintigraphy before surgery and mark the location of the sentinel node on the patient's skin. Others do not request imaging but use a radiation detector probe at surgery to find the sentinel node, on which they then perform biopsy. The combination of the two methods is common. Lymphoscintigraphy allows the surgeon to anticipate the drainage pattern.

Four to six injections of 100 μCi in tuberculin syringes are made intracutaneously around the lesion or surgical site. Sequential imaging is performed every 5 minutes for 60 to 90 minutes until the sentinel node is detected. The location of the node can then be noted with an indelible marker pen. Alternatively, no skin marking is needed and an intraoperative gamma probe is used to locate the site at surgery.

*Breast cancer* On the day of surgery several (four to six) intracutaneous or subcutaneous injections of the radiopharmaceutical, 100 μCi each, are made around the biopsy site. Imaging may or may not be performed. An intraoperative gamma probe is used to detect the sentinel node so that biopsy can be performed.

## SUGGESTED READINGS

Alazraki NP, Eshima D, Eshima LA, et al: Lymphoscintigraphy, the sentinel node concept, and the intraoperative gamma probe in melanoma, breast cancer, and other potential cancers, *Semin Nucl Med* 27:55-67, 1997.

Al-Suigar A, Coleman RE: Applications of PET in lung cancer, *Semin Nucl Med* 28:303-319, 1998.

Balaban EP, Walker BS, Cox JV, et al: Detection and staging of small cell lung carcinoma with a technetium-labeled monoclonal antibody (Verluma): a comparison with standard staging methods, *Clin Nucl Med* 17:439-445, 1992.

Collier BD, Abdel-Nabi H, Doerr RJ, et al: Immuno-scintigraphy performed with In-111-labeled CYT-103 in the management of colorectal cancer: comparison with CT, *Radiology* 185:179-186, 1992.

Delbeke D, Patton JA, Martin WH, Sandler MP: Positron imaging in oncology: present and future. In Freeman LM: *Nuclear medicine annual 1998*, Philadelphia, 1998, Lippincott-Raven.

Front D, Bar-Shalom R, Israel O: Role of gallium and other radiopharmaceuticals in the management of patients with lymphoma. In Freeman LM: *Nuclear medicine annual 1998*, Philadelphia, 1998, Lippincott-Raven.

Haseman MK, Reed NL: Capromab pendetide (ProstaScint) imaging of prostate cancer. In Freeman LM: *Nuclear medicine annual 1998*, Philadelphia, 1998, Lippincott-Raven.

Hoh CK, Schiepers C, Seltzer MA, et al: PET in oncology: will it replace the other modalities? *Semin Nucl Med* 27:94-106, 1997.

Kaplan WD, Jochelson MS, Herman TS: Gallium-67 imaging: a predictor of residual tumor viability and clinical outcome in patients with diffuse large-cell lymphoma, *J Clin Oncol* 8:1966-1970, 1990.

Krag D, Weaver D, Ashikaga T, et al: The sentinel node in breast cancer: a multicenter validation study, *N Engl J Med* 339:941-946, 1998.

Krenning EP, Kwekkeboom DJ, Bakker WH, et al: Somatostatin receptor scintigraphy with [111 In-DTPA-Dphe-1] and [123I-Tyr-3]-octreotide: the Rotterdam experience with more than 1000 patients, *Eur J Nucl Med* 20:716-731, 1993.

Moffat FL, Pinsky CM, Hammershaimb L, et al: Clinical utility of external immunoscintigraphy with IMMU-4 technetium-99m Fab´ antibody (Tc-99m CEA-SCAN) fragment in patients undergoing surgery for carcinoma of the colon and rectum: results of a pivotal, phase III trial, *J Clin Oncol* 14:2295-2305, 1996.

Taillefer R: The role of 99mTc-sestamibi and other conventional radiopharmaceuticals in breast cancer diagnosis, *Semin Nucl Med* 29:16-40, 1999.

# Hepatobiliary System

Nuclear medicine has played an important role in liver and spleen imaging for more than 25 years, but that role has changed considerably over time. Until the advent of computed tomography (CT), the technetium-99m (Tc-99m) sulfur colloid liver-spleen scan was the primary liver-imaging method. It now has a very limited role because of the alternative abdominal imaging methods of CT, magnetic resonance imaging (MRI), and ultrasonography. Other nuclear medicine liver studies have evolved, however, that provide unique functional and pathophysiological information not available from anatomical imaging methods (Table 10-1).

Cholescintigraphy using Tc-99m iminodiacetic acid analogs (IDAs) is now a well-established hepatobiliary imaging method. Although most often used to diagnose acute cholecystitis, Tc-99m IDA has many other important clinical uses. Tc-99m-labeled red blood cell (RBC) liver imaging has long been used for the diagnosis of

**Table 10-1    Liver radiopharmaceuticals and clinical indications**

| Radiopharmaceutical | Mechanism of uptake | Indication |
|---|---|---|
| Technetium-99m sulfur colloid | Reticuloendothelial system (Kupffer cell) extraction | Focal nodular hyperplasia |
| Tc-99m hepatobiliary iminodiacetic acid analog (HIDA) | Hepatocyte uptake | Cholescintigraphy |
| Tc-99m red blood cells (RBCs) | Blood pool agent | Cavernous hemangioma |
| Tc-99m macroaggregated albumin (MAA) | Blood flow, capillary blockage | Intraarterial chemotherapy |
| Xenon-133 | Lipid soluble | Focal fatty tumor uptake |
| Gallium-67 | Iron binding, lactoferrin binding | Tumor/abscess imaging |
| Fluorodeoxyglucose (F-18 FDG) | Glucose metabolism | Tumor imaging |

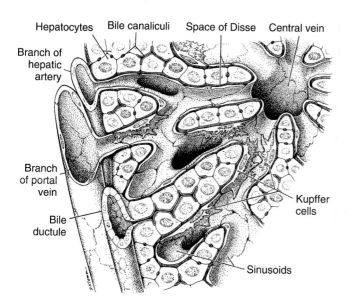

Hepatocytes  Bile canaliculi  Space of Disse  Central vein

Branch of hepatic artery

Branch of portal vein

Bile ductule

Kupffer cells

Sinusoids

**Fig. 10-1**    Anatomy of a liver lobule. Plates of hepatic cells (hepatocytes and Kupffer cells) are distributed radially around the central vein. Branches of the portal vein and hepatic artery located at the periphey of the lobule deliver blood to the sinusoids. Blood leaves through the central vein (proximal branch of hepatic veins). Peripherally located bile ducts drain bile canaliculi that course between hepatocytes.

cavernous hemangiomas of the liver, with high accuracy and rare false positives. Other nuclear medicine liver-imaging modalities with different physiological mechanisms of uptake and distribution make it possible to evaluate various aspects of hepatic physiology and function (Fig. 10-1). These include the use of Tc-99m macroaggregated albumin (MAA) for intraarterial chemotherapy, Tc-99m sulfur colloid for liver-spleen imaging, and xenon-133 for fatty tumor imaging.

## CHOLESCINTIGRAPHY

Cholescintigraphy now has a well-developed methodology with accepted clinical indications, provid-

**Box 10-1    Clinical Indications for Cholescintigraphy**

Acute cholecystitis
Acalculous cholecystitis: acute and chronic
Common duct obstruction
Postcholecystectomy syndrome
  Cystic duct remnant
  Recurrent or retained common duct stone
  Sphincter of Oddi dysfunction
Postoperative leaks
Biliary diversion procedures
Biliary stent follow-up
Focal nodular hyperplasia
Hepatocellular carcinoma
Sclerosing cholangitis
Enterogastric bile reflux

ing unique insight into liver function, patency of the biliary tract, and postoperative hepatobiliary complications.

### Radiopharmaceuticals

Iodine-131-labeled rose bengal, introduced in 1955, was for 20 years the only available liver radiopharmaceutical that was extracted and cleared by hepatocytes. However, its poor imaging characteristics and high radiation dosimetry limited its clinical use. I-123 rose bengal was superior in both regards but never gained widespread use because of its limited availability and the introduction of Tc-99m-labeled hepatobiliary imaging radiopharmaceuticals in the mid-1970s. The Tc-99m IDAs have become important in the diagnosis of various hepatobiliary disorders (Box 10-1). Cholescintigraphy (Tc-99m IDA) is the most frequently performed liver study in nuclear medicine.

## Chemistry

The technetium-labeled IDA radiopharmaceuticals were originally synthesized to develop a heart-imaging agent, based on the structural similarities between IDA and lidocaine molecules (Fig. 10-2). The high liver extraction of one early IDA compound (dimethyl IDA) prompted the acronym *HIDA,* for hepatobiliary IDA. Tc-99m HIDA cleared from blood more rapidly than radioiodinated rose bengal, but with a similar hepatobiliary clearance rate.

A variety of analogs were then developed with different chemical substitutions around the aromatic ring. The newer analogs offered improvements in hepatocellular uptake and more rapid blood clearance. These IDA analogs are known by many acronyms (e.g., BIDA, DIDA, EIDA, PIPIDA). The U.S. Food and Drug Administration (FDA) has approved three: Tc-99m lidofenin (HIDA), Tc-99m disofenin (DISIDA; Hepatolite, DuPont-Merck Pharmaceuticals, Billerica, Mass.), and Tc-99m mebrofenin (BrIDA; Choletec, E.R. Squibb & Sons, New Brunswick, N.J.). Only the latter two are in clinical use in the United States.

The IDA radiopharmaceuticals are organic anions that act as bifunctional chelates. The iminodiacetate ($NCH_2$ COO) attaches at one end to the radioactivity (Tc-99m) and at the other end to an acetanilide analog of lidocaine, which carries the biological function. Relatively minor structural changes in the phenyl ring (N substitutions) result in significant alterations in the IDA pharmacokinetics (Table 10-2).

The final Tc-99m IDA complex exists as a dimer, with two molecules of the chelating agent (IDA) reacting with one atom of Tc-99m. This dimeric configuration, with Tc-99m serving as a bridging atom between the two ligand molecules, confers stability to the technetium complex and determines hepatobiliary excretion.

## Preparation

The Tc-99m IDA radiopharmaceuticals are available as kits that contain the IDA analog and stannous chloride in lyophilized form. The Tc-99m–IDA complex is formed by the simple addition of pertechnetate to the vial. The product is stable for at least 6 hours after reconstitution.

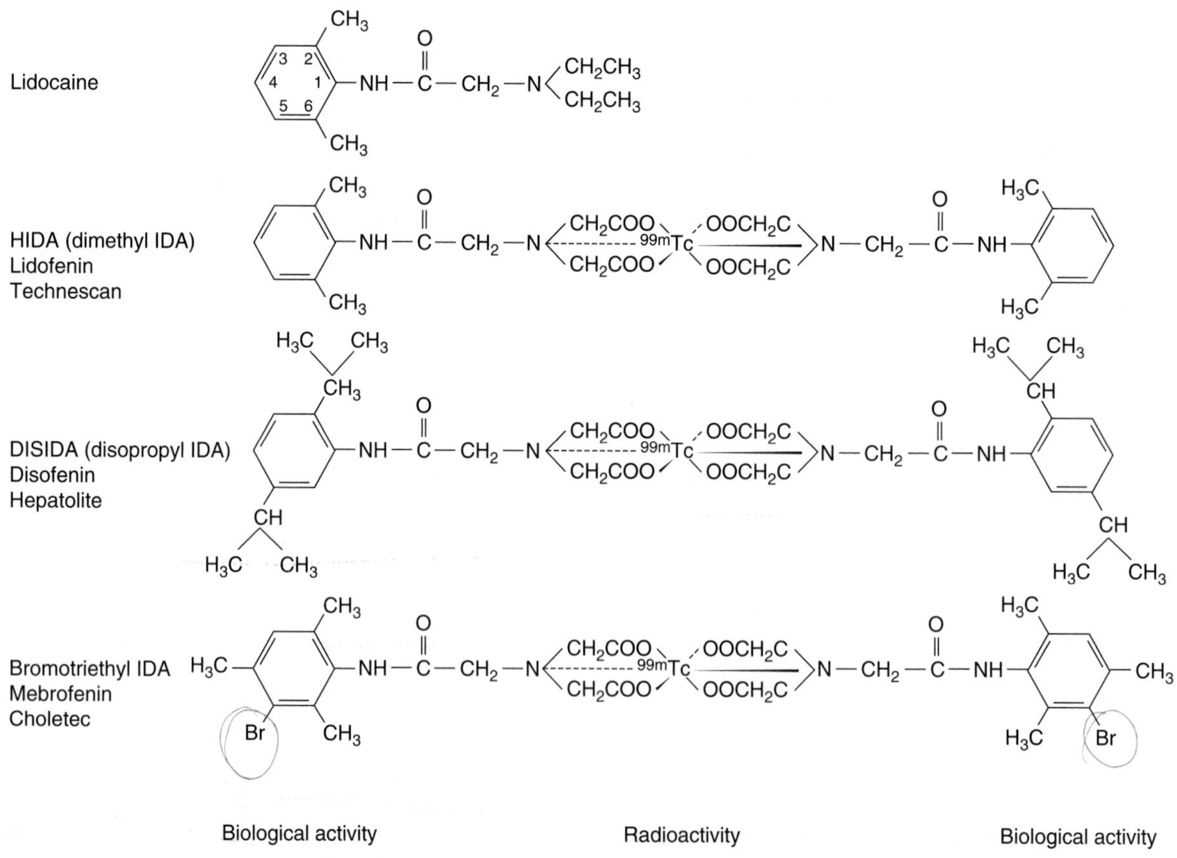

**Fig. 10-2** Chemical structure of hepatobiliary iminodiacetic acid analog (HIDA) radiopharmaceuticals. Note similarity of technetium-99m iminoacetic acid analogs (Tc-99m IDAs) to lidocaine. Radioactivity is located centrally (Tc-99m), bridging two ligand molecules. Iminodiacetate ($NCH_2COO$) attaches to Tc-99m, and the acetanilide analog (IDA) of lidocaine at the periphery carries the biological activity. Substitutions on aromatic rings differentiate the various Tc-99m IDAs and determine their pharmacokinetics.

## Mechanism of Uptake and Clearance

Tc-99m IDA radiopharmaceuticals have the same hepatocyte uptake, transport, and excretion pathways as bilirubin (Fig. 10-3). After intravenous (IV) injection, Tc-99m IDA is tightly bound to protein in the blood, minimizing renal clearance. The radiotracer is transported into the hepatocyte by a high-capacity, carrier-mediated, anionic clearance mechanism. After hepatocellular uptake, the tracer is transported into the bile canaliculi by an active membrane transport system. Tc-99m IDA compounds are stable in vivo and, in contrast to bilirubin, are excreted in their original radiochemical form without being conjugated or undergoing significant metabolism. Because they travel the same pathway as bilirubin, however, these compounds are subject to competitive inhibition by high levels of serum bilirubin.

## Pharmacokinetics

Once Tc-99m IDA reaches the bile canaliculi, the radiopharmaceutical follows the flow of bilirubin into the gallbladder via the cystic duct and into the duodenum via the common duct (Fig. 10-3). The relative flow into each is determined by the patency of the bile ducts, sphincter of Oddi tone, and intraluminal pressures. Bile is concentrated in the gallbladder and stored for later discharge into the intestines. The gallbladder contracts and empties in response to cholecystokinin (CCK), endogenously produced and secreted by the duodenal mucosa in response to fat in an ingested meal. Simultaneously, CCK relaxes the sphincter of Oddi, allowing bile to pass into the small intestine.

Although bilirubin levels greater than 5 mg/dl result in poor image quality with Tc-99m lidofenin (HIDA), Tc-99m disofenin (Hepatolite) and Tc-99m mebrofenin (Choletec) can be effectively used with serum bilirubin levels as high as 20 to 30 mg/dl because of their higher extraction efficiency (Table 9-2). Mebrofenin has an advantage over disofenin at very high serum bilirubin levels because of its greater resistance to displacement by bilirubin and higher hepatic uptake. Renal excretion serves as the alternative route of clearance for all IDA radiopharmaceuticals. Poor hepatic function results in increased renal excretion.

## Dosimetry

Both Tc-99m disofenin and Tc-99m mebrofenin have similar dosimetry. The highest estimated radiation dose (target organ) is to the large bowel, about 2 rads (Table 10-3). The radiation dose to the gallbladder depends on whether the gallbladder fills, its ability to contract, and the length of time after the study before it is stimulated to contract.

## Patient History

The patient's clinical history should be reviewed carefully before beginning cholescintigraphy. The fol-

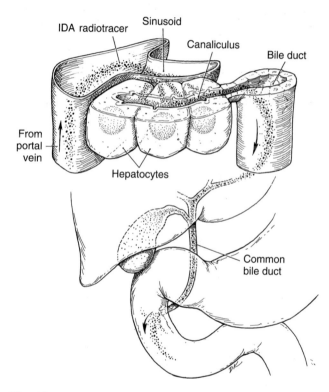

**Fig. 10-3**  Physiology and pharmacokinetics of Tc-99m iminodiacetic acid analog. Hepatic uptake and clearance of Tc-99m IDA are similar to bilirubin except that IDAs are not conjugated or metabolized. Bilirubin is transported in the blood bound to albumin, extracted by the hepatocyte, secreted into the bile canaliculi, and cleared through the biliary tract into the bowel.

**Table 10-2**  Normal pharmacokinetics of technetium-99m iminodiacetic acid analogs (IDAs)

| Agent | Hepatic uptake (%) | Clearance half-life (min) | Renal excretion (2-hr) (%) |
|---|---|---|---|
| Tc-99m lidofenin (HIDA) | 84 | 42 | >14 |
| Tc-99m disofenin (DISIDA) | 88 | 19 | <9 |
| Tc-99m mebrofenin (BrIDA) | 98 | 17 | <1 |

| | Disofenin (Hepatolite) | Mebrofenin (Choletec) |
|---|---|---|
| **Table 10-3** | **Dosimetry for technetium-99m IDA radiopharmaceuticals** | |
| Organ | Rads/5 mCi (cGy/185 MBq) | |
| Liver | 0.19 | 0.24 |
| Gallbladder | 0.60 | 0.69 |
| Large intestine | 1.90 | 2.37 |
| Urinary bladder | 0.46 | 0.14 |
| Ovaries | 0.41 | 0.51 |
| Testes | 0.03 | 0.03 |
| Marrow | 0.14 | 0.17 |
| Total body | 0.08 | 0.10 |

lowing questions help determine proper protocol and interpretation of a Tc-99m IDA study:

What is the clinical question being asked by the referring physician?

Are the symptoms acute or chronic?

When and what did the patient last eat?

Has the patient received any drugs (e.g., morphine, Demerol) that could affect normal biliary physiology and interpretation of results?

Has ultrasonography or other imaging been performed? What did it show?

Has the patient had biliary surgery? With a biliary diversion procedure, what is the anatomy? Are there any intraabdominal tubes or drains? If so, where are they placed, and which tubing drains each? Are they open or clamped?

## Methodology

Box 10-2 summarizes a typical protocol for cholescintigraphy. Specifics of the protocol will vary depending on the clinical situation (see Clinical Applications).

## Image Interpretation

Cholescintigraphy allows visualization of blood flow to the liver, hepatic extraction, biliary excretion, patency of the biliary tract, and gallbladder function (Fig. 10-4).

**Blood flow** The liver does not normally visualize during the arterial blood flow phase because its blood supply is predominantly portal in origin (75% portal vein and 25% hepatic artery). The liver is seen 6 to 8 seconds after the spleen and kidneys (Fig. 10-4, *A*). Early, diffusely increased blood flow may be seen if the liver is arterialized (e.g., cirrhosis, generalized tumor involvement, focal tumor mass or abscess) or in the gallbladder fossa region because of the inflammation of acute cholecystitis.

## Box 10-2   Cholescintigraphy: Protocol Summary

**PATIENT PREPARATION**

1. Nothing by mouth (NPO) for 4 hr before study.
2. If fasting longer than 24 hr: infuse sincalide, 0.02 µg/kg, in 30 ml of normal saline over 30 min using constant infusion pump.

**RADIOPHARMACEUTICAL**

Tc-99m mebrofenin or Tc-99m disofenin, intravenous injection:

Adults: bilirubin  <2 mg/dl    5.0 mCi (185 MBq)
                    2 mg/dl    7.5 mCi (278 MBq)
                   10 mg/dl   10.0 mCi (370 MBq)
Children: 200 µCi/kg (no less than 1 mCi or 35 MBq)

**INSTRUMENTATION**

Camera: large-field-of-view gamma camera
Collimator: low energy, all purpose, parallel hole
Window: 15% over 140-keV photopeak
Computer acquisition: 1-sec frames for 60 sec, then 1-min frames for 60 min
Static film images: 500k to 1000k count immediate anterior image, then images for equal time every 2 to 5 min for 60 min

**PATIENT POSITIONING**

Supine; upper abdomen in field of view.

**IMAGING PROTOCOL**

1. Inject Tc-99m IDA IV as a bolus and start computer.
2. If acute cholecystitis is suspected and there is biliary-to-bowel transit but gallbladder has not filled by 60 min, inject morphine sulfate (MS) intravenously, 0.04 mg/kg over 1 min. Occasionally, Tc-99m IDA reinjection is necessary if liver activity has been washed out.
3. At end of routine study (at 60 min or 30 min after MS), acquire images in right lateral and left anterior oblique views.
4. Perform delayed imaging at 2 to 4 hr *if:*
   a. MS is not administered and gallbladder has not filled. Shielding of bowel activity and a longer acquisition time may be necessary to visualize gallbladder fossa if most tracer has cleared from liver.
   b. Other clinical indications exist (e.g., hepatic insufficiency, partial common duct obstruction, suspected biliary leak).

**CHOLECYSTOKININ (CCK) ADMINISTRATION**

1. Set up computer for 30 1-min frames.
2. Start the computer 1 min before injection.
3. Infuse 0.02 µg/kg of sincalide over 30 min.
4. Calculate percentage of gallbladder emptying (maximum counts minus minimum counts divided by maximum counts, all corrected for background).

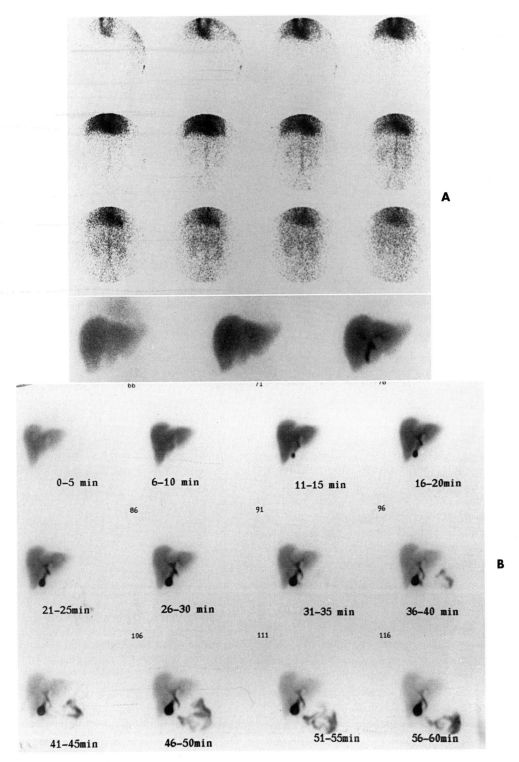

**Fig. 10-4**    Normal technetium-99m IDA studies. **A,** *Top three rows,* Two-second blood flow images. Visualization of the liver is delayed compared with the spleen and kidneys because of the liver's predominantly portal blood flow. *Bottom,* Heart blood pool seen on immediate image clears over next two frames at 5 and 10 minutes, consistent with good hepatic function. **B,** Images acquired every 5 minutes for 60 minutes in another patient. Right, left, and common hepatic ducts are seen by 15 to 20 minutes and common bile duct by 30 minutes; biliary-to-bowel clearance is noted at 36 minutes. Gallbladder is visualized early.

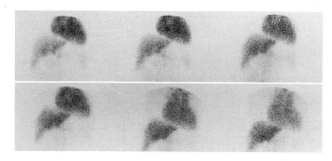

**Fig. 10-5** Hepatic insufficiency. Sequential 5-minute images, with very slow heart blood pool clearance caused by hepatic dysfunction. Biliary ducts are not visualized because of slow hepatic clearance. Biliary-to-bowel clearance was seen on 6-hour images.

---

**Box 10-3 Normal Percentage of Visualization 60 Minutes After Tc-99m IDA Injection**

Common bile duct: 100%
Gallbladder: 100%
Intestine: 80% (no visualization: 20%)

---

**Liver morphology** During the early hepatic phase, before biliary clearance, an assessment can be made of liver size and shape and the presence or absence of intrahepatic lesions.

**Hepatic function** Liver function can be evaluated by comparing the high-count image obtained immediately after the flow phase with the 5- and 10-minute images. The immediate image is that of blood pool distribution before significant Tc-99m IDA extraction has occurred. By 5 minutes, most of the blood pool, best seen in the heart, normally clears because of its rapid hepatic extraction (Fig. 10-4, *A*). Delayed blood pool clearance is a sign of hepatic insufficiency (Fig. 10-5). The kidneys act as an alternative route of excretion. A small amount of renal clearance may normally be seen. Increased amounts of renal clearance occur with poor liver function.

**Biliary clearance** With good hepatic function, biliary excretion usually begins by 10 minutes after injection. The smaller peripheral biliary structures typically cannot be visualized unless enlarged. The left and right hepatic bile ducts, common hepatic duct, and common bile duct are usually seen, particularly with frequent image acquisition and computer cinematic display (Fig. 10-4, *B*). The left hepatic ducts are often more prominent. Although evidence of dilation can be seen on cholescintigraphy, the study cannot accurately determine duct size. On the other hand, it can determine the functional patency of normal-sized or enlarged biliary ducts.

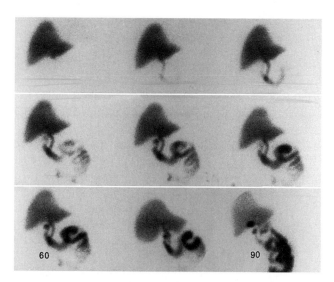

**Fig. 10-6** Delayed gallbladder visualization in patient with chronic cholecystitis. At 60 minutes the gallbladder is not adequately visualized. Focal activity is just lateral to the proximal common duct. Next image in the left anterior oblique view confirms that the focal activity is caused by duodenal clearance. Gallbladder visualization occurs at 90 minutes.

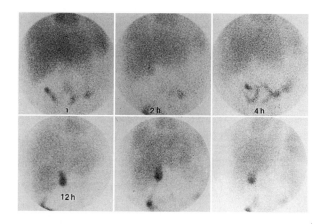

**Fig. 10-7** Delayed gallbladder visualization in patient with severe hepatic insufficiency. Very slow blood pool clearance and poor target-to-background resolution result from liver dysfunction. Gallbladder is not visualized until 12 hours. Last two images are right and left anterior oblique views.

Approximately two thirds of biliary flow travels through the common duct and the sphincter of Oddi into the second portion of the duodenum. The remaining third enters the gallbladder through the cystic duct. The normal gallbladder usually fills by 30 minutes, although visualization by 60 minutes is defined as normal (Box 10-3). Delayed gallbladder visualization (up to 4 hours) is seen most often in patients with chronic cholecystitis, probably from partial cystic duct obstruction (Fig. 10-6), and also occurs in patients with hepatic insufficiency because of delayed uptake and clearance (Fig. 10-7).

Biliary-to-bowel transit also normally occurs by 60 minutes. However, up to 20% of normal subjects have

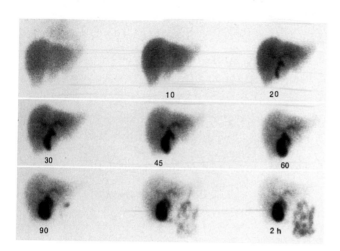

**Fig. 10-8** Delayed biliary-to-bowel clearance. Gallbladder begins to fill by 30 minutes, common duct is defined at 60 minutes, but no biliary-to-bowel clearance is seen. Delayed images show clearance into the bowel starting at 90 minutes and decreased activity in the common duct by 2 hours. This pattern is seen in patients with chronic cholecystitis and those pretreated with cholecystokinin.

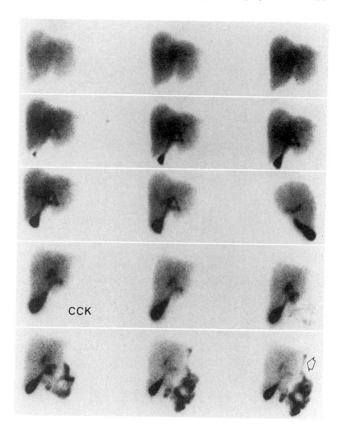

**Fig. 10-9** Delayed biliary-to-bowel transit. *Top three rows,* Sequential images acquired over 60 minutes. Gallbladder begins to fill early. Biliary ducts are visualized, but no biliary-to-bowel clearance is seen at 60 minutes. *Lower two rows,* Cholecystokinin *(CCK)* is infused over 30 minutes. Gallbladder contracts (ejection fraction, 51%), and biliary-to-bowel transit results from concomitant relaxation of sphincter of Oddi. *Arrowhead,* Mild gastric reflux. Study is normal because of functional hypertonic sphincter of Oddi.

common duct visualization but delayed (up to 4 hours) biliary-to-bowel transit because of a functional "hypertonic" sphincter of Oddi (Fig. 10-8). Although delayed imaging can confirm common duct patency, administration of CCK more promptly differentiates this normal variation from partial common duct obstruction (Fig. 10-9).

## Cholecystokinin

**Physiology and pharmacokinetics** CCK is a 33–amino acid polypeptide, with the C-terminal octapeptide as the physiologically active portion. CCK has numerous gastrointestinal effects in addition to stimulating contraction of the gallbladder and relaxation of the sphincter of Oddi (Box 10-4). The timely coordination and release of bile into the bowel are necessary for normal fat absorption.

After ingestion of a fatty meal, CCK is endogenously secreted from the duodenal and proximal jejunal mucosa. The serum CCK level rises rapidly and peaks at about 20 minutes (Fig. 10-10). Gallbladder contraction is threshold dependent and commences once the serum CCK increases above that threshold, a serum level considerably lower than the peak level. The gallbladder remains contracted until the production of CCK declines and the serum level falls below the contraction threshold. This may require several hours until the meal has passed through the stomach and proximal small bowel, with the exact time depending on meal size and content and the rate of gastric emptying.

---

**Box 10-4  Gastrointestinal Actions of Cholecystokinin**

Promotes gallbladder contraction
Relaxes sphincter of Oddi
Stimulates intestinal motility
Inhibits gastric emptying
Reduces gastrointestinal sphincter tone
Stimulates hepatic bile secretion
Stimulates pancreatic enzyme secretion

---

Simultaneous with gallbladder contraction, CCK relaxes the sphincter of Oddi, allowing bile to pass through the common duct and into the small bowel (Box 10-4). Gallbladder tone and function are modulated by numerous endogenous hormones (e.g., gastrin, secretin, motilin) as well as vagal-sympathetic neural interactions.

**Sincalide** Sincalide (Kinevac; Squibb & Sons) is a synthetic C-terminal octapeptide of CCK and the only

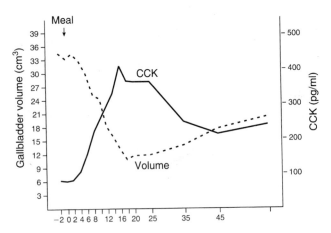

**Fig. 10-10** Physiology of gallbladder contraction. After ingestion of a fatty meal, serum cholecystokinin *(CCK)* rises to a peak at 15 to 20 minutes; time is variable depending on the type of meal and rate of gastric emptying. Gallbladder contraction is threshold dependent and considerably lower than peak CCK serum concentration. Peak gallbladder contraction occurs at peak CCK concentration. CCK continues to be released by the duodenum until food empties from the stomach and proximal bowel. Gallbladder remains contracted until serum CCK falls below contraction threshold.

---

**Box 10-5  Indications for Use of Cholecystokinin**

**BEFORE HIDA STUDY**

Empty gallbladder in patient fasting longer than 24 hr.
Diagnose sphincter of Oddi dysfunction.

**AFTER HIDA STUDY**

Differentiate common duct obstruction from normal variation.
Exclude acute acalculous cholecystitis if gallbladder fills.
Diagnose chronic acalculous cholecystitis.
Confirm or exclude chronic calculous cholecystitis.

*HIDA,* Hepatobiliary iminodiacetic acid analog for cholescintigraphy.

---

**Box 10-6  Advantages of Longer Sincalide Infusion**

More physiological
No side effects
Better emptying
Lower false positive rate

---

form commercially available in the United States. The recommended IV dose is 0.02 µg/kg. The degree of gallbladder contraction depends on three factors: the total dose, dose rate, and length of infusion.

**Clinical indications**  The indications for CCK infusion are discussed under the appropriate clinical application (Box 10-5).

Fatty meal ingestion and CCK have both been used for many years for evaluation of gallbladder function, originally with oral cholecystography and now with cholescintigraphy. Although a fatty meal might seem more physiological, this approach has disadvantages. Meal ingestion to gallbladder contraction requires more time than with CCK infusion and depends on the rate of gastric emptying, which can vary greatly among patients. CCK is quicker, permits better standardization, and is more reproducible. CCK has also been used with ultrasonography for gallbladder evaluation. Cholescintigraphy is simple to perform, is not operator dependent, and is more accurate.

**Methodology**  Bolus infusions of CCK may cause spasm of the gallbladder neck and result in ineffective contraction. Thus the sincalide package insert recommends infusion of 0.02 µg/kg over 30 to 60 seconds. In one common method this dose is infused over 1 to 3 minutes. However, even this dose rate is supraphysiological for some patients and may result in ineffective contraction and a falsely low gallbladder ejection fraction.

Best results are obtained if sincalide, 0.02 µg/kg, is infused over 30 to 60 minutes (Box 10-6); a 30-minute

protocol is recommended (Box 10-2). The slow infusion results in more complete emptying and fewer false positives (poor contraction of a normal gallbladder), without the adverse side effects from the 1- to 3-minute infusion (e.g., 50% of patients have nausea, vomiting, or epigastric cramps).

If indicated, sincalide can be infused intravenously more than once in a patient study because of its 2½-minute half-life. For example, sincalide may be given before the study to a patient who has fasted longer than 24 hours, then again after the study to evaluate gallbladder contraction. Caution is indicated in giving CCK after the patient has received morphine sulfate because morphine's pharmacological effect may last 4 to 6 hours and counteract the effect of CCK.

The normal pharmacokinetics of Tc-99m IDA may change with the infusion of CCK, resulting in delayed biliary-to-bowel transit, that is, no clearance of radiotracer into the bowel by 60 minutes. This is an indication for delayed imaging or, preferably, repeating the CCK infusion. The sphincter should promptly relax, and biliary-to-bowel transit will follow (Fig. 10-9).

When given before cholescintigraphy, Tc-99m IDA should not be injected until 30 minutes after CCK infusion to allow time for full gallbladder relaxation.

## Clinical Applications

**Acute cholecystitis**    The most common clinical indication for Tc-99m IDA cholescintigraphy is patients with suspected acute cholecystitis.

*Pathophysiology*    Acute cholecystitis is caused by obstruction of the cystic duct. An impacted biliary stone is the most common etiology. Immediately after obstruction, a progression of histopathological inflammatory changes ensues in the gallbladder wall: edema, white blood cell infiltration, ulceration, hemorrhage, necrosis, and finally gangrene and perforation. Cholecystectomy is the standard treatment.

*Diagnosis*    Characteristic symptoms include acute colicky right upper quadrant pain, nausea, and vomiting, usually accompanied by leukocytosis. Even for patients with classic symptoms, typical physical findings, and diagnostic laboratory values, a confirmatory imaging study is usually required before surgery. Ultrasonography and cholescintigraphy are the two major diagnostic imaging modalities.

ULTRASONOGRAPHY    Ultrasonography is commonly requested for patients with suspected acute biliary or chronic symptoms. A stone impacted in the cystic duct is diagnostic of acute cholecystitis, but this finding is rare (less than 5%). Although most patients with acute cholecystitis have gallstones, this is not a specific finding. Less than half of patients presenting in the emergency room with acute symptoms who have gallstones on ultrasonography are shown to have acute cholecystitis. Thickening of the gallbladder wall and pericholecystic fluid are also nonspecific findings seen with other acute and chronic diseases. The "sonographic Murphy's sign" (localized tenderness on examination in the region of the gallbladder) is sonographic, operator dependent, and not always reliable because patients with a distended gallbladder without inflammation may have tenderness. Reports on the accuracy of this finding have varied greatly.

Sensitivity and specificity of ultrasonography for detection of cholelithiasis are greater than 90%. In general, the combination of gallstones, intramural lucency (a fairly specific indicator of inflammation), and the sonographic Murphy's sign makes the diagnosis of acute cholecystitis likely. Numerous investigators have reported high accuracy for ultrasonography. The few studies that have directly compared sonography with cholescintigraphy, however, have found cholescintigraphy to be superior (Table 10-4). Ultrasonography can detect other diseases that may be causing the patient's symptoms, such as common duct dilation, pancreatic and liver tumors, renal stones, pulmonary consolidation, and pleural effusion.

TECHNETIUM-99M IDA    Cholescintigraphy is generally considered the study of choice for confirming the diagnosis of acute cholecystitis. It defines the underlying pathophysiology, that is, obstruction of the cystic duct, as manifested by nonfilling of the gallbladder.

**Table 10-4    Accuracy of cholescintigraphy and ultrasonography for diagnosis of acute cholecystitis**

| Study | Cholescintigraphy | | Ultrasonography | |
|---|---|---|---|---|
| | Sensitivity (%) | Specificity (%) | Sensitivity (%) | Specificity (%) |
| Freitas | 100 | 96 | | |
| Szlabick | 100 | 98 | 98 | 78 |
| Weissman | 95 | 99 | | |
| Zeman | 98 | 81 | 67 | 82 |
| Mauro | 100 | 94 | | |
| Samuels | 97 | 93 | 97 | 64 |

The patient must have nothing by mouth for 3 to 4 hours before the study. A recently ingested meal will produce a contracted gallbladder that may prevent radiotracer entry. Although the half-life of CCK in serum is short (2½ minutes), a meal continuously stimulates release of endogenous CCK until the food has emptied from the stomach and proximal small bowel. A false positive study for acute cholecystitis (nonfilling gallbladder) may result.

Fasting for longer than 24 hours can also lead to a false positive study. Without any stimulus to contraction, bile in the gallbladder becomes concentrated and viscous, preventing radiotracer entry. Clear liquid or food without fat and protein is not usually an adequate stimulus for gallbladder contraction. Prolonged fasting is a common problem in hospitalized patients. CCK should be administered before the study to empty the gallbladder.

Nonfilling of the gallbladder by 60 minutes after Tc-99m IDA injection is abnormal. However, some patients who do not have acute cholecystitis will have delayed gallbladder filling (Fig. 10-6). Diagnosis of acute cholecystitis can be made only if the gallbladder has not filled by 3 to 4 hours after injection or by 30 minutes after administration of morphine (see following discussion).

One large study found that cholescintigraphy had a sensitivity of 95% and specificity of 99% for acute cholecystitis (Table 10-3). Although the test's sensitivity for acute cholecystitis is high (95% to 99%), the reported specificity has varied because of the different investigative methodologies used, with a false positive rate ranging from 0.6% to 27%. Differences in methodology involve (1) the patient population (e.g., criteria for surgical selection), (2) the time limit used for gallbladder visualization (1 hour versus 2 to 4 hours), (3) the requirement or lack of requirement for the fasting state, and (4) the surgical and pathological criteria selected for the confirmation of acute cholecystitis. All four factors have a significant impact on the sensitivity and specificity reported. Proper methodology should eliminate factors 2 and 3. Factor 4 relates to the gold standard used to diagnose acute cholecystitis. False positive rates are often inflated because of failure to recognize the fibrotic reparative process that can limit edema and transmural leukocytic infiltration; that is, edema and leukocyte infiltration should be the standard. False positive rates fall greatly when these factors are considered, and specificity increases to approximately 95%.

Although false positives are inevitable, most can be avoided or at least anticipated (Box 10-7). The most common cause for a false positive study is chronic cholecystitis. Less than 1% of patients with chronic cholecystitis have a totally obstructed cystic duct, and another 5% have delayed gallbladder visualization because of a partial cystic duct obstruction secondary to recurrent inflammation and cellular debris. If CCK is administered before the HIDA study, patients who would otherwise have delayed gallbladder visualization will have a filled gallbladder within the first hour (Box 10-5). This has not been routinely done, however, because it would (1) require administering CCK to all patients and (2) prevent differentiation of patients without gallbladder disease from those with chronic cholecystitis. A preferable method is to obtain delayed images for up to 4 hours.

MORPHINE AUGMENTATION   The 3- to 4-hour delay required to diagnose acute cholecystitis when the gallbladder does not visualize in the first hour is not desirable for an acutely ill patient, who may need prompt surgical intervention. As an alternative to delayed imaging, morphine sulfate is now often routinely used to shorten the duration of cholescintigraphy.

Morphine sulfate increases intraluminal pressure by constricting the sphincter of Oddi, thus producing a 10-fold increase in resting common bile duct pressure. This results in preferential bile flow to and through the cystic duct, if it is patent. The dose of morphine required to constrict the sphincter of Oddi is less than that required for pain relief. Morphine (0.04 mg/kg, approximately 2 mg) is infused intravenously if the gallbladder has not filled by 60 minutes. With cystic duct patency

the gallbladder fills promptly, and the study is complete by 30 minutes after morphine injection. Thus the entire Tc-99m IDA study requires 90 minutes (Fig. 10-11).

Morphine should not be administered if common bile duct obstruction is suspected (e.g., prominent common duct, retention of activity in common duct, lack of biliary-to-bowel transit). Morphine produces a functional partial common duct obstruction, and thus a pathological obstruction cannot be differentiated from

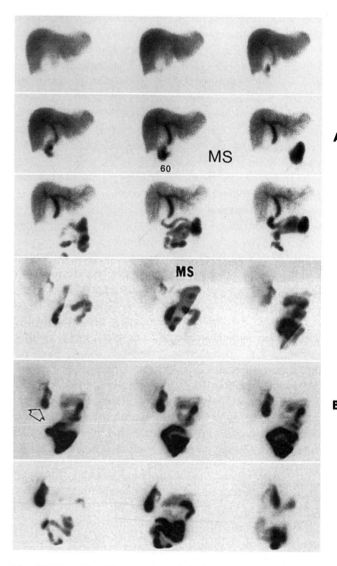

**Fig. 10-11**   Morphine-augmented cholescintigraphy. **A,** Patient with clinically suspected acute cholecystitis. Technetium-99m iminoacetic acid analog (Tc-99m IDA) images for 60 minutes show good visualization of common hepatic and common bile ducts, biliary clearance into the duodenum, but no gallbladder visualization. Morphine sulfate *(MS)* is given. Gallbladder is not visualized, confirming diagnosis of acute cholecystitis by 90 minutes. **B,** Another patient shows no gallbladder filling at 60 minutes *(upper left),* so MS is given. Gallbladder filling begins within 5 minutes and is definite by 10 minutes *(arrowhead).* Acute cholecystitis is ruled out.

---

**Box 10-7   Causes of False Positive Cholescintigraphy for Acute Cholecystitis**

Fasting <4 hr
Fasting >24 hr
Concurrent severe illness
Chronic cholecystitis
Hepatic insufficiency
Hyperalimentation
Alcoholism (?)
Pancreatitis (?)

morphine's physiological effect. These patients should have delayed imaging rather than morphine. Morphine-augmented cholescintigraphy for the diagnosis of acute cholecystitis has a proven high accuracy (Table 10-5), at least similar to the results reported with delayed imaging (Table 10-3).

FALSE POSITIVE STUDIES   Patients who have been fasting for more than 24 hours may have a false positive study because the lack of stimulus to contraction allows the gallbladder to fill with concentrated viscous bile, preventing radiotracer entry. Administration of CCK before the study to empty the gallbladder reduces false positive results. CCK is effective only if the gallbladder is capable of contracting. Patients with symptomatic chronic cholecystitis may have a nonfunctioning gallbladder, and CCK may not produce the desired result, with some false positives.

False positive studies also may occur in hospitalized patients who have concurrent serious illness. These patients often have had nothing by mouth for days and may be receiving hyperalimentation. Patients with hepatic insufficiency have altered uptake and clearance of Tc-99m IDA, which can delay or prevent visualization of the gallbladder (Fig. 10-7). Pancreatitis and alcoholism may be associated with an increased incidence of false positive studies.

RIM SIGN   Increased hepatic uptake in the region of the gallbladder fossa is seen in about 25% of patients with acute cholecystitis (Fig. 10-12). This finding identifies patients who are at a later stage of acute cholecystitis, such as with hemorrhage and necrosis of the gallbladder wall. These patients are at increased risk for complications of gallbladder perforation and gangrene. Although cited as a specific finding for acute cholecystitis, the rim sign is seen in some patients with chronic cholecystitis.

The pathophysiological mechanism producing the rim sign is probably twofold. First, blood flow increases to the inflamed liver adjacent to the gallbladder, and the inflammatory process in the gallbladder wall can spread to the adjacent normal liver. The increased blood flow and the high liver extraction efficiency of the radiopharmaceutical result in increased uptake. Second, regional clearance may be delayed because of the edema and inflammation of biliary canaliculi.

IMAGE INTERPRETATION   Differentiating gallbladder filling from radiotracer in the adjacent or overlapping common duct and duodenum may be problematic. Right lateral and left anterior oblique (LAO) views after 60 minutes can confirm or rule out gallbladder filling (Fig. 10-13). In

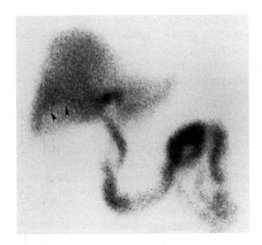

**Fig. 10-12**   Rim sign. Increased uptake is seen in the liver in area of the gallbladder fossa. Normal biliary-to-bowel transit, but no gallbladder visualization on 60-minute image.

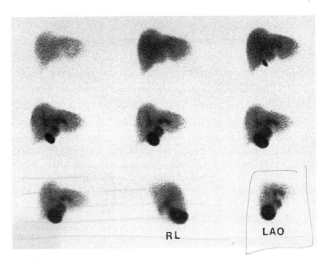

**Fig. 10-13**   Differentiating gallbladder from common duct and duodenum. In this study, separating the gallbladder from the common bile duct and duodenum is a problem *(middle row)*. Right lateral *(RL)* view confirms gallbladder filling since it is anterior. Left anterior oblique *(LAO)* view demonstrates the common bile duct, but no biliary-to-bowel clearance has occurred and therefore no duodenal activity. In the LAO view the gallbladder moves to the right (anteriorly), and the common bile duct and duodenum move to the left (posteriorly).

| Table 10-5 | Accuracy of morphine-augmented cholescintigraphy | |
| --- | --- | --- |
| **Study** | **Sensitivity (%)** | **Specificity (%)** |
| Choy | 96 | 100 |
| Kim | 100 | 100 |
| Keslar | 100 | 83 |
| Vasquez | 100 | 85 |
| Fig | 94 | 69* |
| Flanebaum | 97 | 95 |
| Fink-Bennett | 95 | 96 |
| Kistler | 93 | 78* |

*High percentage of patients with concurrent illness.

the right lateral projection the gallbladder is usually seen anteriorly. In the LAO projection the gallbladder (anterior structure) moves to the patient's right, and the common duct and duodenum (more posterior structures) move to the left. Upright imaging or ingestion of water may help to clear duodenal activity. Morphine sulfate also may assist, since contraction of the sphincter of Oddi prevents further biliary-to-bowel clearance while duodenal activity moves distally (Fig. 10-11, *A*).

*Acute acalculous cholecystitis* Acute acalculous cholecystitis is a life-threatening disease that typically occurs in hospitalized patients (Box 10-8). Acalculous acute cholecystitis is often caused by cystic duct obstruction secondary to inflammatory debris and inspissated bile. At other times, however, direct infection or ischemia of the gallbladder wall may occur without cystic duct obstruction. Because of high mortality (30%) and morbidity (55%), early diagnosis is imperative. Since the cystic duct may not be obstructed, false negative cholescintigraphy (i.e., gallbladder filling) has been a concern. One study did report a 68% sensitivity, but ultrasonography had a similarly low sensitivity. Subsequent investigations reported greater than 90% sensitivity for cholescintigraphy, only slightly less than for acute calculous cholecystitis (Table 10-6).

If a false negative study is suspected, CCK may be helpful (Box 10-5). An acutely inflamed gallbladder will not contract normally, and normal contraction rules out the disease. Poor contraction is consistent with suspected acute acalculous cholecystitis but is not specific; this finding cannot differentiate acute from chronic cholecystitis. An indium-111 oxine leukocyte study can confirm the diagnosis.

**Chronic cholecystitis** Patients with chronic cholecystitis typically are middle-aged obese women with symptoms of recurrent right upper quadrant pain. Gallstones are usually present, and the gallbladder wall is infiltrated with lymphocytes and is fibrosed. The clinical

diagnosis is usually confirmed by detecting gallstones on ultrasonography or another modality. Routine cholescintigraphy is usually normal. A few patients show abnormalities, such as common duct obstruction (1%), gallbladder filling defects (uncommon), delayed gallbladder filling (less than 5%) (Fig. 10-6), and delayed biliary-to-bowel transit (nonspecific) (Fig. 10-9).

Symptomatic chronic cholecystitis is usually associated with poor gallbladder contraction, as demonstrated by a decreased ejection fraction when stimulated with a fatty meal or CCK. Cholescintigraphy with CCK may differentiate patients with symptomatic cholelithiasis from those with incidental gallstones and chronic abdominal pain from other causes. The primary role of CCK cholescintigraphy in chronic cholecystitis, however, is to confirm the clinically suspected diagnosis of the acalculous form.

*Chronic acalculous cholecystitis* Over the years, chronic cholecystitis without stones has been described by various names (Box 10-9). It occurs in only 5% of patients with symptomatic chronic cholecystitis and otherwise is clinically and pathologically identical to the calculous form.

In the past the diagnosis could not be confirmed preoperatively despite extensive medical workups. Gall-

**Table 10-6  Sensitivity of cholescintigraphy for acute acalculous cholecystitis**

| Study | Patients (no.) | Sensitivity (%) |
|---|---|---|
| Shuman | 19 | 68 |
| Weissman | 15 | 93 |
| Mirvis | 19 | 95 |
| Swayne | 49 | 93 |
| Frazee | 10 | 100 |
| Ramanna | 11 | 100 |

**Box 10-8  Clinical Conditions Associated with Acute Acalculous Cholecystitis**

Surgery
Trauma
Burns
Shock and ischemia
Narcotics
Parenteral nutrition
Acquired immunodeficiency syndrome
Mechanical ventilation
Multiple transfusion
Vasculitis

**Box 10-9  Terminology for Recurrent Pain Syndromes of Biliary Origin**

**CHRONIC ACALCULOUS CHOLECYSTITIS**

Acalculous biliary disease
Gallbladder spasm
Cystic duct syndrome

**SPHINCTER OF ODDI DYSFUNCTION**

Papillary stenosis
Biliary spasm
Biliary dyskinesia

stones are the imaging requisite for chronic cholecystitis. Surgeons are reluctant to perform surgery without objective evidence of cholecystitis, since other nonsurgical diseases can have similar symptoms (e.g., irritable bowel syndrome).

Patients with chronic cholecystitis have poor gallbladder contraction. Past studies with CCK or fatty meal cholecystograms demonstrated this, but the data were inconsistent. With the introduction of the Tc-99m IDA radiopharmaceuticals, many investigations have proved that CCK cholescintigraphy can confirm the diagnosis of chronic acalculous cholecystitis. A low gallbladder ejection fraction (less than 35%) after sincalide infusion can preoperatively predict symptomatic relief with cholecystectomy and provide histopathological evidence of chronic cholecystitis (Fig. 10-14). The positive predictive value of CCK cholescintigraphy is greater than 90%.

Poor gallbladder function is not synonymous with chronic cholecystitis. A variety of drugs and nonbiliary diseases have been associated with poor gallbladder function (Box 10-10). However, the accuracy of CCK cholescintigraphy is high when used in the proper clinical setting.

The diagnosis of chronic acalculous cholecystitis should not be made in sick or hospitalized patients; too many other causes are likely. CCK cholescintigraphy should be performed for outpatients with a history of recurrent abdominal pain who have had thorough workups to rule out other diseases and who have been followed over time. These patients have a high likelihood of chronic cholecystitis, and CCK cholescintigraphy can confirm the clinical diagnosis.

A misconception holds that reproduction of the patient's pain with CCK is diagnostic of chronic acalculous cholecystitis. The pain of patients with irritable bowel syndrome is also aggravated by CCK. Whether the patient experiences pain with infusion of CCK depends on the rate of administration, not on the presence or absence of disease. Half of patients receiving 0.02 µg/kg over 1 to 3 minutes may have abdominal cramps or nausea. Patients receiving the same dose over 30 minutes do not experience pain, whether or not they have chronic cholecystitis.

**Common duct obstruction** The terms *surgical jaundice, biliary obstruction,* and *bile duct dilation* are not synonymous. Biliary obstruction can be seen in the absence of hyperbilirubinemia or jaundice. Jaundice is usually a late manifestation of biliary obstruction. Obstruction does not always result in dilation of the bile ducts, and dilation can occur in the absence of obstruction.

*High-grade obstruction*

The sequence of pathophysiological events in high-grade obstruction progresses in a predictable manner: obstruction, increased intraductal pressure, reduced bile flow, biliary duct dilation, increased cellular permeability, and fibrogenesis leading to hepatocellular damage (biliary cirrhosis). Because these events require time, ductal dilation may not become evident until 24 to 72 hours after the initiating event, even in high-grade obstruction.

The causes for common duct obstruction include choledocholithiasis, neoplasm, and inflammatory stricture. The clinical presentation is variable, depending on

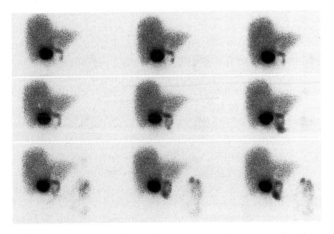

**Fig. 10-14** Chronic acalculous cholecystitis. Extremely poor contraction of the gallbladder is evident after sincalide infusion (ejection fraction, 20%). Biliary-to-bowel transit is delayed, a nonspecific finding of chronic cholecystitis.

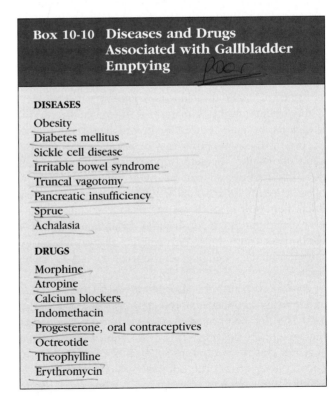

**Box 10-10 Diseases and Drugs Associated with Gallbladder Emptying**

**DISEASES**

Obesity
Diabetes mellitus
Sickle cell disease
Irritable bowel syndrome
Truncal vagotomy
Pancreatic insufficiency
Sprue
Achalasia

**DRUGS**

Morphine
Atropine
Calcium blockers
Indomethacin
Progesterone, oral contraceptives
Octreotide
Theophylline
Erythromycin

the etiology and the rapidity of onset. Abdominal pain and fever, with elevated serum bilirubin and alkaline phosphatase levels, are typical findings.

Cancerous and noncancerous causes of biliary tract obstruction produce different findings on hepatobiliary imaging. Tumors typically cause high-grade obstruction and often secondary hepatocyte dysfunction, whereas choledocholithiasis most often produces a picture of partial obstruction with little or no secondary liver dysfunction. On occasion, malignant tumors cause only partial obstruction, and choledocholithiasis can result in complete obstruction. Pancreatitis tends to cause only mild partial obstruction.

The noninvasive imaging workup of patients with suspected biliary obstruction usually starts with ultrasonography. Obstruction can be confirmed by the anatomical observation that the biliary tree is dilated. The amount of dilation varies widely and is directly related to the duration, degree, and etiology of the obstruction. Dilation is most common with long-standing obstruction, especially when secondary to malignant etiologies. Although the degree of dilation is not directly proportional to the serum bilirubin, the largest, most dilated ducts tend to occur in deeply jaundiced patients.

Patients with high-grade common duct obstruction of recent onset usually show good hepatic extraction and uptake, but no excretion of the radiolabeled bile into the biliary tree. There is a persistent hepatogram (Fig. 10-15). The high intraductal backpressure prevents excretion into the biliary ducts. This pattern is characteristic. In very high grade obstructions, imaging up to 24 hours will show no change. With less complete obstruction some slow excretion into biliary ducts may be seen on delayed imaging. More chronic obstruction will show evidence of hepatic dysfunction. Despite this classic appearance, cholescintigraphy is not usually necessary to make the clinical diagnosis.

Cholescintigraphy is necessary, however, in certain situations. In acute obstruction before ductal dilation has occurred, ultrasonography may be normal and the HIDA study shows the characteristic abnormality of common duct obstruction. In patients who have had previous obstruction or biliary tract instrumentation, the biliary ducts may remain permanently dilated. Cholescintigraphy can differentiate obstructive from nonobstructive dilation; for example, nonobstructed dilation will show normal ductal clearance and normal biliary-to-bowel transit.

*Partial obstruction*    The natural history of low-grade and intermittent obstruction (e.g., from choledocholithiasis) has not been as well documented or studied as high-grade obstruction. However, clinical experience suggests that the symptoms, clinical presentation, time course, and perhaps the outcome are different.

Without jaundice, clinical and laboratory exam-

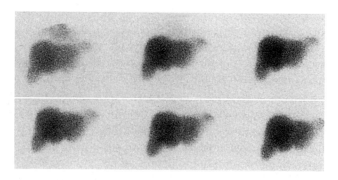

**Fig. 10-15**    High-grade common bile duct obstruction. Good hepatic uptake is seen, but no secretion into biliary ducts. High backpressure prevents tracer from entering biliary system.

inations may be unrewarding in patients with partial obstruction. Ultrasonography may also be normal. Common duct stones are infrequently seen with ultrasonography or even IV cholangiography (less than 10%). In addition, dilated ducts may not be seen in patients with low-grade or intermittent biliary obstruction. Ductal dilation can also be restricted by edema and scarring resulting from infection or cirrhosis. In these cases Tc-99m IDA studies can help determine the need for a more invasive workup, such as endoscopic retrograde cholangiopancreatography (ERCP) or percutaneous cholangiography.

Discordance between anatomical imaging with ultrasonography and functional imaging with cholescintigraphy is well documented. In one report of 125 patients with mild hyperbilirubinemia being evaluated for biliary obstruction, 23% had conflicting sonography and scintigraphy. Thirteen patients with early obstruction did not show sonographic evidence of ductal dilation, whereas cholescintigraphy demonstrated abnormal bile flow, emphasizing that functional abnormalities may precede morphologically evident disease. Seven patients showed ductal dilation on sonography but normal bile flow on cholescintigraphy. These patients had dilated ducts from prior exploration or chronic passage of stones.

Imaging findings with partial common duct obstruction are very different from those seen with high-grade common duct obstruction (Box 10-11). Delayed biliary-to-bowel transit (after 60 minutes) is the least specific finding; up to 50% of patients with partial obstruction have normal transit. On the other hand, delayed transit occurs in up to 20% of normal subjects, so biliary-to-bowel transit alone is neither sensitive nor specific (Box 10-3).

Other scintigraphic findings are more specific for the diagnosis of partial common duct obstruction (Box 10-11 and Figs. 10-16 and 10-17). Intraluminal filling defects (from stones) are usually not seen; they are most likely to be visualized as filling of the duct begins. Segmental

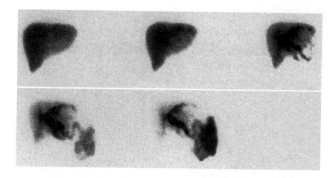

**Fig. 10-17**    Postoperative stricture causing partial common duct obstruction. Images acquired at 5, 10, 20, 40, and 60 minutes. Common hepatic and bile ducts are dilated above an abrupt distal cut-off, but biliary-to-bowel transit is normal.

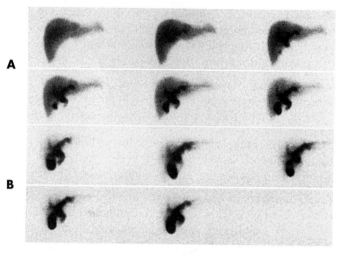

**Fig. 10-16**    Partial common duct obstruction. **A,** Common bile duct appears prominent. Retained or refluxed bile is seen in the left hepatic duct. No biliary-to-bowel transit occurs by 60 minutes. **B,** Cholecystokinin infusion with sequential images up to 30 minutes. No gallbladder contraction and minimal biliary-to-bowel transit occur. Pattern is diagnostic of partial common duct obstruction.

narrowing with proximal ductal prominence is a characteristic finding and may be an abrupt or a gradual cut-off. Delayed clearance from the common duct is noted. Retained activity in the common duct at 1 hour should suggest partial obstruction, and the lack of clearance on delayed images should raise concern.

Functional causes of delayed biliary-to-bowel transit can sometimes be differentiated from true obstruction by having the patient change position or walk around. A more rapid and reproducible method is with CCK administration. Persistent pooling in the common duct after CCK infusion is diagnostic of obstruction, whereas clearance rules out obstruction (Figs. 10-9 and 10-16). With obstruction, reflux of radiotracer may occur into the hepatic ducts after CCK because of the high backpressure.

**Choledochal cyst**    A choledochal cyst often presents clinically as obstruction, although many are asymptomatic. This is not a true cyst but rather dilation that may occur anywhere in the biliary system. Ultrasonography may show a cystic structure but often cannot ascertain whether it connects with the biliary tract. Although complete obstruction would result in nonvisualization of the biliary tract on cholescintigraphy, a partial obstruction can often be confirmed (Fig. 10-18). With partial obstruction, Tc-99m IDA tracer will fill the choledochal cyst, with prolonged retention. Delayed images are frequently helpful.

**Biliary atresia**    Cholescintigraphy has been successfully used for differentiating biliary atresia from other causes of neonatal jaundice, such as hepatitis and cholestasis. Early diagnosis of biliary atresia is critical because surgery must be performed within the first 60 days of life before irreversible liver failure ensues. The congenitally atretic bile ducts produce a picture of high-grade obstruction (Fig. 10-19).

Pretreatment with phenobarbital (5 mg/kg/day for 5 days) before Tc-99m IDA imaging maximizes sensitivity by activating the liver excretory enzymes. Serum phenobarbital should be checked before the study to ensure a therapeutic level.

The lack of biliary clearance into the bowel by 24 hours is predictive of biliary atresia. Patients with nonobstructive causes of neonatal jaundice will show biliary clearance into the bowel in that period. However, false positive studies occur. Cholescintigraphy is probably most accurate in excluding the diagnosis of biliary atresia. Severe forms of parenchymal liver disease may not demonstrate clearance into the intestines by 24 hours.

**Postoperative biliary tract**    Cholescintigraphy has also proved useful in the evaluation of postoperative patients with suspected complications of biliary tract surgery, biliary enteric anastomoses, laparoscopic cholecystectomy, or gallstone lithotripsy and in the differ-

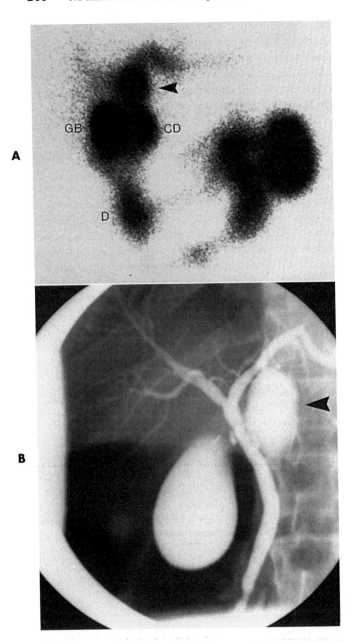

**Fig. 10-18**  Choledochal cyst in 25-year-old woman with abdominal pain. Ultrasound showed a cystic structure adjacent to the common hepatic biliary duct. A definite connection to the biliary system could not be ascertained. **A,** Technetium-99 iminoacetic acid analog (Tc-99m IDA) study shows filling of choledochal cyst in the region of the common hepatic duct *(arrowhead)*. Image acquired at 90 minutes after the liver had cleared most of the tracer. *CD,* Common duct; *GB,* gallbladder, *D,* duodenum. **B,** Cholangiogram confirmed the diagnosis.

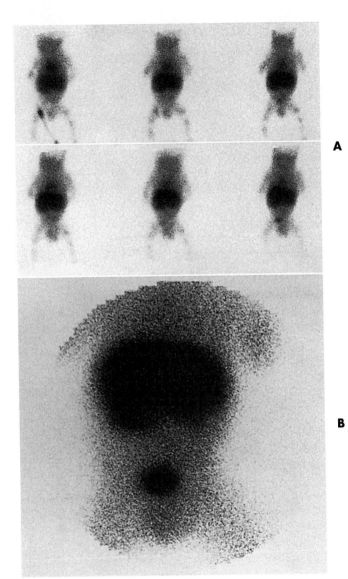

**Fig. 10-19**  Biliary atresia in 4-week-old child. Serum phenobarbital level is in the therapeutic range. **A,** Imaging every 10 minutes for first hour after injection of technetium-99m mebrofenin shows no biliary-to-bowel transit. Very delayed heart blood pool clearance results from hepatic insufficiency. **B,** Images at 24 hours show no bowel activity, only renal clearance into bladder. Surgery confirmed the diagnosis.

ential diagnosis of the postcholecystectomy syndrome. Posttherapeutic evaluation Tc-99m IDA studies are also useful for follow-up of patients treated for obstruction with papillotomy or biliary stents and can be used to confirm patency or diagnose restenosis (Fig. 10-20).

*Biliary leaks and obstruction*  The laparoscopic method has become the procedure of choice for elective cholecystectomy. However, it is associated with a signif-

icantly higher rate of bile duct injury than open cholecystectomy.

Although ultrasonography can demonstrate fluid collections, it cannot determine the etiology and source. Cholescintigraphy can determine whether a fluid collection seen on ultrasonography or CT is of biliary origin, rather than ascites or an abscess, and can determine the site and rate of leakage (Fig. 10-21). Rapid leaks may require surgery, whereas slow ones often resolve spontaneously. This information can help the surgeon decide

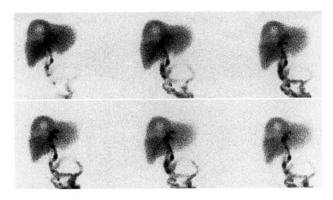

**Fig. 10-20** Patent biliary stent. Common duct stent was placed to relieve tumor obstruction. HIDA study confirms patency of stent. Note the hepatic mass in the liver dome.

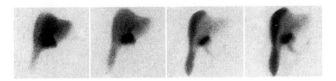

**Fig. 10-21** Postoperative biliary leak. Computed tomography scan 4 days after cholecystectomy showed intraabdominal fluid. HIDA study, ordered to determine if the fluid collection was of biliary origin, confirms the biliary leak. Sequential images are from 60 minutes (*left*) to 6 hours (*right*) after injection. Bile is localized between the liver and chest wall, over the liver dome, and in the portal area.

whether surgical intervention or conservative observation is more appropriate.

Follow-up studies can confirm resolution or persistence of the leakage. Before percutaneous drainage of a biloma, cholescintigraphy can ensure that central biliary obstruction is not present. With obstruction, it is unlikely that bile leakage can be effectively treated by percutaneous drainage without addressing the underlying cause of obstruction.

Bile leakage appears as a progressively increasing pericholecystic collection of radiotracer or as free bile in the abdomen (Fig. 10-21). Bile can accumulate perihepatically, over the dome of the liver, in the subdiaphragmatic space, or in the colonic gutters. Delayed imaging up to 24 hours may be required to detect a small or slow leak. Patient repositioning may be necessary to confirm its presence. Peritoneal tubing, drains, and drainage bags may exhibit trace accumulation and should be imaged as well.

*Biliary diversion surgery* Cholescintigraphy can be useful for the evaluation of postoperative biliary-enteric anastomoses, both for detection of early complications and for long-term follow-up. Biliary leaks can be detected, the functional patency of the anastomosis determined, and recurrent obstruction diagnosed.

Contrast cholangiography is limited in the evaluation of these patients. For example, it may not be possible to reach the biliary tract using ERCP if a long Roux-en-Y

**Box 10-12   Causes of Postcholecystectomy Pain Syndrome**

Cystic duct remnant
Retained or recurrent stone
Inflammatory stricture
Sphincter of Oddi dysfunction
Nonhepatobiliary origin

loop has been created as part of the anastomosis. Percutaneous transhepatic cholangiography is an invasive procedure with associated morbidity.

Ultrasonography has about a 67% incidence of nondiagnostic tests, often caused by gas in the anastomotic bowel segment or refluxed biliary air, a finding that does not guarantee patency of the biliary tree. Biliary dilation may be present in over 20% of patients even when obstruction has been adequately relieved by surgery. Cholescintigraphy is the only noninvasive method that can distinguish obstructed dilated ducts from those that are chronically dilated but not obstructed.

*Postcholecystectomy pain syndrome* Recurrent pain after gallbladder surgery is a clinically perplexing entity with a variety of etiologies. First, symptoms may be of a nonbiliary origin. If hepatobiliary in origin, pain may be caused by partial common duct obstruction secondary to a retained stone, postoperative stricture, or sphincter of Oddi dysfunction (Box 10-12). Occasionally a cystic duct remnant acts like a small gallbladder and becomes diseased, producing symptoms identical to those of acute or chronic cholecystitis.

Retained or recurrent common duct stones and inflammatory fibrosis are common causes of postcholecystectomy pain syndrome. The scintigraphic findings described for partial common duct obstruction apply (Box 10-11). Because the gallbladder is not present to act as an alternate reservoir for bile, duct dynamics directly predicts the adequacy of biliary drainage. With obstruction, unchanging or increasing activity, rather than normal decreasing activity, is seen within the common duct on images obtained 1 to 2 hours after injection.

SPHINCTER OF ODDI DYSFUNCTION Sphincter of Oddi dysfunction (SOD) is poorly understood and has various names (Box 10-9). It occurs in up to 14% of postcholecystectomy patients and presents as intermittent abdominal pain and transient liver function abnormalities. The obstruction may be fixed (*papillary stenosis*) or functional (*biliary dyskinesia*). These patients do not have mechanical obstruction, however, and symptoms often respond to sphincterotomy.

Exploratory laparotomy with the inability to pass a Bakes dilator greater than 3 mm in diameter was originally the surgical criterion for diagnosis. ERCP made it possible to exclude an anatomical cause of obstruction (e.g., stone, fibrosis). Delayed drainage of contrast material beyond 45 minutes is consistent with the diagnosis but not specific.

Endoscopic biliary manometry is considered the best method for the diagnosis of SOD. Pressures greater than 40 mm Hg are considered abnormal. However, this technique is invasive, not widely available, technically difficult, impossible to perform in some patients, and prone to interpretative errors. Also, medications given during ERCP can affect results, reproducibility is a concern, and pancreatitis is a serious complication. Thus a noninvasive alternative is preferable.

Real-time ultrasonography relies solely on duct size, as discussed earlier. After a fatty meal or CCK, ultrasonography has been used to evaluate borderline or marginally dilated bile ducts but has a poor sensitivity of 67%.

Cholescintigraphy allows physiological assessment of duct drainage, which correlates well with the washout of contrast material from the biliary tract observed on ERCP. Scintigraphically, SOD is a partial common duct obstruction. Cholescintigraphy is useful for making the diagnosis, although study results have varied (sensitivity, 67% to 93%; specificity, 64% to 85%). CCK infusion may improve diagnostic accuracy because it increases bile flow and thus stresses the capacity of the biliary ducts, revealing abnormalities that might not otherwise be seen. One recent study reported 100% accuracy in 26 patients when CCK was infused before scintigraphy and a semiquantitative score of visual findings (e.g., bowel visualization, common duct emptying) was used. Although these preliminary results are promising, further data are needed.

**Liver transplants**  The role of cholescintigraphy in the postoperative evaluation of liver transplant patients is surprisingly limited. Differentiation of rejection from other complications is suggested by clinical symptoms and liver function tests, but this is often a diagnosis of exclusion. The findings of rejection on cholescintigraphy are nonspecific signs of liver dysfunction. Liver biopsy is necessary to make the diagnosis. Cholescintigraphy can detect leaks and obstruction, however, and may be useful for monitoring a patient's response to therapy and predicting recovery of poorly functioning grafts.

**Trauma**  Posttraumatic lesions that must be clinically differentiated include hepatic laceration, hematoma, bile duct transection, extrahepatic biliary leakage, intrahepatic biloma formation, and perforation of the gallbladder. CT and ultrasonography are used to detect liver parenchymal injury. However, only biliary scintigraphy can demonstrate communication between the biliary tree and space-occupying lesions that represent biloma formation.

Bile leakage is common after penetrating and blunt trauma. It may initially be occult and detected only after clinical deterioration or discharge of bilious material from surgical bed drains. Cholescintigraphy can be used

### Box 10-13  Differential Diagnosis of Primary Hepatic Tumors with Technetium-99m HIDA

| Lesion | Flow | Uptake | Clearance |
| --- | --- | --- | --- |
| Focal nodular hyperplasia | Increased | Immediate | Delayed |
| Hepatic adenoma | Normal | None | — |
| Hepatocellular carcinoma | Increased | Delayed | Delayed |

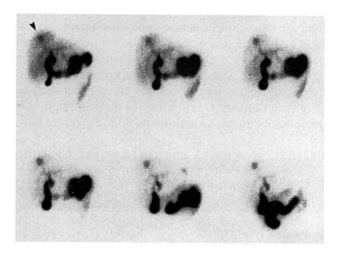

**Fig. 10-22**  Focal nodular hyperplasia. Sequential images every 5 minutes show early uptake by tumor in the liver dome that persists throughout the 60-minute study while the normal liver clears the tracer. Focal uptake persisted on delayed images acquired at 3 hours.

to follow the quantity of bile leakage and assess resolution in patients treated conservatively.

**Primary benign and malignant tumors**  Liver tumors that contain hepatocytes should take up to Tc-99m IDA, and these studies can assist in the differential diagnosis of primary benign and malignant hepatic tumors, including focal nodular hyperplasia (FNH), hepatic adenoma, and hepatocellular carcinoma (Box 10-13).

*Hepatic adenoma and focal nodular hyperplasia*  The natural history and therapy of FNH and hepatic adenoma are quite different. FNH is usually asymptomatic, is often discovered incidentally, and requires no specific therapy, whereas hepatic adenomas are often symptomatic, may result in serious hemorrhage, and can be life threatening. Adenomas have a strong association with oral contraceptive use, and oral contraceptives must be discontinued if adenoma is diagnosed.

FNH is a benign tumor that contains all hepatic cell types, including hepatocytes, Kupffer cells, and bile canaliculi. The characteristic findings with cholescintigraphy are increased blood flow, prompt hepatic uptake, and delayed clearance (Fig. 10-22). Poor

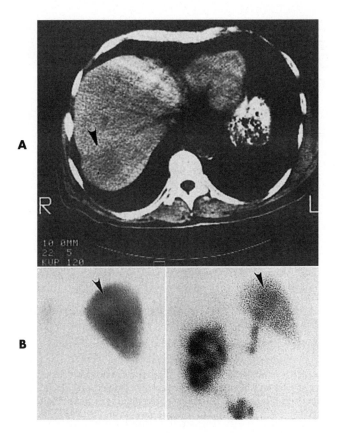

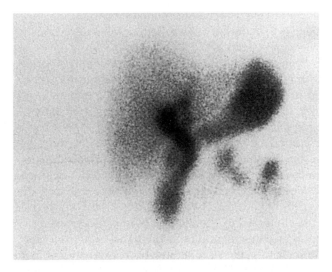

**Fig. 10-24** Enterogastric reflux. Sixty minutes after injection of technetium-99m iminoacetic acid analog, reflux of labeled bile into the stomach is seen. Bile gastritis was confirmed at endoscopy.

**Fig. 10-23** Hepatocellular carcinoma. **A,** Computed tomography shows a large lesion in the posterior aspect of the right lobe *(arrowhead).* **B,** *Left,* Tc-99m HIDA posterior view acquired at 5 minutes shows a cold defect in the same region as seen on CT *(arrowhead). Right,* Posterior view. HIDA at 2 hours shows increased uptake within the lesion *(arrowhead)* and good washout of the remainder of the liver. Surgery confirmed hepatocellular carcinoma.

clearance probably results from abnormal biliary canaliculi. Hepatic adenoma, a benign tumor made up only of hepatocytes, does not usually exhibit uptake on cholescintigraphy.

*Hepatocellular carcinoma* Tc-99m IDA cholescintigraphy also demonstrates characteristic findings for hepatocellular carcinoma *(hepatoma).* The malignant hepatocytes are hypofunctional compared with normal liver. During the first hour of cholescintigraphy, no uptake within the lesion (cold defect) is seen. Delayed imaging at 2 to 4 hours often shows "filling in," or continuing uptake within the tumor and concomitant clearing of adjacent normal liver (Fig. 10-23). This pattern is very specific for hepatoma, although some poorly differentiated hepatomas will not fill in on delayed imaging. Tc-99m IDA uptake can sometimes be seen at sites of hepatocellular metastases.

**Enterogastric bile reflux** Alkaline gastritis occurs secondary to enterogastric reflux, seen most often after gastric resection surgery. Symptoms are identical to those of acid-related disease. Cholescintigraphy can demonstrate the bile reflux (Fig. 10-24). Some bile reflux is commonly seen on cholescintigraphy, particularly if

morphine sulfate or CCK has been administered. The greater the quantity and the more persistent the reflux, the more likely that the reflux is related to the patient's symptoms.

## TECHNETIUM-99M RED BLOOD CELL LIVER SCINTIGRAPHY

*Cavernous hemangiomas* are the most common benign tumor of the liver and the second most common hepatic tumor, exceeded in incidence only by liver metastases. Hemangiomas are usually asymptomatic and discovered incidentally on CT or ultrasonography during the clinical workup or staging of a patient with a known primary malignancy or during evaluation of unrelated abdominal symptoms or disease. Hemangiomas require no specific therapy but must be differentiated from other, more serious liver tumors.

Tc-99m-labeled red blood cell (Tc-99m RBC) scintigraphy is highly accurate for making the diagnosis of hemangioma and can obviate the need for biopsy, which has resulted in hemorrhage-associated morbidity and even mortality. This radionuclide imaging technique has an exceedingly low false positive rate.

### Pathology

Cavernous hemangiomas of the liver are abnormally dilated, endothelium-lined vascular channels of varying sizes separated by fibrous septa. Cavernous hemangiomas are not pathologically related to capillary hemangiomas, angiodysplasia, or infantile hemangioendotheliomas. Ten percent of these benign liver tumors are multiple. Lesions larger than 4 cm are often called giant cavernous hemangiomas.

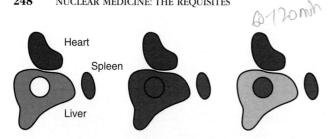

*@-120mh*

**Fig. 10-25** Pharmacokinetics of technetium-99m red blood cells (RBCs) in cavernous hemangioma. *Left,* Immediately after injection the hemangioma is "cold." Blood pool activity within the liver is considerably greater than activity within the large hemangioma. Time is required for injected Tc-99m RBCs to equilibrate with the large number of unlabeled RBCs in enlarged blood pool volume of the hemangioma. *Middle,* As the Tc-99m-labeled cells increasingly enter hemangioma and mix with the unlabeled cells, the relative uptake in the hemangioma becomes equal to the normal liver. *Right,* When RBCs are fully equilibrated (60 to 120 minutes), uptake within the hemangioma exceeds uptake in the surrounding liver and is often equal to activity in the heart and spleen.

## Radiopharmaceutical

Labeling the patient's RBCs with Tc-99m pertechnetate is done by the same methodology as discussed in Chapters 4 and 11 under "Radionuclide Ventriculography" and "Gastrointestinal Bleeding," respectively. The in vitro kit method is now the preferred approach because of its high labeling efficiency and ease of preparation.

## Mechanism of Localization and Pharmacokinetics

After injection, the Tc-99m-labeled RBCs are distributed within the blood pool of the liver. The labeled cells require time to exchange and equilibrate within the large, relatively stagnant, nonlabeled blood pool of the hemangioma (Fig. 10-25). This equilibration time varies from 30 to 120 minutes, depending somewhat on the size of the hemangioma. When the RBCs are fully equilibrated, the radioactivity per pixel within the hemangioma is greater than in adjacent normal liver and usually equal to heart blood pool radioactivity.

## Dosimetry

The total body radiation absorbed dose is about 0.4 rad. The target organ is the heart wall, which receives 1.2 rads; the bladder and spleen radiation dose is slightly less (Table 10-7).

## Methodology

A combined three-phase planar and single-photon emission computed tomography (SPECT) technique is

**Table 10-7   Dosimetry for in vitro technetium-99m red blood cell scintigraphy**

| Target | Rads/25 mCi (cGy/925 MBq) | Rad/mCi |
|---|---|---|
| Heart wall | 1.350 | 0.054 |
| Bladder wall | 1.275 | 0.051 |
| Spleen | 1.025 | 0.041 |
| Blood | 0.875 | 0.035 |
| Liver | 0.650 | 0.026 |
| Kidneys | 0.625 | 0.025 |
| Ovaries | 0.425 | 0.017 |
| Testes | 0.175 | 0.007 |
| Total body | 0.375 | 0.015 |

used (Box 10-14). SPECT is mandatory for state-of-the-art Tc-99m RBC scintigraphy. If SPECT is performed, planar flow and immediate images are optional. Reviewing CT, MR, or ultrasonographic images can help determine the projection for the flow study and the immediate images to visualize the lesion optimally. Careful correlation of the Tc-99m RBC SPECT slices with the imaging modality also can help ensure that small lesions are not missed on the SPECT study. The exact methodology used for image acquisition and processing depends on available instrumentation (e.g., single-, dual-, or triple-headed SPECT camera).

## Image Interpretation

**Normal hepatic vascular anatomy**   The liver has a complex vascular system (Figs. 10-1 and 10-26). It receives approximately two thirds to three fourths of its blood supply from the portal vein and only one third from the hepatic artery. The sinusoids act as the capillary bed for the liver cells. Blood leaves the liver through the hepatic veins, which then empty into the inferior vena cava. The caudate lobe is an exception in that it also has a direct connection with the vena cava. Much of this normal vascular anatomy of the liver is seen with Tc-99m-labeled RBCs (Figs. 10-27 to 10-31).

**Normal distribution**   The organs with the highest activity per pixel are the heart and spleen, followed by the kidney. The normal liver has much less blood pool activity. The aorta, inferior vena cava, and occasionally the portal vein can be seen with planar imaging. Portal branching vessels and hepatic veins can be seen with SPECT.

**Diagnostic criteria**   Cavernous hemangiomas have increased activity within the lesion compared with adjacent liver on 1- to 2-hour delayed imaging. The uptake is usually equal to that of the blood pool of the heart and spleen. Benign and malignant liver tumors,

## Box 10-14   Technetium-99m Red Blood Cell Liver Hemangioma Scintigraphy: Protocol Summary

**PATIENT PREPARATION**

None.

**RADIOPHARMACEUTICAL**

Tc-99m pertechnetate, 25 mCi, labeled to RBCs (in vitro kit method)

Inject intravenously; bolus injection for flow images

**INSTRUMENTATION**

Camera: large-field-of-view gamma with SPECT capability

Energy window: 15% centered over 140-keV photopeak

Collimator: low energy, high resolution, parallel hole

**IMAGE ACQUISITION**
**Planar Imaging**

1. Blood flow: 1-sec frames for 60 sec on computer and 2-sec film images.
2. Immediate images: acquire 750k to 1000k count planar image in same projection and other views as necessary to best visualize lesion(s).
3. Delayed images: acquire 750k to 1000k count planar static images 1 to 2 hr after injection in multiple projections (anterior, posterior, lateral, and oblique views).

**Single-Photon Emission Computed Tomography**

1. Position patient supine on imaging table. Raise patient's arms above head.
2. Center liver in field of view.
3. Rotate camera head around patient to ensure that camera does not come in contact with patient. Liver should remain completely in field of view during test rotation.

|  | Single-headed SPECT | Triple-headed SPECT |
|---|---|---|
| **CAMERA SETUP** | | |
| Window | 15% window centered over 140-keV Tc-99m photopeak | 15% window centered over 140-keV Tc-99m photopeak |
| Setup | Step and shoot | Step and shoot |
| Collimator(s) | High resolution | Ultrahigh resolution |
| **COMPUTER SETUP** | | |
| **Acquisition Parameters** | | |
| Patient orientation | Supine | Supine |
| Rotation | Clockwise | Clockwise as viewed from feet |
| Matrix | 64 × 64 word mode | 128 × 128 word mode |
| Image/arc combination | 128 images/360° | 40 images/120° each detector (120 images/360°) |
| Time/frame | 10 sec/stop | 40 sec/stop |
| **Reconstruction Parameters** | | |
| Filters | Manufacturer specific Personal preference | Manufacturer specific Personal preference |
| Attenuation correction | Yes | Yes |
| Reformatting | Transverse, sagittal, coronal | Transverse, sagittal, coronal |

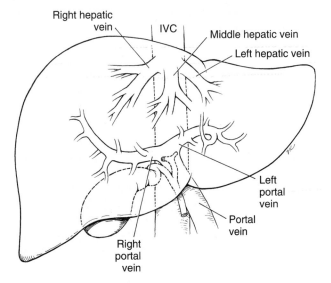

**Fig. 10-26**   Normal vascular anatomy of the liver. Blood supply to the liver is predominantly from the portal vein (75%) and to a lesser extent from the hepatic artery (25%). Both enter the liver in the portal area. Hepatic artery and its branches are not shown here. Portal vein divides into right and left branches and then subdivides. Smaller branches with hepatic artery branches and canaliculi define the periphery of lobules (Fig. 10-1). Hepatic veins originate at lobule center (central veins), feeding into right, middle, and left hepatic veins, which drain into the inferior vena cava (IVC).

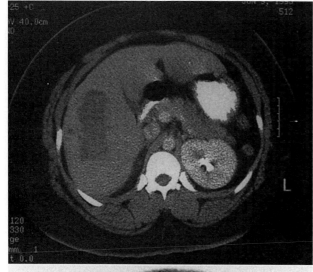

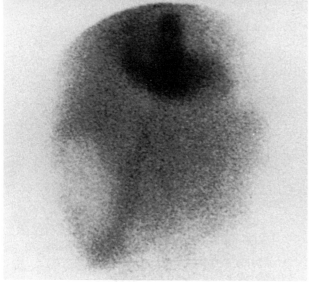

**Fig. 10-27**    Negative technetium-99m red blood cell (RBC) study for hemangioma. **A,** Computed tomography scan shows large lesion in right lobe of the liver. **B,** Planar Tc-99m RBC scan is cold in the same region and therefore negative for hemangioma. Metastatic colon cancer was ultimately diagnosed.

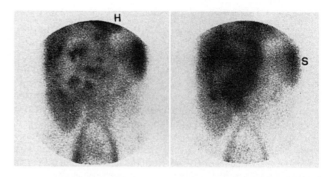

**Fig. 10-28**    Giant cavernous hemangioma. *Left,* Immediate post-injection image shows a large, relatively photopenic area involving most of the left lobe and a large portion of the right lobe. Some focal areas of increased uptake are seen. *Right,* Delayed 1-hour image shows filling of the initial cold area and increased uptake throughout this large hemangioma that is equal to the heart *(H)* and spleen *(S).*

abscesses, cirrhotic nodules, and cysts have decreased activity (Fig. 10-27).

The arterial blood flow to a hemangioma is usually normal. The blood pool, not the blood flow, is increased. Typically, immediate blood pool images show decreased uptake within the hemangioma compared with adjacent liver, although early increased uptake is occasionally seen (Figs. 10-28 and 10-29). Giant cavernous hemangiomas often show heterogeneity of uptake on delayed images, with areas of decreased as well as increased uptake (Fig. 10-28). These cold regions, often located centrally, are caused by thrombosis, necrosis, and fibrosis.

### Other modalities

*Ultrasonography*    The typical sonographic pattern for hemangioma, a homogeneous, hyperechoic mass with well-defined margins and posterior acoustical enhancement, is neither sensitive nor specific for the diagnosis of cavernous hemangioma.

*Computed tomography*    Strict CT criteria for hemangioma include relative hypoattenuation before IV contrast agent injection, early peripheral enhancement during the rapid bolus dynamic phase, progressive opacification toward the center of the lesion, and complete isodense fill-in, usually by 30 minutes after contrast agent administration. Frequently, not all criteria are satisfied. When these criteria are used to maximize specificity, the sensitivity of CT is only 55%; less strict criteria result in a high false positive rate. Accuracy is even poorer with multiple hemangiomas.

*Magnetic resonance imaging*    Cavernous hemangiomas have a characteristic MR appearance, with high signal intensity on T2-weighted spin-echo images (light bulb sign). A gadolinium contrast agent may be used, with findings similar to those with CT. Although MRI is much more accurate than CT or ultrasonography, other benign and malignant tumors may give false positive results, including metastatic adenocarcinoma of the lung, metastatic carcinoid, pheochromocytoma, islet cell carcinoma, pancreatic and uterine adenocarcinomas, and various sarcomas. MRI is particularly helpful in the diagnosis of small lesions and those adjacent to major vessels or vascular organs.

### Accuracy

Tc-99m RBC scintigraphy has a very high positive predictive value (approaching 100%). In other words, a positive test is likely to be a true positive. In more than a decade of clinical use, very few false positive studies have been reported with large hepatomas and angiosarcoma. However, the vast majority of hepatomas are negative on Tc-99m RBC imaging. Angiosarcomas are extremely rare.

Although extensive fibrosis or thrombosis may rarely

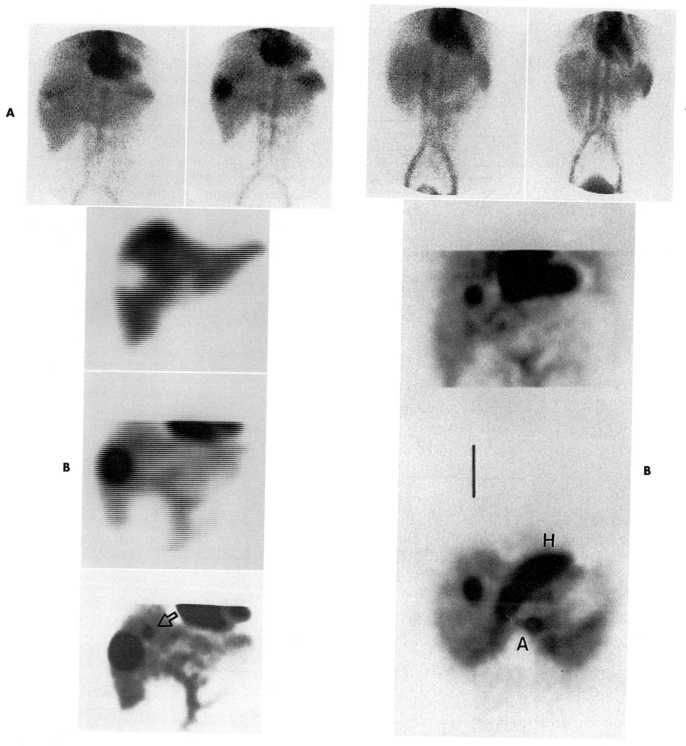

**Fig. 10-29** Comparison of planar images with single-headed and multiheaded SPECT images. **A,** Planar study. *Left,* Immediate postinjection image shows cold defect in superolateral portion of the right lobe. Small area has increased uptake. *Right,* Delayed image acquired at 60 minutes shows complete filling, diagnostic of hemangioma. **B,** SPECT coronal sections. *Top,* Single-headed technetium-99m sulfur colloid SPECT section with well-defined cold defect. *Middle,* Comparable Tc-99m red blood cell coronal section with same camera shows increased uptake in lesion, consistent with hemangioma. Although contrast resolution is improved with SPECT, there is no diagnostic advantage over planar imaging. *Bottom,* Triple-headed SPECT study in same patient shows the hemangioma, as well as a small hemangioma immediately adjacent *(arrow)* not seen with single-headed SPECT. The small hemangioma measured 0.9 cm on computed tomography.

**Fig. 10-30** Improved visualization of small lesion with SPECT. **A,** *Left,* Immediate postinjection planar image shows neither decreased nor increased uptake, probably because of small lesion size. *Right,* After 1½-hour delay, planar study shows mildly increased focal uptake in the liver dome. If lesion had been more central, it likely would not have been seen due to overlying activity. **B,** SPECT coronal *(top)* and transverse *(bottom)* sections are strongly positive for hemangioma with high target-to-background ratio. Note the heart *(H)* and aorta *(A).*

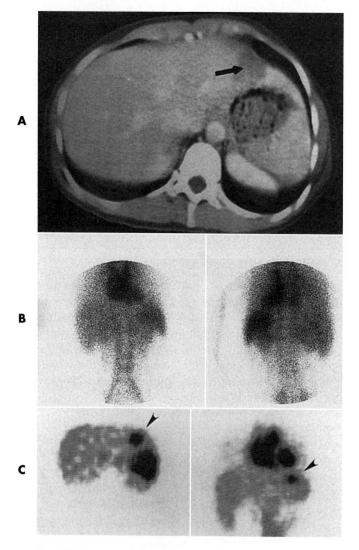

**Fig. 10-31** Negative planar and positive SPECT (technetium-99m red blood cell [RBC]) study. **A,** Liver computed tomography scan shows lesion of uncertain etiology in the left lobe. **B,** Planar anterior *(left)* and posterior *(right)* Tc-99m RBC study is negative, probably because of proximity of lesion to hot spleen. Oblique views were not helpful. **C,** SPECT study performed with a single-headed camera clearly detects the hemangioma *(arrowheads)* adjacent to the spleen and the heart's left ventricle in coronal *(right)* and transverse *(left)* slices.

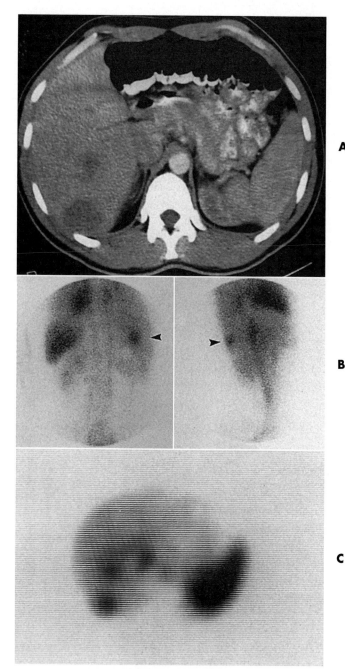

**Fig. 10-32** More lesions detected with SPECT. **A,** Computed tomography scan shows two lesions in middle and posterior aspect of the right lobe. **B,** Only the larger and more posterior lesion is positive on planar imaging *(arrowheads)*. **C,** Both lesions are seen with SPECT. The inferior vena cava and aorta are medial to the hemangiomas.

result in a false negative study, areas of increased uptake are usually seen. The diagnostic sensitivity of Tc-99m RBC imaging depends primarily on lesion size and the camera system. SPECT is clearly superior to planar imaging because of its improved contrast resolution (Figs. 10-29 to 10-32). SPECT is especially useful for the detection of small hemangiomas, those located centrally in the liver, multiple hemangiomas, and those adjacent to the heart, kidney, and spleen (Fig. 10-31). In seven comparison studies performed between 1987 and 1991, the mean overall sensitivity (all studies combined) for planar imaging was 55% and for SPECT, 88% (Table 10-8).

Lesion size and location are critical determinants of detectability (Table 10-9). Generally, planar imaging can demonstrate hemangiomas down to about 3 cm. Single-headed SPECT has good sensitivity for hemangiomas 2 cm and larger, whereas multiheaded SPECT can detect almost all hemangiomas greater than 1.4 cm and may show lesions as small as 0.5 cm, although with lower sensitivity. In multiheaded SPECT the increased sensitivity resulting from multiple detectors can be sacrificed for improved resolution by using ultra-high-resolution collimators (Fig. 10-29).

| Table 10-8 | Planar imaging versus SPECT for technetium-99m red blood cell detection of hemangioma |

| Study | Sensitivity (%) | |
| --- | --- | --- |
| | Planar | SPECT |
| Tumah, 1987 | 43 | 100 |
| Malik, 1987 | 77 | 100 |
| Brodski, 1987 | 44 | 78 |
| Itenzo, 1988 | 88 | 100 |
| Brunetti, 1988 | 69 | 100 |
| Kudo, 1989* | 42 | 74 |
| Ziessman, 1991* | 30 | 71 |
| Overall | 55 | 88 |

*Lower sensitivity in later years is caused by the larger number of small lesions.

| Table 10-9 | Sensitivity for hemangioma detection by lesion size with multiheaded SPECT |

| Lesion (cm) | Sensitivity (%) |
| --- | --- |
| >1.4 | 100 |
| >1.3 | 91 |
| 1.0-2.0 | 65 |
| 0.9-1.3 | 33 |
| 0.5-0.9 | 20 |

# TECHNETIUM-99M SULFUR COLLOID LIVER-SPLEEN IMAGING

Radiocolloids such as gold-198 colloid have been used for liver imaging since the mid-1950s. Tc-99m sulfur colloid was introduced in 1963 and became the preeminent method of liver-spleen imaging until the advent of CT. Although not a frequently requested study today, it still has some useful clinical indications.

## Mechanism of Localization and Pharmacokinetics

After IV injection the small colloid particles of Tc-99m sulfur colloid (0.1 to 1.0 µm) are extracted from the blood by cells of the reticuloendothelial system (RES), with a single-pass extraction efficiency of 95% and a blood clearance half-life of 2 to 3 minutes. After phagocytosis the sulfur colloid particles are fixed intracellularly. Liver uptake is complete by 15 minutes. Tc-99m sulfur colloid localizes within the Kupffer cells of the liver (85%) and the macrophages of the spleen (10%) and bone marrow (5%).

Besides extraction efficiency, factors that influence

| Table 10-10 | Technetium-99m sulfur colloid dosimetry |

| Organ | Rads/5 mCi (cGy/185 MBq) | |
| --- | --- | --- |
| | Normal | Diffuse parenchymal disease |
| Liver | 1.7 | 0.8 |
| Spleen | 1.1 | 2.1 |
| Bone marrow | 0.14 | 0.4 |
| Testes | 0.006 | 0.016 |
| Ovaries | 0.028 | 0.06 |
| Total body | 0.095 | 0.09 |

the distribution of colloid particles include blood flow, particle size, and disease states. For example, increased blood flow to a region of the liver (e.g., in FNH) increases the relative regional delivery of colloid, resulting in focally increased uptake on imaging. The larger the colloid particle size, the greater the proportion taken up by the liver, whereas the smaller the particles, the greater the distribution to bone marrow.

Kupffer cells are found diffusely throughout the liver (Fig. 10-1) but make up less than 10% of liver cell mass. Most liver diseases affect hepatocytes and adjacent Kupffer cells similarly. Disease results in local, diffuse, or heterogeneously decreased uptake because of destruction or displacement of normal liver.

With severe diffuse liver disease there is a generalized reduction in hepatic extraction and relatively increased distribution to the spleen and bone marrow (colloid shift). Colloid shift is most often seen with portal hypertension. However, splenomegaly alone can produce increased Tc-99m sulfur colloid uptake. In immunologically active states, such as systemic tumor without liver involvement (melanoma), increased splenic uptake may be seen.

## Preparation

Tc-99m sulfur colloid is available in kit form and requires 15 minutes to prepare. Acid is added to a mixture of Tc-99m pertechnetate and sodium thiosulfate, which is heated in a water bath (95° to 100° F) for 5 to 10 minutes. The pH is adjusted with a buffer, gelatin is added to control particle size and stabilize the colloid, and EDTA is added to remove any aluminum ions by chelation. Labeling yield is greater than 99%.

## Dosimetry

Estimated radiation dose from Tc-99m sulfur colloid is 1.7 rads to the liver and 1.1 rads to the spleen. The relative liver-to-spleen dosimetry is reversed with diffuse parenchymal disease and colloid shift (Table 10-10).

## Clinical Applications

The clinical role for Tc-99m sulfur colloid is limited to (1) situations in which it can add functional information not available from the usual anatomical imaging methods of CT, ultrasonography, and MRI or (2) situations in which it acts as a template for correlating imaging findings with another radionuclide study (e.g., Ga-67, In-111 leukocytes) (Fig. 8-7) and for splenic imaging (Box 10-15).

## Methodology

No patient preparation is required. Imaging can start within 20 minutes after radiopharmaceutical injection. SPECT is now routine (Box 10-16).

## Image Interpretation

Interpretation of Tc-99m sulfur colloid liver-spleen scans requires an appreciation of normal liver anatomy and its variability, the effect of extrinsic liver compression by normal and abnormal structures, and common artifacts (Figs. 10-33 to 10-37).

Planar imaging with multiple views has been used successfully for many years. However, SPECT improves lesion detection because of its improved contrast resolution (Fig. 10-38). Interpretation requires a knowledge of normal cross-sectional hepatic anatomy (Fig. 10-39).

Abnormal scintigraphic findings include hepatomegaly, inhomogeneity, splenomegaly, colloid shift, and single and multiple focal defects. Hepatomegaly is a

nonspecific finding and may be caused by a variety of disease processes (Box 10-17). Inhomogeneity of uptake suggests hepatic dysfunction or an infiltrating process (Box 10-18). Hepatomegaly and inhomogeneity may be the only findings in early lung and breast cancer because these liver metastases may be small and diffusely infiltrating. On the other hand, colon cancer tumors metastatic to the liver are usually larger and focal at clinical presentation.

Various methods have been used to estimate liver and spleen size. Linear measurements can be obtained using a costal margin marker (e.g., cobalt hot markers with 1-cm intervals, lead cold markers). Generally, the normal liver's longest vertical and midclavicular line dimensions are 17 and 15 cm, respectively. Spleen size greater than 14 cm in its longest axis or greater than 110 cm$^2$ using two perpendicular dimensions is considered enlarged.

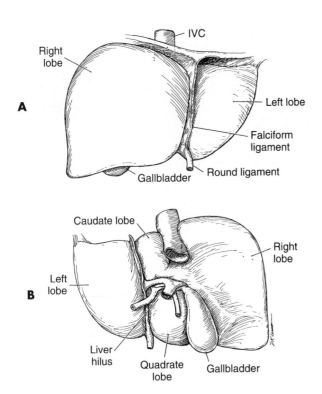

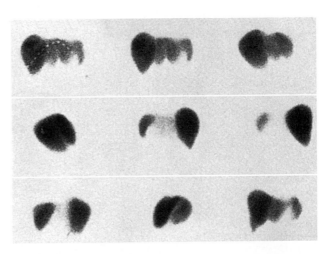

**Fig. 10-35** Normal technetium-99m sulfur colloid liver-spleen scan. Two anterior views, with marker in supine position *(top left)* and without marker in upright position *(top middle)*. In sequence, remaining images are right anterior oblique, right lateral, posterior, right posterior oblique (shallow), left posterior oblique, left lateral, and left anterior oblique.

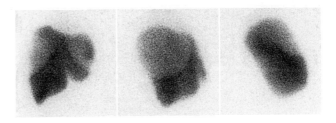

**Fig. 10-36** Breast artifact on anterior, right anterior oblique, and right lateral views. Curvilinear line of increased activity at breast border attributed to soft tissue, short-angle scatter.

**Fig. 10-33** Normal anatomy of liver. **A,** Anterior view. *IVC,* Inferior vena cava. **B,** Posterior view.

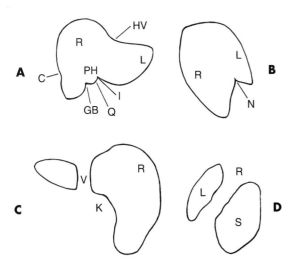

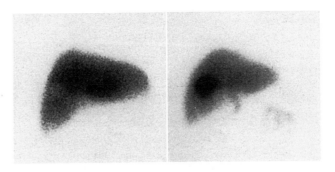

**Fig. 10-37** Liver "lesion" caused by intrahepatic gallbladder. *Left,* Anterior technetium-99m sulfur colloid liver image with photopenic defect in lateral aspect of mid-right lobe. *Right,* Tc-99m iminodiacetic acid analog study performed immediately after sulfur colloid study showed gallbladder filling of the Tc-99m sulfur colloid defect.

**Fig. 10-34** Normal anatomical landmarks and potential interpretative pitfalls for technetium-99m sulfur colloid liver scintigraphy. **A,** Anterior view. *C,* Costal indentation of ribs; *GB,* gallbladder fossa; *HV,* notch from hepatic veins; *I,* incisura umbilicus (ligamentum teres); *K,* kidney impression; *L,* left lobe. **B,** Right lateral view. *N,* Notch between right and left lobes; *PH,* porta hepatis; *Q,* quadrate lobe; *R,* right lobe. **C,** Posterior view. *V,* Vertebral spine attenuation. **D,** Left lateral view. *S,* Spleen.

In properly exposed images, bone marrow uptake is usually not perceptible. The intensity of the spleen on the posterior view is normally equal to or less than that of the liver (Fig. 10-35). Colloid shift is seen with a variety of hepatic diseases (Fig. 10-40). Quantitative spleen-to-liver count ratios greater than 1.5 are abnormal.

**Liver** Lung radiocolloid uptake is uncommon. It may result from improper labeling (excessive aluminum causing large-particle clumping) and is associated with various pathophysiological processes but most often with severe liver dysfunction (Fig. 10-41). Postulated mechanisms include activation of normal lung macro-

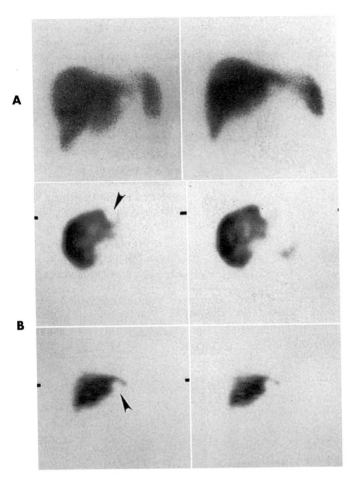

Fig. 10-38   Improved lesion detectability with SPECT. Patient with primary malignant melanoma referred for technetium-99m sulfur colloid study to rule out hepatic metastases. **A,** Anterior planar images in upright *(left)* and supine *(right)* views. Questionable defect at medial inferior aspect of the left lobe was thought to be a normal variation. **B,** Selected SPECT short-axis *(top two)* and coronal *(bottom two)* sections demonstrate well-defined lesion in anterior aspect of the left lobe *(arrowheads).*

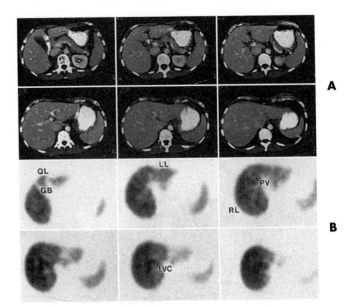

Fig. 10-39   Normal liver anatomy on SPECT correlated with computed tomography (CT). **A,** Selected CT sections. **B,** Corresponding SPECT sections in the same patient. The most inferior images are at the upper left and the most superior images at the lower right. *GB,* Gallbladder fossa; *QL,* quadrate lobe; *PV,* portal vein bifurcation; *IVC,* inferior vena cava; *RL,* right lobe; *LL,* left lobe.

---

**Box 10-17   Causes of Hepatomegaly**

Infiltrative: fatty metamorphosis, alcoholic liver disease,
   amyloidosis, Gaucher's disease, Wilson's disease,
   granulomas
Congestive: heart failure, hepatic vein thrombosis
Neoplastic: primary and secondary tumors
Infectious: hepatitis, sepsis, malaria
Inflammatory: drugs (e.g., methyldopa, isoniazid)
Miscellaneous: cystic disease

---

**Box 10-18   Causes of Liver
               Inhomogeneity**

Metastases (infiltrative, early)
Lymphoma, leukemia
Hepatitis
Fatty metamorphosis
Chronic passive congestion
Parenchymal liver diseases
Cirrhosis

---

phages and stimulation of RES cell migration from other parts of the body to the lung.

*Decreased uptake*   Most benign and malignant lesions of the liver produce "cold" or "photopenic" defects on Tc-99m sulfur colloid liver imaging (Box 10-19; Figs. 10-29, *B,* and 10-42). Radiation therapy results in a characteristic rectangular port–shaped hepatic defect.

Diffusely decreased uptake is usually caused by hepatocellular disease, although early infiltrating tumor involvement appears similar.

Ancillary radionuclide tests are sometimes helpful in making a more specific diagnosis, such as In-111 leukocyte study for infection, Ga-67 citrate for hepatoma, and Tc-99m RBC study for hemangioma (Box 10-15). Xenon-133, an inert gas and fat-soluble radiopharmaceutical, exhibits increased uptake in focal fatty tumors and in generalized fatty metamorphosis of the liver.

*Increased uptake*   Increased hepatic uptake on Tc-99m sulfur colloid imaging is uncommon (Box 10-20). Focal areas of increased uptake can result from (1) increased blood flow to an area, resulting in more radiocolloid delivered to normally functioning Kupffer cells, or (2) normal flow to an area of increased density of Kupffer cells. Increased uptake cannot result from

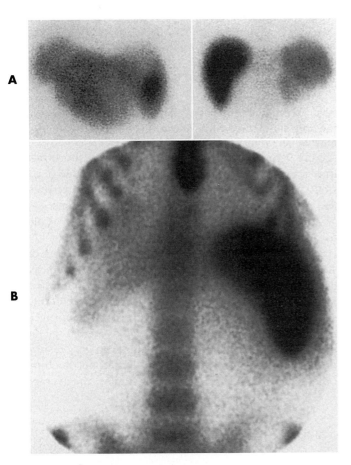

**Fig. 10-40** Hepatic parenchymal disease on technetium-99m sulfur colloid study. **A,** Hyperpigmentation and biopsy-proven hemochromatosis in 52-year-old man. Anterior *(left)* and posterior *(right)* views show small right lobe, hypertrophied left lobe, large spleen, and colloid shift. **B,** Severe cirrhosis. Anterior view shows very small liver with poor uptake, enlarged spleen, and prominent colloid shift to the marrow and spleen.

---

### Box 10-19  Causes of Focal Liver Defects

Cyst
Benign and malignant tumors
Dilated bile ducts
Abscess
Hematoma
Laceration
Localized hepatitis
Radiation therapy
Infarction
Cirrhosis (pseudotumors)
Fatty infiltration

---

increased Kupffer cell activity alone because the extraction efficiency is so high.

In *superior vena cava obstruction*, collateral thoracic and abdominal wall vessels communicate with the recanalized umbilical vein delivering radiocolloid via the

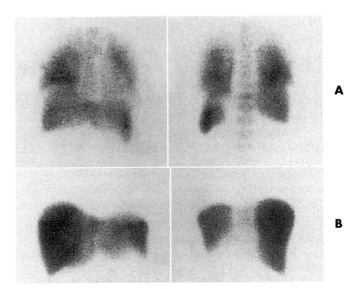

**Fig. 10-41** Technetium-99m sulfur colloid lung uptake. Fatty metamorphosis of the liver during pregnancy. **A,** During the patient's acute illness the liver-spleen scan showed increased lung uptake, colloid shift to the marrow and spleen, and inhomogeneous liver uptake. **B,** Follow-up study after patient clinically recovered. Tc-99m sulfur colloid liver-spleen scan returned to normal.

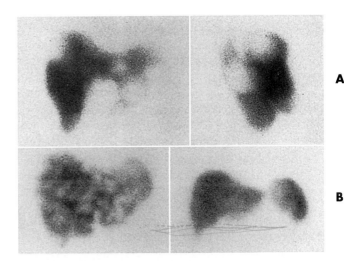

**Fig. 10-42** **A,** Colon cancer metastases on technetium-99m sulfur colloid study. Anterior and right lateral views show large metastases in the right and left lobes. **B,** Good response to chemotherapy. Extensive liver metastases on initial Tc-99m sulfur colloid study *(left)* and definite response to therapy seen on follow-up 4 months later *(right).*

left portal vein to a small volume of tissue, usually in the region of the quadrate lobe, producing a "hot spot" (Fig. 10-43). This collateral blood flow has a relatively increased concentration of colloid compared with blood delivered to the bulk of the liver after systemic mixing. Injection in the lower extremity rather than the upper extremity results in a normal scan.

*Focal nodular hyperplasia* may have increased uptake because of both the vascular nature of this benign

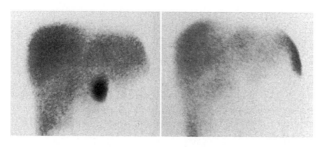

**Fig. 10-43** Superior vena cava syndrome. *Left,* Hot spot in region of quadrate lobe on technetium-99m sulfur colloid liver spleen scan in patient with lung cancer and superior vena cava obstruction. Radiotracer was injected in the arm. *Right,* Repeat study in same patient with radiotracer injected in lower extremity. No hot spot is seen.

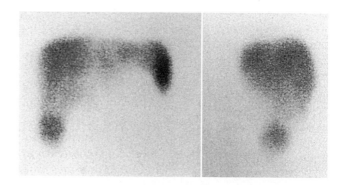

**Fig. 10-44** Focal nodular hyperplasia. Anterior *(left)* and right lateral *(right)* views show increased uptake in lesion at inferior tip of right lobe of liver. Angiography confirmed the diagnosis of focal nodular hyperplasia.

---

**Box 10-20  Causes of Increased Focal Uptake on Technetium-99m Sulfur Colloid Imaging**

Superior vena cava syndrome (arm injection)
Inferior vena cava obstruction (leg injection)
Focal nodular hyperplasia
Budd-Chiari syndrome
Cirrhosis (regenerating nodule)

---

tumor and the increased density of functioning Kupffer cells (Fig. 10-44). FNH can be confirmed with Tc-99m sulfur colloid. Since this tumor has hepatocytes, bile ducts, and Kupffer cells, normal or increased colloid uptake is seen in two thirds of patients. One third are cold, for uncertain reasons. In contrast, hepatic adenoma (hepatocytes only) is always cold.

The *Budd-Chiari syndrome* (hepatic vein thrombosis) is often listed as a cause of increased Tc-99m sulfur colloid uptake. More correctly, the caudate lobe has relatively more uptake than the remainder of the liver (Fig. 10-45). The impaired venous drainage of the majority of the liver results in poor hepatic function. The caudate lobe retains good function as a result of its direct venous drainage into the inferior vena cava. This finding is seen in 50% of patients.

Many diseases affect the liver diffusely (Boxes 10-17 and 10-18). In the Western world, *alcoholic liver disease* is the most common cause and may be seen as fatty infiltration, acute alcoholic hepatitis, or cirrhosis. With mild *fatty infiltration* the liver scan may be normal or show mild inhomogeneity. As the severity increases, hepatomegaly and colloid shift result (Fig. 10-40). *Alcoholic hepatitis* results in hepatic necrosis and wide-

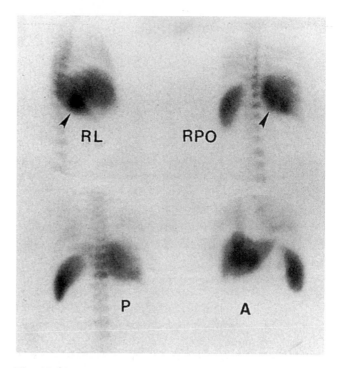

**Fig. 10-45** Budd-Chiari syndrome. Good technetium-99m sulfur colloid uptake in region of caudate lobe *(arrowheads)* in patient with hepatic vein thrombosis. Images were acquired in the right lateral *(RL),* right posterior oblique *(RPO),* posterior *(P),* and anterior *(A)* projections. Note increased marrow uptake.

spread inflammation, particularly around the central efferent veins, causing an irregular distribution of colloid on scans.

*Cirrhosis* may be micronodular, macronodular, or mixed. Scan pattern is related to the degree of pathology and the presence or absence of portal hypertension. With increasing severity the liver, particularly the right lobe, shrinks; the left lobe compensates with hypertrophy, and colloid redistribution becomes more marked (Fig. 10-40). Splenomegaly and marked splenic uptake are seen with portal hypertension.

The inhomogeneous appearance seen in severe cirrhosis, caused by uneven blood flow, shunting, and irregular distribution of the functioning Kupffer cells, may give the impression of focal defects *(pseudotumors)*. This can be a diagnostic dilemma because the incidence of hepatoma is increased in cirrhotic patients. Ga-67 citrate can aid in this differential diagnosis because it is taken up by tumor but not by regenerating nodules (see Fig. 9-7).

*Accuracy*  Cold liver lesions can be detected on planar imaging if they are larger than 2 to 3 cm and on SPECT if greater than 1.5 to 2 cm. Superficial lesions are more easily detected than deep ones. SPECT aids in detecting smaller and more central lesions because of its improved contrast resolution. Multiheaded SPECT cameras using ultra-high-resolution collimators can provide resolution in the range of 1 to 1.2 cm.

Based on combined data from many studies, the average sensitivity for detecting metastatic liver disease with planar Tc-99m sulfur colloid imaging is 81%, and the specificity is 90%. SPECT improves the sensitivity by 10%. Direct comparison studies have not shown a statistical difference between CT and Tc-99m sulfur colloid. However, CT is now the liver-imaging method of choice because of its better image resolution and whole abdomen imaging capability.

**Spleen**  The spleen serves as a reservoir for formed blood elements, as a site for clearance of microorganisms and particle trapping, as a potential site of hematopoiesis during bone marrow failure, and as a source of humor or cellular response to foreign antigens. It plays a role in white blood cell (WBC) production, contributes to platelet processing, and has immunological functions. Thus the spleen can be visualized by various radiopharmaceuticals with different mechanisms of uptake, such as Tc-99m sulfur colloid (RES function), In-111 WBC imaging (leukocyte migration), Tc-99m RBC imaging (erythrocyte distribution), and damaged RBC imaging (sequestration).

Radionuclide splenic imaging is most often requested to detect splenic infarcts (Fig. 10-46), postoperative splenic remnants, accessory spleens, or splenosis (Fig. 10-47, *A*). Although Tc-99m sulfur colloid scintigraphy can often make these diagnoses, liver uptake may obscure adjacent splenic uptake. In addition, the tip of the left lobe often migrates into the splenic bed after splenectomy. Imaging with heat or chemically damaged Tc-99m RBCs provides excellent splenic images with less liver uptake (Fig. 10-47, *B*).

Nonvisualization of the spleen may result from congenital absence or from acquired *functional asplenia*

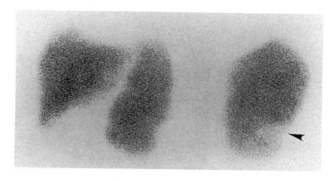

**Fig. 10-46**  Splenic infarct. *Right,* Large, wedge-shaped defect *(arrowhead)* of the spleen in patient with massive splenomegaly and myeloid metaplasia on technetium-99m sulfur colloid study. *Left,* Smaller defects can also be seen on anterior view.

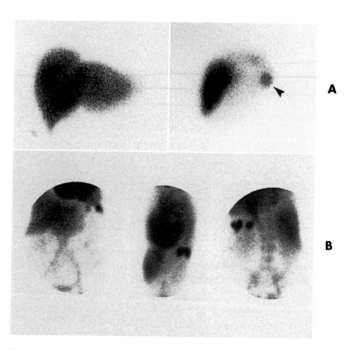

**Fig. 10-47**  **A,** Splenic remnant on technetium-99m sulfur colloid study is best seen in the left lateral view *(arrowhead)*. Patient had a splenectomy. **B,** Splenosis, or autotransplantation of splenic tissue after splenic trauma. Damaged Tc-99m-labeled red blood cell study shows definite splenic tissue in left upper quadrant. *Left* to *right,* Anterior, left lateral, and posterior views.

caused by interruption of the blood supply (splenic artery occlusion) or secondary to RES dysfunction (sickle cell crisis). Functional asplenia may be irreversible (e.g., Thorotrast irradiation, chemotherapy, amyloid) or reversible (e.g., sickle cell crisis). With sickle cell disease, discordance is seen between RES phagocytic function and other splenic functions.

## TECHNETIUM-99M MACROAGGREGATED ALBUMIN HEPATIC ARTERIAL PERFUSION SCINTIGRAPHY

Oncologists have used intraarterial chemotherapy to treat primary and metastatic cancer since the 1960s. Enthusiasm for this form of chemotherapy has varied over the years, waxing with the introduction of new technology that makes administration of the chemotherapy easier, safer, and potentially more effective and waning after disenchantment with the overall results in light of the technical difficulties and expense.

Survival in untreated patients with liver metastases varies from 1 to 22 months. Complete surgical resection is curative but feasible only for a few patients with solitary or unilobar metastases. Conventional IV chemotherapy yields response rates of only 10% to 30%. Response rates with intraarterial chemotherapy range from 34% to 72%.

The advantage of a selective intraarterial approach to chemotherapy is based on the differential blood flow to tumor and normal liver. As tumor in the liver grows, it derives most of its blood supply from the hepatic artery, whereas normal liver cells are supplied predominantly by the portal circulation. Intraarterial chemotherapy delivers the drug preferentially to the tumor, minimizing exposure to normal liver and to drug-sensitive, dose-limiting tissues such as gastrointestinal epithelium and bone marrow, often the source of side effects from conventional IV chemotherapy.

Successful application of intraarterial chemotherapy requires that the drug be reliably and safely delivered to the tumor. After initial arteriographic assessment of the vascular supply of the tumor and liver, a therapeutic catheter is inserted either (1) percutaneously, using a transfemoral or transaxillary approach and attached to an external infusion pump, or (2) surgically, connected to a subcutaneously implanted, constant-infusion pump (Fig. 10-48). Confirmation is needed to ensure that the perfusion distribution from the catheter truly encompasses the entire tumor without perfusion of other visceral organs (Figs. 10-49 to 10-51).

Although angiography is needed before initial catheter placement, it is not a good indicator of blood flow at the capillary level. The high flow rates required for good

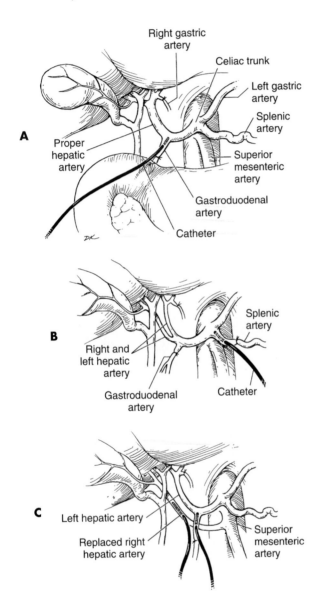

**Fig. 10-48**  Surgical placement of intraarterial catheters. **A,** Standard anatomy. Gastroduodenal artery is ligated and catheter placed at junction of gastroduodenal and common hepatic arteries. Right gastric artery is ligated. **B,** Trifurcation. Right and left hepatic arteries originate too close to gastroduodenal artery to allow equal distribution to all areas of the liver. In this normal variation, gastroduodenal and right gastric arteries are ligated. Splenic artery is ligated and catheter is positioned at junction of splenic artery and celiac axis. **C,** Replaced right hepatic artery originating from superior mesenteric artery requires use of two catheters. Similarly, patient with left hepatic artery arising from left gastric artery requires two catheters.

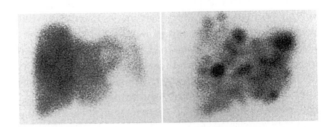

**Fig. 10-49**  Comparison of technetium-99m macroaggregated albumin (MAA) with Tc-99m sulfur colloid. Patient with colon cancer and liver metastases. *Left,* Tc-99m sulfur colloid study shows multiple lesions involving right and left lobes. *Right,* Tc-99m MAA study shows solid tumor nodules involving both lobes of liver in pattern similar to defects seen on Tc-99m sulfur colloid. Perfusion to the liver is good. No extrahepatic perfusion.

contrast angiography often do not reflect the actual perfusion pattern that occurs with the slower infusion rates used in chemotherapy delivery systems. A high-pressure contrast bolus may result in streaming, reflux, or retrograde flow. Contrast angiography cannot be performed through the small-bore, surgically placed catheters, which deliver chemotherapy at a rate of 1 to 5 ml/day.

Incorrect positioning of the intraarterial catheter results in inadequate perfusion of the tumor-involved liver and can cause extrahepatic perfusion to the stomach, pancreas, spleen, and bowel (Fig. 10-52). Suboptimal perfusion may result from difficulties in

placement due to normal vascular anatomical variation. Even if the catheter is properly placed initially, catheter movement, occlusion, or arterial thrombosis may produce a change from the initial perfusion pattern. Tc-99m macroaggregated albumin (MAA) hepatic arterial scintigraphy reliably estimates the adequacy of blood flow to the tumor and determines the presence or absence of extrahepatic perfusion, a frequent cause of gastrointestinal and systemic toxicity.

## Mechanism of Localization and Pharmacokinetics

Tc-99m MAA particles are larger than capillary size (range, 10 to 90 μm; mean, 30 to 50 μm). When injected into the hepatic artery, they are distributed according to

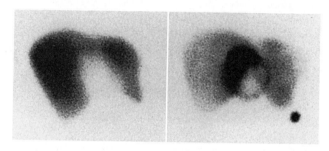

**Fig. 10-50**  Technetium-99m macroaggregated albumin (MAA) hyperperfusion of tumor periphery. *Left,* Large tumor mass in midportion of the liver on Tc-99m sulfur colloid study. *Right,* Tc-99m MAA study shows hyperperfusion of the periphery of the large tumor mass with a large, cold, necrotic center.

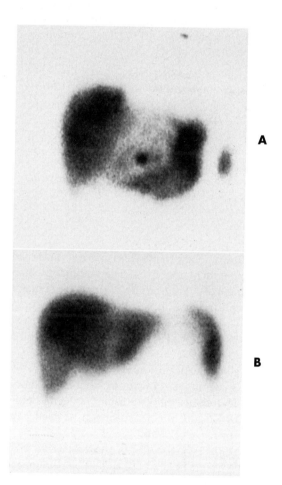

A

B

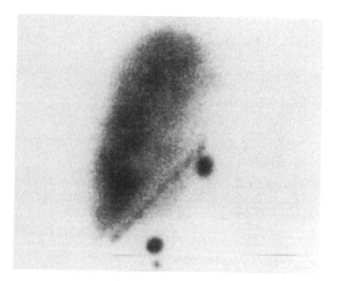

**Fig. 10-51**  Incomplete hepatic perfusion. Only right lobe is perfused on technetium-99m macroaggregated albumin study. Upper hot spot is a clot in the catheter; lower hot spot is infusion pump. Hot marker is placed along costal margin.

**Fig. 10-52**  Extrahepatic perfusion. **A,** Poor perfusion to the left lobe and extrahepatic perfusion to the stomach. Focal hot spot is caused by partial catheter thrombosis. **B,** With catheter replaced, entire liver is well perfused, although some extrahepatic perfusion to spleen occurs.

---

**Box 10-21   Technetium-99m Macroaggregated Albumin Hepatic Arterial Scintigraphy: Protocol Summary**

**PATIENT PREPARATION**

None. Tc-99m sulfur colloid study performed within 24 to 48 hr is helpful for comparison when interpreting Tc-99m MAA study.

**INSTRUMENTATION**

Camera: large-field-of-view gamma
Collimator: low energy, all purpose, parallel hole
Energy window: 15% centered over 140-keV photopeak

**RADIOPHARMACEUTICAL**

Tc-99m MAA, 1 to 4 mCi (37 to 148 MBq) for planar imaging and 5 to 6 mCi (185 to 222 MBq) for SPECT
Infuse in small volume (0.5 to 1 ml) through an intraarterial catheter

**METHOD OF ADMINISTRATION**
**Surgically Implanted Infusion Pump and Catheter**

Insert 22-gauge 1-inch Huber needle into infusion pump side port.
After ascertaining free flow, infuse Tc-99m MAA slowly over 1 to 2 min and flush with 10 ml of saline.
Before removing needle, inject 5 ml of heparin (10 units/ml).

**Percutaneously Placed Catheter and External Infusion Pump**

Place three-way stopcock as close as possible to the site of catheter entry.
With patient positioned under the camera so that entering flow can be monitored, gently flush catheter with 10 to 20 ml of normal saline.
Infuse Tc-99m MAA in 0.2-ml volume via the three-way stopcock.
Increase the external pump flow rate to 200 ml/hr.
Monitor progress of radioactive injectate on the persistence scope. As bolus approaches the liver, decrease flow rate of the pump to rate at which chemotherapy is to be delivered, generally 10 to 20 ml/hr.

**IMAGING PROTOCOL**

Acquire images with the patient lying on the table supine.
Acquire 500k-count anterior image, then posterior, right and left lateral, and anterior chest views for equal time.
If extrahepatic gastric perfusion is suspected, 4 g of sodium bicarbonate–citric acid–simethicone effervescent granules (EZ-gas, Sparkles) should be given in 100 ml of water by mouth. The patient must be encouraged not to eruct. Repeat anterior and left lateral images.
SPECT option: technique similar to Tc-99m sulfur colloid SPECT.

---

blood flow and are trapped on first pass in the arteriolar-capillary bed of the liver. The irregularly shaped and malleable particles occlude a small percentage of the liver capillary bed, break down into smaller particles (effective liver half-life of 4 hours), and are eventually taken up by RES macrophages or cleared through the kidney.

Extrahepatic perfusion is seen on Tc-99m MAA perfusion imaging as uptake in abdominal visceral organs, including the stomach, spleen, and bowel (Figs. 10-52 and 10-53). Although a small amount of arteriovenous (AV) shunting is common (1% to 7%), shunting of 10% to 40% is possible (Fig. 10-54). AV shunting results in less perfusion of the tumor, increased systemic exposure, and increased potential for side effects.

The typical pattern of tumor perfusion on Tc-99m MAA studies is greater uptake in the tumors compared with normal liver (tumor/nontumor ratio, 3:1). Small tumor nodules show uniform uptake (Fig. 10-49), whereas larger tumors often have increased uptake at the periphery of the tumor and relatively decreased uptake centrally because of necrosis (Fig. 10-50). Selective

hepatic angiography has demonstrated that most cancers are hypervascular, particularly at the periphery of the tumor, where active growth occurs (neovascularity). This increased tumor/nontumor flow ratio is a major advantage of the intraarterial technique.

## Methodology

The method of Tc-99m MAA administration depends on the type of intraarterial catheter and whether it is placed percutaneously or surgically (Box 10-21).

## Clinical Applications

The Tc-99m MAA hepatic arterial perfusion study is often performed after initial catheter placement and before courses of chemotherapy, particularly if the patient has symptoms suggestive of gastrointestinal toxicity. Effectiveness of intraarterial chemotherapy is maximized if the entire tumor-involved liver is perfused, and side effects are minimized if there is no extrahepatic perfusion or AV shunting to the lung.

At times symptoms (e.g., pain, nausea, vomiting)

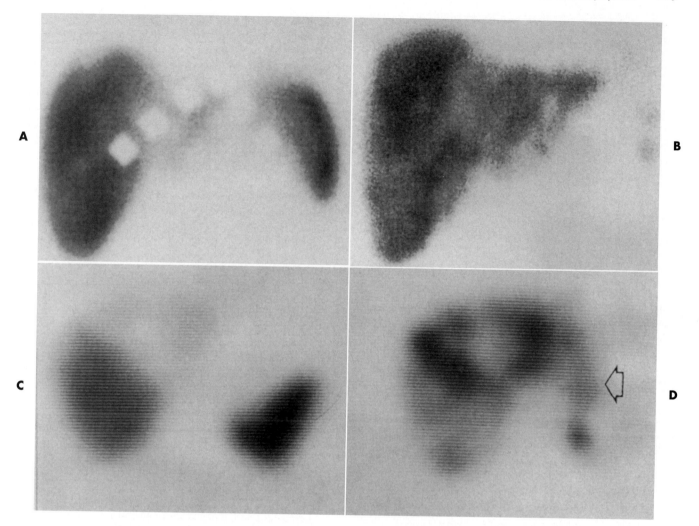

**Fig. 10-53**    Extrahepatic perfusion: utility of SPECT. **A,** Technetium-99m sulfur colloid planar study shows the left lobe replaced by tumor (cold markers overlie left lobe). **B,** Tc-99m macroaggregated albumin (MAA) planar study shows perfusion of the left lobe tumor without definite gastric perfusion. There is a suggestion of splenic perfusion, and activity adjacent to the left lobe could be gastric perfusion. **C,** Tc-99m sulfur colloid SPECT transverse image shows a large tumor defect in the left lobe. **D,** Tc-99m MAA SPECT study shows hyperperfusion of the periphery of the large tumor nodule, which is cold centrally. Definite gastric perfusion is clearly seen on the transverse SPECT slice. Splenic perfusion was seen on other sections not shown here.

caused by tumor involvement can be difficult to differentiate from those caused by extrahepatic perfusion of the stomach and bowel. The latter are associated with a high incidence of adverse symptoms (70%, versus 20% in patients without extrahepatic perfusion), including nausea, vomiting, gastritis, ulceration, and hemorrhage.

## Image Interpretation

Hepatic uptake is often inhomogeneous. Tumor nodules have increased uptake compared with surrounding normal liver. Multiple views (right lateral, anterior, posterior, left lateral) are often helpful for establishing the distribution of perfusion, and comparison with a recent Tc-99m sulfur colloid liver scan can be helpful (Figs. 10-50 and 10-53).

AV shunting is seen on Tc-99m MAA studies as lung uptake (Fig. 10-54). The particles shunted through the tumor bypass the capillary bed and are trapped in the capillary bed of the lung. This gives an estimate of the percentage of drug not delivered to the tumor, which could result in systemic exposure and potential toxicity.

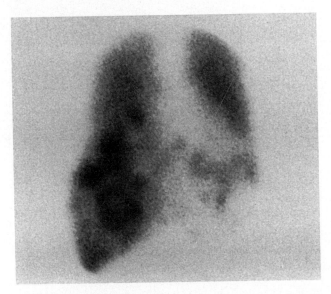

**Fig. 10-54**   Lung uptake of technetium-99m macroaggregated albumin consistent with large amount of arteriovenous shunting (40%).

## SUGGESTED READINGS

Choy D, Shi EC, McLean RG, et al: Cholescintigraphy in acute cholecystitis: use of intravenous morphine, *Radiology* 151:203-207, 1984.

Fig LM, Stewart RE, Wahl RL: Morphine-augmented hepatobiliary scintigraphy in the severely ill: caution is in order, *Radiology* 175:473-476, 1990.

Fink-Bennett D, DeRidder P, Kolozsi WZ, et al: Cholecystokinin cholescintigraphy: detection of abnormal gallbladder motor function in patients with chronic acalculous gallbladder disease, *J Nucl Med* 32:1695-1699, 1991.

Freitas JE, Coleman RE, Nagle CE, et al: Influence of scan and pathologic criteria on the specificity of cholescintigraphy, *J Nucl Med* 24:876-879, 1983.

Krishnamurthy S, Krishnamurthy GT: Cholecystokinin and morphine pharmacological intervention during 99mTc-HIDA cholescintigraphy: a rational approach, *Semin Nucl Med* 26:16-24, 1996.

Sostre S, Kaloo AN, Spiegler EJ, et al: A noninvasive test of sphincter of Oddi dysfunction in postcholecystectomy patients: the scintigraphic score, *J Nucl Med* 33:1216-1222, 1992.

Weissman HS, Freeman LM: The biliary tract. In Freeman LM, editor: *Freeman and Johnson's clinical radionuclide imaging,* New York, 1984, Grune & Stratton.

Yap L, Wycherley AG, Morphett AD, Toouli J: Acalculous biliary pain: cholecystectomy alleviates symptoms in patients with abnormal cholescintigraphy, *Gastroenterology* 101:786-793, 1991.

Zeman RK, Ziessman HA: Correlation of nuclear techniques with other hepatobiliary imaging modalities. In *Diagnostic nuclear medicine,* ed 3, Baltimore, 1996, Williams & Wilkins.

Ziessman HA: Diagnosis of chronic acalculous cholecystitis using cholecystokinin cholescintigraphy: methodology and interpretation. In Freeman LM, editor: *Nuclear medicine annual 1999,* Baltimore, 1999, Williams & Wilkins.

Ziessman HA, Fahey FN, Hixson DJ: Calculation of a gallbladder ejection fraction: advantage of continuous sincalide infusion over the 3-minute method, *J Nucl Med* 33:537-541, 1992.

Ziessman HA, Silverman PM, Patterson J, et al: Improved detection of small cavernous hemangiomas of the liver with high-resolution three-headed SPECT, *J Nucl Med* 32:2086-2091, 1991.

Ziessman HA, Thrall JH, Yang PJ, et al: Hepatic arterial perfusion scintigraphy with Tc-99m MAA, *Radiology* 152:167-172, 1984.

# Gastrointestinal System

Gastrointestinal (GI) radionuclide studies provide unique physiological information about esophageal and GI function. Quantification of esophageal, gastric, and intestinal motility provides clinically useful information not easily available by any other methodology.

Gastroesophageal radionuclide reflux studies are routinely used by pediatricians as a sensitive, noninvasive method to diagnose and quantify reflux. GI bleeding studies have become a standard radionuclide technique to aid in localization of the active bleeding site. Meckel's scan remains clinically useful in the diagnosis of ectopic gastric mucosa.

Nonimaging studies of GI function date back to the

earliest days of nuclear medicine. For example, the Schilling test for vitamin B$_{12}$ malabsorption and diagnosis of pernicious anemia is still unchallenged. More recently, a new understanding of the infectious origin of gastritis and ulcer disease has led to a new therapy and diagnostic radiocarbon-14 (C-14) urea breath test performed to evaluate the effectiveness of antibiotic therapy for *Helicobacter pylori.*

## ESOPHAGEAL TRANSIT

The esophagus transports liquids and solids from the mouth to the stomach, clears regurgitated substances, and prevents tracheobronchial aspiration and acid reflux (Fig. 11-1). Dysphagia is the most common complaint of patients with abnormal esophageal motility. Esophageal motor disorders have been classified as primary (e.g., achalasia) or secondary (e.g., scleroderma) and by the

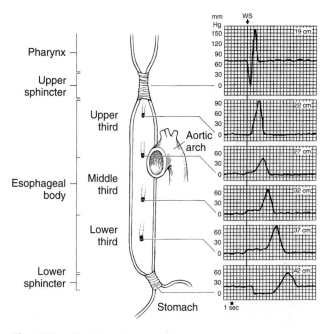

**Fig. 11-1** Esophageal anatomy and function. Swallowing initiates a coordinated peristaltic contraction that propagates down the esophagus. The esophagus is a posterior mediastinal structure with three distinct regions: (1) the upper esophageal sphincter (UES), which allows food to pass from the mouth to the esophagus and prevents tracheobronchial aspiration; (2) the esophageal body, with striated muscle proximally and smooth muscle distally, and the lower esophageal sphincter (LES); and (3) a high-pressure smooth muscle region that prevents gastric reflux but relaxes during swallowing to allow passage of food into the stomach. *Right,* Manometric pressure changes with a water swallow *(WS)* of an 8-ml bolus. Immediately after swallowing, UES pressure falls transiently. Shortly thereafter, LES pressure falls and remains low until the peristaltic contraction passes aborally through the UES and the esophageal body, which closes the LES.

degree of dysfunction (amotility, hypomotility, hypermotility) (Box 11-1).

*Barium radiography* can demonstrate anatomical lesions and mucosal changes and provides a qualitative assessment of motility. *Manometry* is the accepted reference standard for the diagnosis of motility disorders. It provides quantitative information on peristaltic contraction, sphincter pressure, and upper and lower esophageal sphincter (LES) relaxation, but it is invasive and technically demanding.

*Esophageal transit scintigraphy* provides functional information on esophageal motility. The radionuclide procedure is noninvasive, simple to perform, and quantitative, but its clinical role is still being defined. It is most often used to screen symptomatic patients and evaluate the effectiveness of therapy for esophageal motility disorders.

### Esophageal Motor Disorders

**Achalasia** Symptoms of achalasia include dysphagia, weight loss, nocturnal regurgitation, cough, and occasionally aspiration. The etiology is unknown. Achalasia is characterized by an absence of peristalsis in the distal two thirds of the esophagus, increased LES pressure, and incomplete sphincter relaxation with swallowing. Esophageal dilation and retention of food result.

The diagnosis is often confirmed by esophageal manometry. Radionuclide esophageal transit studies have a high sensitivity for diagnosing achalasia and can help determine the effectiveness of therapy.

**Box 11-1 Classification of Esophageal Motility Disorders**

**PRIMARY/SECONDARY**

Primary
  Achalasia
  Esophageal spasm
  Nutcracker esophagus
Secondary
  Scleroderma
  Diabetic enteropathy

**DEGREE OF MOTILITY**

Amotility
  Achalasia
  Scleroderma
Hypomotility
  Presbyesophagus
Hypermotility
  Diffuse spasm
  Nutcracker esophagus

**Diffuse esophageal spasm** Symptoms of esophageal spasm include intermittent chest pain and dysphagia, but with no demonstrable organic lesion. Symptoms result from abnormal nonperistaltic contractions of the esophageal body, as demonstrated by manometry or radiological studies.

**Nutcracker esophagus** This controversial syndrome entity is associated with noncardiac chest pain and normal radiographic studies. Nutcracker esophagus is defined by its manometric manifestations, which include high-amplitude, possibly prolonged peristaltic contractions.

**Scleroderma** A systemic connective tissue disease, scleroderma involves smooth muscle of the esophagus. Contrast radiography reveals a dilated, aperistaltic esophagus, with barium retention and gastroesophageal reflux (GER). Manometry can document the decreased or absent LES pressure and decreased amplitude of contrac-

*patulas GES ( late stricture 20 reflux)*

tions of esophageal smooth muscle. Scintigraphy shows the associated delayed transit.

**Other disorders** Esophageal smooth muscle disease is also seen in systemic lupus erythematosus and polymyositis. Striated muscle abnormalities occur with muscular dystrophy, myasthenia gravis, and myotonia dystrophica. Other diseases associated with abnormalities of esophageal motor function are *diabetes* and *alcoholism*. Esophagitis itself, particularly when severe, may result in disordered motility.

## Radiopharmaceutical

Esophageal transit scintigraphy is performed with technetium-99m (Tc-99m) sulfur colloid (300 μmCi), dispersed in a liquid bolus, usually water. Preliminary reports suggest that semisolid food boluses may be more sensitive than liquid boluses for detecting dysmotility. Transit is faster for less viscous materials, for small versus larger volumes, and in the upright versus the supine position.

## Dosimetry

Tc-99m sulfur colloid is used for studies of esophageal transit, GER, and gastric emptying. The dosimetry described applies to all three (Tables 11-1 and 11-2). The large intestine receives the highest radiation absorbed dose.

## Methodology

Box 11-2 describes a typical protocol. The numerous variations depend on the type of bolus, patient positioning, method of acquisition, and method of analysis.

**Table 11-1   Dosimetry for technetium-99m sulfur colloid gastroesophageal scintigraphy for children**

| Organ | Rad/100 μCi by age (usual dose, 200-500 μCi) | | | |
|---|---|---|---|---|
| | Newborn | 1 yr | 5 yr | 10 yr |
| Stomach | 0.383 | 0.093 | 0.050 | 0.031 |
| Small intestine | 0.372 | 0.164 | 0.090 | 0.058 |
| Large intestine | 0.927 | 0.380 | 0.194 | 0.120 |
| Ovaries | 0.099 | 0.042 | 0.033 | 0.072 |
| Testes | 0.018 | 0.007 | 0.003 | 0.011 |
| Whole body | 0.020 | 0.011 | 0.006 | 0.004 |

**Table 11-2   Adult dosimetry for esophageal and gastric scintigraphy**

| | Millirads/study meal, by organ | | | | | |
|---|---|---|---|---|---|---|
| | Stomach | Small intestine | Large intestine | Ovaries | Testes | Total body |
| **LIQUID** | | | | | | |
| 300 mCi Tc-99m sulfur colloid | 28 | 83 | 160 | 29 | 2 | 5 |
| 1 mCi Tc-99m DTPA | 93 | 280 | 520 | 98 | 5 | 20 |
| 250 μCi In-111 DTPA | 110 | 490 | 2000 | 420 | 27 | 60 |
| **SOLID** | | | | | | |
| 500 μCi Tc-99m sulfur colloid ovalbumin | 120 | 120 | 230 | 42 | 2 | 9 |
| 250 μCi In-111 chicken liver | 240 | 480 | 1900 | 400 | 28 | 58 |
| 500 μCi Tc-99m chicken liver | 120 | 120 | 230 | 42 | 2 | 9 |

*DTPA*, Diethylenetriamine pentaacetic acid, pentetic acid.

---

## Box 11-2   Technetium-99m Sulfur Colloid Esophageal Transit Imaging: Protocol Summary

**PATIENT PREPARATION**

Order an overnight fast.
Place radioactive marker on cricoid cartilage.
Position the patient supine.
Practice swallows with nonradioactive bolus.

**RADIOPHARMACEUTICAL**

Technetium-99m sulfur colloid, 300 μCi in 10 ml of water.

**INSTRUMENTATION**

Camera setup: Tc-99m photopeak with 20% window
Computer setup: 0.8-sec frame × 240; byte mode, 64 × 64

**SWALLOWING PROCEDURE**

Swallow Tc-99m sulfur colloid as a bolus.
Dry swallow at 30 sec, then radiolabeled bolus every 30 sec × 4.
No swallowing between boluses.

**PROCESSING**

Time-activity curves, condensed dynamic images

**QUANTITATION**

Time of 90% emptying
Transit time

---

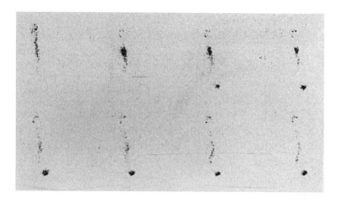

**Fig. 11-2**   Normal esophageal transit study. Images are obtained supine at 2-second intervals. Swallowed bolus travels rapidly through the upper esophagus. Transit time is 11 seconds (normal, 15 seconds).

---

The supine position is preferable because it eliminates the effect of gravity on esophageal emptying. Both anterior and posterior views have been used. Since gravity is the only mechanism of emptying in achalasia, the upright position may be preferable for serial quantitative studies in this disease. In contrast, emptying occurs in both the supine and the upright position in systemic sclerosis, a differential point.

Multiple swallows are often necessary for complete emptying even in normal subjects because of a 25% incidence of "aberrant" swallows, or extra swallows that occur between the two prescribed swallows. This results in inhibition of the initial swallow and a delay in transit. Any normal residual remaining after an initial swallow clears when followed by a dry swallow.

---

### Analysis and Quantification

Analog film images or computer cinematic displays are often adequate to diagnose severe abnormalities of motility (Figs. 11-2 and 11-3, *A*). Quantitative analysis, however, is advocated for diagnosing less severe abnormalities, evaluating the effectiveness of therapy, and comparing serial studies.

Esophageal transit can be quantified by calculating either the transit time or the residual activity in the esophagus (Fig. 11-3, *B*), as follows:

$$\text{Residual esophageal activity (\%)} = [(E_{max} - E_t)/E_{max}] \times 100$$

where $E_{max}$ is the maximum counting rate in the esophagus (15-second intervals), and $E_t$ is the counting rate after dry swallow number *t*. *Transit time* is the time from the initial entry of the bolus into the esophagus until all but 10% of peak activity clears (abnormal, longer than 15 seconds).

Pattern analysis and functional images can assist diagnosis. Time-activity curves (TACs) can be derived for the entire esophagus and for the proximal, middle, and distal thirds. Normally, peak activity is seen in sequence from proximal to distal, but this pattern is often lost in disease states (Fig. 11-4).

Functional images can be helpful for interpreting the many images acquired in a single transit study. Since craniocaudal transit, not lateral motion, is needed, the dynamic data can be condensed into a single image with one spatial (vertical) and one temporal dimension (Fig. 11-5). Characteristic disease patterns have been described (Fig. 11-6).

---

### Accuracy

Esophageal transit studies have a high sensitivity for the diagnosis of achalasia. They have a lower detection rate for other conditions, however, limiting their routine use as screening tests. The quantitative monitoring of a disease process over time and its response to pharmacological, medical, or surgical therapy is a common indication.

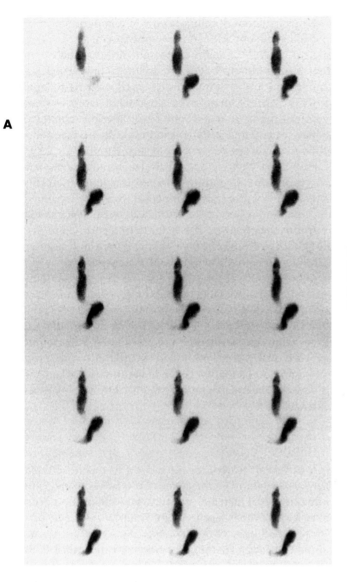

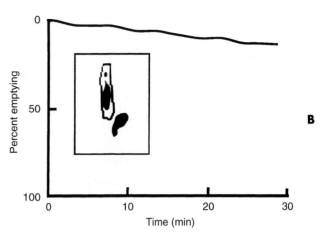

**Fig. 11-3**    Achalasia. **A,** Prominent stasis in the esophagus (1-minute images over 30 minutes). **B,** Quantitative analysis. Region of interest was drawn on computer for the entire esophagus, with resulting time-activity curve. Esophageal emptying over 30 minutes was only 12%.

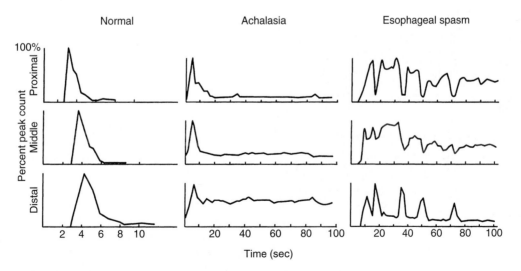

**Fig. 11-4**    Time-activity profiles: normal, achalasia, and esophageal spasm. Three regions of interest are the proximal, middle, and distal esophagus. *Left,* In the normal subject, the bolus proceeds sequentially from proximal to distal esophagus. *Middle,* In the patient with achalasia, retention is seen predominantly in the lower esophagus. *Right,* In the patient with diffuse spasm and uncoordinated contraction, the bolus shows poor progression through the esophagus.

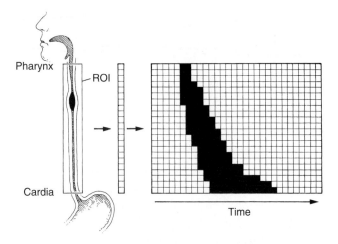

**Fig. 11-5**  Generation of condensed esophageal dynamic images. In each consecutive frame, the data in an esophageal region of interest *(ROI)* are compressed into a single column, displaying the distribution of the tracer from the pharynx to the proximal stomach for each 0.8-second interval. The columns are arranged consecutively, generating a space and time matrix, with vertical and horizontal dimensions representing spatial and temporal activity changes.

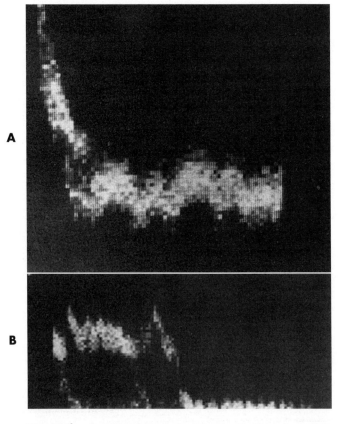

**Fig. 11-6**  Condensed dynamic images. **A,** Normal swallow. Uninterrupted transit of the bolus down the esophagus. **B,** Diffuse esophageal spasm. After the initial swallow, part of the bolus remains in the midesophagus as the remainder is transported to the stomach. A subsequent dry swallow propels the rest of the bolus into the stomach.

# GASTROESOPHAGEAL REFLUX

Symptomatic reflux of gastric contents into the esophagus is a common problem. Heartburn is the usual complaint. Serious complications of gastroesophageal reflux (GER) include esophagitis, bleeding, perforation, and stricture. Clinical presentation in infants and children differs considerably from that in adults. In addition to regurgitation, common pediatric symptoms include respiratory problems, iron deficiency anemia, and failure to thrive.

Reflux occurs in infants as a normal physiological event that usually resolves spontaneously by 7 to 8 months of age. Clinically important reflux often is evident by 2 months of age. Most children have a benign course and are symptom free by 18 months of age. However, approximately one third have persistent symptoms until age 4 and may have significant sequelae, including strictures and even death from inanition or recurrent pneumonia (5% to 10%).

The adequacy of esophageal clearance is important in determining whether GER becomes clinically evident. Delayed clearance increases the duration of mucosal exposure to refluxate. Other factors include the efficacy of the antireflux mechanism, the volume of gastric contents, the potency of refluxed material (acid, pepsin), mucosal resistance to injury, and mucosal reparative ability.

Although LES pressure is reduced in many patients with reflux, overlap exists between healthy and ill subjects. Reflux events can result from (1) a transient LES relaxation not associated with swallowing, (2) stress reflux caused by transient increases in intraabdominal pressure, or (3) free reflux across an atonic sphincter.

Although most patients with moderate to severe esophagitis have a sliding hiatus hernia, the majority of individuals with a hiatus hernia do not have reflux disease.

## Diagnostic Tests

A variety of tests have been used to diagnose GER. *Barium esophagography* can detect severe grades of reflux, mucosal damage, stricture, and tumor, but it has a low sensitivity for detecting reflux. *Endoscopy* provides a direct view of the esophageal mucosa and allows biopsy; however, histological evidence of esophagitis is not particularly sensitive for diagnosing reflux disease.

The *Bernstein acid infusion test* attempts to reproduce the patient's symptoms and confirm their esophageal origin by infusion of 0.1N hydrochloric acid into the distal esophagus. The *Tuttle acid reflux test* is considered the reference standard but is technically demanding. Reflux events are detected by positioning a pH electrode in the distal esophagus. An abrupt drop in esophageal pH (less than 4) is diagnostic of a reflux event. Detection of recurrent events requires clearance of the previous reflux event. Although reflux volume clears within seconds, acid clearance takes several minutes because neutralization by swallowed saliva is necessary.

The radionuclide method for detecting GER has the advantages of being sensitive, physiological, easily performed, well tolerated, and quantitative. It also results in a low radiation dose. The radionuclide GER study and pH monitoring measure different components of refluxate (volume versus acid concentration) and are influenced by different physiological events, such as meal ingestion, gastric emptying, and esophageal acid clearance. Whereas the pH probe cannot detect a second reflux event until acid has cleared the pH probe, the radionuclide study can detect reflux only while the radiolabeled meal remains in the stomach. As stomach volume decreases, reflux events also decrease.

## Methodology

The radionuclide GER study has generally been performed differently in adults and children (Box 11-3). The reason for this is primarily historical, probably without a clinical rationale today. The adult method was developed in a manner similar to the barium contrast study. The pediatric method is more physiological and sensitive for detection of GER.

## Image Interpretation

**Adults** All 30-second frames at each level of abdominal pressure are reviewed for evidence of reflux, using computer enhancement. Greater than 4% reflux of stomach contents into the esophagus is considered abnormal.

**Children** All frames should be reviewed with contrast enhancement. GER is seen as distinct spikes of activity into the esophagus (Fig. 11-7). Reflux events are graded as low level or high level (less or greater than midesophagus), by duration (e.g., less or more than 10 seconds), and by their temporal relationship to meal ingestion. Reflux events of longer duration increase the risk of esophagitis. Events that occur with small gastric volumes have more clinical significance because reflux is occurring without the effect of the increased pressure of a full meal volume and acid buffering.

TACs can be generated and regions of interest (ROIs) drawn for the oropharynx, esophagus, and stomach. A variety of quantitative indices have been used in both adult and pediatric populations (Box 11-4). Peaks greater than 5% generally correspond to reflux. The gastric emptying portion of the study can be quantified by drawing a stomach ROI on computer for the initial

---

### Box 11-3  Gastroesophageal Reflux: Protocol Summaries

**ADULT**
**Patient Preparation**

Order an overnight fast.

**Imaging Procedure**

Patient ingests 150 ml of orange juice, 150 ml of 0.1N HCl, and 300 µCi of Tc-99m sulfur colloid.

Obtain a 30-sec acquisition on computer to ensure that bolus transited the esophagus.

Position patient supine over a wide-field-of-view gamma camera.

Patient performs Valsalva maneuver; acquire a 30-sec image on computer.

Place abdominal binder below rib cage; attach sphygmomanometer to increase the pressure in 20 mm Hg increments from 0 to 100 mm Hg.

Obtain 30-sec images at each pressure gradient.

Calculate GER at each pressure step using the formula $R = (E_t - E_b) \times 100/G_0$, where $R$ is % GER, $E_t$ is esophageal counts at time $t$, $E_b$ is esophageal background counts, and $G_0$ is gastric counts at the start of the study. A value greater than 4% is considered abnormal.

**CHILDREN**
**Patient Preparation**

Order an overnight fast.

**Computer Setup**

Framing rate of 5 to 10 sec/frame for 60 min

**Radiopharmaceutical**

Tc-99m SC, 0.1 to 1 mCi (5 µCi/ml)

**Imaging Procedure**

*Optional:* Esophageal transit study may be performed initially or at end of the study. Give 250 µCi Tc-99m serum colloid in 10 ml of sterile water as bolus through feeding tube placed in the posterior pharynx. Once transit study is completed, the remaining meal volume can be fed.

Feed infant meal that approximates its normal feeding (formula or milk).

After burping infant, place supine with gamma camera positioned posteriorly and the chest and upper abdomen in the field of view. *Abdominal compression is not used because it is considered nonphysiological, is poorly tolerated in infants, and does not increase the detection rate.*

Acquire 2- to 4-hr delayed images of chest. Review for aspiration with computer enhancement.

Calculate reflux.

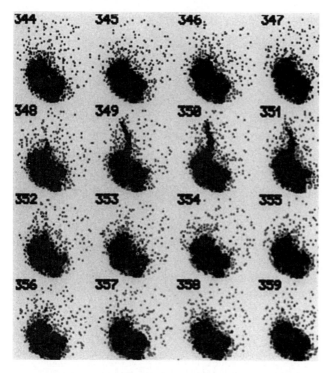

**Fig. 11-7** Gastroesophageal reflux. Sequential 5-second frames show episode of high-grade reflux over 15 seconds.

---

**Box 11-4    Methods Used for Quantifying Gastroesophageal Reflux in Children**

Mean value of the esophageal time-activity curve as a percentage of the initial gastric activity

Reflux index, derived by integrating esophageal TAC over 60 min and dividing by initial gastric activity

Percent activity relative to gastric activity in a specified episode multiplied by duration of the episode

Number of episodes of high-level and low-level reflux and their duration

---

1-hour and 2-hour images and is usually expressed as the percent emptying.

"True" normal values for children are not available because truly normal infants have not been studied. However, 40% to 50% emptying of milk at 1 hour and 60% to 75% at 2 hours is generally considered normal. The 2-hour emptying is more reliable.

Pulmonary aspiration should be looked for carefully, and computer enhancement is essential; however, aspiration is detected infrequently. The *salivagram* is a more sensitive method of detecting aspiration than the reflux study (Fig. 11-8). The salivagram is essentially an esophageal transit study and is performed by placing a labeled bolus of radiotracer in the infant's posterior pharynx and using a rapid acquisition framing rate for imaging the swallow.

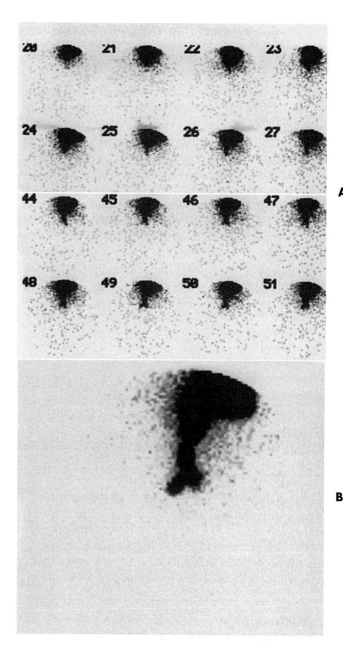

**Fig. 11-8** Salivagram: diagnosis of aspiration. Neonate with neurological deficits and swallowing difficulties with gastroesophageal reflux and aspiration. GER (milk) study performed after feeding by nasogastric tube showed numerous reflux events, but no aspiration. **A,** Salivagram was performed later. After radiotracer was placed in the posterior pharynx, sequential 5-second frames showed transit into the tracheal bifurcation and no evidence of esophageal activity. **B,** High-count image at the end of 60 minutes. Radiotracer remains at the tracheal bifurcation.

---

### Accuracy

**Adults**  Although the sensitivity of GER scintigraphy may be as high as 90%, a lower sensitivity of 60% to 70% is reported. Because of gastroenterologists' perception that this test is not very sensitive and because of competing modalities, scintigraphy is not often used in adults. The poor sensitivity in some studies may result from differences in methodology for adults and children, such as the longer framing rate and the nonphysiological method of relying on external pressure.

**Children** Pediatricians generally consider scintigraphy a useful noninvasive method for confirming the diagnosis of GER in children and determining its severity. The sensitivity is very high, 75% to 100%. Scintigraphy is more sensitive than barium studies or manometry. The gold standard is still pH monitoring. The best sensitivity is achieved by using a combination of scintigraphy, pH monitoring, and manometry.

The detection of aspiration with reflux studies is low, none to 25%. However, the salivagram can often demonstrate aspiration when the GER study is negative.

## GASTRIC MOTILITY

A variety of nonradionuclide techniques have been used for evaluating gastric function, but all have serious limitations. Gastric intubation methods require serial aspiration. Marker-dilution techniques with duodenal recovery are cumbersome and disliked by patients, and the tubing may alter emptying. Radiographic contrast methods can define anatomy and show gross mechanical obstruction but are insensitive to motor disturbances of the stomach and cannot provide quantitative information on emptying.

Radionuclide gastric emptying studies have become the standard method for evaluating gastric motility because the technique is accurate, sensitive, quantitative, and relatively easy to perform.

### Physiology

The stomach is composed of two functionally distinct regions (Fig. 11-9). The proximal stomach, or *fundus,* serves as a reservoir and accepts large fluid volumes with only minimal increases in pressure (receptive relaxation). Regular, slow, tonic muscular contractions produce a pressure gradient between the stomach and duodenum, moving the stomach contents toward the distal stomach. Liquid emptying is accomplished primarily through this fundal mechanism. Liquid emptying is volume dependent and occurs exponentially, that is, the larger the volume, the more rapid the emptying (Fig. 11-10). Nutrients, salts, and acidity all slow the rate of liquid emptying.

The distal stomach, or *antrum,* is responsible for the grinding and sieving of solid food and controls the rate of emptying into the duodenum. After ingestion of solid food, muscular contractions sweep down the antrum in a ringlike pattern, squeezing the food toward the pylorus. Large food particles are not allowed to pass and are retropelled back toward the antrum. The food particles become progressively ground up, and this

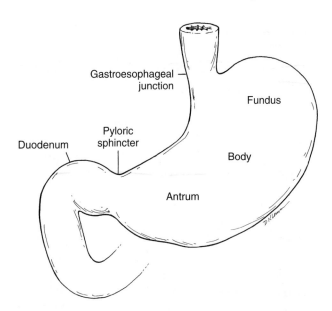

**Fig. 11-9** Gastric anatomy and function. The proximal stomach (fundus) accommodates and stores food. The distal stomach (antrum) acts as a preparatory chamber where mixing and grinding of food occur.

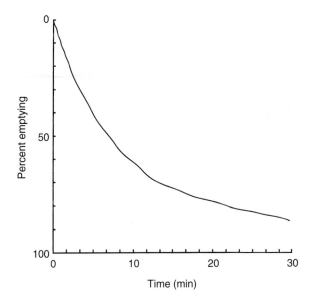

**Fig. 11-10** Liquid-only gastric emptying. The patient ingested 300 ml of water with Tc-99m sulfur colloid, and 1-minute frames were acquired for 30 minutes. A time-activity curve was generated by drawing a whole stomach region of interest on computer. Emptying began immediately, and the clearance curve pattern was exponential. Normal half-emptying time is less than 20 minutes.

chyme mixture eventually is able to pass through the pyloric sphincter (1- to 2-mm particles).

The time required for grinding food into small particles before emptying is the *lag phase*. Solid emptying occurs at a constant, usually linear manner (Fig. 11-11). The rate of emptying depends on the size and contents of the meal. Fat, acid, protein, and high-osmolality foods all act to slow solid emptying (Box 11-5).

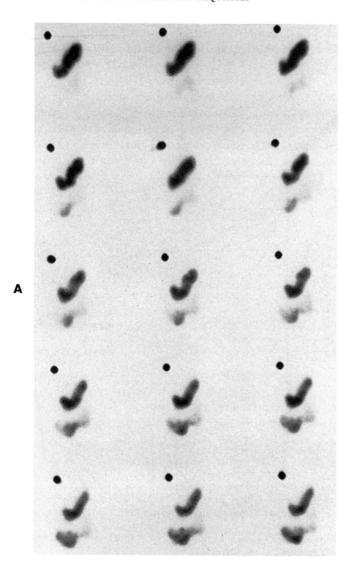

A

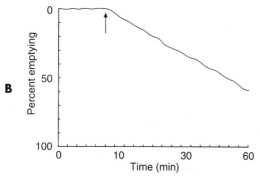

B

**Box 11-5    Factors That Affect Gastric Emptying Results**

**PHYSIOLOGICAL**

Meal content
    Fat, protein, acid, osmolality
    Volume
    Weight
    Caloric density
    Particle size
Time of day
Patient position (standing, sitting, supine)
Gender
Metabolic state
Stress
Drugs

**TECHNICAL**

Radioisotope decay
Attenuation and correction method
Single-isotope versus dual-isotope study
Scatter and septal penetration
Single-head versus dual-head camera
Frequent versus infrequent image acquisition
Method of quantification

In the fasting state between meals, so-called phase III interdigestive contractions empty nondigestible debris from the stomach. These forceful, lumen-obliterating peristaltic waves sweep the gastric contents through the pylorus. *Motilin,* a peptide hormone secreted by the upper small bowel mucosa, is responsible for this interdigestive contraction.

Gastric motility is modulated by sympathetic and parasympathetic neural innervation, as well as by a variety of hormones with complex interactions.

### Stasis Syndromes

Mechanical causes of gastric stasis, such as obstruction by tumor or pyloric channel ulcer, must be excluded by endoscopy or contrast barium radiography. Functional causes of gastroparesis may occur with acute illnesses (e.g., viral gastroenteritis, metabolic derangement), but chronic stasis is a more common clinical problem with serious long-term consequences (Box 11-6).

Early satiety, bloating, nausea, and vomiting are common symptoms of gastric paresis. Although mild to moderate gastroparesis may be asymptomatic, ultimately symptoms become manifest. Rapid gastric emptying can also produce symptoms, at times severe, including palpitations, diaphoresis, weakness, and diarrhea *(dumping syndrome)* (Box 11-7).

**Fig. 11-11**    Solid gastric emptying. **A,** Normal progression of stomach contents during a radionuclide gastric emptying study, with 5-minute sequential images acquired for 60 minutes. Meal moves from the gastric fundus to the antrum in a normal emptying pattern. A radioactive marker has been placed in the right chest as a check for movement. **B,** Solid meal (egg sandwich) computer-generated time-activity curve in a different patient, with an initial delay of 25 minutes before emptying begins. The length of the lag phase *(arrow)* is 9 minutes (normal 5 to 25 minutes). A linear pattern of emptying follows. Greater than 50% emptying occurred by 90 minutes (normal, 40%).

## Box 11-6   Causes of Functional Gastric Stasis Syndromes

**ACUTE DYSFUNCTION**

Trauma
Postoperative ileus
Gastroenteritis
Hyperalimentation
Metabolic disorders: hyperglycemia, acidosis, hypokalemia, hypercalcemia, hepatic coma, myxedema
Physiological effects: labyrinth stimulation, physical and mental stress, gastric distention, increased intragastric pressure
Drugs: anticholinergics, antidepressants, nicotine, opiates, levodopa, progesterone, oral contraceptives, beta-adrenergic agonists, alcohol
Hormones: gastrin, secretin, glucagon, cholecystokinin, somatostatin, estrogen, progesterone

**CHRONIC DISEASES**

Diabetes mellitus
Hypothyroidism
Progressive systemic sclerosis
Systemic lupus erythematosus
Dermatomyositis
Myotonic dystrophy
Familial dysautonomia
Fabry's disease
Amyloidosis
Pernicious anemia
Anorexia nervosa
Bulbar poliomyelitis
Gastric ulcer
Postvagotomy (for obstruction) with or without pyloroplasty
Tumor-associated gastroparesis
Idiopathic

## Box 11-7   Causes of Rapid Gastric Emptying

Postoperative
   Pyloroplasty
   Hemigastrectomy (Billroth I, II)
Diseases
   Duodenal ulcer
   Gastrinoma (Zollinger-Ellison syndrome)
   Hyperthyroidism
Hormones
   Thyroxine
   Motilin
   Enterogastrone
Drugs
   Erythromycin

**Diabetic gastroparesis**  The most common clinical cause of chronic gastric stasis, diabetic gastroparesis usually occurs in patients with long-standing insulin-dependent diabetes. Although gastroparesis is thought to result from vagal damage as part of a generalized autonomic neuropathy, no morphological abnormality in the gastric wall or abdominal vagus has been identified.

In addition to producing disturbing symptoms, poor gastric emptying may make diabetic glucose control difficult, since timing of the insulin dose, food ingestion, and absorption is critical. On the other hand, delayed emptying in the diabetic patient may also be caused by uncontrolled hyperglycemia alone. The latter is reversible with good glucose control.

Because symptoms suggestive of gastric stasis in the diabetic patient are nonspecific and may be from other causes (e.g., infection, poor glucose control), gastric motility studies should be performed when the patient is under optimal diabetic control.

**Pharmacological therapy**  Various drugs have been used to treat chronic gastroparesis. The gastrokinetic properties of these drugs are mediated by different mechanisms.

*Metoclopramide* has both central and peripheral antidopaminergic properties; it also releases acetylcholine from the myenteric plexus. Neurological side effects (e.g., drowsiness, lassitude) occur in up to 20% of patients. Metoclopramide can also improve symptoms in some patients through a central antinausea effect without improving emptying.

*Domperidone* is a peripheral dopamine antagonist that penetrates the blood-brain barrier poorly and therefore rarely produces neurological side effects. *Cisapride* releases acetylcholine from the myenteric plexus. *Erythromycin* acts as an agonist of motilin. All these drugs improve gastric emptying by increasing the amplitude of antral contractions. A repeat study is necessary to determine if symptomatic improvement is indeed due to improved gastric emptying.

### Radiopharmaceuticals

For accurate quantification of solid gastric emptying, the radioactive marker must be tightly bound to the food. Elution of the radiolabel in vivo will result in a part-solid, part-liquid–labeled mixture that will produce an erroneously shortened solid emptying time, since liquids empty faster than solids.

A physiologically superb method for labeling chicken liver in vivo was described by early investigators and used on a clinical and research basis. It involves injecting Tc-99m sulfur colloid into the wing vein of a chicken; the chicken is killed and the liver removed and cooked. Tc-99m sulfur colloid is efficiently extracted by the Kupffer cells and becomes fixed intracellularly. This label is highly stable and does not dissociate after ingestion. The chicken liver is typically mixed with beef or chicken stew for palatability and volume. Although this method is of proven utility, it is not generally used, for obvious practical reasons.

Alternative acceptable in vitro methods of labeling liver have subsequently proved clinically useful. Cooking injected or surface-labeled liver cubes or liver paté traps the radionuclide within the meat. A more common meal used in the majority of nuclear medicine clinics today is eggs labeled with Tc-99m sulfur colloid. Frying the eggs with Tc-99m sulfur colloid results in very good binding to the egg albumin. Often administered as an egg sandwich, this semisolid meal is palatable to most patients and easy to prepare.

Good liquid-phase markers should equilibrate rapidly and be nonabsorbable. Tc-99m sulfur colloid in water meets these criteria and is most often used to evaluate liquid gastric emptying. Two-phase markers, one for the solid meal and another for the liquid phase, can be used. In these dual-isotope, solid-liquid studies, indium-111 diethylenetriame pentaacetic acid (In-111 DTPA) is often used as the liquid marker (171 and 247 keV) in combination with the Tc-99m sulfur colloid (140-keV) solid meal (Fig. 11-12).

## Methodology

No standard protocol exists for performing gastric emptying studies. Meal composition, patient positioning, instrumentation, data acquisition, and quantitative methods vary from laboratory to laboratory. Since all these factors affect the rate of emptying, no applicable normal values apply. Thus the test must be standardized in each laboratory (i.e., performed the same way, at the same time of day, with the same meal, instrumentation, and computer processing). Normal values must be determined in each clinic, or the clinician must closely follow a protocol in the medical literature and use its normal values.

Despite the variable methodologies, the radionuclide study is relatively straightforward. The patient ingests a

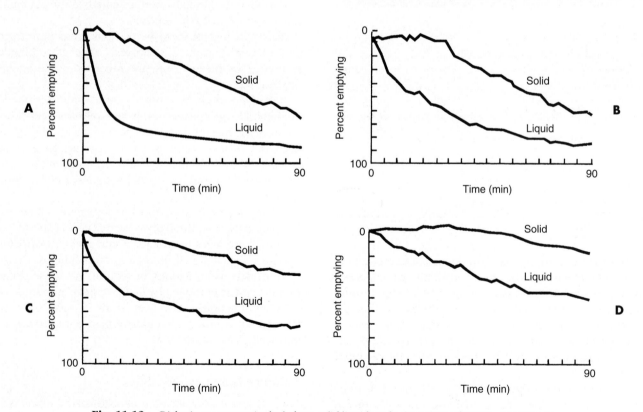

**Fig. 11-12**   Diabetic gastroparesis: dual-phase solid-liquid study. Spectrum of gastric emptying in the diabetic population. **A,** Normal subject. Linear solid emptying after a short lag phase and rapid exponential liquid emptying. **B,** Diabetic patient with normal solid and liquid emptying. **C,** Diabetic with delayed solid emptying but normal liquid emptying. **D,** Diabetic with delay in solid and liquid emptying.

radiolabeled meal and is placed supine under a gamma camera. The gastric emptying study is acquired on computer for a specified time (e.g., 90 to 120 minutes). It is then processed and quantified. Each laboratory must decide how best to perform the study using available instrumentation and software and considering various factors (Box 11-5).

**Meal**   The food content of the ingested meal is a primary factor affecting the rate of gastric emptying. Clear liquids empty faster than liquids with nutrients; liquids empty faster than semisolids, which empty faster than solids; and large meals empty faster than small meals. Increases in volume, weight, caloric density, and particle size all tend to slow the rate of gastric emptying. Therefore normal emptying values for a laboratory that uses labeled paté mixed with stew do not apply to a laboratory that uses a Tc-99m-labeled egg sandwich or even to a laboratory that uses a similar meal but a larger volume or different calorie content.

**Solid versus liquid**   The solid gastric emptying study is more sensitive than liquid emptying for detection of abnormal gastric emptying. Liquid emptying is always normal when solid emptying is normal. When solid emptying is delayed, liquid emptying may be normal or delayed, depending on the severity of the gastroparesis. A liquid-only study should be reserved for patients who cannot tolerate solids.

**Single versus dual isotope**   A dual-isotope study allows simultaneous evaluation of liquid and solid gastric emptying. Although dual-phase studies are useful for the investigation of gastric physiology and pharmacology, they add complexity, cost, and increased radiation exposure to the patient. The dual-isotope study has no added clinical benefit over a single-isotope solid emptying study.

**Study length**   Although ideally the clinician should continue to acquire a gastric emptying study until half-emptying occurs, a practical guideline for the busy clinic is to use a routine study length equal to the normal mean half-emptying time of the method being used. Large, difficult-to-digest meals (stew) empty slowly and may require 2½ to 3 hours for acquisition, whereas smaller, more easily digestible semisolid meals (egg) require a shorter study length, about 1½ hours. Decay correction should be routine.

**Attenuation correction**   The ingested meal moves from the gastric fundus, which is relatively posterior and lateral, to the gastric antrum, which is more anterior and medial. The posterior to anterior movement of the gastric contents results in variable attenuation and detection efficiency of the radioactivity by the gamma camera. A radiolabeled meal is detected with greatest efficiency when the stomach contents are close to the camera, that is, with the least amount of attenuating material between the camera and stomach.

In a study acquired with a single-headed gamma camera placed in the anterior view, the detected radioactive counts rise as the meal moves from the fundus to the antrum, even though the amount of food in the stomach is unchanged. This attenuation effect adversely affects the accuracy of quantification and can result in an underestimation of gastric emptying. The amount of error varies from patient to patient, depending on size and anatomy. This attenuation artifact is a particular problem in obese patients. The average error of gastric emptying quantitation resulting from attenuation is 10% to 15% but can be 30% to 50% in some individuals and is largely unpredictable.

*Geometric mean method*   The accepted gold standard in correcting for attenuation, the geometric mean (GM) method requires acquisition of opposed images, typically the anterior and posterior projections (Fig. 11-13). Mathematical correction for attenuation is then done by calculating the GM (square root of the product of the counts in the anterior and posterior views) at each data point. Ideally, both images are obtained simultaneously, which requires a dual-headed gamma camera. With a single-headed camera the two opposing views must be obtained sequentially.

*Left anterior oblique method*   An alternative method of attenuation compensation that requires only a single-headed gamma camera and allows frequent image acquisition is the left anterior oblique (LAO) method. When the study is acquired in this projection, the stomach contents move roughly parallel to the head of the gamma camera, minimizing the effect of attenuation.

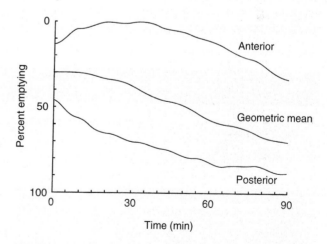

**Fig. 11-13**   Geometric mean (GM) attenuation correction. Anterior and posterior acquisition with GM correction. Both the anterior and the posterior views of the time-activity curve show the effect of attenuation. Anterior data have a rising time-activity curve before it begins to empty. Posterior view shows decreasing counts from time zero. GM corrects for this attenuation effect. Two-phase emptying is seen. Nearly flat early portion of the GM curve confirms good attenuation correction.

This method has the advantages of simple acquisition and no need for mathematical correction. Because of normal anatomical variation, this method is not as accurate in all patients as the GM method, but it is adequate for most clinical purposes and clearly superior to anterior view–only acquisition.

**Frequency of image acquisition**  With infrequent image acquisition, much of the qualitative and quantitative potential of radionuclide gastric emptying studies is lost. For example, solid emptying is biphasic. Delayed emptying may be the result of a prolonged lag phase, a decreased rate of emptying, or both. In addition, the more data points on the emptying TAC, the more accurate the quantification. If a study is acquired every 30 minutes for 2 hours, only five data points result. A lag phase of 15 minutes would be missed completely, and the calculated slope of the resulting emptying curve may be erroneous, depending on whether the first or the second data point was used as the start of emptying. Frequent image acquisition improves accuracy.

In the past, many institutions acquired images every 15, 20, or even 30 minutes. A major reason was difficulty in acquiring frequent images when sequential anterior and posterior images were acquired on a single-headed camera. At present, with dual-headed cameras and computer techniques for acquiring frequent images in the LAO view using a single-headed camera, as well as summed image-processing computer methods, there is no reason for infrequent image acquisition.

**Scatter correction**  With dual-isotope meals (e.g., In-111 and Tc-99m), correction for downscatter (In-111 into the Tc-99m window) and perhaps even upscatter may be necessary. Whether and how much correction is needed can be determined from a simulated phantom study. However, the error is inconsequential when the

dose ratio of Tc-99m/In-111 is at least 4 to 5:1. Again, this is not a factor in single-isotope studies used for clinical purposes.

## Analysis of Gastric Emptying

The method of processing depends to some extent on how the study is acquired (e.g., frequency of image acquisition, anterior and posterior views acquired sequentially or simultaneously). Generally, a gastric ROI is drawn on computer for individual or summed images. After correction for decay and attenuation, a TAC is generated and a parameter of gastric emptying calculated, such as the percent emptying at the end of the study, the half-time of emptying, or an emptying rate (%/min).

**Liquid emptying**  Clear liquids begin to empty immediately, with no lag phase. The computer-generated clearance curve is monoexponential, with a normal half-time of 10 to 20 minutes (Fig. 11-10). Liquids in a dual-phase meal also empty exponentially but considerably more slowly than a liquid-only meal. The emptying rate depends greatly on the type of solid-phase meal (Fig. 11-12).

**Solid emptying**  After an initial delay before emptying begins (lag phase), solid meals usually empty at a constant linear rate. The length of the lag phase is affected by the same factors that affect the rate of emptying.

The clinical importance of the lag phase is uncertain. Studies report that a prolonged lag phase is the cause of delayed emptying in certain diseases (e.g., diabetes, morbid obesity) and that the prokinetic effect of certain drugs (e.g., metoclopramide, erythromycin) improves emptying by shortening the lag phase. Data are limited

**Table 11-3  Gastric emptying protocols**

| | Single-headed camera (LAO method) | Dual-headed camera (geometric mean) |
|---|---|---|
| Preparation | Overnight fast | Overnight fast |
| Meal | Tc-99m sulfur colloid egg white sandwich, 200 ml water | Tc-99m sulfur colloid egg white sandwich, 200 ml water |
| Dose | Tc-99m sulfur colloid, 1 mCi | Tc-99m sulfur colloid, 1 mCi |
| Window | 15% 140 keV | 15% 140 keV |
| Patient position | Semiupright (60°) | Supine |
| Projections | LAO | Anterior and posterior simultaneously |
| Framing rate | 90 sec/frame for 90 min | 60 sec/frame for 90 min |
| Decay correct | Yes | Yes |
| Attenuation correction | LAO nonmathematical method | Geometric mean |
| Computer processing | ROI around summed gastric image | ROI around summed gastric image |
| Data presentation | TAC of counts versus time | TAC of anterior, posterior, and geometric mean counts versus time |
| Quantification | Percent emptying at 90 min | Percent emptying at 90 min |
| Abnormal* | Less than 35% | Less than 30% |

*LAO*, Left anterior oblique; *ROI*, region of interest; *TAC*, time-activity curve.
*Based on Georgetown University methodology and normal values.

and conflicting. For example, other studies have found both a prolonged lag phase and a slow rate of emptying in diabetes mellitus. Different methodologies most likely account for the difference in investigational results.

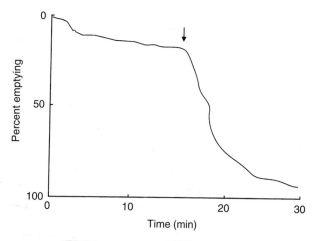

**Fig. 11-14** Metoclopramide intervention. Diabetic patient with very delayed liquid-only gastric emptying. Metoclopramide was infused at 17 minutes *(arrow)*. Prompt, rapid emptying ensued. This study predicts the clinical effectiveness of the drug in this patient.

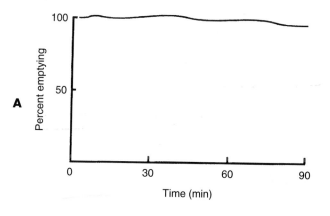

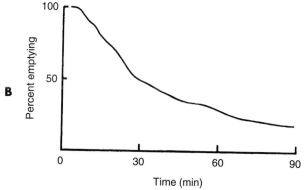

**Fig. 11-15** Pyloric obstruction. Patient with pyloric obstruction secondary to peptic ulcer disease. **A,** Preoperative study shows no gastric emptying. Partial gastrectomy was performed. **B,** Postoperative study shows a short lag phase and relatively rapid emptying.

Although the half-time of emptying has often been used to characterize the rate of solid emptying, it infers an exponential emptying pattern. Since solid emptying is usually linear, calculation of a linear rate of emptying is theoretically preferable (e.g., %/min). The percent gastric emptying at the end of the study is an acceptable alternative method, since it encompasses both the lag phase and the emptying rate.

The specific protocol therefore is determined by factors unique to each laboratory. Table 11-3 describes two typical protocols used at Georgetown University Hospital.

### Evaluation of Interventions

Pharmacological intervention can help predict the effectiveness of a particular therapy. For example, if poor emptying is noted during a gastric emptying study, metoclopramide can be administered intravenously. A change to a steeper emptying slope would demonstrate the anticipated response to the drug (Fig. 11-14). Alternatively, the study can be repeated after oral ingestion of the therapeutic drug, either after a single dose or preferably after several days or weeks of therapy. The effectiveness of various surgical therapies (e.g., gastroplasty, surgical relief of obstruction) can also be effectively evaluated (Fig. 11-15).

## *HELICOBACTER PYLORI* INFECTION

*Helicobacter pylori,* formerly called *Campylobacter pylori,* a gram-negative bacterium, infects the gastric mucosa of most patients with duodenal ulcer disease, gastric ulcer disease, and antral gastritis. *H. pylori* is the causal agent in most cases. Bacterial eradication greatly decreases duodenal ulcer recurrence rates, reverses histological gastritis, and promotes healing of active duodenal ulcers.

### Urea Breath Test

In the presence of the bacterial enzyme urease, orally administered urea is hydrolyzed to carbon dioxide ($CO_2$) and ammonia. If the urea carbon is labeled with either the stable isotope carbon-13 (C-13) or radioactive C-14, it can be detected in the breath as labeled $CO_2$. *H. pylori* is the most common urease-containing gastric pathogen, and therefore a positive urea breath test can be equated with *H. pylori* infection.

The urea breath test is now widely available. An analyzer is not needed, since the gas-filled balloon can be sent for breath analysis. This test is simple to perform, noninvasive, accurate, and inexpensive. False negative results occasionally occur because of the recent use of antibiotics or bismuth-containing medications. False positive results occur in patients with achlorhydria, contamination with oral urease-containing bacteria, and colonization with another *Helicobacter,* such as *H. felis.*

The urea breath test can be used as an alternative to gastric biopsy and as a method to determine the effectiveness of therapy against *H. pylori.* Whether C-13 or C-14 is used will probably depend on the institution's capabilities, the clinicians' interests, and the cost. Serological tests cannot determine the effectiveness of therapy because the antibody titer falls too slowly to be diagnostically useful.

## GASTROINTESTINAL BLEEDING

Effective and prompt therapy for acute GI bleeding depends on accurate localization of the site of hemorrhage. The history and clinical examination can often distinguish upper from lower tract bleeding. Upper tract hemorrhage can be confirmed with gastric intubation and localized with flexible fiberoptic endoscopy. Lower GI bleeding is more problematic. During active hemorrhage, endoscopy and barium radiography are of limited value in the small bowel and colon.

### Angiography

Angiography can be diagnostic but will demonstrate the bleeding site only if the contrast agent is injected during active hemorrhage. Bleeding is typically intermittent, however, and the clinical determination of whether the patient is actively bleeding can be difficult. The clinical signs of active bleeding often develop after the hemorrhage has ceased.

Since repeated angiographic studies are not practical, often the angiographer requests that a radionuclide GI bleeding study be performed before angiography. First, the radionuclide study ensures that the patient is still actively bleeding. Second, the study localizes the bleeding site so that the angiographer can infuse the contrast into the appropriate artery; this limits the duration of the study and the amount of contrast agent used.

### Radionuclide Methods

In 1977, Alavi and associates first described scintigraphic imaging of active GI bleeding using Tc-99m sulfur colloid. In 1979, Winzelberg et al. described the use of Tc-99m-labeled red blood cells (RBCs) for the same purpose.

**Technetium-99m sulfur colloid scintigraphy**    After injection, Tc-99m sulfur colloid is rapidly extracted by the reticuloendothelial cells of the liver, spleen, and bone marrow (3-minute serum half-life). By 15 minutes after injection most of the radiopharmaceutical is cleared from the vascular system. During active bleeding, radio-

tracer extravasates at the bleeding site into the bowel lumen, increasing with each recirculation of blood. Continued extravasation with simultaneous background clearance results in a high target-to-background ratio, permitting visualization of the intraabdominal active bleeding site (Fig. 11-16).

*Methodology*    The Alavi method requires the intravenous injection of 10 mCi of freshly prepared Tc-99m sulfur colloid and acquisition of serial 500k to 750k count images of the abdomen and pelvis every 1 to 2 minutes for 20 to 30 minutes (Box 11-8).

*Image interpretation*    Rapid bleeding may be detected on the 1 sec/frame blood flow images. Vascular blushes of tumors, angiodysplasia, and arteriovenous malformations may be seen in the absence of active bleeding. Active hemorrhage is most often detected in the first 5 to 10 minutes of imaging on the static high-count images. The site of bleeding is seen as a focal

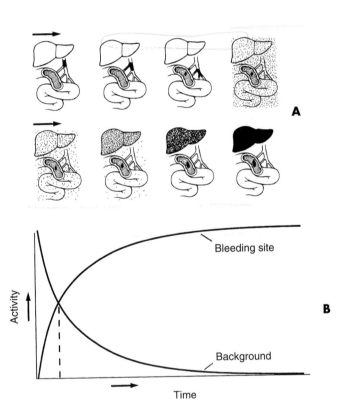

**Fig. 11-16**    Technetium-99m sulfur colloid scintigraphy for diagnosing acute gastrointestinal bleeding. **A,** After injection, Tc-99m sulfur colloid is cleared by the reticuloenthelial system, with a short serum half-life of 3 minutes. By 15 minutes most is cleared from the vascular system. With active bleeding a fraction of the injected radiotracer will extravasate at the site of bleeding; this recurs with each recirculation. Because of rapid background clearance, a high-contrast image of acute bleeding can be produced. **B,** Time-activity curves demonstrate rapid exponential clearance of background and inversely increasing activity at the bleeding site. Contrast improves as the target-to-background ratio increases with time.

area of radiotracer accumulation that increases in intensity and moves through the GI tract (Fig. 11-17).

Because blood acts as an intestinal irritant, intestinal transit can be rapid and even bidirectional. A fixed region of radiotracer accumulation most likely represents Tc-99m sulfur colloid uptake (e.g., ectopic spleen, renal transplants) rather than intraluminal hemorrhage. Asymmetrical bone marrow uptake can be misleading, since marrow replacement by tumor, infarction, or fibrosis may make the adjacent marrow appear as focal uptake and suggest a bleeding site. The critical diagnostic point is that this region of tracer accumulation is fixed and does not move. When the initial study is negative but active bleeding is suspected clinically, a repeat injection is indicated.

Detection of bleeding in the region of the splenic

flexure or transverse colon can sometimes be difficult because of normal liver and spleen uptake. Flow images, frequent repeated static images, and rapid movement of intraluminal contents may allow identification of the bleeding site. As in angiography, a major disadvantage of the Tc-99m sulfur colloid method is that bleeding must be active at injection.

**Technetium-99m red blood cell scintigraphy** Since GI bleeding is intermittent, Tc-99m-labeled RBCs have a major advantage over Tc-99m sulfur colloid for localizing the site of bleeding. If active bleeding is not detected on initial imaging, which normally lasts 60 to 90 minutes, delayed imaging can be performed. The length of the study depends only on the physical half-life of Tc-99m and the stability of the radiolabel. Imaging at 2 to 6 hours after injection is done, and imaging up to 24 hours is possible.

*Labeling techniques* A high labeling efficiency is important for proper interpretation of the Tc-99m RBC bleeding study. Free unbound Tc-99m pertechnetate is taken up by the salivary glands and gastric mucosa and then secreted into the GI tract, potentially complicating interpretation of the study. Various labeling techniques (in vivo, modified in vivo, in vitro) with different

---

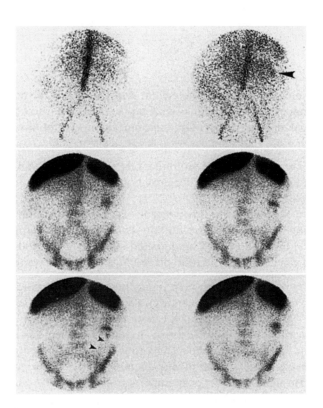

**Fig. 11-17**   Technetium-99m sulfur colloid study of bleeding site in descending colon. *Top,* Two sequential 3-second flow images; the second flow image indicates the site of bleeding *(large arrowhead)*. *Middle* and *bottom,* Four sequential 5-minute images showing the site of bleeding. Lower two images show movement to the more distal left colon *(small arrowheads)*.

## Box 11-9  Methods of Technetium-99m Red Blood Cell Labeling

**IN VIVO METHOD**

(labeling efficiency, 75% to 80%)
1. Inject stannous pyrophosphate.
2. Wait 10 to 20 min.
3. Inject Tc-99m sodium pertechnetate.

**MODIFIED IN VIVO (IN VITRO) METHOD**

(labeling efficiency, 85% to 90%)
1. Inject stannous pyrophosphate.
2. Wait 10 to 20 min.
3. Withdraw 5 to 8 ml of blood into shielded syringe with technetium-99m.
4. Gently mix syringe contents for 10 min at room temperature.

**IN VITRO (BROOKHAVEN) METHOD**

(labeling efficiency, 98%)
1. Add 4 ml of heparinized blood to reagent vial of 2 mg $Sn^{+2}$, 3.67 mg Na citrate, 5.5 mg dextrose, and 0.11 mg NaCl.
2. Incubate at room temperature for 5 min.
3. Add 2 ml of 4.4% EDTA.
4. Centrifuge tube for 5 min at 1300 *g*.
5. Withdraw 1.25 ml of packed RBCs and transfer to sterile vial containing 1 to 3 ml of Tc-99m.
6. Incubate at room temperature for 10 min.

**IN VITRO COMMERCIAL KIT**

(labeling efficiency, 98%)
1. Add 1 to 3 ml of blood (heparin or acid citrate dextrose as anticoagulant) to reagent vial (50 to 100 µg stannous chloride, 3.67 mg Na citrate) and mix. Allow 5 min to react.
2. Add syringe 1 contents (0.6 mg sodium hypochlorite) and mix by inverting four or five times.
3. Add contents of syringe 2 (8.7 mg citric acid, 32.5 mg Na citrate, dextrose) and mix.
4. Add 370 to 3700 MBq (10 to 100 mCi) of Tc-99m to reaction vial.
5. Mix and allow to react for 20 min, with occasional mixing.

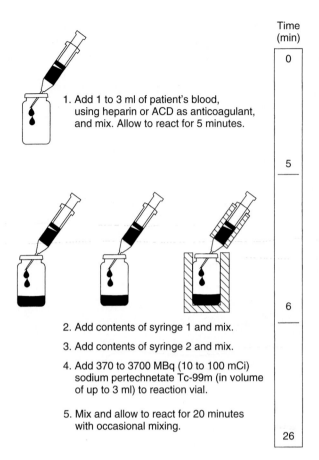

1. Add 1 to 3 ml of patient's blood, using heparin or ACD as anticoagulant, and mix. Allow to react for 5 minutes.

2. Add contents of syringe 1 and mix.

3. Add contents of syringe 2 and mix.

4. Add 370 to 3700 MBq (10 to 100 mCi) sodium pertechnetate Tc-99m (in volume of up to 3 ml) to reaction vial.

5. Mix and allow to react for 20 minutes with occasional mixing.

**Fig. 11-18**  Kit technique for labeling technetium-99m red blood cells in vitro (UltraTag RBC, Mallinckrodt, St. Louis). Each kit consists of three nonradioactive components: a 10-ml vial containing stannous chloride; syringe 1, containing sodium hypochlorite; and syringe 2, containing citric acid, sodium citrate, and dextrose *(ACD)*. Typical labeling efficiency is 98%.

labeling efficiencies have been used (Box 11-9). An in vitro method is clearly preferable because of its superior labeling efficiency (greater than 98%).

A simple kit technique for labeling RBCs in vitro is commercially available (Fig. 11-18). This method uses whole blood and does not require centrifugation or transfer of RBCs. The in vivo and modified in vivo method depended on biological clearance of undesirable extracellularly reduced stannous ion; the original in vitro method removed it by centrifugation. However, the in vitro kit method prevents extracellular reduction of stannous ion by adding an oxidizing agent (sodium hypochlorite), which cannot enter the RBCs.

*Methodology*  An initial flow study may be helpful for a Tc-99m-labeled RBC study (Box 11-10). Frequent image acquisition (1-minute frames) on computer allows a cinematic mode. Initial study duration is usually 60 to 90 minutes. If negative, a 30-minute acquisition can be repeated (e.g., at 2, 4, or 6 hours and up to 24).

*Image interpretation*  The flow phase can be helpful for detecting the site of bleeding even if the bleeding is not active. For example, a vascular blush may be seen with angiodysplasia or tumors (Fig. 11-19). In addition, vascular structures can be defined (e.g., kidneys, ectatic vessels, uterus) to help interpret images later. The radionuclide angiogram also occasionally detects a site of active bleeding that is difficult to see on later dynamic imaging, such as adjacent to the bladder.

Active bleeding is most often diagnosed by review of the sequential images obtained during the first 90 minutes of the study (Figs. 11-20 and 11-21). Approximately 75% of bleeding site localizations are made during the initial imaging time.

## Box 11-10  Technetium-99m Red Blood Cell Scintigraphy: Protocol Summary

**PATIENT PREPARATION**

None

**RADIOPHARMACEUTICAL**

Tc-99m labeled RBCs

**INSTRUMENTATION**

Camera: Large-field-of-view gamma.

Collimator: high resolution, parallel hole.

Computer setup: 1-sec frames for 60 sec; 1-min frames for 60 to 90 min.

If needed: 2-4-hr delayed image sequence as 1-min frames for 20 to 30 min.

Static images: 2- to 3-sec flow images and 1000k count images every 2 to 5 min.

Set intensity so that aorta, inferior vena cava, and iliac vessels are well visualized.

**PATIENT POSITION**

Supine; anterior imaging, with abdomen and pelvis in field of view.

**IMAGING PROCEDURE**

Inject patient's Tc-99m-labeled RBCs intravenously.

Acquire flow images, followed by static images for 60 to 90 min.

If study is negative or bleeding is recurrent, repeat 30-min acquisition.

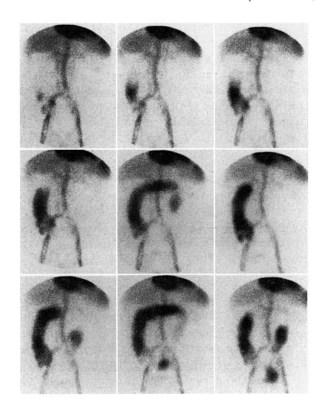

**Fig. 11-20**  Hepatic flexure bleeding. The active bleeding transits a low-lying transverse colon and then enters the left colon by the end of the 60-minute study. A tortuous aorta is noted. The source of bleeding in this elderly patient was cancer of the colon.

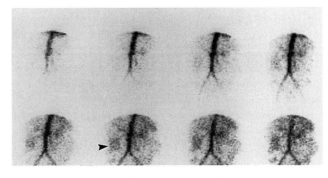

**Fig. 11-19**  Positive flow study for source of bleeding. Study shows increased flow to a circumscribed area in the region of the hepatic flexure *(arrowhead)*. Routine technetium-99m red blood cell study was negative after 90 minutes of acquisition and after a second acquisition for 30 minutes at 3 hours. Colonoscopy with biopsy was used to diagnose colon cancer in the region of interest.

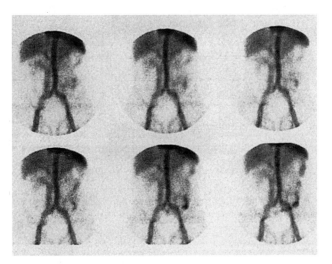

**Fig. 11-21**  Left colonic bleeding. Dynamic images acquired over 60 minutes show increasing activity in the region of the sigmoid colon that moves distally.

DIAGNOSTIC CRITERIA  Since the clinician refers the patient to determine the site of bleeding, it is not sufficient to interpret the study as positive for bleeding, which was already known. The study might be considered an expensive alternative to a stool guiac study. Specific criteria should be used to diagnose the site of bleeding (Box 11-11). The extravascular activity must be intraluminal, and the focus must be increasing over time. An important criterion: movement must be seen through the GI tract. Activity that is not moving should not be diagnosed as an active bleeding site and usually results from a fixed vascular struc-

---

**Box 11-11  Criteria for Positive Technetium-99m Red Blood Cell Scintigraphy**

"Hot spot" appears and conforms to intestinal anatomy.
Abnormal activity increases over time.
Abnormal activity moves antegrade or retrograde through bowel (essential criterion).

---

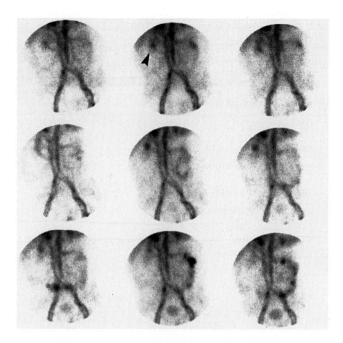

**Fig. 11-23**  Duodenal bleeding and small bowel transit. The bleeding source *(arrowhead)* is in the region of the duodenum, and sequential images show transit through the small intestines.

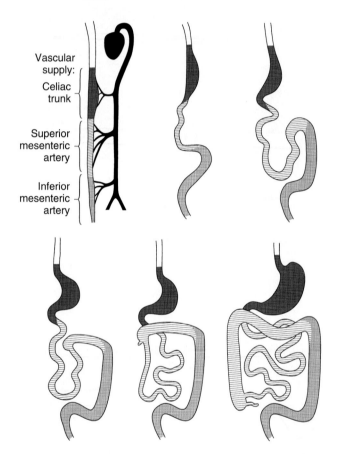

**Fig. 11-22**  Vascular supply of gastrointestinal tract. The embryological development of the gastrointestinal tract explains both its anatomical configuration and its vascular supply. An understanding of this schematic diagram is helpful for following the transit of radiolabeled red blood cells through the bowel and determining the bleeding site's origin and vascular supply (celiac, superior mesenteric, and inferior mesenteric arteries), which is ultimately what the angiographer needs to know.

ture (e.g., hemangioma, accessory spleen, ectopic kidney).

Because of scintigraphic limitations in anatomical localization of the bleeding site, clinicians generally refer to the general region, such as the hepatic flexure, transverse colon, splenic flexure, and rectosigmoid. This is usually sufficient for the angiographer to determine which vessel to inject with contrast, such as the superior mesenteric, inferior mesenteric, or celiac artery. Carefully noting GI transit of the radioactivity is critical for determining the anatomical bleeding site. An understanding of GI vascular anatomy and its embryological development is helpful in pinpointing the vascular bed for the angiographer (Fig. 11-22).

Frequent image acquisition can be important for localizing the site of bleeding because hemorrhage may be rapid and may move both antegrade and retrograde. Although the bleeding site can often be identified by viewing static images acquired every 5 to 10 minutes, review of 1-minute dynamic frames displayed on computer in a cinematic mode is most helpful in confirming and better defining the site of bleeding.

Localization of the site of bleeding to the small intestine may be difficult (Fig. 11-23). The cecum is often the site for pooling of more proximal small bowel bleeding, but the original source (duodenum, jejunum, ileum) is not always certain. Glucagon has been advocated to assist in the diagnosis of small bowel bleeding. After injection, bowel peristalsis is inhibited, resulting in pooling of the radiotracer in the small bowel at the site of active bleeding.

PITFALLS  Some interpretive pitfalls may lead to misinterpretation (Box 11-12). Pitfalls are normal, pathological, or technical findings that can usually be distinguished from active hemorrhage if the potential problems are known. A normal anatomical pitfall is focal activity in the genitourinary tract, the most common

## Box 11-12  Pitfalls in Interpretation of Technetium-99m Red Blood Cell Scintigraphy

**PHYSIOLOGICAL**
**Common**

Gastrointestinal (free technetium-99m pertechnetate)
Stomach, small and large intestine
Genitourinary
Pelvic kidney
Ectopic kidney
Renal pelvic activity
Ureter
Bladder
Uterine blush
Penis

**Uncommon**

Accessory spleen
Hepatic hemangioma
Varices, esophageal and gastric

**RARE**
**Vascular**

Abdominal aortic aneurysm
Gastroduodenal artery aneurysm
Abdominal varices
Caput medusae and dilated mesenteric veins
Gallbladder varices
Pseudoaneurysm
Hemobilia from false hepatic artery aneurysm
Arterial grafts
Cutaneous hemangioma
Duodenal telangiectasia
Angiodysplasia

**Miscellaneous**

Gallbladder (heme products)
Gluteal hematoma
Nonhemorrhagic gastritis
Factitious gastrointestinal bleeding

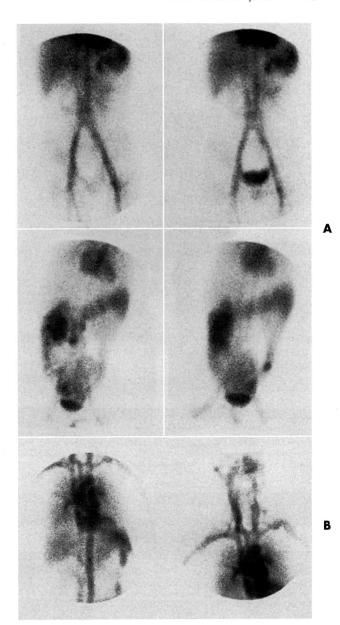

**Fig. 11-24** Hemorrhagic gastritis versus free technetium-99m pertechnetate. Hemorrhagic gastritis may occasionally be diagnosed with a labeled–red blood cell study; however, evidence of free pertechnetate should be vigorously sought. **A,** Images obtained at 10, 20, 60, and 90 minutes show prominent gastric uptake at 10 and 20 minutes. On the later images, however, gastric activity is no longer present and activity has transited to the colon. **B,** Images of the neck show no thyroid or salivary activity, which rules against free Tc-99m pertechnetate. Endoscopy confirmed hemorrhagic gastritis.

cause of a false positive study. A pathological pitfall is abdominal varices.

A technical pitfall is the presence of free Tc-99m pertechnetate because of poor radiolabeling. Free Tc-99m pertechnetate can be particularly troublesome because gastric uptake may simulate gastric bleeding or delayed images may suggest more distal bleeding (Fig. 11-24, *A*). Images of the thyroid and salivary glands are helpful in excluding free Tc-99m pertechnetate as a source of gastric activity (Figs. 11-24, *B*, and 11-25). Free Tc-99m pertechnetate is now a less common problem with the availability of the in vitro kit for labeling erythrocytes.

Although upper tract bleeding should be detected clinically by aspiration through a nasogastric tube placed in the stomach before scintigraphy, this does not always happen. Upper GI bleeding can be diagnosed with radiolabeled RBCs, but normal uptake in the liver, heart, and spleen sometimes makes interpretation difficult (Fig. 11-23).

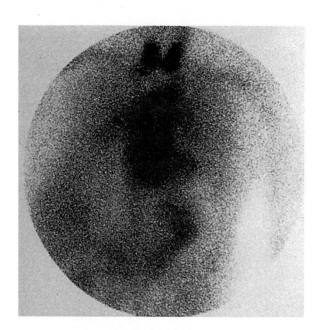

**Fig. 11-25** Free technetium-99m pertechnetate. In contrast to Fig. 11-24, there is not only gastric but also thyroid uptake. Poor target-to-background ratio results from free Tc-99m pertechnetate.

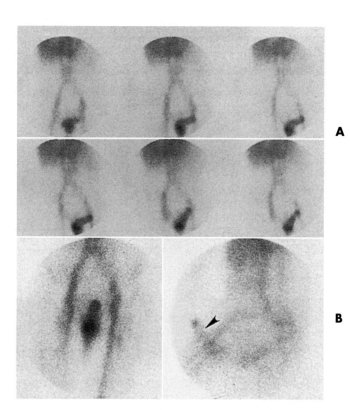

**Fig. 11-26** False positive gastrointestinal bleeding study. **A,** Images acquired every 10 minutes over 1 hour show changing, increasing activity in the lower left and middle pelvis. **B,** Anterior *(left)* and left lateral *(right)* images acquired 90 minutes after tracer injection show the activity to be the penile blood pool *(arrowhead).* Not recognizing a potentially false positive study can be serious and embarrassing. Left lateral views should be obtained whenever pelvic activity is seen with separate rectal, bladder, and penile activity.

A serious pitfall is the misinterpretation of activity seen in the lower pelvis. The differential diagnosis should include rectal hemorrhage, bladder activity from free Tc-99m pertechnetate, uterus, and penis. A left lateral view is mandatory to make the differentiation (Fig. 11-26).

Intraluminal radioactivity first detected on delayed images can be a diagnostic dilemma. Blood first seen in the sigmoid colon or rectum on a single delayed image obtained at 12 to 24 hours may have originated from anywhere in the GI tract and could even be caused by the transit of free Tc-99m pertechnetate from the stomach. Misinterpretation of this isolated finding can be avoided by acquiring dynamic 1-minute images whenever delayed imaging is performed. An active bleeding site can be diagnosed only by using the criteria described earlier.

**Accuracy** Experimental animal studies show that bleeding rates as low as 0.05 to 0.1 ml/min can be detected. Only 2 to 3 ml of extravasated blood is necessary for detection. This compares favorably with the ability of contrast angiography to detect bleeding rates of about 1 ml/min or greater, a 10-fold difference.

Early investigations showed high accuracy for the radionuclide method, but subsequent studies have not found the study helpful. The clinical community is divided on the utility of GI bleeding studies. Many reasons

exist for differences in the literature. The scientific validity of many studies is difficult to judge because no good gold standard exists. Not all patients have angiography, which may be negative because of the intermittent nature of bleeding. Barium enema or endoscopy may locate a pathological condition, but with no active bleeding, proving that this is the site of bleeding is difficult. The persistence of the imagers also plays a role.

Another important variable is how soon after arrival at the emergency room or admission the study is ordered. The earlier that imaging commences, the greater the likelihood of detecting the bleeding site. At some institutions radionuclide imaging is done only after every other method of diagnosis has been unsuccessful. The patient is sometimes admitted and stabilized so that endoscopy can be performed the next day, followed by barium enema if negative. By the time the radionuclide study is done, bleeding has long stopped, and the study is deemed unhelpful. Being available when needed and having good communication with referring physicians are critical.

**Table 11-4    Comparison of technetium-99m sulfur colloid and Tc-99m red blood cells (RBCs) for gastrointestinal bleeding**

|  | Tc-99m sulfur colloid | Tc-99m RBCs |
|---|---|---|
| Dose | 10 mCi (may be repeated) | 25 mCi |
| Dosimetry |  |  |
| Whole body | 0.2 rad | 0.4 rad |
| Target organ | 3.6 rads (liver) | 1.2 rads (heart) |
| Minimal bleeding detectable | 0.1 ml/min | 0.05-0.4 ml/min |
| Labeling | Commercial kit | Commercial kit |
| Imaging duration | 20-30 min (repeat once) | 60-90 min (repeat as needed for 24 hr) |
| Advantages | Short imaging time | Repeat imaging up to 24 hr |
|  | High target-to-background ratio |  |
| Disadvantages | Difficulty detecting hepatic and splenic flexure bleeding | False positive studies due to excretion of free Tc-99m pertechnetate |
|  | Detects bleeding only over short time |  |

**Table 11-5    Dosimetry for technetium-99m red blood cells (RBCs) and Tc-99m sulfur colloid**

|  | Tc-99m RBCs | | Tc-99m sulfur colloid | |
|---|---|---|---|---|
|  | Rad/mCi | Rads/25 mCi (cGy/925 MBq) | Rad/mCi | Rads/25 mCi (cGy/925 MBq) |
| Heart wall | 0.054 | 1.4 |  |  |
| Bladder wall | 0.051 | 1.3 |  |  |
| Spleen | 0.041 | 1.0 | 0.210 | 2.10 |
| Lung | 0.041 | 1.0 |  |  |
| Blood | 0.035 | 0.9 |  |  |
| Liver | 0.026 | 0.7 | 0.340 | 3.40 |
| Kidney | 0.025 | 0.7 |  |  |
| Red marrow | 0.019 | 0.5 | 0.027 | 0.27 |
| Ovaries | 0.017 | 0.5 | 0.006 | 0.06 |
| Testes | 0.007 | 0.2 | 0.001 | 0.01 |
| Whole body | 0.015 | 0.4 | 0.019 | 0.19 |

**Red blood cells versus sulfur colloid** For many years, controversy surrounded which radiopharmaceutical, Tc-99m sulfur colloid or Tc-99m-labeled RBCs, was better for detection of acute GI bleeding (Table 11-4). Consensus now clearly favors Tc-99m RBCs.

A large multicenter study compared the results of these two approaches in 100 patients referred with clinical evidence of acute bleeding. A Tc-99m sulfur colloid study was performed first, followed by in vitro labeled Tc-99m RBCs. Tc-99m sulfur colloid showed only five sites of hemorrhage, whereas Tc-99m RBC imaging accurately disclosed the source of bleeding in 38 cases. The sensitivity of the Tc-99m RBC study was 93% and the specificity 95%. Continuous imaging for 90 minutes revealed 83% of all active hemorrhages. Delayed imaging revealed the remainder. Smaller comparison studies have found similar results.

The obvious advantage of Tc-99m RBC scintigraphy is the ability to image over a prolonged period. Tc-99m sulfur colloid still has a limited role; for example, in a patient who is actively bleeding and clinically unstable, the 20-minute Tc-99m sulfur colloid study will likely be positive and the information valuable to the angiographer.

**Dosimetry** The radiation absorbed dose to the patient using the Tc-99m sulfur colloid technique and the Tc-99m-labeled RBC method is relatively low, particularly when compared with contrast angiography. The target organ for Tc-99m sulfur colloid is the liver and for Tc-99m RBCs the myocardial wall. The whole body dose for labeled RBCs is 0.4 rad/25 mCi (Table 11-5).

## ECTOPIC GASTRIC MUCOSA

Ectopic gastric mucosa presents most often as a Meckel's diverticulum but may be associated with duplication of the GI tract and Barrett's esophagus. After partial gastrectomy for peptic ulcer disease, a retained gastric antrum may inadvertently be left behind. In all these clinical situations, acid and pepsin secretion from the gastric mucosa can produce ulceration of adjacent tissue and result in serious complications. Tc-99m pertechnetate scintigraphy has been used to help make these diagnoses.

## Mechanism of Uptake

Normal mucosa of the gastric fundus contains parietal cells, which secrete hydrochloric acid and intrinsic factor, and chief cells, which secrete pepsinogen. The antrum and pylorus contain G cells, which secrete the hormone gastrin. Columnar mucin-secreting epithelial cells are found throughout the stomach.

Gastric secretions in both normal and ectopic gastric mucosa are stimulated by neural and hormonal mechanisms that respond to the ingestion of food and increase the volume and acidity of gastric secretions over the basal fasting state. The presence or absence of symptoms, the clinical presentation (e.g., bleeding versus obstruction), and the ability of Tc-99m pertechnetate to image ectopic gastric mucosa depend on the gastric mucosal cell types present.

Logically, parietal cells might be responsible for gastric mucosal uptake and secretion. Chloride would be expected to compete for formation of acid by the parietal cell. Although some experimental evidence supports this hypothesis, most evidence lies with the mucin-secreting cells. These cells excrete an alkaline juice that protects the mucosa from the highly acidic gastric fluid.

Tc-99m pertechnetate uptake has been found in gastric tissue with no parietal cells, such as in patients with pernicious anemia, retained gastric antrum, and Barrett's esophagus. Animal studies confirm this, and several autoradiographic studies localize Tc-99m pertechnetate uptake to the mucin cell rather than the parietal cell.

A hypothesis explaining the conflicting data suggests that the predominant mechanism is specific mucin cell uptake and secretion, which is suppressible by sodium perchlorate in a manner similar to iodide, whereas parietal cell uptake is a minor factor, nonspecific, secondary, and as in chloride uptake, not suppressed by perchlorate.

## Dosimetry

The target organ for Tc-99m pertechnetate is the stomach, followed by the thyroid gland (Table 11-6). Sodium perchlorate should *not* be given for thyroid radiation protection before the study because it will prevent uptake in the gastric mucosa.

**Table 11-6  Radiation absorbed dose for technetium-99m pertechnetate**

| Target organ | Rad/mCi | Rad/5 mCi (Cgy/185 MBq) |
|---|---|---|
| Bladder wall | 0.053 | 0.265 |
| Stomach wall | 0.250 | 1.250 |
| Large intestine wall | 0.068 | 0.340 |
| Ovaries | 0.022 | 0.110 |
| Red marrow | 0.019 | 0.095 |
| Testes | 0.009 | 0.045 |
| Thyroid | 0.130 | 0.650 |
| Total body | 0.014 | 0.070 |

**Box 11-13  Epidemiology of Meckel's Diverticulum**

1%-3% incidence in the general population.
50% occur by age 2 yr.
10%-30% have ectopic gastric mucosa.
25%-40% are symptomatic; 50%-67% of these have ectopic gastric mucosa.
95%-98% of patients with bleeding have ectopic gastric mucosa.

## Clinical Indications

**Meckel's diverticulum**  Meckel's diverticulum is the most common congenital anomaly of the GI tract, occurring in 1% to 3% of the population. The diverticulum results from failure of closure of the omphalomesenteric duct of the embryo. (The omphalomesenteric duct connects the yolk sac to the primitive foregut through the umbilical cord.) This true diverticulum arises on the antimesenteric side of the small bowel, usually 80 to 90 cm proximal to the ileocecal valve. It is typically 2 to 3 cm in size but may be considerably larger. Ectopic gastric mucosa is present in 10% to 30% of cases, in approximately 60% of symptomatic patients, and in 98% of those with bleeding (Box 11-13).

*Clinical manifestations*  Gastric mucosal secretions can cause peptic ulceration of the diverticulum or adjacent ileum, resulting in pain, bleeding, or perforation. About 60% of patients with complications of Meckel's diverticulum are under age 2 years. Bleeding accounts for most cases.

Other manifestations of Meckel's diverticulum, seen most often in adults, include intussusception, obstruction, infection, and abnormal fixation of the diverticulum. Bleeding from Meckel's diverticulum after age 40 is unusual.

*Diagnosis* Preoperative diagnosis of Meckel's diverticulum was difficult before scintigraphy. It is often missed on small bowel follow-through films because the diverticulum may have a narrow or stenotic ostium; diverticula are often not well filled and have rapid emptying. Small bowel enteroclysis is a better method for detection because the higher pressure of the barium column more reliably fills the diverticulum. Angiography is useful only with brisk active bleeding and is rarely used. Tc-99m pertechnetate scintigraphy *(Meckel's scan)* is considered the standard method for initial diagnosis of Meckel's diverticulum.

*Methodology* Attention to patient preparation is important (Box 11-14). A full stomach or urinary bladder may obscure an adjacent Meckel's diverticulum. Therefore fasting for 3 to 4 hours before the study or continuous nasogastric aspiration to decrease the size of the stomach is recommended. Voiding before, during, and after the study is also important. Sodium perchlorate is not used to block thyroid uptake before scintigraphy because it will also block uptake of Tc-99m pertechnetate by the gastric mucosa. However, perchlorate may be administered after the study to wash out the radiotracer from the thyroid, minimizing radiation exposure.

Barium studies should not be performed for several days before scintigraphy because attenuation by the contrast material may prevent lesion detection. Procedures (e.g., proctoscopy) or drugs (e.g., laxatives) that irritate the intestinal mucosa and result in nonspecific Tc-99m pertechnetate uptake should be avoided. Certain drugs (e.g., ethosuximide [Zarontin]) may also cause unpredictable uptake.

*Pharmacological augmentation* Various pharmacological maneuvers have been reported to improve the detection of Meckel's diverticulum, including pentagastrin, glucagon, and cimetidine.

PENTAGASTRIN Pretreatment with pentagastrin experimentally increases the rapidity, duration, and intensity of Tc-99m pertechnetate uptake. In one reported case an initially false negative scan was converted to positive with use of the drug. The mechanism is uncertain but may be the result of increased acid production, leading to increased activity of the mucin-producing cells and increased tracer uptake. However, pentagastrin also increases intestinal motility, leading to rapid movement into the small bowel.

GLUCAGON The antiperistaltic effect of glucagon has been used to prevent washout of the tracer from the stomach and from Meckel's diverticulum. One study reported optimal visualization of Meckel's diverticulum with a combination of pentagastrin and glucagon.

CIMETIDINE The histamine $H_2$ receptor antagonist cimetidine also improves the detection of ectopic gastric mucosa because of more intense and prolonged uptake of Tc-99m pertechnetate by the mucosa. This effect is

likely caused by inhibition of cimetidine's release from the gastric mucosa. Although no controlled studies have been performed, some investigators recommend routine use of cimetidine because it does not have significant risks or side effects.

EVALUATION No large series has evaluated the diagnostic effectiveness of these pharmacological maneuvers. Although some authors recommend routine premedication with one or a combination of these drugs, others reserve their use for a suspected false negative Meckel's scan.

*Image interpretation* Meckel's diverticulum is seen as a focal area of increased intraperitoneal activity in the abdomen, most frequently in the right lower quadrant (Fig. 11-27). Abnormal activity is usually first seen 5 to 10 minutes after tracer injection, and uptake increases over time at a rate similar to normal gastric uptake.

## Box 11-14  Meckel's Diverticulum: Protocol Summary

**PATIENT PREPARATION**

4 to 6 hr fasting before study to reduce size of stomach.
No pretreatment with sodium perchlorate; may be given after completion of study.
No barium studies should be performed within 3 to 4 days of scintigraphy.
Void before, during if possible, and after study.

**PREMEDICATION**

None. Alternatively:
Pentagastrin: 6 µg/kg subcutaneously 5 to 15 min before study
Cimetidine: 20 mg/kg orally for 2 days before study
Glucagon: 50 µg/kg intravenously 10 min before study

**RADIOPHARMACEUTICAL**

Tc-99m pertechnetate
    Children: 30 to 100 mCi/kg
    Adults: 5 to 10 mCi intravenously

**INSTRUMENTATION**

Camera: large-field-of-view gamma.
Collimator: low energy, all purpose or high resolution.

**PATIENT POSITION**

Supine under camera with xiphoid to symphysis pubis in field of view

**IMAGING PROCEDURE**

Obtain flow images: 60 1-sec frames.
Obtain static images: 500k counts for first image, others for same time every 5 to 10 min for 1 hr.
Erect, right lateral, posterior, or oblique views may be helpful at 30 to 60 min.
Obtain postvoid image.

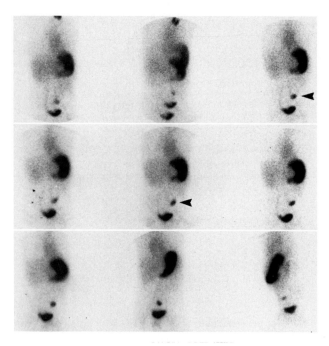

**Fig. 11-27** Meckel's diverticulum. This 7-year-old boy had rectal bleeding. Sequential images show focal uptake in left lower quadrant confirmed at surgery to be Meckel's diverticulum *(arrowheads)*. Note simultaneous rate of uptake of the Meckel's diverticulum and stomach. Motion artifact can be seen in second image.

Lateral or oblique views are sometimes helpful in confirming the anterior position of the diverticulum versus the posterior location of renal or ureteral activity. Upright views can help distinguish fixed activity (e.g., duodenum) from ectopic gastric mucosa, which moves inferiorly in response to the altered position; it also serves to empty renal pelvic activity. The intensity of activity within the lesion may fluctuate because of intestinal secretions, hemorrhage, or increased intestinal motility that washes out the radiotracer. Postvoid images are suggested to help empty collecting system activity and better see uptake adjacent to the bladder.

*Accuracy* False negative studies may result from poor technique, washout of the secreted Tc-99m pertechnetate, or lack of sufficient gastric mucosa. Experimentally, an area smaller than 2 $cm^2$ may not be detected scintigraphically. Meckel's diverticulum with impaired blood supply from intussusception, volvulus, or infarction may also result in a false negative study.

A variety of causes of false positive studies have been reported (Box 11-15). Normal structures can be confused with ectopic gastric mucosa if careful technique is not followed. False positives are often the result of inflammatory or obstructive lesions. Lesions with increased blood pool, such as arteriovenous malformations and tumors, may be seen on flow and blood pool

---

## Box 11-15   Causes of False Positive Meckel's Scan

**URINARY TRACT**

Ectopic kidney
Extrarenal pelvis
Hydronephrosis
Vesicoureteral reflux
Horseshoe kidney
Bladder diverticulum

**VASCULAR**

Arteriovenous malformation
Hemangioma
Aneurysm of intraabdominal vessel
Angiodysplasia

**OTHER AREAS OF ECTOPIC GASTRIC MUCOSA**

Gastrogenic cyst
Enteric duplication
Duplication cysts
Barrett's esophagus
Retained gastric antrum
Pancreas
Duodenum
Colon

**HYPEREMIA AND INFLAMMATORY**

Peptic ulcer
Crohn's disease
Ulcerative colitis
Abscess
Appendicitis
Colitis

**NEOPLASM**

Carcinoma of sigmoid colon
Carcinoid
Lymphoma
Leiomyosarcoma

**SMALL BOWEL OBSTRUCTION**

Intussusception
Volvulus

imaging but do not take up Tc-99m pertechnetate; therefore they are seen early and then fade.

The reported accuracy of scintigraphy in the detection of Meckel's diverticulum has varied considerably and depends on the referral population studied (children or adults), the presenting symptom (rectal bleeding or abdominal pain), and the technology used (traditional rectilinear scanners or modern gamma cameras). One report, however, summarizing the results in 954 patients (mostly children) who had undergone scintigraphy for suspected Meckel's diverticulum using modern imaging methods, found an overall sensitivity of 85% and a specificity of 95%.

Experience in differentiating nonspecific accumulation of pertechnetate from true ectopic gastric mucosa makes this high specificity possible. Earlier studies, often using rectilinear scanners, noted sensitivities and specificities in the range of 78%. Scintigraphy for Meckel's diverticulum in adults appears to have a poorer sensitivity than in children; one series reported a sensitivity of only 63%. There were 10 false positive studies, although seven of the subjects had surgically treatable disease. The lower sensitivity is probably related to the lack of gastric mucosa in the many adult diverticula.

**Gastrointestinal duplications**    Duplications are cystic or tubular lesions of congenital origin composed of GI muscular walls with mucosal linings. Half occur in the small bowel, most in the ileum and 20% in the mediastinum. Although most are symptomatic by age 2 years, some remain asymptomatic into adulthood. The presenting symptoms are similar to those of Meckel's diverticulum because 30% to 50% of patients have ectopic gastric mucosa.

The diagnosis is usually made at surgery. Occasionally a preoperative diagnosis is made after barium radiography or ultrasonography. Scintigraphy occasionally may be helpful; for example, mediastinal GI cysts have been diagnosed with Tc-99m pertechnetate. Duplications often appear as large, sometimes multilobulated areas of increased activity.

**Retained gastric antrum**    The gastric antrum is occasionally left behind in the afferent loop after a Billroth II gastrojejunostomy for peptic ulcer disease. The antrum continues to produce gastrin, which is no longer inhibited by acid in the stomach because it has been diverted through the gastrojejunostomy. The resulting high acid production often leads to marginal ulcers. Other causes of recurrent ulcers after a partial gastrectomy include an incomplete vagotomy and the Zollinger-Ellison syndrome. In the latter a pancreatic tumor causes continued production of gastrin. The clinical diagnosis is usually based on the response of serum gastrin to intravenous calcium or secretin infusions.

Endoscopy or barium radiography can often demonstrate the retained gastric antrum. However, Tc-99m

pertechnetate scintigraphy can be confirmatory. The protocol used is similar to that for imaging Meckel's diverticulum. Uptake in the gastric remnant occurs simultaneously with gastric uptake and is seen as a collar of radioactivity in the duodenal stump of the afferent loop. The retained antrum usually lies to the right of the gastric remnant. In one series, Tc-99m pertechnetate uptake was demonstrated in 16 of 22 patients with a retained antrum.

**Barrett's esophagus**    In patients with Barrett's esophagus the distal esophagus becomes lined by columnar epithelium rather than the usual esophageal squamous epithelium. Thought to result from chronic GER, Barrett's esophagus is associated with ulcers, high strictures, and an 8.5% incidence of esophageal adenocarcinoma.

Although Tc-99m pertechnetate scanning first demonstrated Barrett's esophagus in 1973, the diagnosis is now usually made with endoscopy and mucosal biopsy. Scintigraphy should be performed with the patient erect to minimize reflux. LAO views may be helpful. Although the normal esophagus ends at the esophagogastric junction, a positive scan shows intrathoracic uptake contiguous with the stomach but conforming to the shape and posterior location of the esophagus.

A potential problem is differentiating Barrett's esophagus from a simple hiatal hernia. To avoid problems, the scan should be interpreted in conjunction with an upper GI series. False negative results have been reported, and the scan does not replace endoscopic biopsy. At best, scintigraphy is a complementary or confirmatory procedure.

## INTESTINAL FUNCTION AND TRANSIT

### Protein-Losing Enteropathy

Excessive protein loss through the GI tract has been associated with a variety of gastrointestinal and nongastrointestinal diseases, including intestinal lymphangiectasia, Crohn's disease, Menetrier's disease, amyloidosis, and intestinal fistula. The resulting hypoproteinemia can be a serious clinical problem.

Albumin labeled with chromium-51 (Cr-51) has been used to confirm the diagnosis of protein-losing enteropathy. An endogenously produced macromolecule, $\alpha_1$-antitrypsin, has been used as a nonradioactive fecal marker of malabsorption and is as accurate and reproducible as Cr-51-labeled albumin. Since both require daily stool collection for 48 to 72 hours and fecal quantification, however, they have not been well accepted.

Two imaging radiopharmaceuticals used to diagnose protein-losing enteropathy are *Tc-99m human serum albumin* (THSA) and *In-111 transferrin*. With Tc-99m

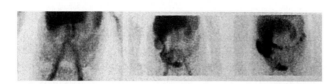

**Fig. 11-28** Protein-losing enteropathy. Patient received Tc-99m human serum albumin. *Left* to *right,* Immediate, 1-hour, and 2-hour images. Increasing activity is seen in the small bowel initially *(middle),* with subsequent transit to the colon *(right),* consistent with protein-losing enteropathy.

HSA, serial abdominal images show radiotracer collection in the small bowel in the first 30 minutes and increasing amounts over 24 hours (Fig. 11-28). In-111 chloride binds in vivo to serum proteins, most notably transferrin, and abdominal imaging can be used to visualize the protein leak.

## Schilling Test

Although most often ordered to diagnose pernicious anemia, the Schilling test evaluates vitamin $B_{12}$ (methylcobalamin) absorption. Vitamin $B_{12}$ can be absorbed from the ileum only if it is complexed with intrinsic factor (IF), which is produced by gastric parietal cells in the stomach. After absorption, vitamin $B_{12}$ is bound to storage sites in various tissues and very slowly metabolized.

Vitamin $B_{12}$ deficiency manifests clinically as a megaloblastic anemia and neurological disease. The cause is rarely inadequate intake, except in strict vegetarians. The most common cause is an IF deficiency in patients with pernicious anemia and associated gastric atrophy. Intestinal causes of vitamin $B_{12}$ malabsorption include Crohn's disease, ileal resection, gluten enteropathy, and tropical sprue. Vitamin $B_{12}$ malabsorption can also result from competition for vitamin $B_{12}$ in bacterial overgrowth syndromes and fish tapeworm *(Diphyllobothrium latum)* infestation. Pancreatic insufficiency can also cause vitamin $B_{12}$ malabsorption.

After oral administration of vitamin $B_{12}$ labeled with cobalt-57 (Co-57) or Co-58 and an intramuscular flushing dose of unlabeled vitamin $B_{12}$, the healthy person will absorb the labeled vitamin and excrete it in the urine through glomerular filtration. The Schilling test measures the fraction of the administered dose that is excreted in the urine (normal, greater than 9% in 24 hours). The purpose of the flushing dose of vitamin $B_{12}$ is to saturate tissue and plasma binding sites, maximizing the renal excretion of absorbed Co-labeled vitamin $B_{12}$.

The traditional approach first measures Co-57-labeled vitamin $B_{12}$ excretion (stage I). If it is abnormal, the study is repeated (stage II) with the addition of IF. If excretion is abnormal without IF but increases signifi-

cantly with IF, the diagnosis of pernicious anemia is made. If both are abnormal, pernicious anemia is ruled out, and the cause is small bowel malabsorption or pancreatic insufficiency. An alternative stage II can be performed (e.g., after antibiotic therapy) for assumed bacterial overgrowth or with pancreatic enzyme replacement.

The second approach to the Schilling test administers vitamin $B_{12}$ and IF simultaneously, with Co-58-labeled vitamin $B_{12}$ and Co-57-labeled vitamin $B_{12}$ bound to IF. The advantage of this method is convenience.

## Intestinal Transit

Small and large intestinal transit scintigraphy is relatively new, and optimal methods are still being developed. Unique technical problems exist. The radiolabeled meal must be able to withstand the acidic environment of the stomach and the alkaline milieu of the small bowel. Quantification is a greater problem than for gastric emptying because the input into the intestine is not a single food bolus, but rather a protracted infusion from the stomach, with no single time zero. In quantification of gastric emptying, all the radiolabeled meal resides in the stomach at the beginning of the study; quantification depends only on the rate of clearance.

Most of the work to date is investigational. The clinical role of intestinal transit tests still must be defined.

**Nonscintigraphic tests** Transit of barium through the small bowel during a routine barium follow-through study is qualitative, not quantitative. Mixing barium with food and plotting its movement on a monitor using image intensification provides an index of the transit rate through the small bowel into the colon. Radiation dosimetry is relatively high, however, and the meal is nonphysiological.

The *hydrogen breath analysis test* measures hydrogen produced when a carbohydrate (C-14 lactose) is fermented by colonic bacteria. The test measures the transit time of the leading edge of the meal from the mouth to the cecum and is not an index of the transit of the meal's bulk. Also, the lactose alters transit, the transit time is affected by the gastric emptying rate, and the test requires fermentative bacteria in the colon, which may be absent in one fourth of the population. The hydrogen breath test is not widely available.

Various radiographic methods have been used for studying large bowel transit, including cineradiography, fluoroscopy to estimate transit times, and use of radiopaque plastic cuttings. All give relatively large radiation doses to the patient and are not physiological.

**Radionuclide scintigraphy** Radiomarkers such as Tc-99m sulfur colloid or Tc-99m DTPA in water or mixed with a semisolid meal have been used because of their simplicity. However, study of the semisolid phase of the intestinal contents is complex, and accurate measurement requires a stable, nondigestible meal.

Fiber is the only normal dietary constituent that is unaffected by gastric antral grinding and that progresses along the small intestine in solid form without hydrolytic ingestion. Labeled with iodine-131 (I-131), fiber is stable in acid and alkaline environments, but synthesis is laborious and the dosimetry relatively high. Other radiopharmaceuticals include Tc-99m-labeled cellulose fiber and In-111-labeled plastic particles and resin pellets. Various quantitative methods have been used.

To obtain the most accurate results and to minimize the length of the study, direct placement of the radiotracer through intubation at the site of interest (proximal small bowel for small bowel transit studies, distal small bowel or cecum for colonic studies) is optimal. Tc-99m DTPA, I-131 fiber cellulose, and In-111 DTPA encapsulated in nondigestible capsules have been used. Cecal or jejunal instillation ensures a clear starting time. Oral ingestion would require a prolonged imaging time. However, intubation methods are not practical for routine clinical performance because they are invasive, technically demanding, and unpleasant for the patient.

An interesting alternative approach is the use of In-111 polystyrene cation exchange resin pellets. They are placed in a gelatin capsule coated with a pH-sensitive polymer that resists disruption at pH levels found in the stomach and proximal small bowel but is disrupted at the ileocecal valve because of the increasing pH. A large-field-of-view camera is used for imaging. The frequency and duration of image acquisition depend on the methodology, the length of the study, and the information needed. Different quantitative methods have been used.

*Clinical results* Normal small bowel transit times vary widely. Patients with diarrhea tend to have rapid mean transit times, whereas those with constipation have longer transit times, although normal values overlap. More data are needed.

## SUGGESTED READINGS

Datz FL: Considerations for accurately measuring gastric emptying, *J Nucl Med* 32:881-884, 1991.

Emslie JT, Zarnegar K, Siegel ME, et al: Technetium-99m-labeled red blood cell scans in the investigation of gastrointestinal bleeding, *Dis Colon Rectum* 39:750-754, 1996.

Fahey FH, Ziessman HA, Collin MJ, Eggli DF: Left anterior oblique projection and peak-to-scatter ratio for attenuation compensation of gastric emptying studies, *J Nucl Med* 30:233-239, 1989.

Heyman S: Pediatric nuclear gastroenterology: evaluation of gastroesophageal reflux and gastrointestinal bleeding. In Freeman LM, Weissman HS, editors: *Nuclear medicine annual 1985,* New York, 1985, Raven Press.

Klein HA, Wald A: Esophageal transit scintigraphy. In Freeman LM, Weissman HS, editors: *Nuclear medicine annual 1985,* New York, 1985, Raven Press.

Malmud LS, Vitti RA, Fisher RS: Gastroesophageal reflux. In Freeman LM, editor: *Freeman and Johnson's clinical radionuclide imaging,* vol III, New York, 1986, Grune & Stratton.

Sfakianakis GN, Haase GM: Abdominal scintigraphy for ectopic gastric mucosa: a retrospective analysis of 143 studies, *AJR Am J Roentgenol* 138:7-12, 1982.

Vitti RA, Malmud LS, Fisher RS: Gastric emptying. In Freeman LM, editor: *Freeman and Johnson's clinical radionuclide imaging,* vol III, New York, 1986, Grune & Stratton.

Winzelberg GG: Radionuclide evaluation of gastrointestinal bleeding. In Freeman LM, editor: *Freeman and Johnson's clinical radionuclide imaging,* vol III, New York, 1986, Grune & Stratton.

Ziessman HA: Gastrointestinal scintigraphy: esophagus and stomach. In Neumann R, Harbert J, Eckelman W, editors: *Nuclear medicine: diagnosis and therapy,* New York, 1996, Thieme.

Ziessman HA: Keep it simple—it's only gastric emptying. In Freeman LM, editor: *Nuclear medicine annual 2000,* Philadelphia, 2000, Lippincott Williams & Wilkins.

Ziessman HA, Fahey FH, Collen MJ: Biphasic solid and liquid gastric emptying in normal controls and diabetics using continuous acquisition in LAO view, *Dig Dis Sci* 37:744-750, 1992.

# Central Nervous System

Brain scintigraphy has long played an important role in the practice of nuclear medicine. Until the advent of computed tomography (CT) in the 1970s, conventional nuclear medicine brain scans were the only noninvasive clinical method available for imaging the brain and represented a large portion of nuclear medicine practice. In current practice, magnetic resonance imaging (MRI) and CT play preeminent roles in clinical brain imaging, producing superb anatomical images of the central nervous system (CNS).

The role of nuclear medicine is now functional brain imaging. Positron emission tomography (PET) led the way by imaging physiological and biochemical processes in the brain, including cerebral blood flow (CBF), glucose metabolism, and oxygen utilization, which had both important research and clinical impact. Subsequently, single-photon blood flow radiopharmaceuticals became available for use with single-photon emission computed tomography (SPECT) cam-eras. Clinical diagnoses based on abnormalities of CBF and glucose metabolism are now made routinely using various

## Box 12-1  Brain SPECT and PET Radiopharmaceuticals Used Clinically

| RADIOPHARMACEUTICAL | RADIONUCLIDE PHOTOPEAK (keV) |
|---|---|
| **Conventional Brain Scintigraphy** | |
| Technetium-99m glucohepto-nate (GH) | 140 |
| Tc-99m DTPA | 140 |
| **Brain Perfusion Scintigraphy** | |
| Iodine-123 iodoamphetamine (IMP) | 159 |
| Tc-99m HMPAO | 140 |
| Tc-99m methyl cysteinate dimer (ECD) | 140 |
| **Positron Emission Tomography** | |
| Fluorine-18 fluorodeoxyglucose (FDG) | 511 |
| **Brain Tumor Imaging** | |
| Thallium-201 | 69-83, 167 |
| Tc-99m sestamibi | 140 |
| **Cisternography** | |
| Indium-111 DTPA | 173, 247 |

*DTPA,* Diethylenetriamine pentaacetic acid, pentetic acid; *HMPAO,* hexamethyl-propylenamine oxime.

single-photon and positron radiopharmaceuticals with both PET and SPECT instrumentation (Box 12-1).

## BLOOD-BRAIN BARRIER SCINTIGRAPHY

The role of blood-brain barrier scintigraphy is limited in modern nuclear medicine. However, an understanding of the radiopharmaceuticals used, the resulting images, and its clinical applications allows the student of nuclear medicine to put in proper perspective present-day neurological imaging with MRI, PET, and SPECT cerebral perfusion studies.

### Radiopharmaceuticals

The BBB is both an anatomical and a physiological barrier that prevents most substances in the blood from entering the CNS. Normally, selective movement of substances across this barrier occurs predominantly by active transport. However, diseases of the brain cause a breakdown in the BBB.

Conventional brain scans are not really brain scans. The BBB radiopharmaceuticals are distributed within the extracellular space and enter brain tissue only when there is a break in the barrier.

Technetium-99m (Tc-99m) pertechnetate was the first radiopharmaceutical used for BBB scintigraphy. Although inexpensive and readily available, Tc-99m pertechnetate has prolonged blood pool activity and is concentrated in the salivary glands and choroid plexus, which adversely affects image interpretation.

Tc-99m diethylenetriamine pentaacetic acid (DTPA) and Tc-99m glucoheptonate (GH) are the preferred agents. They have fast clearance from the blood via urinary excretion, no salivary or choroid plexus uptake, a higher target-to-background ratio, and better lesion detection. With breakdown of the BBB, these agents diffuse into the altered tissue and bind by uncertain mechanisms. Tc-99m GH has higher uptake in tumors, perhaps because it is a glucose analog and serves as a substrate for tumor metabolism. Prior corticosteroid administration may diminish uptake of these radiopharmaceuticals because steroids decrease BBB permeability.

### Dosimetry

The highest radiation dose of Tc-99m DTPA and Tc-99m GH is to the bladder and kidneys (see Table 13-3). The whole body radiation dose from both radiopharmaceuticals is quite low, 0.1 and 0.2 rad, respectively.

### Methodology

In a typical protocol for BBB imaging, dynamic flow images are routinely acquired (Box 12-2). Certain vascular lesions, such as early stroke (cerebrovascular accident [CVA]), carotid occlusion, and arteriovenous malformations (AVMs), may be better seen on the flow phase. Immediate high-count blood pool images can help in the diagnosis of AVMs or venous sinus occlusions and confirm a hypervascular abnormality noted on an initial dynamic flow study.

The flow phase is usually performed in the anterior view, although the posterior view may be preferable for children and patients with cerebellar, occipital, or posterior parietal symptoms and signs. Delayed planar images are acquired in multiple views 1½ to 2 hours after tracer injection. SPECT is optional.

### Image Interpretation

In the conventional brain scan, peripheral activity corresponds to the outer scalp and inner meninges (Fig. 12-1). The normal cerebral cortex is devoid of activity. Venous structures define most of the anatomical regions seen on the scan. Cerebral veins include an external group of veins that course over the surface of the calvarium and an internal group from which the great vein of

## Box 12-2 Blood-Brain Barrier Scintigraphy: Protocol Summary

**PATIENT PREPARATION**

None.

**RADIOPHARMACEUTICAL**

Technetium-99m glucoheptonate or Tc-99m DTPA, 20 mCi (740 MBq)

**INSTRUMENTATION**

Collimator: high resolution, low energy. Camera setup: large-field-of-view gamma.

Window: 15% over 140-keV photopeak

Camera formatter setup: 2- to 3-sec flow images for 30 sec, then immediate and delayed static images in multiple views

Computer setup: 1-sec flow images for 60 sec (64 × 64 byte mode), then static images (128 × 128 frame mode)

**IMAGING PROCEDURE**

1. Inject radiopharmaceutical as an intravenous bolus.
2. Acquire dynamic flow study.
3. *Immediate* 750k static images in the anterior, posterior, right lateral, and left lateral views (optional).
4. Starting 2 hours after injection, acquire *delayed* 750k static images in the anterior, posterior, right lateral, and left lateral views. Vertex view if needed.
5. SPECT (optional).

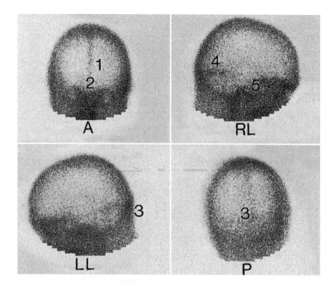

**Fig. 12-1**    Normal blood-brain barrier scan. Anterior *(A)*, right lateral *(RL)*, left lateral *(LL)*, and posterior *(P)* projections. The cerebral hemispheres are surrounded by peripheral activity of the scalp, bone, and superficial cerebral vessels. The superior sagittal sinus *(1)* is seen in the anterior and posterior views. The floor of the frontal sinus *(2)* is the inferior border in the anterior view. The confluence of the sinuses, the torcular Herophili *(3)*, is seen on the left lateral and posterior views. The transverse sinuses *(4)* and sphenoid sinus *(5)* are seen on the lateral views. Compare these images with the schematic diagram in Fig. 12-2.

Galen drains the deep structures of the brain (Fig. 12-2). All drain into the sinuses of the dura mater and carry blood to the internal jugular vein.

An understanding of the normal cerebral anatomy and arterial distribution of the brain and associated perfusion patterns is necessary for the accurate diagnosis of cerebrovascular disease (Figs. 12-3 to 12-6). Two internal carotid arteries and two vertebral arteries perfuse the brain. The internal carotid arteries deliver blood to the majority of the cerebral cortex, whereas the vertebral arteries supply the inferior portion of the cerebrum, cerebellum, and brainstem.

## Clinical Applications

**Brain tumors**    Brain tumor detectability depends on size and location. Tumors less than 2 cm in size and those that are deep seated, centrally located, or adjacent to areas of normally high activity (e.g., base of skull and vascular structures) may be missed. Tumor type is also a factor. Meningiomas and malignant gliomas are detected with high sensitivity, whereas pituitary and parasellar tumors, low-grade gliomas, and brainstem tumors are detected with relatively low sensitivity.

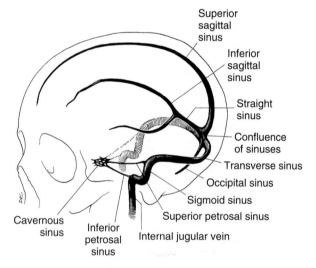

**Fig. 12-2**    Cerebral venous anatomy. The superior sagittal sinus runs along the falx within the superior margin of the interhemispheric fissure. The inferior sagittal sinus is smaller, courses over the corpus callosum, and joins with the great vein of Galen to form the straight sinus, which drains into the superior sagittal sinus at the confluence of sinuses (torcular Herophili) at the occipital protuberance. Transverse sinuses drain the sagittal and occipital sinuses into the internal jugular vein.

The appearance on conventional brain scintigraphy is often not specific for malignancy; however, features suggestive of tumor include a spherical configuration, extension across vascular distributions, and a "doughnut" appearance (Fig. 12-7). The scintigraphic

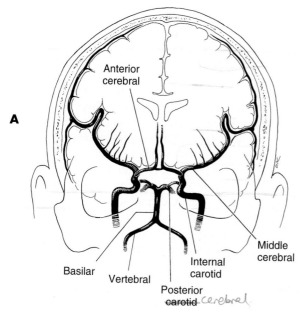

A

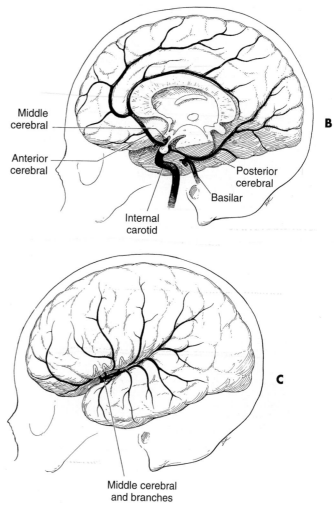

B

C

**Fig. 12-3** Cerebral arterial anatomy. **A,** Coronal section shows circle of Willis and course of the middle and anterior cerebral arteries. Internal carotids divide at the base of the brain (circle of Willis) into the anterior and middle cerebral arteries. The middle cerebral artery runs laterally in the sylvian fissure, then backward and upward on the surface of the insula, where it divides into branches to the *lateral* surface of the cerebral hemisphere and to portions of the basal ganglia. **B,** Midline sagittal view shows distribution of anterior, middle, and posterior cerebral arteries. The anterior cerebral artery supplies the cerebrum along its *medial* margin above the corpus callosum and extends posteriorly to the parietal fissure as well as to the anterior portion of the basal ganglia. Vertebral arteries fuse into the basilar artery, which branches at the circle of Willis into the two posterior cerebral arteries supplying the occipital lobe and the inferior half of the temporal lobe. **C,** Left lateral view shows distribution of the middle cerebral artery over the cerebral cortex.

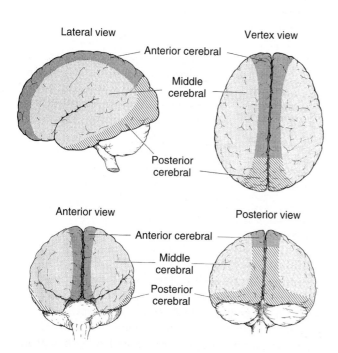

**Fig. 12-4** Regional cerebral cortex perfusion of the anterior, middle, and posterior cerebral arteries.

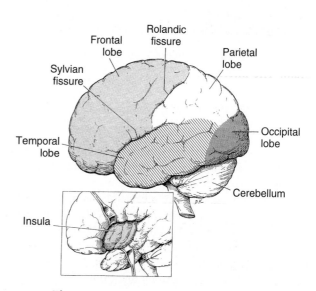

**Fig. 12-5** Cerebral cortex lobar anatomy.

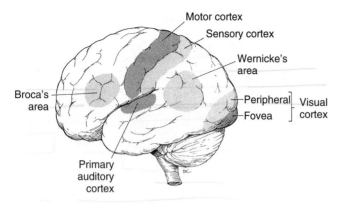

**Fig. 12-6**    Motor, sensory, visual, speech, and auditory functional and associative centers of the brain.

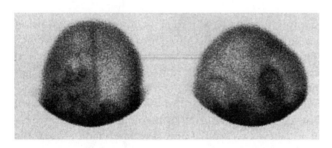

**Fig. 12-7**    Glioblastoma imaging with Tc-99m glucoheptonate. Increased uptake on the brain scan is seen in the right frontal parietal region on both the anterior and right lateral views.

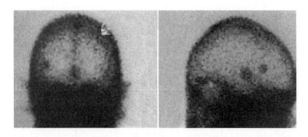

**Fig. 12-8**    Metastatic brain tumor imaging with Tc-99m DTPA. Several focal areas of increased uptake are seen on the anterior and right lateral views in a patient with lung cancer metastatic to the brain.

findings are increased blood flow, localization on blood pool, and focal uptake on delayed imaging after 1 to 2 hours.

Although the pattern for metastatic brain tumor is not specific, multiple lesions are typical (Fig. 12-8). Infection and infarcts may be difficult to differentiate from tumor. Discrete rounded lesions that cross vascular boundaries are more likely to be tumor. CT and MRI are superior to brain scintigraphy for the demonstration of most intracranial tumors.

### Cerebrovascular disease

*Carotid stenosis*    With high-grade carotid stenosis, a characteristic "flip-flop" phenomenon is seen on the radionuclide flow study, with delayed unilateral regional cortical blood flow and clearance compared with the opposite normal side (Fig. 12-9, *A*). This pattern is seen with or without concomitant cerebral infarction.

*Cerebral infarction*    Increased blood flow to an infarcted region may be seen after a recent stroke. This *luxury perfusion* is caused by an uncoupling of blood flow from metabolism and typically occurs 1 to 10 days after the acute event.

After cerebral infarction, delayed static images may be normal during the first week, become positive by 2 to 3 weeks, and return to normal by 2 to 3 months. Characteristic wedge-shaped patterns of increased uptake in the infarcted vascular distribution are typical of strokes (Fig. 12-9, *B* to *D*). Variations in the pattern include central necrosis (doughnut appearance), associated hemorrhage producing a spherical abnormality crossing vascular distributions, occlusion of multiple branches, and *watershed infarctions* (cortical regions at the edge of two different vascular sources).

*Accuracy*    The sensitivity for stroke detection with BBB scintigraphy is approximately 80%. The spectrum of patterns seen on static images overlaps with that of tumor and infection, limiting specificity.

Bone scan agents can be taken up in cerebral infarctions, and the infarct pattern may be seen (Fig. 12-10). CT and MRI can demonstrate acute cerebral infarctions during the first week. They are more specific in distinguishing ischemic from hemorrhagic infarction and can detect intracerebral hematomas, tumors, and brain herniation, as well as estimate ventricular size.

**Subdural hematoma**    The major application of BBB scintigraphy in trauma has been for suspected subacute or chronic subdural hematomas when other studies are negative or equivocal (e.g., during the CT isodense phase).

Dynamic flow images typically show peripherally decreased activity because of the hematoma's mass effect (Fig. 12-11, *A*). Delayed images show increased activity in the same distribution *(crescent sign)* (Fig. 12-11, *B*). Although characteristic, this finding is not specific and can be seen in peripherally located lesions from other causes (e.g., infarction, scalp trauma). Delayed imaging may be helpful, since uptake in the hematoma increases with time.

### Infection

*Intracerebral abscess*    Increased flow is characteristic, and focal increased radionuclide accumulation is seen on delayed imaging. With disease progression a doughnut pattern (hot lesion with cold center) may result. These findings may be seen with other benign and malignant brain lesions.

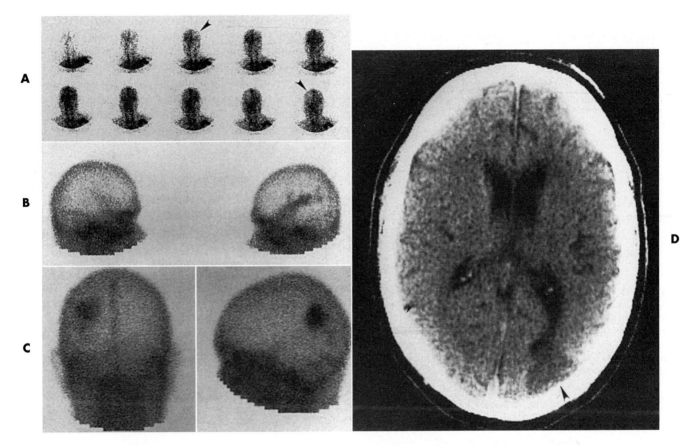

**Fig. 12-9**    Cerebrovascular insufficiency and stroke on conventional brain scans. **A,** Flow study (anterior view) shows a "flip-flop" pattern. Decreased cerebral perfusion is seen on the left *(arrowhead)* compared with the right in the early arterial parenchymal phase; this pattern then reverses on later images, showing delayed perfusion on the left while the right has cleared *(arrowhead)*. **B,** Different patient presenting with stroke and right hemiparesis. Note left parietal uptake in a vascular pattern strongly suggestive of a left middle cerebral artery infarct. **C,** Posterior and left lateral views of technetium-99m DTPA brain scan showing uptake in the posterior parietal region in a patient with a recent cerebrovascular accident. **D,** Computed tomography scan of patient in **C** confirmed a stroke in that cortical region *(arrowhead)*.

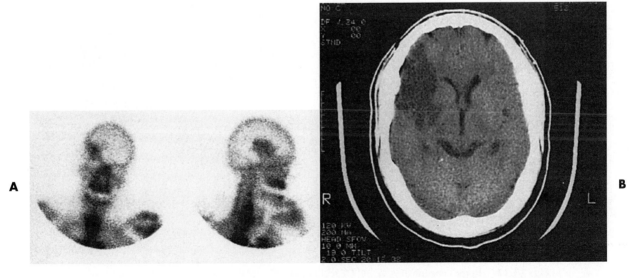

**Fig. 12-10**    Technetium-99m methylene diphosphonate (MDP) uptake in cerebrovascular accident. **A,** Planar Tc-99m MDP bone scan shows intense uptake in a right parietal cortex stroke. **B,** Computed tomography confirmed this finding.

*Herpes encephalitis*   Early diagnosis of herpes encephalitis is essential for effective treatment. Because brain biopsy is required to confirm the diagnosis, imaging localization is critical. Radionuclide imaging is more sensitive than CT for demonstrating encephalitis in its early phase, and the combination of the two has a higher sensitivity than either study alone. However, MRI is now the study of choice. On scintigraphy, increased flow and uptake within the temporal lobe are the typical findings. At present, Tc-99m hexamethylpropylene amine oxime (HMPAO) cerebral perfusion imaging is the superior scintigraphic method (Fig. 12-12; see later discussion).

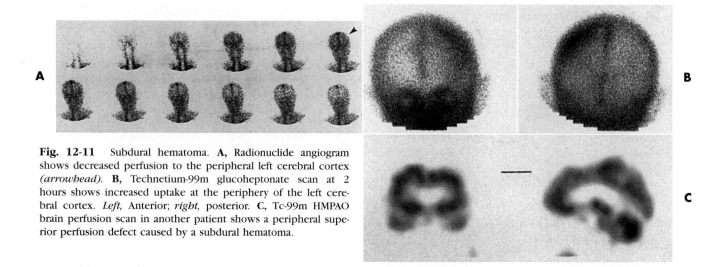

**Fig. 12-11**   Subdural hematoma. **A,** Radionuclide angiogram shows decreased perfusion to the peripheral left cerebral cortex *(arrowhead)*. **B,** Technetium-99m glucoheptonate scan at 2 hours shows increased uptake at the periphery of the left cerebral cortex. *Left,* Anterior; *right,* posterior. **C,** Tc-99m HMPAO brain perfusion scan in another patient shows a peripheral superior perfusion defect caused by a subdural hematoma.

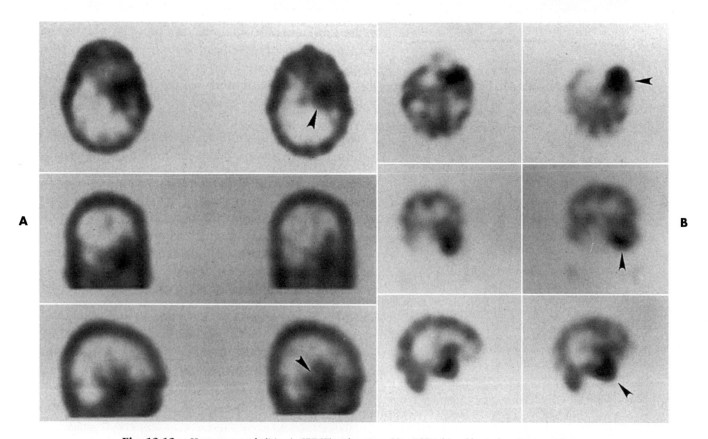

**Fig. 12-12**   Herpes encephalitis. **A,** SPECT technetium-99m DTPA blood-brain barrier scan shows left temporal lobe uptake *(arrowheads)* in patient with biopsy-proven herpes encephalitis. Selected transverse *(top),* coronal *(middle),* and sagittal *(bottom)* sections. **B,** Similar cross-sectional SPECT slices using Tc-99m HMPAO in the same patient. Increased uptake in the left temporal lobe *(arrowheads).*

*Cerebritis and ventriculitis* BBB imaging has been used to diagnose inflammatory lesions of the brain. With viral cerebritis and ventriculitis, increased blood flow is characteristic. On delayed images a pattern of bilaterally increased activity in the lateral ventricles is seen with ventriculitis.

**Vascular abnormalities** The diagnosis of *venous thrombosis* can be made with blood flow and immediate static imaging using BBB agents. However, Tc-99m-labeled red blood cell (RBC) scintigraphy is superior. Good visualization of the sinuses excludes thrombosis.

Diagnosis of cerebral *venous angiomas* can also be confirmed with Tc-99m-labeled RBC imaging. Increased uptake on delayed imaging is diagnostic (Fig. 12-13). Follow-up scintigraphy can evaluate therapeutic effectiveness.

The diagnosis of *arteriovenous malformation* can best be made during the dynamic flow phase. A focal area of intense blush and rapid washout is seen. Although the pattern is characteristic, hypervascular tu-

mors occasionally look similar. Because the BBB is intact in uncomplicated AVM, delayed static brain imaging is often negative. Immediate static images are more likely to be positive.

## Accuracy

The overall sensitivity of conventional brain scintigraphy is good (Box 12-3). However, CT and MRI are superior for most clinical indications.

## POSITRON EMISSION TOMOGRAPHY

A new era in nuclear medicine brain imaging emerged with the development of PET. This unique tool allows in vivo imaging of brain biochemistry and physiology. The potential of PET is that virtually any compound of biological interest (e.g., protein, sugar, fat, receptors, enzymes) can theoretically be labeled with radioactive oxygen, nitrogen, or carbon and used as a radiotracer (Table 12-1). Most efforts in the clinical arena to date have focused on imaging and quantifying glucose metabolism with fluorine-18 (F-18) fluorodeoxyglucose (FDG) and blood flow with oxygen-15 water (O-15 $H_2O$).

Clinical studies have found PET with F-18 FDG useful for making the diagnosis of a variety of neurological disorders, including stroke, epilepsy, dementia, and seizure disorders. Until recently, cost and regulatory issues had hindered the widespread availability of PET. However, the era of F-18 FDG imaging has arrived.

## Instrumentation

Advances in PET instrumentation have made this imaging modality not only a formidable research instrument but also a useful clinical tool. Modern PET cameras have excellent resolution. Unlike traditional SPECT instrumentation, no collimator is needed and attenuation correction can be accurately performed.

**SPECT** Dual-headed SPECT cameras are now used to image positron radionuclides. One method uses

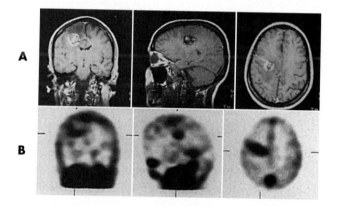

**Fig. 12-13** Venous hemangioma. **A,** Magnetic resonance imaging (MRI) shows a lesion in the right parietal cortex on coronal, sagittal, and transverse sections *(right to left)*. Angioma was suspected clinically. **B,** Technetium-99m red blood cell (RBC) study confirms the diagnosis of hemangioma (corresponding SPECT and MRI sections). RBC study could also be used to confirm the effectiveness of ablative therapy.

| Box 12-3 | Sensitivity of Blood-Brain Barrier Scintigraphy |
| --- | --- |
| **DISORDER** | **SENSITIVITY (%)** |
| Arteriovenous malformations | 95 |
| Brain abscess | 90 |
| Encephalitis | 90 |
| Brain tumors | 85 |
| Stroke | 80 |
| Subdural hematoma | |
| Chronic | 90 |
| Less than 10 days' duration | 50 |

| Table 12-1 Cyclotron-produced positron emission tomography radionuclides | | |
| --- | --- | --- |
| Radiopharmaceutical | Half-life (min) | Maximum beta + energy (MeV) |
| Fluorine-18 | 110 | 0.635 |
| Carbon-11 | 20 | 0.970 |
| Nitrogen-13 | 10 | 1.2 |
| Oxygen-15 | 2 | 1.7 |

## Box 12-4    Nuclear and Physical Properties of Fluorine-18

| | |
|---|---|
| Physical half-life | 110 min |
| Decay mode | Beta (+) decay (97%), electron capture (3%) |
| Principal emission | Positron |
| Energy (yield) | 511 keV (194%) |

## Box 12-5    Positron Emission Tomography Radiopharmaceuticals for Neurological Imaging

| COMPOUND | APPLICATION |
|---|---|
| 0-15 H$_2$O | Blood flow |
| F-18 fluorodeoxy-glucose (FDG) | Glucose metabolism |
| 0-15 O$_2$ | Oxygen metabolism |
| C-11 methionine | Amino acid metabolism |
| C-11 methylspiper-one | Dopamine receptor activity |
| C-11 carfentanil | Opiate receptor activity |
| C-11 flunitrazepam | Benzodiazepine receptor activity |
| C-11 scopolamine | Muscarinic cholinergic receptors |
| F-18 fluoro-L-DOPA | Presynaptic dopaminergic system |
| C-11 ephedrine | Adrenergic terminals |
| C-11 or O-15 car-boxyhemoglobin | Blood volume |

O, Oxygen; F, fluorine; C, carbon.

specially designed high-energy collimators, although the preferable approach uses specially adapted coincidence detection circuitry. With the coincidence detectors resolution rivals many PET cameras, although camera sensitivity is considerably poorer. Although the images are not of the same quality as with PET, this new technology allows positron imaging with cameras available in most nuclear medicine clinics.

**Cyclotron**    Production of positron radiopharmaceuticals requires a cyclotron. In the past, this required a large, expensive facility with extensive shielding and many support personnel. However, cyclotrons are now relatively small, self-contained, automated, and less costly.

For clinical F-18 FDG imaging, on-site cyclotrons are no longer required. Because of its relatively long half-life (110 minutes) (Box 12-4) and increasing clinical demand, the radiopharmaceutical is now provided on a regional basis.

## Radiopharmaceuticals

A variety of positron radiopharmaceuticals with different biochemical and physiological mechanisms are used on an investigational basis (Box 12-5) and offer great promise. Current PET research efforts focus on receptor imaging, tumor metabolism, and drug pharmacokinetic research. At present, however, F-18 FDG is the only positron radiopharmaceutical used routinely on a clinical basis.

**Mechanism of uptake**    The metabolism of the brain is based exclusively on glucose. Several glucose analogs have been investigated, but they are rapidly cleared from the brain. For example, carbon-11 (C-11) glucose is rapidly taken up by the brain cells but is quickly metabolized, and significant activity begins to leave the brain by 5 minutes as C-11 lactate and carbon dioxide.

F-18 FDG is handled differently by the brain. Once taken up, it is phosphorylated by hexokinase to deoxyglucose-6-phosphate. Unlike glucose-6-phosphate, FDG is not metabolized further and cannot diffuse

from the brain; it is metabolically trapped intracellularly. This and the relatively long half-life of F-18 make it an excellent radiopharmaceutical for imaging cerebral metabolism.

**Pharmacokinetics**    Localization of FDG in the brain occurs with an uptake half-time of about 8 minutes. By 35 minutes after injection, 95% of peak uptake is achieved. Brain uptake in human subjects averages approximately 4% of the administered dose. FDG, unlike glucose, is freely filtered by the glomerulus but partially reabsorbed by the tubules. Urinary elimination is variable, ranging from 10% to 40% of the injected dose in the first 2 hours. The distribution of FDG depends directly on regional cerebral metabolism.

**Normal and abnormal distribution**    Relative uptake of F-18 FDG is directly related to regional glucose consumption (Fig. 12-14). Uptake in gray matter is three to four times that in white matter. Increased focal or regional uptake relative to normal brain occurs with increased metabolism, as seen with malignant tumors and ictal seizure foci. Decreased uptake is seen in areas of reduced regional glucose metabolism (e.g., stroke, organic dementia).

## Dosimetry

The radiation absorbed dose of F-18 FDG is similar to those of other clinically used imaging radiopharmaceuticals. The target organ is the urinary bladder, with 4.1 rads/10 mCi. The whole body dose is 0.4 rad (Table 12-2).

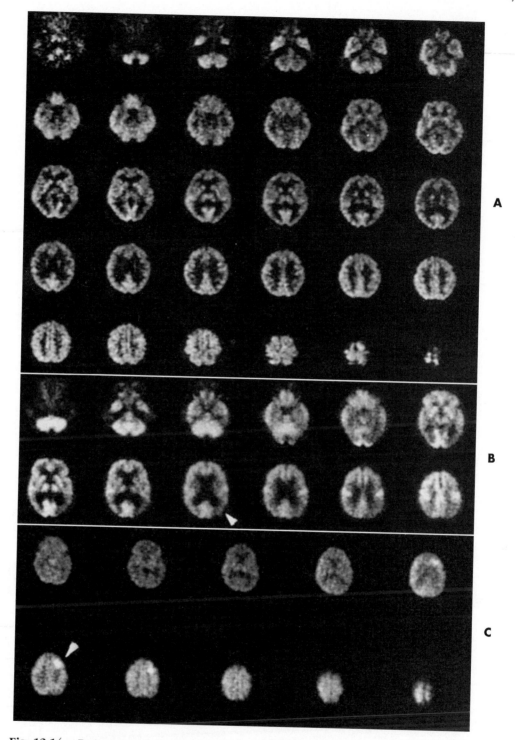

**Fig. 12-14**  Positron emission tomography. **A,** Normal fluorine-18 fluorodeoxyglucose scan with high-resolution cross-sectional images. **B,** Alzheimer's disease. Note bilateral parietal temporal hypoperfusion *(arrowheads),* although it is somewhat asymmetrical, with more decrease on the left than the right. **C,** Seizure disorder. Focally increased uptake in the left frontal parietal region *(arrowhead)* during a seizure *(ictal).*
*Continued*

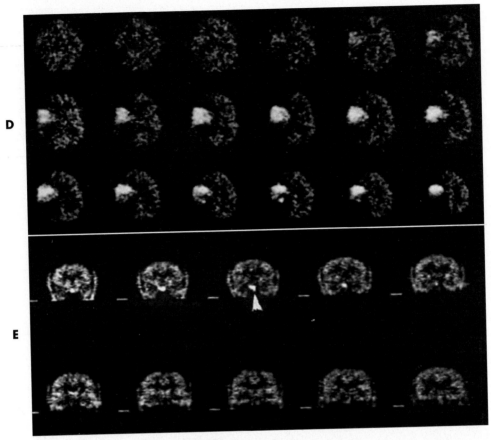

**Fig. 12-14, cont'd    D,** Astrocytoma. Focal uptake is greatly increased in this high-grade tumor.
**E,** Pituitary adenoma. Coronal sections show increased uptake in this tumor *(arrowhead).*

**Table 12-2    Radiation absorbed doses**

| Organ | 1-123 IMP<br>Rads/6 mCi<br>(cGy/222 MBq) | Tc-99m HMPAO<br>Rads/20 mCi<br>(cGy/740 MBq) | Tc-99m ECD<br>Rads/20 mCi<br>(cGy/740 MBq) | F-18 FDG<br>Rads/10 mCi<br>(cGy/370 MBq) |
|---|---|---|---|---|
| Brain | 0.4 | 0.5 | 0.4 | 0.7 |
| Lens and retina | 0.3 | 0.5 | | 1.5 |
| Heart | | | 0.2 | 0.6 |
| Lung | 0.8 | | 0.2 | 0.6 |
| Liver | 0.8 | 1.1 | | 1.4 |
| Spleen | | 3.8 | 4.0 | |
| Gallbladder | | 2.6 | 0.5 | 0.7 |
| Kidney | | 1.6 | 1.1 | |
| Large bowel | | 0.9 | 2.2 | **4.1** |
| Bladder | **1.4** | 0.1 | 0.3 | |
| Testes | 0.3 | 0.5 | 0.6 | |
| Ovaries | 0.3 | | 0.2 | |
| Red marrow | 0.3 | | 0.2 | 0.4 |
| Total body | 0.3 | 0.3 | 0.2 | |

Target organ in **bold** numbers.

## Methodology

Imaging protocols depend greatly on specific instrumentation and software. Patients are studied in the fasting state because hyperglycemia results in decreased cerebral uptake of FDG. The dose of F-18 FDG is typically 5 to 10 mCi (185 to 370 MBq). Imaging begins 30 to 60 minutes after injection. A scan time of 15 to 30 minutes is typical. To correct for attenuation, a transmission scan using an external source is also acquired. Reconstruction is now typically done using an iterative algorithm, although older systems still use filtered backprojection.

## Clinical Applications

PET first demonstrated the clinical utility of functional brain imaging for diagnosis of stroke, Alzheimer's disease, as well as localization of partial complex seizure disorder and brain tumors (Fig. 12-14). SPECT with Tc-99m-labeled cerebral perfusion agents has replicated much of the PET data. The clinical indications, scintigraphic pattern, and interpretation of the two techniques are similar.

Tc-99m-labeled cerebral perfusion agents give images similar to F-18 FDG because blood flow follows metabolism (F-18 FDG) in most disease states. Specific PET and SPECT applications are discussed with the Tc-99m-labeled brain perfusion agents; any differences are noted.

One important exception to the similarity in clinical information is with brain tumors. F-18 FDG is taken up in malignant tumors because of their increased glycolysis. The Tc-99m cerebral perfusion agents typically show decreased uptake in tumors, probably owing to the lack of receptors. However, SPECT thallium-201 (Tl-201) and Tc-99m sestamibi give clinical information and images similar to PET.

### SPECT CEREBRAL PERFUSION IMAGING

Both F-18 PET and SPECT Tc-99m-radiolabeled cerebral perfusion studies often detect functional abnormalities before morphological abnormalities are seen with CT or MRI (Box 12-6).

## Radiopharmaceuticals

**Iodine-123 isopropyl iodoamphetamine**    I-123 IMP was the first single-photon brain perfusion radiopharmaceutical approved for clinical use (1980). Although it showed the utility of cerebral perfusion agents and had unique properties, it also had limitations because of its I-123 radiolabel. Images were suboptimal because of scatter from high-energy photons (1.1% 529 keV) and the relatively low doses (3 to 6 mCi) dictated by dosimetric

---

**Box 12-6    Clinical Indications for Cerebral Perfusion Scintigraphy**

Stroke
Dementia
    Alzheimer's disease
    Multiinfarct dementia
    Acquired immunodeficiency syndrome–dementia
        complex
    Pick's disease
Epilepsy
Head trauma
Movement disorders
    Parkinson's disease
    Huntington's chorea
Psychiatric disorders
    Obsessive-compulsive disorder
    Schizophrenia
Brain death

---

considerations. I-123 IMP has been replaced on a clinical basis by the Tc-99m-labeled agents and is not generally available.

Being lipophilic, I-123 IMP rapidly crosses the BBB, diffuses through the interstitial space, and binds to amphetamine receptors on the brain cells. It has a high first-pass extraction fraction of greater than 95%. Peak brain activity is reached by 20 minutes. From 6% to 9% of the intravenous (IV) dose localizes in the brain (Table 12-3). Good correlation exists between initial IMP distribution and regional cerebral blood flow (rCBF), as determined by labeled microspheres.

Delayed cerebral uptake occurs because of IMP's slow release from the lungs and subsequent uptake by the brain. This delayed uptake by the cortex does not necessarily occur in the distribution of rCBF (redistribution). Intracranial washout also occurs. Therefore imaging must be done promptly because definition between cortex and white matter is lost within 1 hour.

**Technetium-99m agents**    A new family of Tc-99m-based CBF radiopharmaceuticals was introduced in the mid-1980s. These newer agents share several characteristics that make them useful for cerebral perfusion imaging.

The Tc-99m-labeled cerebral perfusion agents are lipophilic, permitting rapid diffusion across the BBB. They have a small molecular size, a neutral charge, and high degree of brain extraction proportional to blood flow. They distribute in the brain according to CBF, with a 3:1 to 4:1 ratio of gray/white matter uptake. The radiopharmaceuticals become fixed in brain cells with little redistribution and clear from the blood at a rate that

**Table 12-3    Pharmacokinetics of brain blood flow radiopharmaceuticals**

| Radiopharmaceuticals | Peak brain activity (min) | Blood half-life | First-pass extraction (%) | Brain uptake (%) | Washout |
|---|---|---|---|---|---|
| I-123 IMP | 20 | Slow | >90 | 6.5-8.3 | Redistribution 15% over 15 min |
| Tc-99m HMPAO | 5 | Slow | 70-80 | 3.5-7.0 | 6% per hr |
| Tc-99m ECD | 5 | Rapid | >70 | 5.0-7.0 | |

*ECD,* Ethyl cysteinate dimer; *HMPAO,* hexamethylpropyleneamine oxime; *IMP,* isopropyl iodoamphetamine.

provides a good brain/blood ratio within 1 to 2 hours after injection.

*Technetium-99m hexamethylpropyleneamine oxime* Tc-99m HMPAO (exametazime; Ceretec, Medi-physics, Inc., Paramus, N.J.) was the first Tc-99m-labeled cerebral perfusion agent to be approved and used clinically. It has a first-pass extraction fraction of 80%. Brain uptake reaches a maximum within 10 minutes after IV injection, and 3.5% to 7% of the injected dose remains within the brain (Table 12-3). Most remains fixed in the brain for several hours. Within cerebral cortical cells, HMPAO is converted by glutathione to a more hydrophilic complex that cannot diffuse back across the BBB.

The distribution of Tc-99m HMPAO within the brain is proportional to rCBF. The gray/white matter ratio is 2.5:1. If CBF and metabolism are uncoupled (e.g., in the luxury perfusion of acute stroke), Tc-99m HMPAO uptake may be normal or even increased, in contrast to I-123 IMP uptake, which always shows the metabolic defect of decreased uptake.

The original form of Tc-99m HMPAO was chemically unstable, with a shelf life of only 30 minutes, and thus had to be injected promptly after preparation. A more stable formulation with a 4-hour shelf life is now available.

*Technetium-99m ethyl cysteinate dimer* Tc-99m ECD (bicisate; Neurolite, DuPont, Billerica, Mass.) was approved for clinical use in the mid-1990s. It has a shelf life of 6 hours after preparation. After IV injection Tc-99m ECD rapidly enters the brain through passive diffusion. In the brain it is converted to a negatively charged complex that cannot diffuse back across the BBB.

As with Tc-99m HMPAO, Tc-99m ECD has moderately good first-pass extraction and somewhat underestimates rCBF. Peak activity occurs within 5 minutes after injection, and 6% to 7% of the injected dose is retained within the brain (Table 12-3). Brain uptake is rapid, and clearance from the brain is very slow. Blood clearance is rapid, resulting in a higher brain-to-background activity ratio than with Tc-99m HMPAO.

## Methodology

Functional brain imaging requires strict adherence to a standard protocol. The radiopharmaceutical should always be injected under the same environmental circumstances (e.g., room lighting, background noise, patient position). Standardization is important for proper interpretation. Otherwise, functional differences in metabolism and thus perfusion may be seen. For example, occipital parasagittal visual center activation depends on whether the eyes are open or closed.

SPECT is mandatory for diagnostic cerebral perfusion imaging. Although single-headed cameras can produce diagnostic images, dedicated brain SPECT and multi-headed cameras are preferable because of their superior image resolution. State-of-the-art SPECT systems can now give 6- to 9-mm resolution with imaging times of 10 to 20 minutes (Box 12-7).

## Dosimetry

The target organ with the greatest uptake of I-123 IMP is the lung (Box 12-8). Animal studies suggested that I-123 IMP had considerable eye uptake, although this has not been proved in humans. Sodium or potassium perchlorate should be given to prevent thyroid uptake of free I-123.

Whole body uptake of Tc-99m HMPAO is low (0.3 to 0.4 rad/20 mCi). The target organ is the gallbladder. Tc-99m ECD has a similar low dosimetry (Box 12-8).

## Image Interpretation

**Anatomy**    The cerebral cortex is composed of gray matter and anatomically divided into lobes (Fig. 12-5).

The *frontal lobe* extends from the anterior portion of the brain to the central sulcus (fissure of Rolando). Extending along the central gyrus anteriorly is the precentral gyrus, which is the motor center of the cortex. The postcentral gyrus, the sensory center of the

## Box 12-7  SPECT Cerebral Perfusion Imaging: Protocol Summary

**PATIENT PREPARATION**

None.

**RADIOPHARMACEUTICAL**

20 mCi technetium-99m HMPAO (Ceretec) or Tc-99m ECD (Neurolite)

**INSTRUMENTATION**

Camera: triple-headed SPECT
Collimators: ultra-high resolution
Computer setup: SPECT acquisition parameters
  Matrix size: $64 \times 64$
  Zoom: 2
  Rotation: step and shoot
  Orbit: circular
  Angle step size: $3°$
  Stops: 40 per head
  Time per stop: 40 sec (total time, 1600 sec or 27 min)

**IMAGING PROCEDURE**

Prepare dose according to package insert. Note shelf life.
Position patient so that brain is entirely within field of view of all detectors.
Position collimators as close as possible to patient's head.
Begin scanning 15 min or later after radiopharmaceutical injection.

**PROCESSING**

Filtered backprojection
Filter: Hamming, 1.2 high-frequency cut-off
Attenuation correction: $0.11 \text{ cm}^{-1}$

## Box 12-8  Effectiveness of SPECT for Brain Applications

| APPLICATION | RATING |
|---|---|
| Stroke (cerebrovascular accident) | |
| Detection of acute ischemia | Established |
| Determination of stroke subtype | Promising |
| Vasospasm after subarachnoid hemorrhage | Promising |
| Prognosis and recovery from stroke | Investigational |
| Monitoring therapies | Investigational |
| Diagnosis of transient ischemic attack | Investigational |
| Prognosis of transient ischemic attack | Investigational |
| Neoplasm | |
| Grading gliomas | Investigational |
| Differentiating radiation necrosis from tumor recurrence | Investigational |
| Human immunodeficiency virus encephalopathy | Investigational |
| Head trauma | Investigational |
| Epilepsy | |
| Presurgical ictal detection of seizure focus | Established |
| Localization of seizure focus | Promising |
| Differential diagnosis of ictus | Investigational |
| Interictal detection of seizure subtype | Investigational |
| Receptor studies | Investigational |
| Monitoring therapy | Doubtful |
| Alzheimer's disease: supporting clinical diagnosis | Established |
| Huntington's chorea | Investigational |
| Persistent vegetative state | Investigational |
| Brain death | Promising |

Data from Assessment of brain SPECT: report of the Therapeutics and Technology Assessment Subcommittee of the American Academy of Neurology, *Neurology* 46:278-285, 1996.

cortex, runs along the posterior margin of the central sulcus. The *parietal lobe* lies behind the central (rolandic) fissure. The most posterior segment of the cortex is the *occipital lobe,* with the right and left visual cortices on either side of the fissure.

A large, deep fissure, the lateral sulcus or sylvian fissure, divides the frontal and parietal lobes from the *temporal lobe.* If the temporal lobe is removed, its most medial margin is seen to lie adjacent to another series of gyri, the *insula* or *central lobe,* which lies hidden in the depths of the lateral sulcus. Each cerebral hemisphere is associated with sensory and motor function for the opposite side of the body. Discrete associate areas are (1) *Broca's area,* situated in the lateral portion of the frontal lobe and controlling coordination of mouth movements into coherent speech, and (2) *Wernicke's area,* located in the temporal lobe and controlling the sensory component of speech and word selection (Fig. 12-6).

Beneath the gray matter of the cerebral cortex lies the white matter, composed of myelinated fibers connecting the cortex with other parts of the brain and spinal cord. The *basal ganglion* (caudate nucleus, putamen, and globus pallidus) is the central gray matter of the cerebrum and lies between the insula and the thalamus, separated by the internal capsule of the cortical white matter. The components of the basal ganglion are important for the initiation of movement. The cerebellum occupies the posterior cranial fossa and lies between the brainstem and the occipital lobes of the cerebrum. It is involved in the regulation of muscle tone and the initiation and coordination of voluntary movements.

**Normal distribution** SPECT cerebral perfusion radiopharmaceuticals are distributed throughout the gray matter of the brain, and uptake reflects the distribution of rCBF. Uptake appears somewhat heterogeneous as a result of the normal irregular convolutions of the gyri and sulci and the resolution limits of SPECT instrumentation. Uptake is highest in the cerebellum, followed by the temporal, parietal, and frontal lobes and the basal ganglia, which have slightly lower cortical uptake (75% to 85% of the cerebellar uptake) (Fig. 12-15). Uptake in

white matter is considerably less because of the lower CBF. As a result, white matter is not seen on SPECT imaging because it fades into the background. The appearance of a central cold area seen on cross-sectional SPECT images is caused by not only the ventricular cavities, but also white matter.

## Quantification

Quantification of regional cerebral metabolism and blood flow can add greatly to the understanding of brain function and provide valuable clinical information. Al-

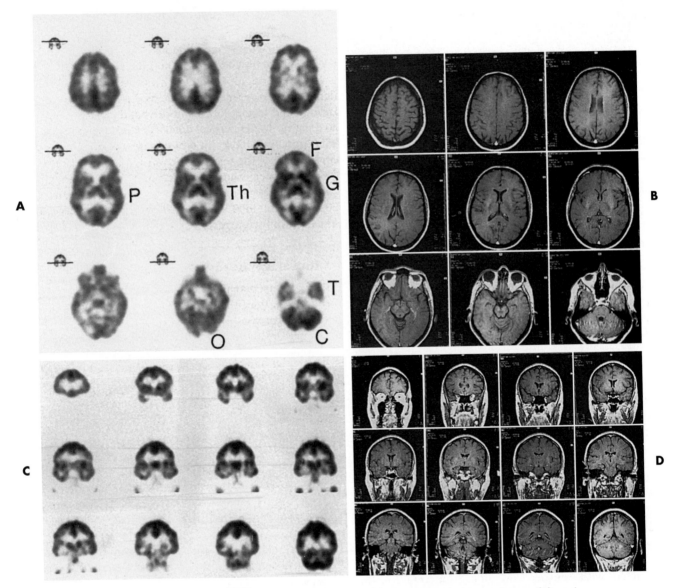

**Fig. 12-15** Normal technetium-99m HMPAO perfusion. High-resolution transverse **(A)** and coronal **(C)** cross-sectional images acquired with a three-headed camera. The frontal *(F)*, parietal *(P)*, occipital *(O)*, and temporal *(T)* lobes are delineated, as well as the thalamus *(Th)* and basal ganglion (caudate, putamen) *(G)*. Comparable transverse **(B)** and coronal **(D)** computed tomography sections in the same patient made for anatomical correlation. Relatively photopenic areas in the SPECT study are caused by not only ventricles but also white matter.

though absolute quantification is still used primarily on an investigational basis, regional quantification can be helpful in selected clinical circumstances.

Mean CBF in the normal person is 50.5 ± 6.2 ml/min/100 g. Children 3 to 10 years old have greater mean CBF, about 100 ml/min/100 g. Substantial differences exist in normal regional perfusion. Mean gray matter CBF is approximately 80 ml/min/100 g, whereas white matter CBF is 20 ml.

Blood flow increases in regions of increased metabolic demand. For example, with unilateral hand exercise, blood flow increases greatly in the contralateral motor area of the precentral gyrus. Similarly, blood flow is increased by 30% in the occipital lobes when the eyes are open versus closed. Hypoxia and hypercapnia at the tissue level increase flow by local vasodilation. The increased metabolism associated with a seizure results in increased flow. Decreased blood flow may be seen diffusely (senile dementia) or regionally (occlusive cerebrovascular disease and severe brain injury).

The standard test for quantification of CBF experimentally is the microsphere method. However, microsphere injection directly into the carotid artery is invasive and not practical clinically. PET, using oxygen-labeled water ($H_2^{15}O$) or carbon dioxide ($C^{15}O_2$), computer modeling, and arterial blood sampling, allows accurate quantification of CBF but is complex and not widely available.

Blood flow can be measured by quantifying the clearance of xenon-133 from the brain. Xenon-133 is an inert gas administered by inhalation or IV injection. The lipid-soluble gas diffuses rapidly into tissues. Washout is also rapid and directly proportional to CBF that can be calculated in ml/min/100 g.

Xenon-133 multiprobe detectors have been used for quantifying cortical blood flow. However, these systems had poor spatial resolution and measured only surface blood flow. Dynamic SPECT has been used to quantify CBF. Xenon's fast brain clearance requires very rapid acquisition capability and special instrumentation and software. Stable nonradioactive xenon has been used with CT to measure CBF, but technical difficulties, low count rates, and toxicity from pharmacological levels of xenon have limited its clinical use.

Quantification of CBF with Tc-99m HMPAO and I-123 IMP can be done but with difficulty. It requires arterial sampling and careful modeling to account for incomplete extraction, reflux from the brain, and other deviations from the theoretical model. For clinical purposes, absolute quantification is not practical. Relative quantification, however, such as right-to-left parietal cortex uptake ratio, can be clinically helpful as an aid to image interpretation.

## Clinical Applications

SPECT cerebral perfusion imaging and F-18 FDG PET can provide valuable functional and diagnostic information for a variety of neurological disorders. However, the neurological community differs regarding the clinical indications for perfusion imaging. A panel of neurological experts analyzed the clinical utility of SPECT in different disease states based on published data (Box 12-8).

**Cerebrovascular disease** Strokes (CVAs) can be categorized as (1) thrombotic, with occlusion of large vessels or branches and lacunar infarcts; (2) embolic, with thrombi originating from ulcerated carotid atheromas or diseased heart valves; and (3) hemorrhagic, including intraparenchymal hemorrhage and subarachnoid hemorrhage (SAH) produced by rupture of an aneurysm. SAH may give rise to major arterial spasm, which may result in a stroke. Less common causes include neoplasms, lupus, Moyamoya disease, fibromuscular hyperplasia, and migraine.

*Acute cerebral infarction* Stroke was the first application for SPECT cerebral perfusion imaging. Decreased rCBF can be seen immediately after the acute cerebrovascular event (Figs. 12-16 and 12-17). During the first 8 hours after infarction, only 20% of CT scans are positive, whereas 90% of SPECT scans are abnormal. With MRI several hours must pass before changes can be detected; its false negative rate is 7% to 20%.

The sensitivity of SPECT is 85% for nonlacunar strokes but somewhat less for lacunar strokes. Specificity is 88% to 98%. A wedge-shaped defect is typically seen with

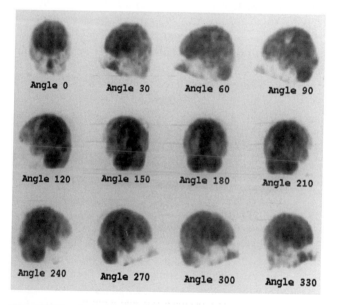

**Fig. 12-16** Reconstructed SPECT volume display of cerebral infarct with technetium-99m HMPAO shows left parietal stroke in a 65-year-old male.

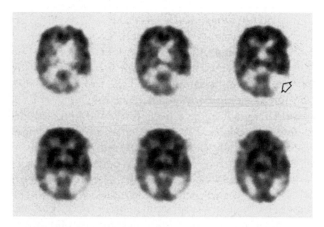

**Fig. 12-17**    Cerebral infarct with technetium-99m HMPAO. Left posterior parietal perfusion defect *(arrowhead)* is seen on sequential transverse cross-sectional SPECT images in a patient with an acute right-sided stroke.

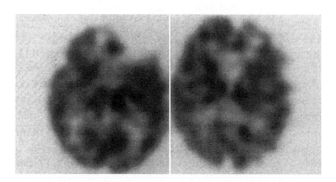

**Fig. 12-18**    Iodine-123 isopropyl iodoamphetamine (IMP) redistribution. *Left,* Immediate postinjection I-123 IMP SPECT study shows cerebral perfusion defect in the left frontal cortex. *Right,* Repeat SPECT 4 hours later shows much improved perfusion in a comparable transverse section, consistent with at least partially reversible ischemia.

embolic infarction. A normal SPECT with a lacunar syndrome is predictive of small vessel disease.

The need for a rapid and accurate method to differentiate stroke subtypes is becoming increasingly important as more specific therapies become available. Classifying stroke patients based on clinical information and anatomical imaging has significant limitations.

Defects seen on SPECT are often larger than those seen on CT, suggesting an area of ischemic brain tissue surrounding the infarction at risk for infarction (penumbra). One study predicted a good prognosis for patients who have a SPECT defect larger than that seen on CT and a poor prognosis when the two are equal in size. The explanation is that a high SPECT/CT defect ratio indicates the presence of viable but dysfunctional tissue that retains the capacity for subsequent improvement. If defect size is equal, no such capacity exists.

Imaging during the subacute phase of a stroke should be interpreted cautiously. Luxury perfusion is nonnutritive flow when there is decoupling of metabolism and rCBF in infarcted brain, thought to result from local accumulation of radicals such as potassium ions and lactate. This CBF is seen 1 to 10 days after stroke onset. Decreased cerebellar perfusion contralateral to the cortical infarct *(crossed cerebellar diaschisis)* is often noted during the acute and subacute phases of stroke and is thought to result from metabolic inhibition from direct neuroconnections.

*Transient ischemic attack*    Signs and symptoms of a stroke can be caused by transient hypoperfusion or ischemia. Rather than progressing to a completed stroke, the event resolves completely within 24 hours. Approximately 60% of patients who have had transient ischemic attacks (TIAs) later have a completed stroke. More than 80% of CT studies are normal in patients with a TIA. SPECT perfusion studies may be abnormal in up to 60% of patients during the first 24 hours, 40% by day 2, and

decreasing over 1 week. The defects seen may predict the area of eventual stroke.

*Cerebrovascular reserve*    SPECT has the potential for detecting low flow states and for evaluating cerebrovascular reserve. Specially performed SPECT studies and drug interventions may be able to identify patients who might benefit from intervention, such as carotid endarterectomy, temporal–middle cerebral artery bypass procedures, or IV thrombolytic therapy.

As CBF decreases, the normal compensatory tissue response to increased oxygen extraction is local vasodilation. This increases the blood volume/blood flow ratio to that region. The rCBF/blood volume ratio has been quantified with SPECT using combined brain perfusion (e.g., I-123 IMP) and blood volume studies (Tc-99m-labeled RBCs). An increased blood volume/perfusion ratio suggests ischemia and tissue at risk for infarction.

A less demanding method for determining the adequacy of cerebrovascular reserve is to challenge the vasculature's ability to vasodilate using acetazolamide (Diamox), a carbonic anhydrase inhibitor. In the past, neurologists have used carbon dioxide ($CO_2$) for this purpose. Normally, CBF increases fourfold with the administration of $CO_2$ or Diamox. Regions of the brain with a perfusion reserve deficit cannot increase flow normally because vasodilation is already maximal. This results in a Diamox-induced regional perfusion deficit when compared to a baseline study.

I-123 IMP, because of its property of "redistribution," may be able to demonstrate viable brain tissue in resting, low-perfusion states. Studies suggest that delayed (4-hour) uptake in regions of early hypoperfusion is an indication of viable and potentially reversible ischemia (Fig. 12-18). The hypothesized mechanism is that I-123 metabolites are taken up by viable brain cells. Although

## Box 12-9   Causes of Dementia

| DISEASE | INCIDENCE (%) |
|---|---|
| Alzheimer's disease | 50-60 |
| Parkinsonism | 15 |
| Multiinfarct dementia | 5-10 |
| Drugs and alcohol | 10 |
| Pick's disease | <1 |
| Creutzfeldt-Jakob disease | <1 |
| Progressive supranuclear palsy | <1 |
| Huntington's chorea | <1 |
| Multiple sclerosis | <1 |
| Vitamin $B_{12}$ deficiency | <1 |
| Endocrine (hypothyroid) disease | <1 |
| Chronic infection (e.g., tuberculosis, syphilis) | <1 |
| Human immunodeficiency virus encephalopathy | |

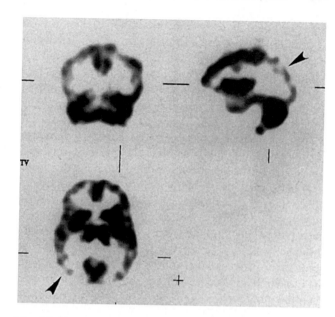

**Fig. 12-19**   Alzheimer's disease. The patient had dementia, and Alzheimer's disease was clinically suspected. The three-view display of selected coronal, sagittal, and transverse technetium-99m HMPAO sections shows a classic pattern of Alzheimer's disease with bilateral temporal-parietal hypoperfusion *(arrowheads)*. This is best seen in the sagittal view.

the mechanism differs, it is similar to T1-201 redistribution in the heart.

Although preliminary data are encouraging for tests evaluating vascular reserve, particularly the Diamox challenge test, the clinical role of these tests is uncertain and more investigation is needed.

*Subarachnoid hemorrhage*   One half of intracranial hemorrhages occur secondary to SAH, with a mortality rate approaching 50%. The cause is rupture of an intracranial aneurysm. The acute hemorrhage results in stroke symptoms, and an abnormal rCBF pattern is seen with SPECT. Delayed symptoms and signs may occur secondary to major vessel spasm for up to 2 weeks after SAH, resulting in ischemia and stroke. SPECT perfusion studies can detect these areas of spasm, which often are not evident on CT, and can guide therapy.

**Dementia**   The diagnosis of dementia implies loss of mental faculties sufficient to interfere with social and occupational functioning. Deficits include memory, language, and visual-spatial perception. Psychiatric symptoms may occur. The differential diagnosis is extensive, and the entities are not always clinically distinguishable (Box 12-9). SPECT cerebral perfusion imaging has shown clinical utility in the differential diagnosis.

*Alzheimer's disease*   Alzheimer's disease is now recognized as a common cause of dementia. In the past the diagnosis was associated with a relatively young age group (presenile dementia). It is now appreciated that many patients previously classified as having multiinfarct dementia actually had Alzheimer's disease. On the other hand, approximately 25% of patients in whom Alzheimer's disease is diagnosed are found to have other diseases at autopsy. Clinical neurological criteria can often differentiate these diseases, but considerable overlap exists. Clinical accuracy in histologically confirmed

cases is reported to be only 60% to 80%. Brain biopsy is the only definitive method of diagnosis but is rarely used.

Alzheimer's disease has characteristic pathological findings. Abnormal *tangles* of nerve fibers and degenerative neuritic *plaques* are seen, usually in the temporal and parietal lobes bilaterally. The patient's degree of dysfunction is related to the number of these abnormal cortical structures.

The classic scintigraphic pattern for Alzheimer's disease on SPECT perfusion imaging is bilateral posterior temporal and parietal hypoperfusion (Fig. 12-19). The areas of reduced perfusion are secondary to the reduced brain metabolism in areas of neuronal depletion. With severe disease, frontal lobe hypoperfusion is seen as well.

This scintigraphic pattern of bilateral decreased posterior parietal-temporal perfusion has a predictive value of greater than 80% for Alzheimer's disease, although it may be seen in other diseases (e.g., severe Parkinson's disease and associated dementia). Less frequent and less specific patterns seen with Alzheimer's disease include unilateral temporal-parietal and anterior perfusion defects. The occipital lobes, sensory motor cortex, and cerebellum are generally spared.

*Other dementias*   Other causes of dementia have characteristic patterns as well. *Pick's disease* is characterized by frontal lobe hypoperfusion (Fig. 12-20). The scintigraphic pattern of *multiinfarct dementia* shows multiple asymmetrical perfusion defects, often involving the primary cortex and deep structures. Patients with

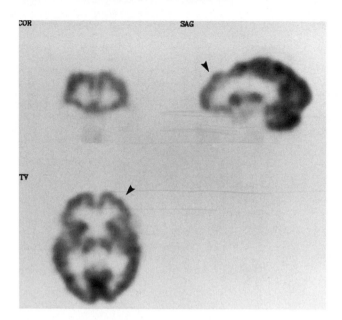

**Fig. 12-20** Pick's disease. SPECT technetium-99m ethylcysteinate dimer shows typical hypoperfusion of frontal lobes *(arrowheads)*. Patient had dementia.

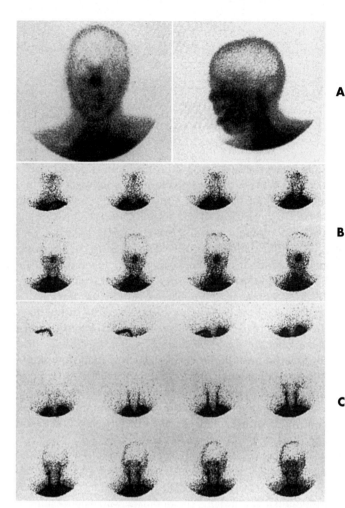

**Fig. 12-21** Brain death. **A,** Flow study with technetium-99m HMPAO shows no cerebral perfusion. **B,** Planar images obtained 15 minutes after injection of Tc-99m HMPAO show no cortical uptake. The images appear similar to a normal blood-brain barrier study (Fig. 12-1). This is diagnostic of brain death (Fig. 12-22). **C,** Tc-99m DTPA late blood flow study shows activity transiting the internal carotids but no intracerebral blood flow. The "hot nose" is caused by shunting of flow from the internal to the external carotid system that supplies the face and scalp. Hot nose can also be seen in *B*.

depression and systemic metabolic etiologies typically have normal perfusion.

**Brain death**  Diagnosis of brain death is primarily clinical. Accuracy and speed in making the diagnosis become critical when organ donation for transplantation is considered and life support systems must be used.

*Clinical diagnosis*  Specific criteria are necessary to make the diagnosis of brain death, as follows:

1. The patient must be in deep coma with total absence of brainstem reflexes or spontaneous respiration.
2. Potentially reversible causes must be excluded, such as drug intoxication, metabolic derangement, or hypothermia.
3. The cause of the brain dysfunction must be diagnosed (e.g., trauma, stroke).
4. The clinical findings of brain death must be present for a defined period of observation (6 to 24 hours).

*Confirmatory tests*  Ancillary tests are used by clinicians to increase certainty, but the diagnosis of brain death is still primarily a clinical one. An isoelectric electroencephalogram (EEG) by itself does not establish brain death, and at least one repeat study is required. In the patient with intoxication from barbiturates and other depressive drugs or with hypothermia, the EEG may be flat, even though cerebral perfusion is still present and recovery is possible.

*Pathology*  Edema, softening, necrosis, and autolysis of brain tissue lead to increased intracranial pressure sufficient to overcome arterial pressure and prevent CBF. Lack of blood flow to the brain is diagnostic of brain death. This can be demonstrated with four-vessel arteriography, but the test is invasive, usually impractical, and unnecessary.

*Radionuclide studies*  The radionuclide brain death study is usually performed when the patient meets clinical criteria for brain death but the EEG is equivocal. It is simple and rapid, can be performed at the bedside, and serves as an important ancillary test for confirming brain death. Scintigraphy is not affected by drug intoxication or hypothermia. An abnormal radionuclide angiogram showing no cerebral perfusion is more specific for brain death than an isoelectric EEG.

RADIOPHARMACEUTICALS  Brain death can be diagnosed using a radionuclide flow study alone. The lack of intracerebral blood flow is diagnostic (Fig. 12-21, *A*). Any technetium-labeled radiopharmaceutical can be used, since interpretation is based only on the flow phase. Tc-99m DTPA is often used because it is cleared rapidly from the blood, allowing a repeat study if

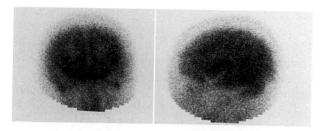

**Fig. 12-22**    Planar images of normal technetium-99m HMPAO cerebral perfusion. *Left,* Anterior; *right,* left lateral. Cortical uptake is normal. SPECT is not needed to diagnose or exclude brain death.

necessary. Diagnosis depends on a good bolus. However, Tc-99m HMPAO and Tc-99m ECD are preferred, although more expensive. Flow images can be obtained but are not really necessary, since cortical uptake of these agents depends on CBF. If no CBF is present, no cerebral uptake will occur (Fig. 12-21, *B*). Planar images are adequate, and SPECT is not necessary to diagnose brain death (Fig. 12-22).

METHODOLOGY    The radionuclide angiogram protocol for CBF is used in brain death (Box 12-2). A scalp tourniquet may be used to minimize flow through the external carotid arteries, facilitating image interpretation of brain perfusion. A tourniquet is contraindicated in children, however, because it could increase intracranial pressure. Adults also probably do not require a tourniquet, since peripheral scalp activity can usually be differentiated from cerebral perfusion.

IMAGE INTERPRETATION    An adequate radiopharmaceutical dose, 10 mCi or 370 MBq, and good bolus are required to ensure a diagnostic flow study. Diagnostic findings of brain death include the lack of intracranial arterial flow and no visualization of major venous sinuses on subsequent static images. Flow to both common carotid arteries is seen to the level of the base of the skull.

Often the "hot nose" sign is seen (Fig. 12-21, *C*). Diversion of flow from the intracranial to extracranial circulation results in relatively increased flow to the face and nose. This pattern can also be seen in internal carotid artery occlusion without brain death. Faint visualization of the venous sagittal or transverse sinus in the absence of intracranial perfusion is also sometimes seen.

Although most interpret these findings as equivocal and recommend a repeat follow-up study (hours to days), others believe that these represent part of the spectrum of decreasing cerebral perfusion and that brain death can be diagnosed if there is unequivocal lack of arterial flow. These patients typically progress to death within days.

**Seizure disorders**    Many patients with partial complex seizures unresponsive to anticonvulsant drug therapy may be helped by temporal lobectomy. The most common pathological finding is mesial temporal sclerosis, thought to result from a glial scar after resolution of a disease process. Excision of well-localized foci can lead

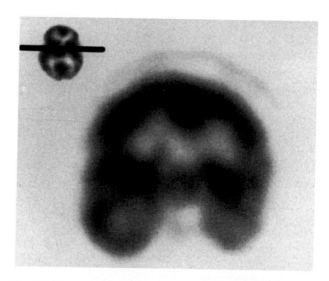

**Fig. 12-23**    Seizure disorder with technetium-99m HMPAO. The patient had partial complex seizures poorly responsive to conventional anticonvulsant therapy and was being considered for temporal lobectomy. The electroencephalogram and clinical history favored a left temporal focus. If the Tc-99m HMPAO study could confirm this, subdurally placed depth electrodes could be avoided. The interictal study shows hypoperfusion of the left temporal lobe, consistent with a left temporal lobe focus.

to elimination of seizures or significantly improved pharmacological control in 80% of surgical patients. Only a few undergo surgery, however, partly because of the difficulty of adequate seizure focus localization.

Surface EEG has poor spatial resolution, depends on cortical surface effects, and is limited by the area of brain sampled. As a result, EEG may not always be diagnostic and can be misleading. CT and MRI have low sensitivity for seizure focus detection, 17% and 34%, respectively. Although surgically placed depth EEG electrodes can confirm a suspected site of seizure focus, only limited regions can be sampled, and the technique is invasive and associated with some risk.

F-18 FDG PET and SPECT perfusion agents can localize *epileptic foci*. Seizure foci are seen as areas of hypometabolism and hypoperfusion *interictally* (Fig. 12-23) and hypermetabolism and hyperperfusion *ictally* (Fig. 12-14, *C*), usually in the temporal lobes. Extratemporal seizure foci, such as in the frontal lobe, can also be identified, although surgical results have been less successful.

Concurrence of the clinical picture, surface EEG pattern, and radionuclide localization can obviate the need for more invasive diagnostic procedures. PET and SPECT studies have a similar sensitivity for detection of interictal seizure foci (65% to 75%). Sensitivity for localizing the seizure focus ictally is considerably higher (greater than 90%).

For ictal identification of seizure focus the patient must be under continuous EEG monitoring, the radiopharmaceutical must be on hand to inject at the time of the seizure, and imaging must be performed soon after.

FDG PET is particularly a problem because of the short half-life of F-18. SPECT is also limited by radionuclide half-life, as well as by the shelf life of the pharmaceutical. This approach has been successful at a few institutions but poses logistical and radiation safety problems at most hospitals.

**Head trauma**   Tc-99m HMPAO SPECT is more sensitive than CT in detecting abnormalities in patients with a history of closed traumatic brain injury and can detect the changes earlier, particularly in patients with minor head injuries.

In addition to acute evidence of injury in the form of direct and contrecoup rCBF deficits, SPECT studies can demonstrate residual flow defects in patients with remote trauma. In one study, SPECT showed rCBF defects in 80% of patients with head trauma versus 55% on CT and 45% on MRI. With minor head injuries, 60% showed deficits on SPECT and only 25% on CT.

**Huntington's chorea**   The symptoms of the hereditary disorder Huntington's chorea, also called Huntington's disease, develop insidiously and usually are manifested between ages 35 and 50 years, inevitably progressing to uncontrollable choreiform movements and dementia. Basal ganglia atrophy, especially the caudate nuclei. The caudate and putamen are deficient in the inhibitory neurotransmitter gamma-aminobutyric acid (GABA) and in glutamic acid decarboxylase. Although the disease can begin asymmetrically, symmetrical involvement eventually develops. Both PET and SPECT imaging can show decreased uptake in the caudate nucleus, which often precedes the atrophy seen on CT, in patients with moderate to severe Huntington's chorea.

**HIV encephalopathy and AIDS-dementia complex**   Early clinical signs involving human immunodeficiency virus (HIV) and acquired immunodeficiency syndrome (AIDS) are frequently subtle and may be difficult to distinguish from depression, psychosis, or focal neurological disease. Because treatment (e.g., with AZT) can improve cognitive function, early detection is helpful. Findings on CT and MRI are not specific.

Cerebral perfusion SPECT is highly sensitive for AIDs-dementia complex and shows a typical scintigraphic pattern of multifocal or patchy cortical and subcortical regions of hypoperfusion, most frequently in the frontal, temporal, and parietal lobes. Basal ganglia involvement is common. Many patients also have focal areas of increased activity. The perfusion pattern can improve with therapy. A similar brain perfusion pattern has been described in chronic cocaine and polydrug users.

**Psychiatric diseases**   The role of PET and SPECT brain perfusion imaging in psychiatric diseases is uncertain. Diagnostic or prognostic functional abnormalities have not been identified in psychiatric diseases. Although frontal lobe hypometabolism and hypoperfusion have been described in *schizophrenia*, the findings are nonspecific. Studies in patients with *depression* have yielded conflicting results, although patients with depression and metabolic disturbances usually have normal perfusion. Limited studies in patients with *obsessive-compulsive disorder*, mostly with PET, have shown increased metabolism in the orbital region of the frontal cortex and caudate nuclei. At present, functional scintigraphy may be of most value in identifying patients with psychiatric symptoms in whom underlying organic disease is suspected.

## BRAIN TUMORS

Primary intracranial tumors constitute 5% to 10% of all cancers, and gliomas represent 50% of all intracranial tumors. Median survival is about 1 year. F-18 FDG PET can play a role in the clinical management of brain tumors, including the preoperative grading of tumors, determination of prognosis, and differentiation of recurrent tumor from radiation necrosis.

High-grade primary brain tumors are hypermetabolic, as seen with F-18 FDG, whereas low-grade tumors are hypometabolic. FDG PET can more accurately predict the degree of malignancy of a tumor than CT or MRI. Similarly, FDG can predict survival in patients with glioma. Survival of patients with hypermetabolic tumors is 7 to 11 months, compared with 1 to 7 years for low-grade tumors. In addition, PET, unlike CT or MRI, can distinguish radiation necrosis from tumor recurrence (Fig. 12-24). Areas of radiation necrosis are hypometabolic, whereas tumor recurrence appears hypermetabolic. Metastatic brain tumors can also be detected with brain PET. Pituitary adenomas, although benign, can also be detected with FDG PET (Fig. 12-14, *E*).

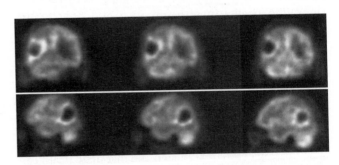

**Fig. 12-24**   Recurrent glioblastoma. A 53-year-old man with a tumor in the parietal lobe received gamma knife therapy. Follow-up magnetic resonance imaging showed enhancement of the left temporal lobe area. Follow-up fluorine-18 fluorodeoxyglucose positron emission tomography study (*top,* coronal; *bottom,* sagittal) was ordered to evaluate therapeutic effectiveness. Intense uptake is seen at the periphery of the cold parietal lobe defect, consistent with residual or recurrent viable tumor.

In contrast, the SPECT cerebral perfusion agents I-123 IMP and Tc-99m HMPAO show decreased uptake in most primary and metastatic tumors. Tumors rarely show increased uptake on SPECT with Tc-99m HMPAO or Tc-99m ECD and never with I-123 IMP, probably because of the lack of normal receptors on the tumor cells. If early dynamic SPECT acquisition is performed, increased flow to the tumor can usually be demonstrated, confirming that these tumors have increased blood flow, but the tumor cannot retain the tracer.

*Thallium-201* (Tl-201), used for myocardial perfusion imaging, is also taken up by a variety of human tumors. SPECT Tl-201 imaging can be used to image brain tumors. As with FDG PET, studies have shown that the degree of uptake in glioblastomas is proportional to the malignant grade of the tumor. Tumors with the highest grade have the most uptake, which has prognostic implications.

The most important clinical use of Tl-201 has been for determining tumor viability after radiation therapy. It is often difficult to differentiate residual or recurrent viable tumor from tumor necrosis and fibrosis on CT or MRI. Both F-18 FDG PET (Fig. 12-24) and Tl-201 SPECT (Fig. 12-25) can reliably distinguish the two with similar high accuracy.

Tl-201 SPECT and FDG PET have been used to evaluate an intracerebral mass lesion in AIDS patients. In this patient group the differential diagnosis is lymphoma (30% incidence) versus toxoplasmosis (60% incidence) and other atypical infectious agents. Lym-

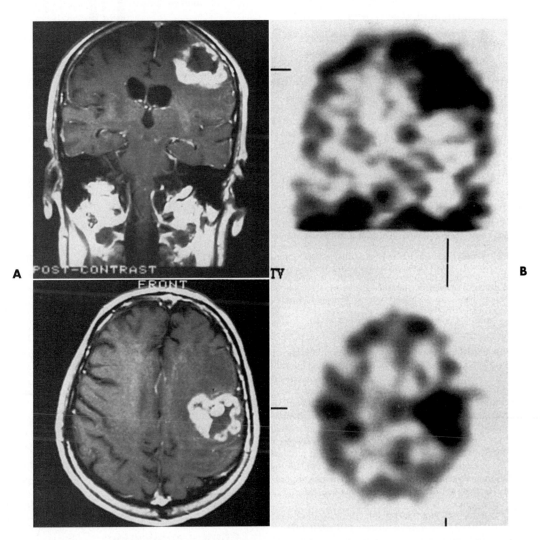

**Fig. 12-25**    Brain tumor imaged with thallium-201. **A,** Magnetic resonance imaging (MRI) shows an astrocytoma in the left parietal region of the brain on selected coronal and transverse sections. **B,** Corresponding sections of a Tl-201 SPECT study in the same patient. The intense uptake is consistent with a high-grade malignant tumor. This test can be used to differentiate viable residual tumor from postradiation therapy fibrosis and necrosis, often not distinguishable on computed tomography or MRI.

phoma in AIDS patients is usually an aggressive tumor and requires prompt therapy. Usually a clinical trial of antitoxoplasmosis therapy is undertaken. However, 2 to 3 weeks or longer is necessary to determine the effectiveness of therapy, often delaying appropriate therapy in patients with other causes of an intracerebral mass lesion. Intracerebral lymphoma in AIDS patients avidly takes up F-18 FDG and Tl-201, unlike infection.

*Tc-99m sestamibi* is similarly taken up by a variety of tumors, but its uptake in the choroid plexus may not be ideal for imaging some brain tumors.

## CISTERNOGRAPHY

Study of cerebrospinal fluid (CSF) dynamics using radiotracers has been used for many years to diagnose the site of CSF leakage, to determine shunt patency, and to diagnose and manage hydrocephalus. Although CT and MRI are now often used, radionuclide cisternography can still play an important role because of the unique physiological information it provides.

### Radiopharmaceuticals

Various radiotracers have been used over the years, including iodine-131 serum albumin, Tc-99m HSA, and yterbium-169. However, *indium-111 DTPA* is now the agent of choice because of its better imaging characteristics, shorter half-life, and lower dosimetry.

**Cerebrospinal fluid**  CSF, which fills the ventricles and subarachnoid space surrounding the brain and spinal cord, is secreted in the choroid plexus of the ventricles and to a lesser extent in extraventricular sites. The CSF normally drains from the lateral ventricles through the interventricular foramen of Monro into the third ventricle (Fig. 12-26). With the additional CSF produced by the choroid plexus of the third ventricle, it then passes through the cerebral aqueduct of Sylvius into the fourth ventricle and then leaves the ventricular system through the median foramen of Magendie and the two lateral foramina of Luschka.

The CSF then enters the subarachnoid space surrounding the brain and spinal cord. Along the base of the brain the subarachnoid space expands into a number of lakes called *cisterns.* The subarachnoid space extends over the surface of the brain. The CSF bathes the brain and is absorbed through the pacchionian granulations of the pia arachnoid villi into the superior sagittal sinus.

**Pharmacokinetics**  Radiopharmaceuticals injected intrathecally into the lumbar subarachnoid space are small molecules that follow the flow of the CSF without affecting the dynamics. The radiotracer normally reaches

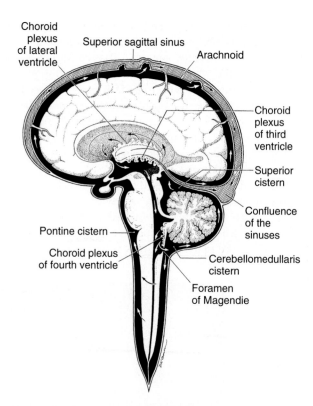

**Fig. 12-26**  Flow dynamics of cerebrospinal fluid (CSF). Originating in the choroid plexus of the lateral ventricle, CSF flows through the third and fourth ventricles into the basal cisterns, moves over the cerebral convexities, and finally is reabsorbed in the superior sagittal sinus.

the basal cisterns by 1 hour, the frontal poles and sylvian fissure area by 2 to 6 hours, the cerebral convexities by 12 hours, and the arachnoid villi in the sagittal sinus by 24 hours. Flow to the parasagittal region occurs through both central and superficial routes. The radiotracer does not normally enter the ventricular system because physiological flow is in the opposite direction.

### Dosimetry

The radiation absorbed dose depends to some extent on the clearance dynamics of a particular patient. The spinal cord receives the highest dose, followed by the kidney and bladder, since the radiopharmaceutical undergoes renal excretion (Box 12-10).

### Clinical applications

**Hydrocephalus**  Hydrocephalus is enlargement of the ventricular cavities with a pathological increase in CSF volume (Table 12-4).

*Generalized nonobstructive hydrocephalus* refers to patients with cerebral atrophy. CT shows ventricular

## Box 12-10  Dosimetry for Indium-111 DTPA Cisternography

| ORGAN | Rads/500 µCi (cGy/18.5 MBq) |
|---|---|
| Total body | 0.04 |
| Kidneys | 0.22 |
| Spinal cord | |
| Surface | 5.00 |
| Average | 1.50 |
| Brain | |
| Surface | 4.10 |
| Average | 0.50 |
| Bladder | 0.50 |
| Testes | 0.05 |
| Ovaries | 0.06 |

## Table 12-4  Classification of hydrocephalus

| Classification | Site of obstruction | Scintigraphy type |
|---|---|---|
| **OBSTRUCTIVE** | | |
| Noncommunicating | Intraventricular, between lateral ventricles and basal cisterns | I, II |
| Communicating | Extraventricular, affecting basal cisterns, cerebral convexities, and arachnoid villi | IIIA, IIIB, IV |
| **NONOBSTRUCTIVE** | | |
| Generalized | Cerebral atrophy | II |
| Localized | Porencephaly | |

## Table 12-5  Cerebrospinal fluid flow patterns in hydrocephalus

| Type | Pattern | Etiologies |
|---|---|---|
| I | Basal cistern, 2-4 hr; Sylvian fissure, 6 hr; Over convexities, 24 hr; Decreased activity, 48 hr | Normal; Intraventricular obstructive hydrocephalus |
| II | No ventricular activity; Delayed migration | Cerebral atrophy; Increased intracerebral pressure; Advanced age; Noncommunicating hydrocephalus |
| IIIA | Transient ventricular activity; Clearance by usual migration (often) | Cerebral atrophy; Evolving or resolving communicating hydrocephalus |
| IIIB | Transient ventricular activity, clearance without usual migration | Communicating hydrocephalus with alternative pathway of resorption (transependymal) |
| IV | Persistent ventricular activity, inadequate clearance | Communicating hydrocephalus |

dilated out of proportion to the cortical sulci and basal cisterns are prominent.

*Normal-pressure hydrocephalus* (NPH) is a common cause of a communicating hydrocephalus. It manifests clinically with dementia, ataxia, and incontinence. The etiology and cisternographic findings do not differ from those of communicating hydrocephalus with elevated pressure. Radionuclide cisternography is usually performed to differentiate NPH from hydrocephalus ex vacuo (generalized brain atrophy). Diagnosis can sometimes be made with MRI based on the size of the ventricles, cisterns, and convexity sulci, but the findings overlap with cerebral atrophy.

Radionuclide cisternography is often needed to confirm the diagnosis of NPH. A spectrum of CSF flow patterns is seen with NPH (Table 12-5 and Fig. 12-27). The common denominators, however, are ventricular reflux that does not clear by 24 hours and delayed clearance over the cerebral hemispheres, consistent with a convexity block (Fig. 12-28). Atrophy alone will cause delayed tracer movement through the enlarged subarachnoid space, sometimes with transient ventricular reflux, but normal clearance over the hemispheres is seen by 24 hours.

NPH is a progressive disease. Surgical shunting of CSF can potentially cure this cause of dementia, but not all patients improve with surgery. Predicting which patients will respond is a diagnostic problem. Radionuclide cisternography, when used in conjunction with clinical

dilation and wide cortical sulci. Porencephaly is a *localized nonobstructive hydrocephalus.*

*Obstructive noncommunicating hydrocephalus* refers to an intraventricular obstruction between the lateral ventricles and the basal cistern, caused by such conditions as a colloid cyst, aqueductal stenosis, Arnold-Chiari malformation, and neoplasm. The diagnosis is usually made by MRI. Lumbar radionuclide cisternography demonstrates a normal flow pattern.

*Obstructive communicating hydrocephalus* refers to an extraventricular obstruction in the basal cisterns, cerebral convexities, or arachnoid villi. Common causes of the latter include a previous SAH, chronic subdural hematoma, leptomeningitis, and meningeal carcinomatosis. On anatomical imaging the ventricular system is

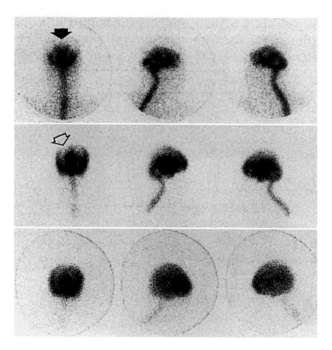

**Fig. 12-27**   Normal-pressure hydrocephalus. Tc-99m DTPA cisternogram images acquired at 24 hours *(top),* 48 hours *(middle),* and 72 hours *(bottom)* in the anterior *(left),* right lateral *(middle),* and left lateral *(right)* views. Ventricular reflux *(closed arrowhead)* is present, as is very delayed flow *(open arrowhead)* over the cerebral convexities. The intracerebral activity at 72 hours was caused by transependymal uptake.

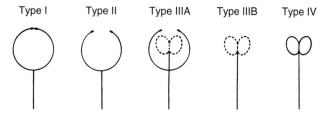

Type I   Type II   Type IIIA   Type IIIB   Type IV

**Fig. 12-28**   Abnormal patterns of cerebrospinal fluid flow (Table 12-5).

findings, such as a response (mental clearing) to CSF fluid reduction, can be helpful. Patients with the type IV cisternographic pattern are most likely to benefit from shunting.

In the cisternography protocol, proper lumbar puncture technique is critical and should be done by an experienced clinician to ensure subarachnoid injection (Box 12-11).

**Surgical shunt patency**   Diversionary CSF shunts (ventriculoperitoneal, ventriculoatrial, lumboperitoneal) are used to treat obstructive forms of hydrocephalus. Many types of shunts and numerous variations have been used over the years. Complications may include catheter blockage, infection, thromboembolism, subdural or epidural hematomas, disconnection of catheters, and bowel perforation.

---

**Box 12-11   Cisternography: Protocol Summary**

**PATIENT PREPARATION**
None.

**RADIOPHARMACEUTICAL**
Indium-111 DTPA, 250 μCi

**INSTRUMENTATION**
Camera: large-field-of-view gamma
Collimator: medium energy

**IMAGING PROCEDURE**
Inject slowly into lumbar subarachnoid space using a 22-gauge needle with the bevel positioned vertically.
Patient should remain recumbent for at least 1 hr after injection.
All images should be obtained for 50k counts.
Imaging times:
   1 hr: thoracic-lumbar spine for evaluation of injection adequacy.
   3 hr: base of the skull to visualize basilar cisterns.
   24 and 48 hr: evaluation of ventricular reflux and arachnoid villi resorption.
Obtain anterior, posterior, and both lateral views of the head at 3, 24, and 48 hr.

---

The diagnosis of shunt patency and adequacy of CSF flow can often be made by examination of the patient and inspection of the subcutaneous CSF reservoir. When this assessment is uncertain, radionuclide studies with In-111 DTPA or Tc-99m DTPA are useful for confirming the diagnosis. Familiarity with the specific type and configuration of shunt is helpful when performing a CSF shunt study. For example, the valves may allow bidirectional or only unidirectional flow.

Shunt injection should be performed by a physician familiar with the type of shunt in place, preferably the neurosurgeon (Box 12-12). Proximal patency into the ventricles can be evaluated before checking distal patency in patients with two-way valves by initially occluding the distal catheter flow.

Images should show prompt flow into the ventricles and then spontaneous distal flow through the shunt catheter (Figs. 12-29 and 12-30). The shunt tubing is usually seen. Catheters draining into the peritoneum show accumulation of radiotracer freely within the abdominal cavity.

**Cerebrospinal fluid leak**   Trauma and surgery (transsphenoidal and nasal) are the most common causes for CSF rhinorrhea. Nontraumatic causes include hydrocephalus and congenital defects. CSF rhinorrhea may occur at any site, from the frontal sinuses to the temporal

bone (Fig. 12-31). The cribriform plate is most susceptible to fracture and rhinorrhea. Otorrhea is much less
common.

Accurate localization of CSF leaks can be clinically
difficult. Although glucose oxidase test strips are used
to confirm CSF leak, both lacrimal and nasal secretions
contain glucose. The false positive rate may be as high
as 50%.

Radionuclide studies are sensitive and accurate methods of detection. The site is most likely to be identified
during heavy leakage. Imaging in the appropriate projection is important for identifying the site of leak; lateral
and anterior imaging is used for rhinorrhea and posterior
imaging for otorrhea.

To maximize the sensitivity of the test, nasal pledgets
are placed in the anterior and posterior portion of each
nasal region and then removed and counted 4 hours
later (Fig. 12-32). A ratio of nasal-to-plasma radioactivity

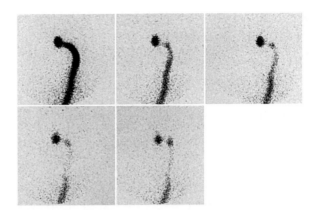

**Fig. 12-29**    Cerebrospinal fluid shunt patency. After injection of
Indium-111 DTPA into the shunt reservoir, rapid clearance occurs
over 30 minutes. Anterior abdominal view can confirm clearance
through the ventriculoperitoneal shunt into the abdominal cavity.

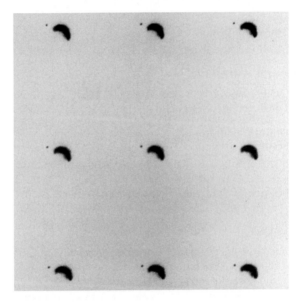

**Fig. 12-30**    Obstructed cerebrospinal fluid shunt. After injection of technetium-99m DTPA into the reservoir, good reflux into
ventricles is seen, consistent with patency of the proximal portion
of the shunt. However, no distal drainage occurs over 60 minutes,
consistent with obstruction.

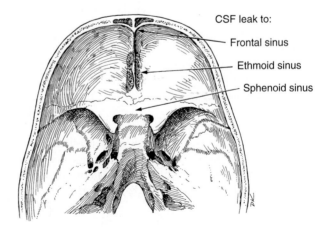

CSF leak to:
- Frontal sinus
- Ethmoid sinus
- Sphenoid sinus

**Fig. 12-31**    Common sites of cerebrospinal fluid *(CSF)* leakage.

## Box 12-13 Cerebrospinal Fluid Leak Detection: Protocol Summary

**PATIENT PREPARATION**

Nasal pledgets should be placed and labeled as to location. The pledgets should be weighed before placement.

After intrathecal injection, place patient in Trendelenburg position to pool the radiotracer in the basal regions until imaging begins.

Once radiotracer reaches basal cisterns, position patient in a position that increases cerebrospinal fluid leakage.

    Rhinorrhea: incline patient's head forward and against camera face with the camera positioned in the lateral position.

    Otorrhea: obtain posterior images instead of lateral views.

**RADIOPHARMACEUTICAL**

In-111 DTPA, 250 µCi

**INSTRUMENTATION**

Camera: large-field-of-view gamma
Collimator: medium energy

**IMAGING PROCEDURE**
**Setup**

Inject intrathecally 500 µCi of In-111 DTPA in 5 ml of dextrose 10% in water.

Begin imaging when activity reaches the basal cisterns (1 to 4 hr).

**Acquisition**

Acquire 5 min/frame for 1 hr in the selected view, then acquire anterior, left lateral, right lateral, and posterior views.

Obtain 50k images every 10 min for 1 hr in the original view.

Remove pledgets and place in separate tubes. Draw a 5-ml blood sample.

Count pledgets and 0.5-ml aliquots of plasma.

Repeat views may be indicated at 6 and 24 hr.

Calculate the ratio of pledgets-to-plasma activity: pledget counts/pledget capacity divided by serum counts/0.5 ml.

**Interpretation**

Positive for CSF leakage if the pledget/plasma activity ratio is greater than 2-3:1

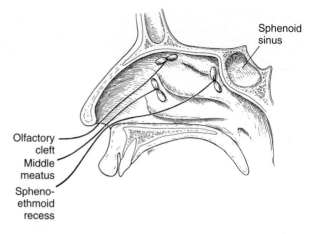

**Fig. 12-32**   Placement of pledgets for cerebrospinal fluid leak study. The labeled cotton pledgets are placed by an otolaryngologist at various locations within the anterior and posterior nares to detect leakage from the frontal, ethmoidal, and sphenoidal sinuses.

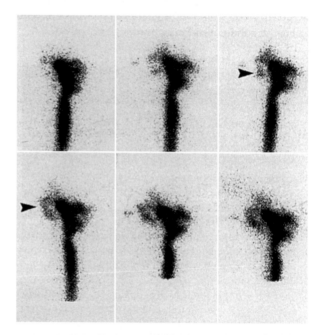

**Fig. 12-33**   Radionuclide cerebrospinal fluid leak study, left lateral view. Positive indium-111 DTPA study with radioactivity increasing over time, originating from the nares, and leaking into the nose and mouth *(arrowheads)*.

CSF leaks are seen on scintigraphy as an increasing accumulation of activity at the site (Fig. 12-33). The pledgets are more sensitive than imaging for detecting CSF leaks. Pledgets are also helpful in determining the origin of the leak (anterior versus posterior).

## SUGGESTED READINGS

Assessment of brain SPECT: report of the Therapeutics and Technology Assessment Subcommittee of the American Academy of Neurology, *Neurology* 46:278-285, 1996.

greater than 2 or 3:1 is considered positive. Nose packing for CSF leak studies should be performed by an otolaryngologist. Often, the patient position associated with greatest leakage is reproduced during imaging (Box 12-13).

Bonte FJ, Devous MD, Holman BL: Single photon emission computed tomographic imaging of the brain. In Sandler MP, Coleman RE, Wackers FJTh, et al, editors: *Diagnostic nuclear medicine,* ed 3, vol 2, Baltimore, 1996, Williams & Wilkins.

Holman BL, Devous MD: Functional brain SPECT: the emergency of a powerful clinical method, *J Nucl Med* 33:1888-1904, 1992.

Mazziotta JC, Gilman S, editors: *Clinical brain imaging: principles and applications,* Philadelphia, 1992, FA Davis.

Mountz JM, Deutsch G, Kuzniecky R, Rosenfeld SS: Brain SPECT: 1994 update. In Freeman LM, editor: *Nuclear medicine annual 1994,* New York, 1994, Raven Press.

Nagel JS, Garada BM, Holman BL: Functional brain imaging in dementia. In Freeman LM, editor: *Nuclear medicine annual 1993,* New York, 1993, Raven Press.

Newberg AB, Alavi A: The role of positron emission tomography in the investigation of neurological disorders. In Sandler MP, Coleman RE, Wackers FJTh, et al, editors: *Diagnostic nuclear medicine,* ed 3, vol 2, Baltimore, 1996, Williams & Wilkins.

Van Heertum RL, Tikofsky RS: *Cerebral SPECT imaging,* ed 2, New York, 1995, Raven Press.

# Genitourinary System

Radionuclides have been used to evaluate renal function since the early 1950s (Table 13-1). Early studies using external probe detector systems produced no images, only time-activity histograms that showed the uptake and clearance of the renal radiotracer. These nonimaging studies did not permit evaluation of renal blood flow or differentiation of renal parenchyma from collecting system.

Probe studies have given way to gamma camera-based evaluations that employ computers to acquire and process dynamic imaging studies. These contemporary studies provide sophisticated examinations of renal blood flow, function, anatomy, and collecting system integrity. Reflecting these various categories of diagnostic interest, different radiopharmaceuticals have been used.

In the lower urinary tract, radionuclide cystography has proved useful for evaluating ureteral reflux, especially for children. Scrotal scintigraphy has played an

important role over the years in the differential diagnosis of the acute scrotum.

## RENAL ANATOMY AND PHYSIOLOGY

The kidneys are paired, bean-shaped organs that measure 9 to 11 cm in length, extend from the first to third lumbar (L1 to L3) vertebral bodies, and weigh about 150 g each. The right kidney is often lower than the left. The outer cortex contains the glomeruli and proximal convoluted tubules. The renal pyramids, consisting of collecting tubules and the loops of Henle, make up the medulla. At the apex of the pyramids, papillae drain into the renal calyces. Cortical tissue between the pyramids is known as the columns of Bertin (Fig. 13-1, *A*).

The kidney is a complex organ with several functions. In addition to regulating water and electrolyte balance, it excretes products of metabolism and foreign chemicals, secretes hormones (renin, erythropoietin), and activates vitamin D.

Approximately 25% of cardiac output is delivered to

**Table 13-1  Historical perspective on radionuclides used for renal function evaluation**

| Year | Radiopharmaceutical | Method |
|---|---|---|
| 1952 | Iodine-131 Iopax | Urine counting |
| 1956 | I-131 Diodrast | Renogram |
| 1960 | I-131 hippuran | Renogram |
| 1968 | I-131 hippuran | Lasix renography |
| 1968 | Mercury-203 chloride | Individual renal function |
| 1969 | Technetium-99m gluconate | Renal scan |
| 1970 | Tc-99m DTPA | Renal scan, GFR |
| 1971 | I-131 hippuran | Single sample GFR |
| 1974 | Tc-99m DMSA | Renal scan |
| 1984 | I-131 hippuran | Captopril renography |
| 1986 | Tc-9m MAG3 | Renal scan |

*GFR*, Glomerular filtration rate.

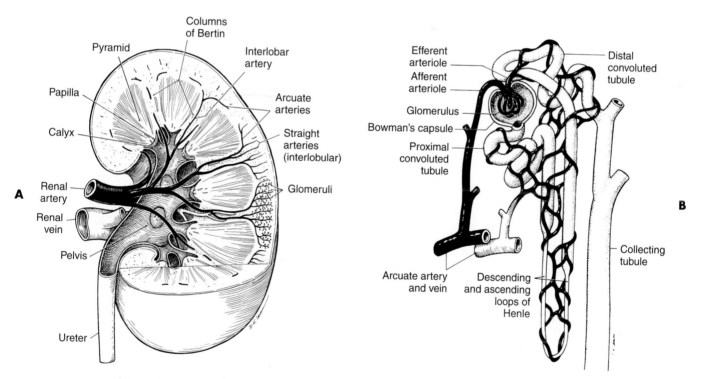

**Fig. 13-1**  Renal anatomy. **A,** The outer layer, or *cortex,* is made up of glomeruli and proximal collecting tubules; the inner layer, or *medulla,* contains the pyramids, made up of distal tubules and loops of Henle. The tubules converge at the papillae, which empty into calyces. The columns of Bertin, between the pyramids, are also cortical tissue. The renal artery and vein enter and leave at the hilus. The interlobar branches of the renal artery divide and become the arcuate arteries, which give rise to straight arteries, from which arise the afferent arterioles that feed the glomerular tuft. **B,** The nephron consists of the vascular afferent and blood vessels leading to a tuft of capillaries, the glomerulus, and efferent vessels. Bowman's capsule surrounds the glomerulus and connects to the proximal and distal renal tubules and loops of Henle.

the kidney by the renal artery and its tributaries. End arterioles lead to tufts of capillaries forming glomeruli, which lie within the renal cortex (Fig. 13-1, *B*). Bowman's capsule surrounds the glomerulus and is the closed end of a long, tortuous renal tubule making up the *nephron,* the basic functional unit of the kidney.

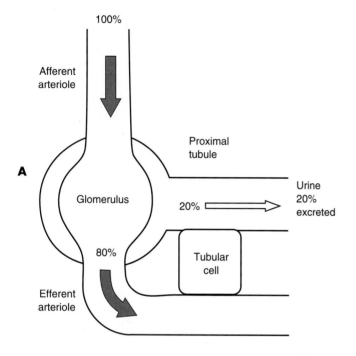

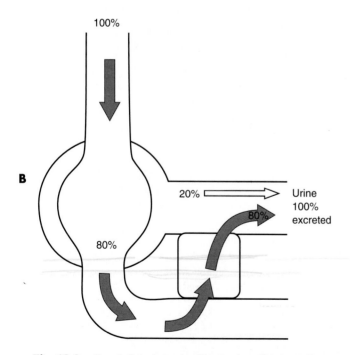

**Fig. 13-2**   Renal function. **A,** Glomerular filtration. Twenty percent of renal blood flow to the kidney is filtered through the glomerulus. **B,** Tubular secretion. The remaining 80% of renal plasma flow is secreted into the proximal tubules from the peritubular fluid space.

Each kidney has more than 1 million functioning nephrons.

Average renal plasma flow (RPF) is about 600 ml/min. Of this, 20% (120 ml/min) is filtered through the glomerulus. The relatively high RPF and resistance provided by the efferent arteriole combine to maintain a pressure gradient that provides the driving force for filtration (Fig. 13-2, *A*). The resulting ultrafiltrate, consisting of water and crystalloids but no colloids or cells, enters into the renal tubule. Nephrologists use *inulin* as a standard measure of the glomerular filtration rate (GFR), since it is entirely filtered through the glomerulus.

The remaining 80% of plasma not filtered enters the peritubular fluid and is actively secreted by the tubular epithelial cells into the renal tubules (Fig. 13-2, *B*). *Paraaminohippurate* (PAH) is the classic example of a drug that, after being partially filtered at the glomerulus (20%), is secreted into the renal tubules (80%). Therefore PAH serves as the standard for quantification of RPF.

Clearance from the plasma of a substance that is maintained in the blood in a steady state (e.g., inulin, PAH, endogenous creatinine) can be used to quantify specific aspects of renal function. Clearance is a measure of the volume of plasma completely cleared of the substance each minute, as follows:

$$\text{Clearance (ml/min)} = UV/P = \frac{\begin{array}{c}\text{Urine concentration (mg/ml)}\\ \times \text{ Volume of urine (ml)}\end{array}}{\text{Plasma concentration (mg/ml)}}$$

As urine passes along the tubule, the filtrate is concentrated and essential substances are conserved. The tubular epithelium actively reabsorbs water and selected substances (glucose, sodium, amino acids) into the blood. This is an energy-dependent process. Water is passively reabsorbed by the osmotic gradient set up by solutes, chiefly sodium. Sixty-five percent of sodium and water filtered at the glomerulus is reabsorbed in the proximal convoluted tubule.

The renal tubules empty formed urine into the calyces through the papillae of the medullary pyramids. From there the urine passes to the renal pelvis, ureter, and bladder.

## RENAL RADIOPHARMACEUTICALS

Various radiopharmaceuticals have been used over the years to evaluate renal function (Box 13-1). They can be conveniently classified by the mechanism that the kidney uses to deal with them physiologically. A functional classification of the major agents is based on their mechanisms of uptake (Table 13-2 and Fig. 13-3). This section discusses only the agents that have been used clinically.

## Mechanisms of Renal Uptake

**Glomerular filtration** A radiopharmaceutical with glomerular filtration as its primary method of renal uptake and clearance is neither reabsorbed nor secreted by the renal tubules. To be freely filtered, the agent must have minimal or preferably no protein binding. Approximately 20% of renal function is the result of glomerular filtration (Fig. 13-2, *A*). A number of different glomerular agents have been used for investigative (e.g., inulin) and quantitative purposes (e.g., I-125 iodothalamate) (Box 13-2). However, clinically the most important imaging agent is *technetium-99m diethylenetriamine pentaacetic acid* (Tc-99m DTPA). This agent is almost totally filtered through the glomerulus.

**Tubular secretion** The remaining 80% of renal function is the result of tubular secretion. The portion of RBF not filtered through the glomerulus is secreted into the proximal tubules from the peritubular fluid space (Fig. 13-2, *B*).

*Iodine-131 orthoiodohippurate* (I-131 OIH, I-131 hippuran), a radiopharmaceutical chemically and pharmacokinetically similar to PAH, has been used as a tubular agent in nuclear medicine since the 1960s (Box 13-3). As with PAH, I-131 OIH is cleared primarily by tubular secretion (80%), but 20% is filtered by the glomerulus. I-131 OIH has been particularly useful in patients with renal insufficiency. In addition, it has been used clinically to calculate effective renal plasma flow

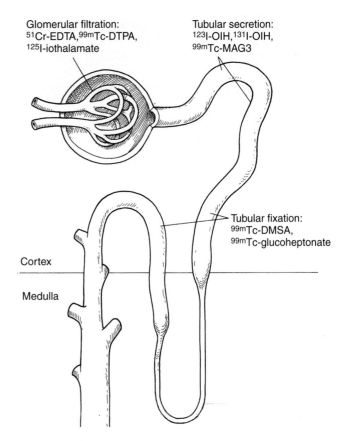

**Fig. 13-3** Radiopharmaceuticals have different mechanisms of renal uptake and excretion, including glomerular filtration, tubular secretion, and cortical tubular binding.

---

| Box 13-1 | Mechanisms of Uptake for Renal Scintigraphic Agents |
|---|---|
| **UPTAKE** | **AGENT** |
| Glomerular filtration (100%) | Tc-99m DTPA |
| Tubular (100%) | Tc-99m MAG3 |
| Tubular (80%) and glomerular (20%) | I-131 and I-123 OIH |
| Cortical binding (50%) | Tc-99m DMSA |
| Glomerular filtration (80%) and cortical binding (20%) | Tc-99m glucoheptonate |

| Box 13-2 Agents Used to Quantify Glomerular Filtration |
|---|
| C-14 or H-3 inulin |
| I-125 diatrizoate |
| I-125 iothalamate |
| Co-57 vitamin $B_{12}$ |
| Cr-51 EDTA |
| In-111 DTPA |
| Yb-169 DTPA |
| Tc-99m DTPA |

*EDTA,* Ethylenediamine tetraacetic acid; *DTPA,* diethylenetriamine pentaacetic acid (pentetic acid).

---

**Table 13-2   Radiation dosimetry for renal radiopharmaceuticals**

| Organ | I-123 OIH (rad/1 mCi) | I-131 OIH (rads/300 mCi) | Tc-DTPA (rads/20 mCi) | Tc-MAG3 (rads/8 mCi) | Tc-DMSA (rads/5 mCi) | Tc-GH (rads/20 mCi) |
|---|---|---|---|---|---|---|
| Bladder | 0.95 | 1.55 | 5.40 | 4.80 | 0.42 | 2.4 |
| Kidneys | 0.05 | 0.05 | 1.80 | 0.14 | 3.78 | 4.8 |
| Ovaries | 0.05 | 0.03 | 0.31 | 0.26 | 0.04 | 0.2 |
| Testes | 0.03 | 0.02 | 0.21 | 0.16 | 0.04 | 0.2 |
| Whole body | 0.02 | 0.01 | 0.12 | 0.07 | 0.09 | 0.2 |

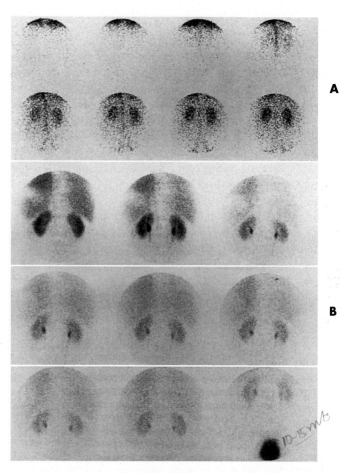

**Box 13-3  Renal Tubular Radiopharmaceuticals Used to Quantify Effective Renal Plasma Flow**

H-2 or C-14 paraaminohippurate (PAH)
I-125, I-131 iodopyracet
I-125, I-123, or I-131 orthoiodohippurate (OIH)
Tc-99m mercaptylacetyltriglycine (MAG3)

(ERPF). However, the I-131 label makes it a suboptimal agent from a dosimetry and imaging standpoint.

*Tc-99m mercaptylacetyltriglycine* (Tc-99m MAG3) became clinically available in the early 1990s and has become the tubular agent of choice. Its mechanism of renal clearance is almost totally tubular secretion. The major advantage Tc-99m MAG3 over I-131 OIH lies in its Tc-99m radiolabel. This results in better images with lower dosimetry and provides valuable information on ERPF and collecting system patency in addition to renal cortical function. A tubular agent, it is particularly useful for imaging patients with renal insufficiency.

**Cortical binding**  Two radiopharmaceuticals demonstrate prolonged retention in the kidney, *Tc-99m glucoheptonate* (Tc-99m GH) and *Tc-99m dimercaptosuccinic acid* (Tc-99m DMSA). Both bind to proximal tubular cells in the renal cortex, allowing excellent planar and single-photon emission computed tomography (SPECT) functional imaging of the renal parenchymal cortex. Uptake and binding require functioning renal cellular elements. Cortical imaging is most often used to diagnose renal scarring in pediatric patients with reflux and recurrent urinary tract infection (UTI) and to differentiate upper from lower UTI. Pyelonephritis produces a cortical tubular dysfunction, manifested by impaired binding of the radiopharmaceuticals to the tubules and thus cortical defects on imaging.

## Technetium-99m Diethylenetriamine Pentaacetic Acid

Tc-99m DTPA is a versatile renal imaging agent that can help evaluate prerenal blood flow, renal parenchymal function, and postrenal collecting system integrity (Fig. 13-4). The 20-mCi intravenous (IV) dose results in good blood flow images (radionuclide angiogram). During the tissue (nephrogram) phase, scintigraphy shows parenchymal uptake and renal anatomy. With renal excretion, good images of the collecting system permit assessment of its patency and thus can be used for evaluation of suspected obstructive uropathy.

**Fig. 13-4**  Normal technetium-99m DTPA study, posterior views. **A,** Blood flow 3-second frames show prompt perfusion to both kidneys. **B,** Dynamic images for 25 minutes. The first image was acquired for 500,000 counts immediately after the 60-second flow study. Subsequent images were acquired for equal time every 3 minutes. The immediate blood pool image shows radiotracer in the liver, spleen, heart, and lungs, as well as the kidneys. By the second image, cortical uptake is maximum, and Tc-99m DTPA is already seen in the pelvis and ureters. Renal and background clearance is prompt, consistent with good renal function. The distal ureters are never well visualized, a typical finding. In the final image the field of view has been moved up to include the bladder.

**Chemistry and radiolabeling**  Radiolabeling is accomplished in commercial preparations by using stannous ion as a reducing agent. The DTPA molecule is a powerful chelating agent that binds Tc-99m avidly in reduced form. As with all Tc-99m-radiolabeled agents, radiopharmaceutical contaminants may result from oxidation of Tc-99m and unlabeled reduction products. In vitro these contaminants are readily detected by radiochromatography.

Unsatisfactory radiolabeling can be recognized in vivo by the uptake of unlabeled free Tc-99m pertechnetate by the thyroid, salivary glands, and stomach. Colloidal impurities may be recognized by increased uptake and prolonged retention of activity in the liver and other reticuloendothelial system (RES) components. Although some protein binding occurs in some commercial preparations, this becomes important only in accurate quantification of GFR and has little consequence for routine scintigraphy.

**Pharmacokinetics**  Tc-99m DTPA pharmacokinetics are similar to those of radiographic contrast media (e.g., diatrizoate, iothalamate) because they are also "glomerular" agents. I-125-radiolabeled iothalamate is commercially available in the United States for nonimaging quantitative measurement of GFR.

After bolus IV injection the initial arterial vascular phase permits an assessment of renal perfusion at the capillary level (Fig. 13-4, *A*). The first-pass filtration fraction is 10% to 20% in patients with normal renal function, although less with poor function. Peak cortical uptake normally occurs 3 to 4 minutes after tracer administration.

Clearance is a function of the GFR, which is normally 120 ml/min. The biological half-life of Tc-99m DTPA is about 2½ hours, with approximately 95% of the dose cleared from the body of normal subjects in 24 hours. During the parenchymal uptake phase the renal cortical outlines are well visualized (Fig. 13-4, *B*). By 5 minutes, tracer appears in the renal collecting system, with visualization of the calyces and then the pelvis. The ureters are not always visualized in normal subjects with normal urine flow rates. Bladder activity is usually seen by 10 to 15 minutes. The half-time of renal clearance is 15 to 20 minutes.

---

## Iodine-131 Orthoiodohippurate

I-131 OIH has been a valuable tool over the years for the evaluation of cortical function in patients with renal insufficiency, particularly renal transplant patients. This is an excellent tubular agent. However, the high-energy I-131 photons are suboptimal for imaging and result in a relatively high radiation dose in patients with renal insufficiency (Tables 13-2 and 13-3). Because of its relatively poor dosimetric characteristics, a low dose (200 to 300 μCi) is used. Also, because of the resulting poor count rate, flow images cannot be obtained, and cortical–collecting system discrimination is often not distinct (Fig. 13-5).

For years it was assumed that the I-131 label would eventually be replaced by I-123 because of its superior image quality and lower radiation exposure to the patient. However, the short half-life of I-123 (15 hours) and the long half-lives of its radionuclide impurities (I-124 or I-125), with their poor dosimetric characteristics, necessitate use on the day of calibration and limit the administered dose. Thus the dose of I-123 OIH is also relatively low (1 to 2 mCi) and insufficient for adequate flow studies. Because of its greater cost, production and

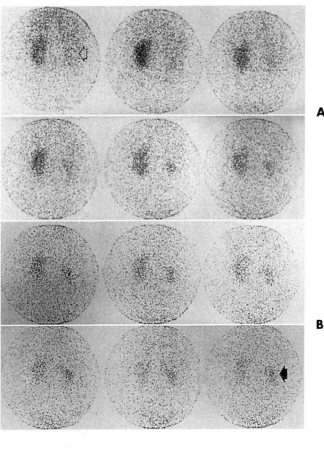

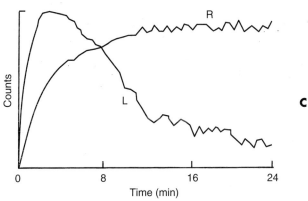

**Fig. 13-5**  Renovascular hypertension with iodine-131 hippuran imaging, posterior views. Image quality is inferior to that achieved with technetium-99m DTPA (Fig. 13-4), but kidney/background ratio is high. No renal flow study is possible because of the low administered dose (250 μCi). **A,** Note the initially decreased uptake in the right kidney *(open arrowhead)*. **B,** With sequential 2-minute images, the normally functioning left kidney has completely cleared by the end of the study, whereas the poorly functioning right kidney is better seen ("flip-flop" pattern) *(closed arrowhead)* because of delayed uptake and clearance of I-131 hippuran. **C,** Time-activity curves confirm the visual impression. The left kidney *(L)* exhibits normal uptake and clearance, whereas the right kidney *(R)* has delayed uptake and very poor clearance.

distribution problems, and the arrival of Tc-99m MAG3, I-123 OIH was never widely used.

**Chemistry and radiolabeling** OIH can be radiolabeled with either I-131 or I-123 by an exchange reaction. The agent tends to degrade with time and should be stored at $4°$ C or less and protected from light. Stabilizing and buffering agents are added for pH adjustment.

**Pharmacokinetics** Because I-131 OIH is cleared by both tubular and glomerular mechanisms, the biological half-life in the body is less than that of Tc-99m DTPA. In subjects with normal renal function, this is 1 hour or less. More than 98% of I-131 OIH is cleared within 24 hours, with a small amount excreted heterotopically in bile. The normal renal clearance half-time is about 10 to 15 minutes.

After IV administration the kidneys are rapidly visualized, with peak cortical concentration in 2 to 4 minutes. The sequence of pelvicocalyceal and bladder visualization is similar and slightly faster than with Tc-99m DTPA. The first-pass extraction fraction of OIH is approximately 85% in subjects with normal renal function and less in those with renal insufficiency.

Patients should receive saturated solution of potassium iodide (SSKI) or Lugol's solution before administration of the radioiodinated agent to prevent any unlabeled radioiodine from being taken up by the thyroid. *United States Pharmacopeia* (USP) standards for OIH call for less than 3% free iodide. Free iodine can be assessed by radiochromatography. Because radioiodine crosses the placenta and is excreted in breast milk, additional precautions should be taken in women who are pregnant or breast-feeding. Breast-feeding should be discontinued for at least 5 days.

I-131 OIH has been used to quantify effective RPF. The term *effective* refers to urinary clearance of OIH being lower than that of PAH (approximately 85%). The lower clearance has been attributed to the presence of free I-131 in the preparation, differences in plasma protein binding, and tubular transport. This has only a small effect on the calculation.

## Technetium-99m Mercaptylacetyltriglycine

In patients with normal renal function, either glomerular or tubular radiopharmaceuticals can be used and provide similar information. For evaluating renal function in patients with renal insufficiency, however, the tubular agents are clearly superior because of their higher extraction efficiency.

**Radiolabeling** Tc-99m MAG3 is available in kit form. The labeling procedure entails the addition of sodium pertechnetate to a reaction vial. A unique feature of the labeling process is that a small amount of air is added to the reaction vial to consume excess stannous ion for

increased stability. Radiolabeling efficiency is 95% or greater.

**Pharmacokinetics** Because it is a tubular agent, Tc-99m MAG3 has a much higher first-pass extraction than Tc-99m DTPA, a glomerular agent, but is not an OIH analog. MAG3 is nearly a pure tubular agent (less than 3% glomerular filtration), with higher protein binding, slower plasma clearance, and a smaller volume of distribution than OIH. Its overall clearance is approximately 60% that of OIH. The alternative route of excretion for Tc-99m MAG3 is hepatobiliary.

Because of its pharmacokinetic differences from I-131 OIH, Tc-99m MAG3 cannot be used to directly calculate ERPF, although a "correction factor" has been used to translate MAG3 clearance into estimated ERPF values.

Tc-99m MAG3 has many advantages over I-131 OIH, especially superior image quality (Fig. 13-6). The better dosimetry allows a larger administered dose with resulting good blood flow images. Parenchymal versus collecting system contrast is excellent, making it useful for evaluating obstructive uropathy. Tc-99m MAG3 is particularly useful for patients with renal insufficiency. Scintigraphic images and time-activity histograms (renograms) are functionally superior in quality to those achieved with OIH because of the much higher counting statistics.

## Technetium-99m Dimercaptosuccinic Acid and Technetium-99m Glucoheptonate

The original agents for imaging the renal cortex were based on radiolabeling of the diuretic chlormerodrin with mercury-203 and then mercury-197. These agents have long been abandoned in favor of the technetium-labeled radiopharmaceuticals Tc-99m DMSA and Tc-99m GH.

The principal advantage of the renal cortical agents is their relatively prolonged and stable retention in the kidney after background and urinary clearance. This allows high-resolution imaging with pinhole collimators or SPECT (Fig. 13-7). The rapid transit of Tc-99m DTPA, OIH, and MAG3 is not suited for the longer imaging times required for SPECT.

**Chemistry and radiolabeling** Both Tc-99m DMSA and Tc-99m GH are supplied in kit form and employ stannous ion for reducing Tc-99m pertechnetate.

**Pharmacokinetics** About 80% of Tc-99m GH is filtered through the glomerulus; the remaining 20% becomes fixed to the proximal renal tubular cells by sulfhydryl-group binding. Uptake depends on adequate RPF and renal tubular function. Cortical images are obtained 1½ to 2 hours after injection to allow maximal cortical uptake and clearance from background soft

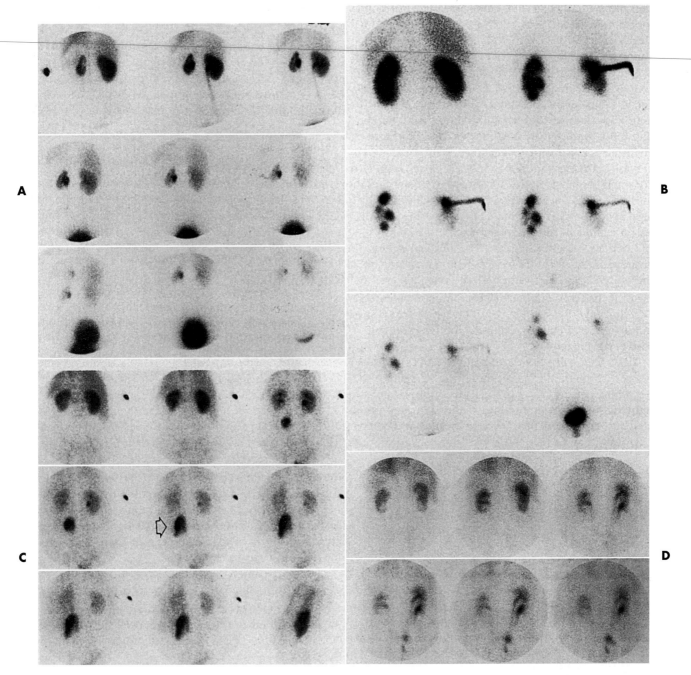

**Fig. 13-6**  Technetium-99m mercaptylacetyltriglycine. **A,** Small scarred left kidney secondary to vesicoureteral reflux. Differential function: 85% (right) and 15% (left). Good cortical definition and clearance are seen. The normal right ureter is visualized. The mildly increasing hepatic uptake over time is normal. Some residual left pelvis activity clears after voiding. Patient movement is noted in the lower left image. **B,** Obstruction of the right kidney secondary to cervical carcinoma. A nephrostomy tube was placed and is draining well. Bilateral renal function is good. Prominent calyces on the left and the pelvis mostly cleared by the end of the study. This shows hydronephrosis, but obstruction is not significant. Last image is taken with bladder in view. **C,** Ureteral leak. Postoperative patient with cervical carcinoma. Rapid ureteral leak was detected early in the imaging sequence *(arrowhead).* **D,** Duplicated right collecting system. This congenital abnormality is often associated with reflux and infection of the lower pole and obstruction of the upper pole.

tissue and the renal collecting structures. A dynamic imaging sequence similar to that used with Tc-99m DTPA and MAG3 can be used for Tc-99m GH during the first 25 to 30 minutes after injection, giving additional information about RPF, dynamic function, and collecting system patency (Fig. 13-8). The liver serves as the alternative route of excretion, and gallbladder filling may occur.

Compared with Tc-99m GH, a significantly higher fraction of the dose of Tc-99m DMSA is bound to the cortex by a similar mechanism (40% to 50%), and a smaller fraction is excreted into the urine (25%). Maximal renal cortical uptake of Tc-99m DMSA is reached within 3 hours of radiotracer administration. Because of the different administered doses (5 mCi for DMSA and 15 to 20 mCi for Tc-99m GH), the absolute amount that binds to the kidneys is similar.

### Radiation Dosimetry

The radiation absorbed dose to the patient from renal radiopharmaceuticals is quite low in subjects with normal renal function (Table 13-2). With renal insufficiency the absorbed dose of Tc-99m-labeled agents is limited by its 6-hour half-life; however, with I-131-labeled agents the absorbed dose can rise significantly (Table 13-3).

| Table 13-3 | Renal dosimetry for iodine-131 orthoiodohippurate with renal insufficiency | |
|---|---|---|
| **Condition** | **Rads/mCi** | **Rads/300 μCi** |
| Normal | 0.1 | 0.03 |
| Tubular necrosis | 6.0 | 1.80 |
| Glomerulonephritis | 67.5 | 20.25 |
| Outflow obstruction (50% uptake) | 400.0 | 120.00 |

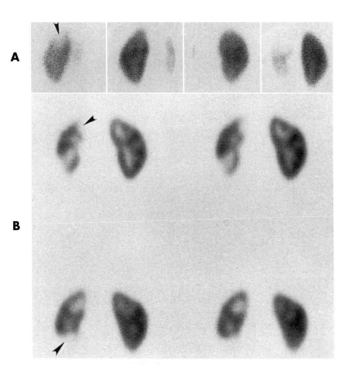

**Fig. 13-7** Technetium-99m dimercaptosuccinic acid planar and SPECT studies in two patients with cortical scars caused by reflux. **A,** Planar images were acquired using a pinhole collimator. *Left to right,* Left posterior oblique (LPO), posterior (left kidney), posterior (right kidney), and right posterior oblique views. Cortical defect in the superior pole on the left *(arrowhead)* is best seen in the LPO view. **B,** High-resolution SPECT. Sequential 3.5-mm coronal sections show a cortical defect in right upper pole and a larger defect in right lower pole *(arrowheads).* Note distinct separation of cortex from medulla and collecting system with SPECT imaging.

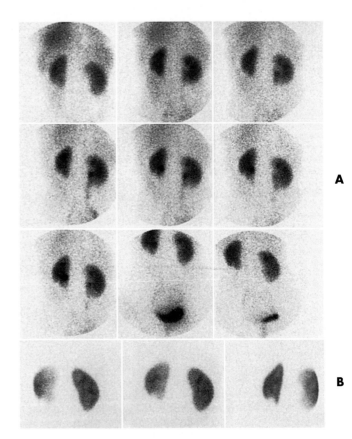

**Fig. 13-8** Technetium-99m glucoheptonate imaging in a patient with vesicoureteral reflux, posterior views. Blood flow is not shown. **A,** Dynamic phase study. **B,** Delayed cortical imaging. Both phases show a cortical defect in the lower pole of the left kidney. Delayed images were acquired using a pinhole collimator, which resulted in improved resolution. *Left to right:* Right posterior oblique, posterior, and left posterior oblique views.

## RENAL IMAGING TECHNIQUES

Renal protocols are modified or tailored for specific clinical applications. This section presents a basic approach to imaging with each of the three major classes of renal radiopharmaceuticals. Modifications and interventions are discussed under their respective clinical applications.

Many of the terms used in this chapter have developed historically. They can be somewhat confusing, since they are often used interchangeably and may refer to instrumentation and methodologies no longer generally used. For example, the term *scan* derives from the early days of nuclear medicine when rectilinear scanners were used for imaging. The term *renogram* originally applied to the time-activity curves (TACs) obtained from nonimaging probe studies (Box 13-4).

## Dynamic Renography

**Methodology**   Similar protocols can be used for Tc-99m DTPA, Tc-99m GH, and Tc-99m MAG3 (Box 13-5).

---

### Box 13-4   Terminology for Radionuclide Renal Studies

**RENOGRAM OR RENOGRAPHY**

Historically, renograms, or time-activity curves (TACs, counts/time), were generated from renal nonimaging probes positioned posterior in the right and left flank. In current practice, renograms are derived from dynamic renal imaging studies by drawing kidney regions of interest (ROIs) on the computer, from which the histograms are generated.

**RENAL SCAN OR RENAL SCINTIGRAPHY**

The term *scan* originated with the first nuclear medicine imaging devices, rectilinear scanners, which scanned back and forth over an ROI, incrementing a short distance between scan passes. The term is still used to refer to any nuclear medicine image. The term *scintigraphy* comes from current scintigraphic gamma cameras. Common use of these terms refers to static or dynamic images obtained from various renal studies.

**RELATIVE RENAL FUNCTION**

Differential or individual renal function is a quantitative measure of relative left-to-right renal cortical uptake. It represents relative functioning of the renal mass. Relative rate of uptake and clearance of a radiopharmaceutical of one kidney is compared to the other kidney on dynamic renography.

**QUANTITATIVE GLOMERULAR FILTRATION RATE OR EFFECTIVE RENAL PLASMA FLOW**

Clearance (ml/min) calculations are derived from either (1) blood sampling after radiotracer injection to determine blood clearance of the radiotracer or (2) computer-derived quantitative estimates of renal cortical uptake from scintigraphy. Both methods, when the appropriate radiopharmaceutical is used, can provide GFR or ERPF estimates.

---

### Box 13-5   Dynamic Renal Scintigraphy: Protocol Summary

**PATIENT PREPARATION**

Hydration
 Adults: drink 300-500 ml of water by mouth.
 Children: intravenous hydration with dextrose 5% in water, 15 ml/kg over 30 min.
Patient must void before starting study.

**RADIOPHARMACEUTICAL**
**Tc-99m DTPA**

Adult: 15 mCi
Child: 200 mCi/kg, 2 mCi minimum, 10 mCi maximum

**Tc-99m GH**

Adult: 20 mCi
Child: same as for Tc-99m DTPA

**Tc-99m MAG3**

Adult: 8 mCi
Child: 100 mCi/kg, 1 mCi minimum, 5 mCi maximum

**INSTRUMENTATION**

Camera: large-field-of-view gamma
Collimator: low energy, all purpose, parallel hole
Photopeak: 15% to 20% window centered over
 140 keV (Tc-99m)

**PATIENT POSITION**

Routine renal imaging: supine, *posterior*
Renal transplant patients: supine, *anterior*

**COMPUTER ACQUISITION**

1-sec frames for 60 sec, then 30-sec frames for 25 min

**STATIC OR ANALOG IMAGE FORMAT**

Flow: 2-sec frames.
Dynamic: immediate image for 500k count, then every
 5 min for equal time.
Obtain postvoid image.

**PROCESSING**

Draw regions of interest on computer for kidneys and
 background.
Generate time-activity curves for 60-sec flow phase and
 for 25-min dynamic study.

Patients should be hydrated before the study. Dehydration can result in delayed uptake and excretion of the radiopharmaceutical, simulating poor function. Imaging is routinely performed posteriorly, preferably with the patient supine, since ptotic kidneys move inferiorly and anteriorly when the patient is upright. The anterior view is used for imaging transplant patients, because the allograft is typically located in the extraperitoneal iliac fossa, and for imaging patients with a suspected or known horseshoe kidney.

Typical adult doses are 15 mCi for Tc-99m DTPA, 20 mCi for Tc-99m GH, and 8 mCi for Tc-99m MAG3. Pediatric administered doses are adjusted downward. Various methods for estimating pediatric doses have been used, including those based on age (*Webster's rule:* [age + 1]/[age + 7] × adult dose) or nomograms based on weight or body surface area.

The study is usually performed in two phases: a 60-second flow study or perfusion phase (radionuclide angiography) (Fig. 13-4, *A*) followed by a 25- to 30-minute dynamic functional imaging phase demonstrating uptake and clearance of the radiotracer (Figs. 13-4, *B*, and 13-6). In contemporary practice, computer acquisition and analysis are mandatory. For the flow phase, 1- to 3-second frames are acquired for 60 seconds, then 30- to 60-second frames are acquired, for a total of 25 to 30 minutes. Computer acquisition permits improved qualitative and quantitative analysis.

Patient preparation and positioning are similar for OIH studies. The protocol for OIH is similar to the Tc-99m studies except that flow studies cannot be performed owing to the low administered dose, and I-131 OIH requires a high-energy collimator.

### Image interpretation

*Flow phase* After IV injection, image acquisition begins when the bolus reaches the level of the abdominal aorta. Blood flow to the kidneys can normally be seen within 4 to 6 seconds of aortic visualization (Fig. 13-4, *A*), immediately after splenic visualization. Any significant asymmetry in tracer flow suggests decreased renal perfusion to that side (Fig. 13-9, *A*). TACs comparing kidney perfusion to aortic flow can be used to confirm the visual interpretation (Fig. 13-9, *B*).

Delayed visualization of both kidneys may be caused by either a bilateral flow abnormality or poor bolus injection. The adequacy of the bolus can be assessed visually and confirmed with TAC histograms. Splenic perfusion must not be confused with left renal perfusion, as in a patient with no left renal function because of disease or surgery.

*Cortical function phase* During the parenchymal tissue phase (1 to 3 minutes), normal kidneys accumulate radiopharmaceutical (Figs. 13-4, *B*, and 13-6). The normal renal cortex appears homogeneous. Images with

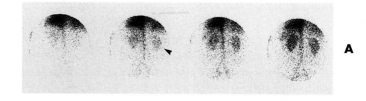

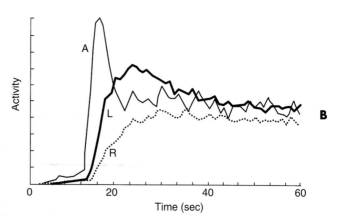

**Fig. 13-9** Unilateral decreased renal blood flow. **A,** Sequential 2-second frames show moderately delayed and decreased blood flow to the right kidney *(arrowhead).* **B,** Sixty-second time activity curves confirm the imaging findings. Initial upslope of the right kidney *(R)* is delayed compared with the aorta *(A)* and the left kidney *(L).*

good resolution show the calyces and pelvis as photopenic areas during this initial uptake phase.

Relative renal function can be judged visually in two ways. First, the clinician can subjectively estimate the relative uptake of the two kidneys by merely looking at the cortical images before their excretion into the collecting system (1- to 3-minute images). With experience the clinician can accurately estimate relative function, a measure of relative renal mass. The differential function of a kidney may be abnormal (less than 45%) because of disease, surgery, or congenital disparity in size. Computer quantification of differential renal function is now routine.

The second important method for evaluating renal function is to compare the temporal sequence of uptake and excretion between the two kidneys. With asymmetrical dysfunction, uptake and excretion are delayed in one kidney relative to the better-functioning kidney. This produces a "flip-flop" pattern; the poorly functioning kidney has less uptake initially, but on later images its cortical activity is higher than the better-functioning kidney, which has already excreted the radiotracer (Fig. 13-5). These subjective evaluations can be corroborated with the renal histograms and quantification of differential function.

*Clearance phase* The calyces and pelvis usually begin filling by 3 minutes. Over the next 10 to 15 minutes, net activity in the kidney and the collecting

**RADIOPHARMACEUTICAL**

**Tc-99m DMSA**

Adult: 5 mCi

Child: 50 mg/kg (minimum dose, of 600 mCi)

**Tc-99m GH**

Adult: 15-20 mCi

Child: 200 mCi/kg

**INSTRUMENTATION**

Camera: large-field-of-view gamma with LEAP collimator
    for anterior and posterior images in quantification of
    differential renal function

Collimator: pinhole for cortical imaging. Converging
    collimator may be used for adults and large children.

SPECT: dual- or triple-headed camera

**IMAGING PROCEDURE**

Patient should void before starting.

Inject radiopharmaceutical intravenously.

Image at 2 hours after injection.

Acquire pinhole images for 100k counts per view. Po-
    sition patient to image each kidney separately in the
    posterior and right and left posterior oblique views.

On computer, acquire anterior and posterior views for
    500k counts using a parallel-hole collimator to
    include both kidneys for quantification of differential
    function.

Quantify differential function by drawing regions of
    interest on anterior and posterior views for both
    kidneys. Calculate the geometric mean (square root
    of the product) counts for each kidney and differ-
    ential function.

**SPECT**

Camera: dual- or triple-headed with low-energy,
    ultra-high-resolution collimator

Matrix: 128 × 128

Zoom: as needed

Orbit: noncircular body contour, rotate 180°, step and
    shoot 40 views/head, 3° per stop, 40 sec per stop

Reconstruction: 64 × 64

Hamming filter with high cut-off

Smoothing kernel

Attenuation correction

Persistent pooling or visualization of pyelocalyceal structures overlapping the cortex or projecting well outside
the renal outlines suggests hydronephrosis.

The normal ureter may or may not visualize, depending on the urinary flow rate. Prolonged and especially
unchanging visualization suggests ureteral dilation. The
bladder is well seen in normal subjects. In small children
and infants the bladder can appear quite large and may
project close to the kidneys, even occasionally overlapping the lower poles.

## Renal Cortical Imaging

**Methodology**  With Tc-99m DMSA, dynamic imaging is not performed; background clearance is slow, and
only a small percentage of the radiotracer (25%) is
cleared by the kidney. Only delayed cortical planar or
SPECT imaging is acquired. Planar imaging is performed
in multiple views, usually the posterior and the left
posterior oblique (LPO) and the right posterior oblique
(RPO) views, using a pinhole or converging collimator
for magnification and improved resolution (Fig. 13-8 and
Box 13-6). High-resolution SPECT affords excellent
cortical imaging, even in small children, although a
multiheaded camera with high-resolution collimators is
required to acquire sufficient counts for quality images.
Small children may need sedation for SPECT.

With Tc-99m GH, similar delayed imaging methodology is used. In contrast to Tc-99m DMSA, dynamic renal scintigraphy can be acquired first, giving
additional information on blood flow and collecting
system patency.

**Image interpretation**  Evidence of infection or scarring is manifested by renal cortical defects. The magnified pinhole or converging collimator images result in
high-resolution images and allow detection of regions of
cortical dysfunction (Figs. 13-7, *A,* and 13-8, *B*). Multiheaded SPECT is more sensitive for detection of small
cortical defects because of its better contrast resolution (Fig. 13-7, *B*). Specificity may be somewhat lower,
however, because some smaller abnormalities may represent normal variation (e.g., fetal lobulation). Experience with either technique can give excellent clinical
results.

## COMPUTER PROCESSING
## OF RENAL STUDIES

Computer processing of renal studies is a valuable
adjunct in the evaluation renal blood flow, cortical function, and collecting system patency. Mentally integrating
all the information in the many images can be challenging, even for the experienced clinician. Computer-
processed TACs provide a dynamic visual presentation of

structures decreases. With good function, most of the
radiotracer clears into the bladder by the end of the
study. In some healthy subjects, pooling of activity in
the calyces results in focal hot spots because imaging
with the patient supine makes some calyces dependent
with respect to the level of the ureteropelvic junction.

temporal changes in flow and function that can aid in assimilating and interpreting these data.

## Dynamic Renography

In the early days of nuclear medicine, renal function studies were performed using two gamma-detector, nonimaging probes placed posteriorly in both flanks. These produced two TACs, or renograms. Current renograms are generated on computer after an appropriate renal region of interest (ROI) is chosen for the dynamic sequential images (Fig. 13-10). TACs can be generated for the 60-second flow phase and the 25- to 30-minute dynamic renal function and clearance phase (Figs. 13-9 and 13-11, *A*).

The TACs and quantitative indices should be interpreted in conjunction with a review of the images, never alone. Any discrepancies must be reconciled.

**Renal blood flow**   To generate TACs for the initial 60-second flow study, ROIs are drawn on computer for the kidney and the adjacent artery, that is, the aorta for subjects with two kidneys and the aorta or iliac artery for renal transplant patients. The computer-generated TACs can help confirm unilateral or bilateral flow disturbances noted on the 2- to 3-second images (Fig. 13-9, *B*). TACs are particularly useful for comparing serial studies (e.g., postoperative course of renal transplant patients).

*Quantification*   Absolute flow, measured in milliliters per kilogram per minute, cannot be calculated using the radiotracers discussed; however, relative flow can be estimated and semiquantitative indices derived from the TACs. It is relatively easy to assess renal blood flow subjectively by comparing the initial upslopes of the

TACs (Fig. 13-9, *B*). The relative upslopes can be quantified with a kidney/aorta (K/A) slope ratio. An alternative method uses a ratio of the total counts integrated under the two curves. Although not absolutely necessary, these indices can be helpful for following the course of an individual subject undergoing serial studies. Both methods are subject to technical errors, and attention to detail is needed to obtain useful data.

**Renal cortical function**   TAC renograms are routine for evaluation of dynamic renal function with Tc-99m DTPA, Tc-99m MAG3, Tc-99m GH, I-123 OIH, and I-131 OIH. Curves are generated for the entire 25- to 30-minute study. Function, as manifested by uptake and excretion of the radiopharmaceutical over sequential images, can be quickly integrated and understood. The curve can be conceptualized by dividing it into three phases (Fig. 13-11, *B*): (1) the *blood flow phase,* characterized by a sharp rise (30 to 60 seconds); (2) the *uptake phase,* in which the TAC rises, but less sharply, because of cortical accumulation of tracer (1 to 3 minutes in normal kidneys, longer with renal insufficiency); and (3) the

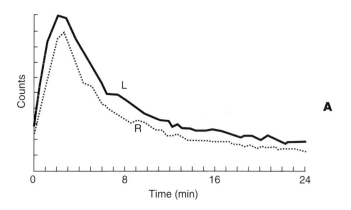

**A**

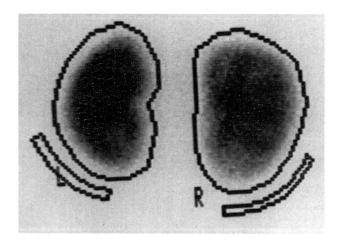

**Fig. 13-10**   Background region of interest selection. Curvilinear ROI around the inferior lateral aspect of both kidneys is most often used for background selection in dynamic renal scintigraphy.

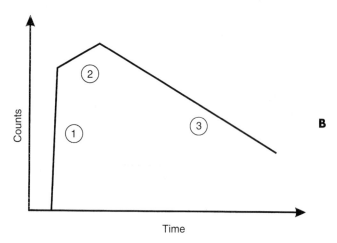

**B**

**Fig. 13-11**   **A,** Normal renogram. Bilateral renogram curves show phases. **B,** Three phases of a renogram: *1,* initial blood flow phase (30 to 60 seconds); *2,* cortical uptake phase, normally 1 to 3 minutes; *3,* clearance phase, representing cortical excretion and collecting system clearance.

*excretory phase,* in which the TAC falls as tracer leaves the cortex and urinary collecting system.

The uptake and clearance of the radiopharmaceutical are a dynamic process. The tracer bolus is progressively extracted from the blood pool at a rate dependent on its extraction ratio. At any point in time the renogram represents a summation of uptake and excretion. For example, the point of maximal uptake represents the point at which uptake equals clearance. In the uptake phase, extraction exceeds excretion, and in the excretion phase, excretion exceeds uptake.

*Region of interest selection* Proper ROI selection is critical and depends on the information needed. Whole kidney ROIs can be used for cortical function curves if collecting system activity clears promptly. With collecting system retention, however, the renogram represents a summation of cortical function and collecting system activity. The ability to discern cortical function is thus hindered. In these cases two-pixel-wide peripheral cortical ROIs may more accurately represent parenchymal function. Calculation of differential renal function requires ROIs that include the entire kidney, because excluding the pelvis and calyces will inevitably exclude some cortex, making quantification erroneous. The TACs of renal insufficiency and renal obstruction may look identical. Only by viewing the images can they be differentiated.

*Quantification* Various quantitative parameters of function have been derived from these TACs, including the time to peak activity, uptake slope, rate of clearance, and percent clearance at 20 minutes. No general standard exists. Personal preference and experience determine the use of quantitative parameters. Only the calculation of differential function is standard.

*Differential renal function* Individual or differential renal function is routinely assessed for patients with two kidneys. This information cannot easily be obtained from any nonradionuclide method. Individual renal function is defined as the percentage of radiotracer extracted by each kidney compared with the other. It represents the percent functional mass of each kidney. Normal differential function ranges from 45% to 55%.

Differential function is calculated using the cortical uptake counts after the flow phase but before arrival of the radioactive tracer into the collecting system, usually 1 to 3 minutes after tracer administration (parenchymal phase, phase 2) (Fig. 13-11, *B*). The total counts from one kidney are divided by the total counts of both kidneys, after correction for background.

*Background selection* Appropriate choice of background ROIs is important for accurate quantification. Unfortunately, true background cannot be determined, since there is soft tissue background anterior and posterior to the kidney. Thus regions adjacent to the kidney must be used. Opinions differ as to the ideal

background ROI. Typically, two-pixel semilunar ROIs adjacent and inferolateral to the kidneys are chosen (Fig. 13-10). Caution is necessary when the liver and spleen overlap the kidneys. This is a special problem with Tc-99m MAG3 because of its alternative hepatobiliary route of excretion. The accuracy of background subtraction decreases with increasing renal dysfunction.

With Tc-99m DMSA and Tc-99m GH cortical imaging, background correction is also performed but is usually less critical owing to the relatively high uptake in the cortex compared with background at the 2-hour imaging period. Background becomes more critical in subjects with renal insufficiency. Imaging may be delayed for up to 24 hours to maximize background clearance.

Again, blood flow TACs, renograms, and quantification should always be interpreted in conjunction with image analysis.

## Filtration Rate and Plasma Flow

Clinical assessment of renal function is relatively crude. Patients may have a significant reduction in renal function before the serum blood urea nitrogen (BUN) or creatinine levels rise. The 24-hour urinary creatinine clearance rate (CrCl) is more accurate but requires urine collection with its associated difficulties. Accurate quantification of GFR or ERPF with nonradioactive inulin or PAH, respectively, requires a constant infusion technique, multiple blood and urine samples, and chemical analysis; none of these tests is routinely performed on a clinical basis.

Quantitative radionuclide methods for measuring renal function can be divided into blood-sampling techniques and camera-based methods. Tc-99m DTPA is typically used in the United States to calculate GFR because of its low cost and widespread availability. I-125 iothalamate is commercially available in the United States, and chromium-151 ethylenediamine tetraacetic acid (Cr-51 EDTA) is available in Europe. I-131 OIH can be used to calculate ERPF.

Accurate renal function can be quantified from the plasma disappearance curve derived from multiple blood samples. The more samples, the more accurate the analysis. However, simplified methods using one or two blood samples have been validated. A popular one-sample technique for determining GFR that uses Tc-99m DTPA as the tracer requires a single sample drawn at 3 hours. For I-131 OIH determination of the ERPF, 44 minutes appears to be the optimal time.

Camera-based methods require no blood sampling and only 15 minutes of imaging time (Fig. 13-12). The basis for this technique is that early radiotracer uptake by each kidney is directly proportional to its clearance. Once the mathematical relationship between uptake and some measurement of renal function (GFR, CrCl, or ERPF) has

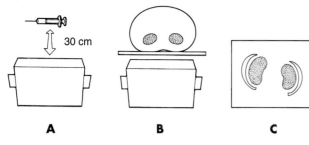

**Fig. 13-12** Gamma camera technique for quantitative calculation of glomerular filtration rate (GFR). **A,** One-minute image of the Tc-99m DTPA syringe acquired before and after injection, 30 cm from the center of the collimator. **B,** After injection, 15-sec/frame images are acquired for a total of 6 minutes. **C,** Kidney and background regions of interest are selected. The background-corrected net renal cortical uptake as a percentage of the injected dose for each kidney is determined. Attenuation is corrected for by using the patient's height and weight. To estimate GFR, data are inserted into a regression analysis formula derived from studying, in an identical manner, a group of patients who also had GFRs calculated by a standardized method.

been established over a range of renal function, it can be applied clinically. The appropriate software is available on most nuclear medicine computer systems.

The simplified radionuclide methods for quantifying renal function are estimates of function, with clinically acceptable levels of error. The error of the estimate typically increases in patients with poor renal function, but so does the error associated with biochemical tests (e.g., CrCl).

To be useful clinically, a method need not be highly accurate; it is more important that the method be reproducible. For example, CrCl is often used clinically to estimate GFR, but creatinine is reabsorbed and secreted by the renal tubules, besides being filtered through the glomerulus. Thus the GFR so determined is not an "accurate" measurement but an approximation. Normal GFR is 100 ml/min, whereas the normal CrCl is 120 ml/min. The method is not very accurate, but it is reproducible and has been found clinically useful for following patients over time.

One problem limiting the more general acceptance of radionuclide methods is cost, which is often greater than that of the biochemical tests. Radionuclide methods are most useful clinically for patients in whom urine collection is difficult, such as poorly cooperative patients, children, and those with renal insufficiency. Camera-based methods offer another advantage: quantification of *individual* renal function.

## CLINICAL APPLICATIONS OF RENAL SCINTIGRAPHY

The clinical uses for renal scintigraphy are numerous. Dynamic renal scintigraphy with computer-derived TAC histograms permits evaluation of blood flow, renal morphology and size, parenchymal function, and collecting system patency. Nuclear medicine studies are often ordered for evaluating pediatric renal problems because of the low radiation dose, lack of toxicity, and valuable information regarding renal function.

### Etiology of Renal Failure

Renal scintigraphy can be useful in the evaluation of renal failure. Prerenal, renal, and postrenal causes can be diagnosed or excluded. Blood flow to the kidneys is routinely evaluated. Decreased perfusion to the kidneys, unilateral or bilateral, may be seen with renal artery stenosis, thrombosis, avulsion, venous thrombosis, and renal infarction.

Approximate renal size, morphological features, and differential renal function are easily determined with scintigraphy. Functional abnormalities of uptake and clearance can be demonstrated with acute and chronic renal disease. However, the findings are not specific for etiology.

Renal scintigraphy is also used to determine the functional significance of dilation seen on other imaging modalities, for example, whether surgical intervention is required. Obstructive nephropathy is discussed later.

### Renovascular Hypertension

Hypertension is a common clinical problem affecting over 50 million people in the United States. More than 90% of patients have no identifiable cause of "essential hypertension" and no prospect for cure. Hypertension requires lifelong medical management with drug therapy. In a minority of patients, however, hypertension is secondary to a potentially curable cause, such as coarctation of the aorta, an endocrine-related etiology, or renovascular hypertension.

Renovascular hypertension refers to hypertension caused by renal arterial hypoperfusion secondary to vascular stenosis of the renal artery or one of its major branches. Renal stenosis may or may not cause sufficient hypoperfusion to trigger the process that leads to hypertension. For example, almost half of normotensive patients over age 60 have atherosclerotic lesions in their renal vessels, and many hypertensive patients have renal artery stenosis not associated with their hypertension.

In a nonselected hypertensive population the prevalence of renovascular hypertension is less than 1%. Among patients referred for renal diagnostic studies, 2% to 4% have renovascular hypertension. However, of patients referred to a subspecialty center for refractory hypertension, 15% to 45% prove to have renovascular hypertension.

**Pathogenesis** Much research and controversy have surrounded the etiology of renovascular hypertension since 1934, when Goldblatt first induced hypertension in dogs by partially occluding one renal artery. Whereas renal sodium retention is the primary mechanism for hypertension resulting from loss of renal parenchyma, increased renin secretion is responsible for the hypertension caused by renal hypoperfusion.

The two main causes of renovascular hypertension are atherosclerosis and fibromuscular dysplasia. Repair of any form of *functional* renovascular disease is indicated. The earlier an arterial stenosis causing hypertension is corrected, the greater is the chance for cure. Otherwise, widespread arteriolar damage and glomerulosclerosis in the contralateral kidney can result from prolonged exposure to hypertension and high levels of angiotensin II.

**Diagnostic tests** The patient's history and physical examination help in selecting patients with an increased likelihood of renovascular hypertension. These selection criteria include an abrupt or recent onset of hypertension, hypertension refractory to therapy, generalized systemic vascular disease, abdominal bruits, young patients with significant hypertension, and patients who experience renal failure during treatment with angiotensin-converting enzyme (ACE) inhibitors. These selection criteria are not specific, however, and the false positive rate would be extremely high if all these patients were subjected to angiography, an invasive procedure.

Researchers have attempted to find a noninvasive screening test that could predict which patients might benefit from surgery or angioplasty. In the past, peripheral blood renin levels and contrast urography were advocated as screening tests for renovascular hypertension. Serum renin is not specific, however, and the "hypertensive intravenous urogram" has an unacceptably high percentage of false positive and false negative results, approximately 25% each. The use of conventional radionuclide renography to diagnose renovascular hypertension was abandoned because of similar poor specificity. Subsequently the recommendation was to screen fewer patients, with renal arteriography only for those with suggestive clinical features.

*Radionuclide evaluation of renal artery stenosis* Although the radionuclide angiogram may show decreased blood flow on the stenotic side, the sensitivity for detecting asymmetrical flow is not high. The primary focus for making a diagnosis of renal hypertension has been the second phase of the renogram. In patients with renovascular hypertension, uptake and clearance of the radiopharmaceutical are delayed (Fig. 13-5). The second phase of the classic renogram is often flattened, with a less steep upslope. The peak of the curve may be blunted and the third phase prolonged without a crisp, concave appearance. This pattern is not specific, however, and is seen in other causes of renal dysfunction. The accuracy of this finding is only slightly better than that of the hypertensive IV urogram.

The development of an interventional pharmacological maneuver, ACE inhibition renography, has led to a renaissance in the use of radionuclide renography to make the noninvasive diagnosis of a renin-dependent renovascular hypertension. ACE-stimulated plasma renin levels have also been advocated, but the specificity is poor.

**Angiotensin-converting enzyme inhibition renography** Early clinical investigations with captopril found that some patients treated for hypertension developed renal failure, which was usually reversible with discontinuation of the medication. These patients had bilateral renal artery stenosis. This observation led to the hypothesis that ACE inhibitors with renography might be used as a noninvasive pharmacological intervention to diagnose renovascular hypertension.

*Mechanism* Glomerular filtration is driven by pressure at the renal glomerulus. When perfusion pressure drops, renal filtration, as measured by GFR, also decreases. Because of the normal compensatory response, renin is released by the juxtaglomerular apparatus. Renin converts angiotensinogen made in the liver to angiotensin I, which is converted to angiotensin II in the lungs by ACE. Some angiotensin II is produced locally within the juxtaglomerular apparatus of the kidney as well. Angiotensin II is a powerful vasoconstrictor that, in addition to peripheral vasoconstriction, produces constriction of the efferent arterioles of the glomerulus (Fig. 13-13). This raises the filtration pressure, thus maintaining GFR. However, this normal compensatory mechanism has limits. If renal blood flow continues to decrease, GFR will deteriorate, and with time the kidney will become scarred and contracted.

ACE inhibitors work by blocking the conversion of angiotensin I to angiotensin II (Fig. 13-14), preventing this normal compensatory mechanism. Postglomerular resistance decreases, and thus the transcapillary driving force that maintains filtration is decreased in kidneys with renin-dependent, hemodynamically significant renal artery stenosis. GFR falls in the involved kidney. This decrease in renal glomerular filtration can be assessed noninvasively with renal scintigraphy.

*Captopril* (Capoten) was the first ACE inhibitor to be used successfully to diagnose renovascular hypertension in combination with I-131 OIH, Tc-99m DTPA, and Tc-99m MAG3. More recently, another ACE inhibitor, IV enalapril (Vasotec), has been advocated. Its main advantage is an interval of 15 minutes before drug administration and renography, versus 60 minutes with captopril.

Conventionally, two radionuclide studies are performed, with and without captopril stimulation. Patients with hemodynamically significant renal artery stenosis have reduced function of the affected kidney. This reduction in GFR can be seen on renal scintigra-

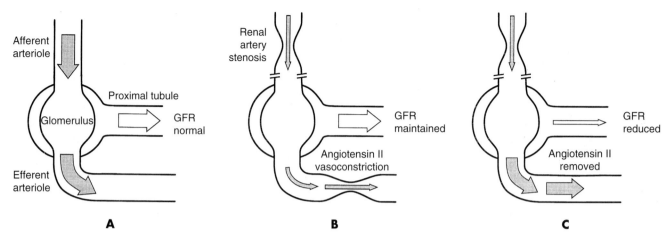

**Fig. 13-13** Pathophysiology of renin-dependent renovascular disease: pharmacological effect of captopril. **A,** Normal glomerular filtration rate *(GFR)*. **B,** Renovascular hypertension. Because of reduced renal plasma flow, filtration pressure and GFR fall. Increased renin and resulting angiotensin II produces vasoconstriction of the efferent glomerular arterioles, raising glomerular pressure and maintaining GFR. **C,** Captopril blocks the normal compensatory mechanism, and GFR falls.

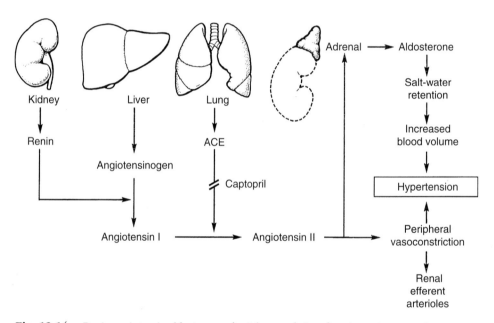

**Fig. 13-14** Renin-angiotensin-aldosterone physiology and site of angiotensin-converting enzyme *(ACE)* inhibitor (captopril) blockage. See text for details.

phy as delayed uptake and cortical retention (Figs. 13-15 and 13-16).

*Indication* Because of cost-effectiveness, ACE inhibition renography should be performed primarily in patients with moderate to high risk of renovascular hypertension. This includes patients with severe hypertension, abrupt or recent onset, onset under age 30 or over age 55, hypertension resistant to medical therapy, abdominal or flank bruits, unexplained azotemia, worsening renal function during therapy with ACE inhibitors, end-organ damage (e.g., left ventricular hypertrophy, retinopathy), or occlusive disease in other vascular beds.

*Imaging protocol* In a typical protocol, ACE inhibition renography is performed first (Box 13-7). If it is normal, no baseline study is required. If any abnormality is noted, however, a baseline study without captopril is performed on a separate day.

The diuretic furosemide is often given simultaneously with the radiopharmaceutical to ensure clearance of the collecting system, which could otherwise affect visual and renographic interpretation. Furosemide is a loop diuretic, acts distal to the proximal tubules where MAG3 and OIH are secreted, and therefore does not affect cortical retention.

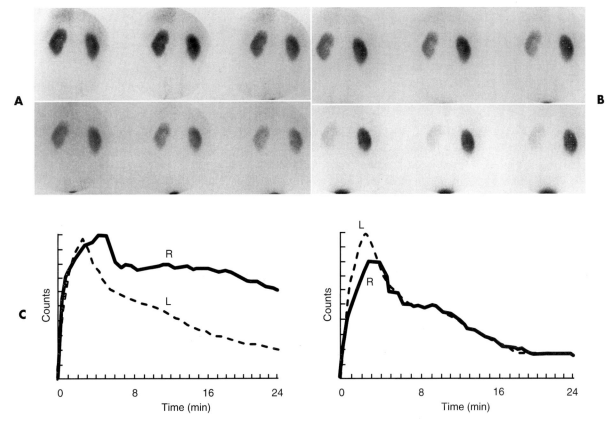

**Fig. 13-15**   Positive captopril study with technetium-99m mercaptylacetyltriglycine (MAG3). **A,** Captopril study was performed first. Note prompt symmetrical initial uptake. Over the length of the study the left kidney washes out normally, but the right kidney shows no washout, with almost all the activity remaining in the cortex. **B,** Baseline study without captopril shows normal uptake and clearance of both kidneys. **C,** Time-activity curves confirm the visual impression of renin-dependent cortical retention of the right kidney.

The diagnostic imaging pattern seen with patients with renin-dependent renovascular hypertension usually occurs without a concomitant drop in blood pressure. Each patient should have an IV line, however, so that fluids can be promptly administered should hypotension occur.

*Diagnostic pattern*   The classic pattern with renin-dependent renovascular hypertension is an abnormal ACE inhibition study but a normal baseline study without ACE inhibition. In patients with unilateral renovascular disease and functional asymmetry on the baseline renogram, the administration of captopril often results in greater asymmetry. In patients with bilateral renovascular disease, ACE inhibition is seen bilaterally, although often asymmetrically. ACE inhibition has no effect on the flow phase of the study. In normal subjects and patients with hypertension unrelated to renal artery stenosis, the renogram curve remains unchanged compared with baseline after administration of the ACE inhibitor. A severely diseased and shrunken kidney may not respond to ACE inhibition because it is no longer renin dependent.

The scintigraphic pattern of renin-dependent renovascular hypertension differs depending on whether glomerular or tubular radiopharmaceuticals are used. Positive ACE inhibition with a glomerular agent (Tc-99m DTPA) shows decreased absolute or relative uptake on the affected side compared with a baseline study. With a tubular-secreted radiopharmaceutical (e.g., Tc-99m MAG3), however, uptake is often unchanged after ACE inhibition. Instead, cortical retention persists on the affected side (Figs. 13-15 and 13-16). This results from the decrease in GFR induced by ACE inhibition on the affected side; the reduced GFR leads to decreased urine flow in the renal tubules and delayed washout of the radiopharmaceutical. With severely reduced tubular flow, cortical retention of Tc-99m DTPA may be seen.

*Quantification*   Various quantitative indices have been used diagnostically to aid in the diagnosis of renin-dependent renovascular hypertension. Because of different clearance mechanisms and imaging patterns of glomerular versus tubular agents, different quantitative parameters are indicated. Tc-99m DTPA is best quantified by using the change in relative or absolute

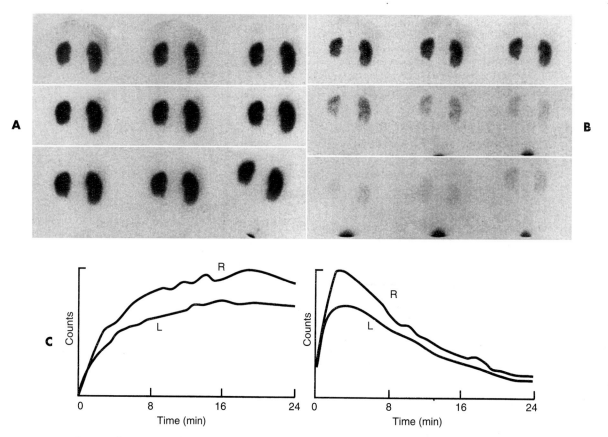

**Fig. 13-16** Bilateral renal artery stenosis. **A,** Captopril-stimulated study with technetium-99m mercaptylacetyltriglycine (MAG3). There is bilateral cortical retention and minimal urinary bladder clearance over 30 minutes. **B,** Baseline study without captopril shows normal cortical function and good clearance into the bladder. This is diagnostic of bilateral renovascular hypertension, although dehydration, hypotension, or functional bladder obstruction could produce a similar pattern. **C,** Time-activity curves confirm the imaging findings. *Left,* Captopril-stimulated study; *right,* baseline study.

individual kidney function. Tc-99m OIH or Tc-99m MAG3 is best quantified by a change in the 20-minute/maximum count ratio or a prolongation of the peak time. In patients with normal renal function and in the absence of pelvicocalyceal retention, a normal 20-minute/maximum count ratio is less than 0.3. A 0.15 change (e.g., 0.3 to 0.45) after ACE inhibition is considered significant. A 0.1 to 0.15 change is borderline (Fig. 13-17).

*Accuracy* Numerous studies have reported high accuracy for ACE inhibition renography. Sensitivity is about 90% and specificity 95%. False positive results are rare. The accuracy with Tc-99m DTPA, I-131 hippuran, and Tc-99m MAG3 seems to be equally high. The sensitivity of the test is lower (75%) in patients receiving long-term ACE inhibitor therapy. If possible, ACE inhibitors should be discontinued for 3 to 5 days before the study, as determined by the drug's half-life. The sensitivity of the test is also less in patients with renal insufficiency.

ACE inhibition renography is often not useful in evaluating small, poorly functioning kidneys, since they may no longer be renin dependent. In these patients, captopril renography can be used to evaluate the contralateral kidney.

## Urinary Tract Obstruction

The diagnosis and management of urinary tract obstruction are issues for both pediatric and adult urology. The clinician is often confronted with evidence of a dilated collecting system and must determine whether there is obstruction or merely dilation, such as from muscular atony or a structural abnormality. The distinction between mechanical obstruction and dilation not associated with obstruction is critical to patient management. Uncorrected obstruction can lead to recurrent infection and ultimately to loss of renal function and parenchymal atrophy.

## Box 13-7 Angiotensin-Converting Enzyme (Captopril) Renography: Protocol Summary

**PATIENT PREPARATION**

Liquids only on morning of study.
No ACE inhibitors for 3 to 5 days before study.
Supine position.

**RADIOPHARMACEUTICAL**

Tc-99m MAG3, 8 mCi

**IMAGING PROCEDURE**

Provide hydration: orally, 7 ml of water/kg body weight 30 to 60 min before the study, or intravenously, half-normal saline, 10 ml/kg over 1 hr to a maximum of 500 ml before radionuclide injection. Keep vein open during entire study so that fluids can be administered promptly in case of hypotension.

Administer ACE inhibitor: captopril (Capoten), 25 mg orally 1 hr before starting the radionuclide study; children: 0.5 mg/kg (maximum, 25 mg). Alternate: enalapril (Vasotec), 40 µg/kg (maximum, 2.5 mg) intravenously infused over 3 to 5 min.

Monitor blood pressure and record every 15 min before and during study with oral dose and at shorter intervals with intravenous drug. A large decrease in pressure may require saline infusion.

Administer 20 to 40 mg furosemide intravenously at the time of radionuclide injection.

Inject radiopharmaceutical intravenously 60 min after oral captopril or 15 min after enalapril.

Imaging is similar to that described for dynamic renal scintigraphy.

**INTERPRETATION**

If the images and time-activity curves are normal, a renin-dependent renovascular hypertension is excluded.

Evidence of delayed uptake or cortical retention on scintigrams and an abnormal TAC require a repeat study without captopril for comparison.

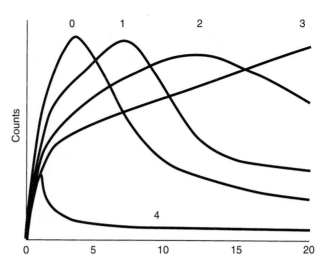

**Fig. 13-17** Renogram pattern changes with ACE inhibition. Time-activity curves illustrate the spectrum from normal to severe renal insufficiency: *0,* Normal; *1,* minor renal insufficiency with mildly delayed uptake and excretion phases (peak time >5, 20-minute/maximum count ratio >0.3); *2,* marked insufficiency with very delayed uptake phase but some washout; *3,* extremely delayed uptake with no washout phase; *4,* renal failure pattern without uptake phase. See text for interpretation of diagnostic changes.

The sequence of pathophysiological events leading to renal atrophy is complex. The effects on renal function are determined by whether obstruction is unilateral or bilateral, acute or chronic, and partial or complete. Preexisting renal disease or coexisting infection accentuates the effects of obstruction on renal function. Obstruction leads to increased pressure within the collecting structures. This pressure is transmitted through the luminal structures to the renal parenchyma, decreasing parenchymal blood flow and GFR. With continued obstruction a progressive loss of nephrons and renal function results.

The changes caused by obstruction can be arrested and even reversed after surgical intervention. Early surgical relief of total obstruction usually restores normal renal function. On the other hand, high-grade obstruction for longer than 1 week is invariably followed by only partial return of function. Low-grade obstructions may exist for weeks, months, or even years with no or mild functional impairment.

Contrast IV urography, ultrasonography, and conventional radionuclide renography are unreliable for differentiating obstructive from nonobstructive causes of hydroureteronephrosis because of the overlap in findings between the conditions. Dilation, delayed opacification, and delayed washout are the hallmarks of obstruction on contrast-enhanced urography but may also be seen secondary to virtually any cause of collecting system dilation. Ultrasonography is a sensitive technique for detecting hydroureteronephrosis but does not depict urodynamics.

**Whitaker test** First described in the early 1970s, the Whitaker test has been used to measure pressure-flow relationships in the renal pelvis. The technique entails fluoroscopically guided insertion of a trocar or more recently a 22-gauge spinal needle into the renal pelvis and bladder catheterization (Fig. 13-18). Pressure in the renal pelvis and bladder is measured under basal conditions and after perfusion of a dilute solution of contrast

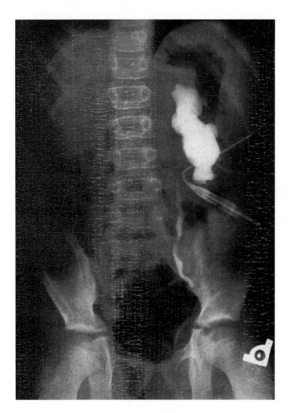

**Fig. 13-18** Whitaker test. Dilute solution of contrast medium is infused into a dilated renal pelvis at the rate of 10 ml/min. Pressure measurements are obtained to evaluate for suspected obstruction.

medium at the rate of 10 ml/min. In a dilated, nonobstructed collecting system the differential pressure between kidney and bladder remains low, less than 10 to 12 cm $H_2O$. In obstructed systems the equilibrium perfusion pressure exceeds 15 cm $H_2O$ and is frequently much higher.

The percutaneous perfusion technique is contraindicated in patients with acute pyelonephritis. Pyelotubular backflow may occur with pelvic pressures greater than 30 cm $H_2O$ and result in systemic infection. The technique is also contraindicated in patients with bleeding diatheses. It is associated with a significant radiation dose when performed fluoroscopically. Because a cannula in the renal pelvis is necessary, the technique is not conducive to frequent follow-up studies. In addition, variable results may be obtained, depending on technical factors such as needle size, volume of the hydronephrotic collecting system, and flow rates. Diuresis renography is a common noninvasive alternative to the Whitaker test.

**Diuresis renography**   For the study of urinary tract obstruction, conventional radionuclide renography has been modified to include a pharmacological intervention, the administration of a potent diuretic. The fundamental hypothesis underlying diuresis renography

is that the prolonged retention of radioactivity seen in nonobstructed, dilated systems is caused by a reservoir effect. Increased urine flow, as produced by a diuretic, produces a prompt washout of activity in a dilated, nonobstructed system. In cases of mechanical obstruction with a narrowed and fixed luminal cross-sectional area at the ureteropelvic or ureterovesical junction, the capacity to augment washout is much less, resulting in prolonged retention of tracer proximal to the obstruction.

For this method to be successful, renal function must be sufficient to promote a significant diuresis. Response patterns depend on the timing of diuretic injection, the amount and type of diuretic, the route of administration, and the patient's state of hydration.

*Methodology*   The imaging protocol for diuresis renography has a number of variations (Box 13-8). An attempt has been made to standardize the methodology for evaluating pediatric patients, for comparing data between institutions, and for evaluating the same patient when studies are done serially over time.

*Radiopharmaceuticals*   The original agent used for diuresis renography was I-131 OIH. A Tc-99m-labeled radiopharmaceutical is more suited to studies with the gamma camera. Tc-99m DTPA has been used successfully, particularly in patients with good renal function. Tc-99m MAG3 has become the agent of choice, however, because of its high clearance rate, excellent images, and utility in patients with renal insufficiency or immaturity.

*Diuretic administration*   Furosemide, the diuretic routinely used, acts through inhibition of sodium and chloride reabsorption in the proximal and distal tubules and the ascending loop of Henle. IV administration of furosemide is required because the peak effect after oral ingestion may not occur for an hour or longer. The injection is given slowly over 1 to 2 minutes. Onset of action occurs within 30 to 60 seconds, with maximal effect at 15 minutes. Side effects are rare.

Patients must be well hydrated so that fluid is available for mobilization in response to diuresis and to prevent dehydration. Urinary catheterization is recommended. Without a catheter, increased pressure from bladder filling can be transmitted retrograde, blunting the diuretic effect. Children and infants must be catheterized, as well as older subjects who cannot void voluntarily. If no catheter is used, the subject must void immediately before the diuresis study, and a postvoid picture is obtained after the acquisition.

The time of diuretic administration varies between laboratories. The diuretic may be given when pelvic filling is seen on the oscilloscope or computer monitor, typically at 15 to 20 minutes (Fig. 13-19). Others give furosemide simultaneous with injection of the radiopharmaceutical because maximal diuretic effect occurs about 15 minutes later. For standardization, many institutions

## Box 13-8  Diuresis Renography: Protocol Summary

**INDICATION**

Evidence of pelvicocalyceal radiotracer retention after routine renal scintigraphy.

**PATIENT PREPARATION**

Provide hydration, as described in protocol for dynamic renal scintigraphy.

Place Foley catheter in children; optional for adults.

If catheter is not used, complete bladder emptying is necessary before diuretic injection and after 20-min study.

**FUROSEMIDE DOSE**

Approximate adult furosemide dose based on patient's creatinine:

| Serum Creatinine (mg/dl) | Creatinine Clearance (ml) | Furosemide Dose (mg) |
|---|---|---|
| 1.0 | 100 | 20 |
| 1.5 | 75 | 40 |
| 2.0 | 50 | 60 |
| 3.0 | 30 | 80 |

Furosemide dosage for children with normal renal function: 1 mg/kg.

**INSTRUMENTATION**

Camera: same as for dynamic renal scintigraphy

Computer setup: 30-sec frames for 60 sec

**IMAGING PROCEDURE**

Start computer and run for at least 60 sec before diuretic injection.

Slowly infuse furosemide intravenously over 60 sec.

Acquire for 20 min on computer after injection.

Obtain postvoid image in patients without catheters.

**IMAGE PROCESSING**

On computer, draw a region of interest around the entire kidney and pelvis.

Generate time-activity curves.

Calculate a half-emptying time or fitted half-time.

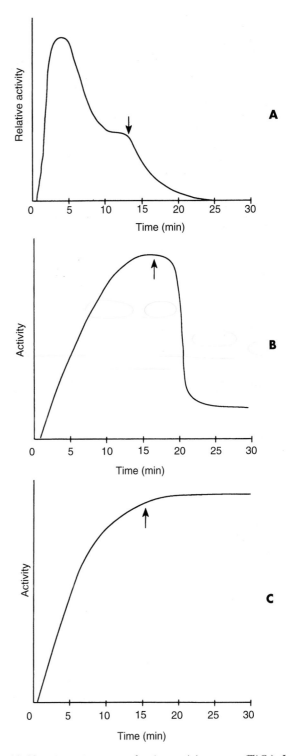

**Fig. 13-19**  Diuresis renography time-activity curves (TACs). In these examples the diuretic is given at the time of peak collecting system filling. **A,** Normal kidney response to diuretic. The short plateau before further emptying represents diuretic-induced flow just before rapid clearance. **B,** Dilated nonobstructed kidney. The slowly rising curve represents progressive pelvicocalyceal filling. With diuretic administration *(arrow),* rapid clearance occurs. **C,** Obstructed kidney. The diuretic has no effect on the abnormal TAC.

have adopted a two-phase study, particularly for children. First, routine dynamic renal scintigraphy of 25 to 30 minutes is performed. The second phase, diuretic renography, requires a second computer setup and acquisition for an additional 20 minutes after furosemide in infused. Digital acquisition of data by computer is mandatory to generate TACs for qualitative and quantitative analysis.

*Image analysis*   The scintigraphic findings of renovascular hypertension depend on the degree and duration of obstruction. With total obstruction of several days' to a week's duration, no renal function may be visible. With high-grade obstruction of shorter duration or lesser obstruction, scintigraphy may show poor blood flow, decreased function, and no evidence of radiotracer entering the collecting system (Fig. 13-20). With lower-

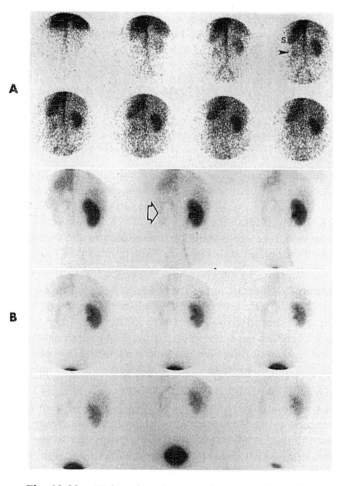

**Fig. 13-20**   High-grade vesicoureteral junction obstruction secondary to a tumor. **A,** Flow study shows very decreased perfusion of the left kidney *(arrowhead).* Do not confuse the spleen *(S)* with the kidney. **B,** Dynamic sequential images acquired every 5 minutes show only a thin rim of cortex with poor uptake *(open arrowhead)* and a very large central photopenic collecting system consistent with hydronephrosis. Diuresis renography would not be indicated or useful, since no tracer fills the collecting system.

grade obstruction the kidney retains good blood flow and function and the radiotracer empties into a hydronephrotic collecting system. During the 25 to 30 minutes, however, little or no pelvicocalyceal clearance occurs (Fig. 13-21).

Obstruction usually cannot be differentiated from a nonobstructed hydronephrosis 25 to 30 minutes after injection with conventional renography (Fig. 13-22). Delayed imaging at 2 to 4 hours shows little change with an obstructed kidney, but a nonobstructed kidney clears of tracer during that interval. However, a more rapid and quantitative method with diuresis renography is preferable. After furosemide infusion, prompt clearance occurs in a nonobstructed kidney, with poor or no clearance in an obstructed kidney. Since this is not an all-or-none phenomenon, computer-generated TACs can be valuable for interpretation of diuresis renography (Figs. 13-21 to 13-23).

*Data analysis*   Each kidney and, if indicated, the ureter are analyzed separately by computer. The entire study is first inspected frame by frame to assess renal cortical and collecting system morphology and to select appropriate ROIs. This step is also useful to make sure the patient has not moved during the study, which can invalidate TAC data. Then a whole kidney ROI that includes the entire collecting system is drawn on computer. A TAC is generated.

*Interpretation*   The significance of TAC response patterns is based on empirical correlations with both surgical results and long-term clinical follow-up. The literature is replete with attempts to refine and quantify response patterns. Conservatively, the diuresis renogram should be taken as only one indicator of renal function and obstruction. It has limitations (discussed later) and sometimes must be interpreted as indeterminate or nondiagnostic. Serial studies can be done to determine whether change occurs over time.

NORMAL PATTERN   In normal pelvicocalyceal systems the conventional radionuclide TAC shows increasing activity that reaches a sharp peak within several minutes after radiotracer injection. This is followed by a spontaneous, rapid decline in activity. Furosemide diuresis accelerates the rate of tracer washout (Fig. 13-19, *A*).

In the normal ureter the TAC histogram is usually flat, indicating a small, constant amount of activity. Frequently a transient spike of activity occurs after diuretic injection, indicating passage of a bolus of accumulated activity from the renal pelvis.

DILATED NONOBSTRUCTED PATTERN   In dilated but nonobstructed kidneys with good function the initial portion of the TAC may be similar to that seen in normal kidneys, but accumulation is progressive, without a sharp, narrow peak. The TAC frequently reaches a plateau 20 to 30 minutes after tracer injection. After furosemide diuresis the level of activity decreases rapidly, indicating diuresis-induced washout (Fig. 13-19, *B*). The rate and degree of decrease 20 minutes after diuretic injection are variable, but a brisk response to diuresis is consistent with a nonobstructed system.

The larger the collecting system, the less "crisp" the response. The relationship between volume and flow is given by the equation $\bar{t} = V/F$, where $\bar{t}$ is the time the tracer transits through a system, $V$ is the volume of the system, and $F$ is the flow through it. According to this formula, the larger the volume, the more prolonged the transit time at a given flow rate; for any given volume the transit time will be longer at lower rates of flow. Thus extremely large, hydronephrotic systems may appear to exhibit delayed washout regardless of whether they are obstructed or not. Likewise, renal units with impaired function and diminished response to the diuretic exhibit prolonged washout, whether they are obstructed or not. In these two situations indeterminate or nondiagnostic patterns may occur.

TACs for dilated, nonobstructed ureters are similar to those for kidneys. After diuretic injection there is a lag in response because of the serial nature of the washout phenomenon from renal pelvis to ureter.

OBSTRUCTED PATTERN   The initial slope of the TAC in obstructed kidneys is frequently less steep than in normal kidneys, and either accumulation of activity is progressive or a plateau is reached within 20 to 30 minutes. After furosemide diuresis the TAC of the obstructed kidney most frequently shows a flat response without significant washout (Figs. 13-19, *C,* and 13-20). In some cases, progressive accumulation actually continues, and in a few cases a transient decrease in activity is followed by reaccumulation. The pattern for obstructed ureters is similar; activity fails to decrease after diuresis.

QUANTIFICATION   Using the standardized two-phase study, a washout half-time of less than 10 minutes generally indicates no significant mechanical obstruction. A half-time of washout greater than 20 minutes is consistent with obstruction, whereas a half-time be-

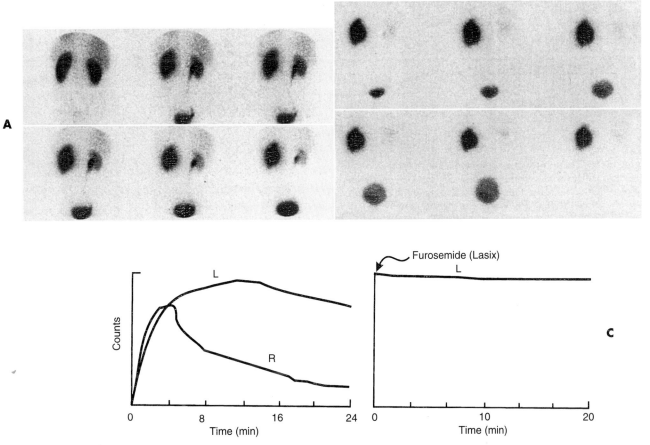

**Fig. 13-21**   Obstructive hydronephrosis on technetium-99m mercaptylacetyltriglycine (MAG3) study. **A,** Progressive filling of an enlarged collecting system is seen on the left, whereas the right kidney clears normally. **B,** Diuresis renography shows almost no clearing of hydronephrotic left kidney after furosemide administration. This is a clinically significant obstruction and requires intervention. **C,** Time-activity curves before *(left)* and after *(right)* furosemide administration confirm the imaging findings, showing extremely poor response to the diuretic.

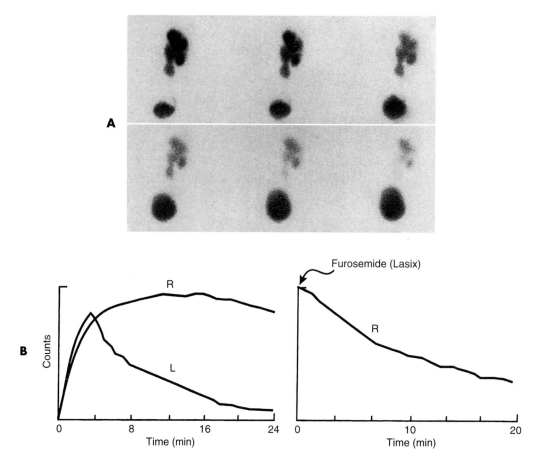

**Fig. 13-22** Nonobstructive hydronephrosis. Diuretic renogram of a patient with surgically treated vesicoureteral obstruction of the right kidney. **A,** Postfurosemide images show that the prominent hydroureteronephrosis responds promptly to the diuretic, with almost complete clearance. **B,** Time-activity curves. Before diuretic administration *(left),* curve of the hydronephrotic kidney rises slowly and plateaus. After furosemide administration *(right),* curve promptly declines, signifying no significant obstruction.

tween 10 and 20 minutes is considered an indeterminate response, and obstruction cannot be excluded.

*Other clinical applications* The most common clinical problem studied by diuresis renography is suspected ureteropelvic junction obstruction (Box 13-9). When dilated collecting systems referred for evaluation are shown not to be obstructed, this eliminates the need for more invasive procedures or a prolonged follow-up series.

Although diuresis renography is often done to differentiate obstructive from nonobstructive hydronephrosis, it also is used to determine the clinical significance of a known partial obstruction, as in patients with pelvic tumors (e.g., cervical carcinoma). A high-grade obstruction results in renal damage and dysfunction, whereas a lower grade obstruction may be compensated for and cause only dilation, without an adverse affect on renal function. Diuresis renography can determine whether

aggressive intervention is indicated (e.g., stenting or surgery).

A kidney from which tracer does not wash out with furosemide is significantly obstructed. Thus renal function can be predicted to deteriorate without intervention. In contrast, a collecting system from which tracer is washed out with furosemide is not at risk for imminent renal deterioration. Serial studies every few months can be used to follow the course of the partial obstruction.

Other, less frequently encountered conditions also can be evaluated by diuresis renography (Box 13-9). For example, some degree of hydronephrosis and hydroureter is common in patients with long-standing ileal loop diversions. The degree of hydronephrosis may be alarming and also associated with reflux. Other conditions, such as prune-belly syndrome, are associated with structural dysmorphism and flaccidity of the collecting structures.

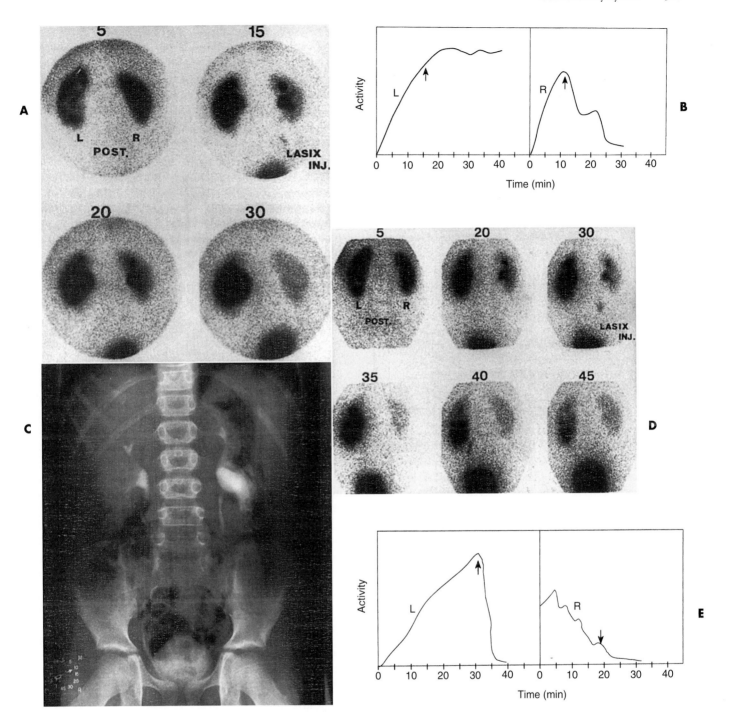

**Fig. 13-23**   Preoperative and postoperative diuresis renography: utility of follow-up. **A,** Eight-year-old boy with history of abdominal pain. Images obtained with technetium-99m DPTA at 15 minutes (before Lasix injection) reveal minor retention in collecting structures on the right but marked retention on the left. After Lasix, there is prompt washout from the right kidney but progressive accumulation on the left (30 minutes). **B,** Time-activity curves (TACs) confirm imaging findings. No response to Lasix injection *(arrows)* is seen on the left, confirming the diagnosis of obstruction. **C,** Patient had a left pyeloplasty and returned 2 months later for follow-up intravenous urography. The postoperative IVU shows dilation on the left, with contrast material accumulating in the pelvis and calyces, especially inferiorly. The adequacy of surgery was uncertain. **D,** Diuresis renography demonstrates persistent urinary retention on the left before Lasix injection. After Lasix, there is prompt washout, except for minimal residual tracer in the left inferior pole. **E,** TACs confirmed prompt bilateral clearance.

*Pitfalls and limitations*   The indeterminate diuresis renogram is neither positive nor negative and does not rule out obstruction. The Whitaker test had a similar category. Some nonobstructed patients with very large collecting systems will always have an indeterminate response because of the reservoir effect.

RENAL INSUFFICIENCY   A flat response or failure to respond after diuretic injection in a patient with significantly impaired renal function is moot, since renal function may be inadequate for effective diuresis.

Good criteria are not available to determine definitively when renal function is adequate to meet the rationale of diuresis renography. If the uptake in the kidney is poor or the collecting structures are not clearly visualized, however, caution should be used in interpretation. The serum creatinine level may be normal in the patient with unilateral renal impairment and is not a reliable indicator with unilateral disease. Increased doses of furosemide can be given to the patient with renal insufficiency, but the dose selected as adequate is only an estimate. Therefore renal insufficiency is a definite limitation of the test.

BLADDER   In infants and children younger than 5 years, radioactivity in the bladder may overlap and obscure the lower ureters and in some cases reach the level of the kidneys. Increased backpressure in the collecting system because of a filled bladder may alter the washout response pattern. Therefore the bladder should be catheterized before the study is initiated. A special problem arises with low-lying or pelvic kidneys where overlap is invariable and catheterization is required.

---

### Box 13-9   Urological Conditions Studied by Diuresis Renography

Ureteropelvic junction obstruction
Megaureter
   Obstructive
   Nonobstructive
   Refluxing
Horseshoe kidney
Multicystic and polycystic kidney
Upper collecting system duplication
Prune-belly syndrome
Ectopic ureterocele
Urethral valves
Ureteral injury
Postoperative states
Pyeloplasty
   Ureteral reimplantation
   Urinary diversion
Renal transplant ureteral obstruction
Obstructing pelvic mass
Ileal loop diversion

---

NEONATAL HYDRONEPHROSIS   Determining the cause of neonatal hydronephrosis can be particularly problematic. Neonates have functionally immature kidneys. Since renal function is still developing, cortical uptake and clearance of radiotracer may be delayed, especially in premature infants. This poses a problem similar to patients who have renal insufficiency. Lasix renography may falsely suggest obstruction. Patients without clearcut obstruction are often followed over time with serial diuresis renograms. Surgeons prefer to perform surgery when the infant and the genitourinary system are larger and more mature.

REFLUX   In some patients with hydroureteronephrosis, dilation is associated with reflux rather than obstruction. Reintroduction of tracer in the upper tracts as a result of reflux is a theoretical problem that can cause an upward deflection on the time-activity histogram. In practice, this is generally recognized by reviewing the sequential images and by assessing the bladder TAC, which shows a reciprocal downward deflection as significant reflux occurs.

TECHNICAL ERRORS   Because infiltration of the diuretic dose can be painful, it is generally recognized in adult subjects but may not be as easily confirmed in infants and small children. From a practical standpoint an IV line should be maintained in children and checked for free flow just before the diuretic is injected. This also reduces the chance for patient motion during the venipuncture.

MOTION ARTIFACTS   Subjects must remain still for the duration of the procedure, which may be difficult for children. Motion artifacts can be minimized by ensuring that the patient's position is comfortable before starting the examination. Motion is easily recognized by rapid sequential viewing of the images on the computer screen and should be suspected if the renal TACs are irregular.

---

### Renal Transplant Evaluation

Radionuclide methods have been used extensively in the evaluation of renal allografts after transplantation. Radiotracer techniques are noninvasive and are easily repeated to clarify the evolving clinical findings.

Kidneys for transplantation come from either living related donors or cadavers. Potential donors typically undergo extensive anatomical and functional evaluation as well as immunological matching. Cadaveric kidneys are carefully preserved and stored in regional organ banks, then distributed to transplantation centers when needed. The surgical technique is well established (Fig. 13-24). The superficial placement of the graft in the anterior iliac fossa allows palpation for assessment of change in size as well as easy access for biopsy and surgical repair.

Renal allografts from living related donors are considerably more successful than cadaveric grafts but represent only 35% of transplanted kidneys. Most kidneys come from unrelated donors who have died of head injuries. One-year graft survival rates are 86% for HLA-identical siblings, 82% for living related donors, but only 56% for cadaver transplants.

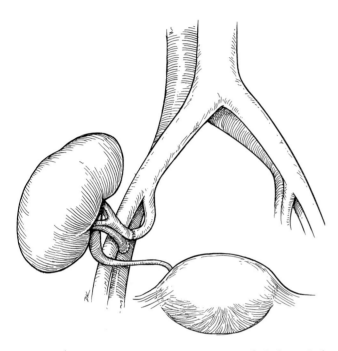

**Fig. 13-24** Renal transplant surgery. For technical surgical reasons the initial allograft is usually placed in the right iliac fossa. The donor renal artery is anastomosed end-to-end to the hypogastric artery and the renal vein end-to-side to the external iliac vein. The allograft ureter is attached to the recipient's ureter or, more often, implanted directly into the bladder. After initial failures, second grafts are usually placed in the left iliac fossa. When a pancreas is transplanted simultaneously with the kidney in a diabetic patient, the transabdominal approach is used.

The length of time after transplantation is a key factor in determining the choice of nuclear medicine procedure and in interpreting the significance of the findings.

**Medical complications**

*Acute tubular necrosis*  An early complication, acute tubular necrosis (ATN) occurs almost invariably with cadaver allografts and much less often with living related donor grafts (Table 13-4). A prolonged time between the donor's death and transplantation increases the severity of ATN. The damage occurs before transplantation. This historical terminology is not a correct description of the usual pathological process, since there is little if any destruction of tubular elements. The more current term is *vasomotor nephropathy,* since the pathophysiological process is a reflex ischemic response within the kidney caused by local activation of the renin-angiotensin axis. ATN is used here because of its common usage.

ATN is characterized scintigraphically by well-preserved perfusion but poor renal function and decreased urine excretion (Fig. 13-25). In severe cases no urine is produced. These findings are usually seen on renal scintigraphy performed within 24 hours of surgery. The severity of ATN varies considerably. ATN usually resolves over 1 to 3 weeks, with return of renal function and urine excretion. The condition may be superimposed on other complications.

*Hyperacute rejection*  Preformed antibodies in the recipient's circulation result in an immediate posttransplantation reaction. The surgeon typically recognizes this event as soon as the vascular clamp is released after anastomosis because the kidney turns blue. The renal vasculature thromboses, resulting in irreversible destruction of the donor kidney. This complication occurs infrequently in contemporary practice because of comprehensive immunological donor and recipient screen-

## Table 13-4  Complications after renal transplantation

| Complication | Usual time of occurrence | Comments |
|---|---|---|
| Acute tubular necrosis | Minutes to hours postoperatively | Cadaveric transplant |
| Rejection | | |
|   Hyperacute | Minutes to hours | Preformed antibodies; irreversible |
|   Accelerated | 1-5 days | Occurs after previous transplant or transfusions |
|   Acute | After 5 days; most common during first 3 months | Cell mediated; responsive to treatment |
|   Chronic | Months to years | Humoral; irreversible |
| Cyclosporin toxicity | Months | Reversible with drug withdrawal |
| Surgical | | |
|   Urine leak | Few days or weeks | |
|   Hematoma | First few days | |
|   Wound infection | First few days | |
|   Obstruction | Days, months, years | Clots, scar, calculi |
|   Lymphocele | 2nd to 4th month | |
|   Renal artery stenosis | After 1st month | |

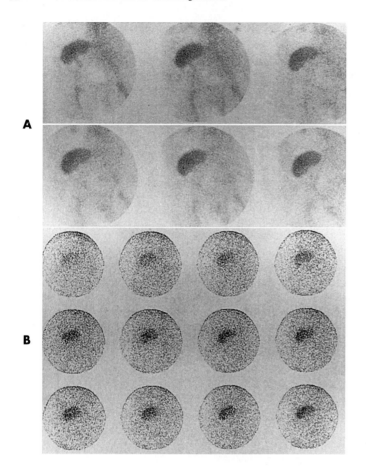

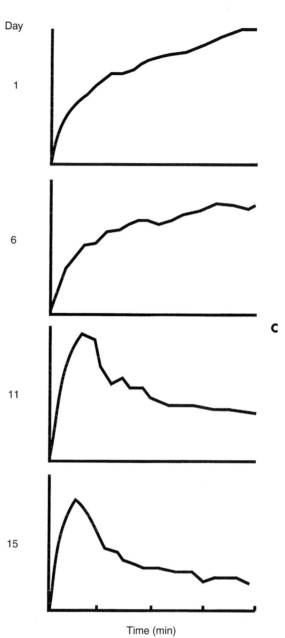

**Fig. 13-25**   Acute tubular necrosis (ATN) after renal transplantation. Blood flow to the kidney is normal *(not shown).* **A,** Technetium-99m DTPA study shows poor renal uptake and no excretion, resulting in high persistent background activity for the 30-minute study. **B,** Iodine-131 hippuran study in the same patient performed immediately after first study shows delayed uptake and no clearance. Unlike Tc-99m DTPA, no vascular structures are seen. **C,** Time-activity curves (TACs) for I-131 OIH on day 1 (this imaging study) and follow-up studies on days 6, 11, and 15. ATN resolved over 2 weeks. As function improves, the TACs change from a gradual upslope without a plateau to a definite early peak and good clearance.

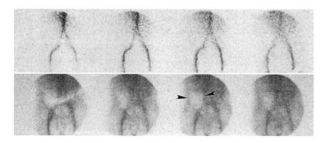

**Fig. 13-26**   Renal artery thrombosis. *Top,* Radionuclide angiogram demonstrates no perfusion to the renal transplant. *Bottom,* Dynamic images acquired immediately after the flow study and sequentially every 5 minutes show a photopenic defect *(arrowheads)* resulting from a nonviable allograft causing attenuation but having no radiopharmaceutical uptake.

ing. Risk factors include prior transplantation and multiple blood transfusions.

Although rarely seen, the scintigraphic appearance of hyperacute rejection is absent perfusion to the transplanted kidney and no function. The kidney appears as a photon-deficient area with high background activity because of tracer retained in the extracellular fluid space. This pattern is similar to that seen in acute arterial or venous thrombosis (Fig. 13-26). The clinical significance of renal vein thrombosis is much greater in the newly transplanted kidney than in native kidneys because the allograft has no venous collaterals. Thus venous thrombosis has the same significance as arterial obstruction in the immediate transplant period.

*Acute rejection*   A common complication, acute rejection typically occurs 5 to 7 days after transplantation, although it may occur at any time, usually during the first 3 months. The cause is a cell-mediated immunological process. Clinically, acute rejection manifests with symptoms of fever, transplant tenderness, and enlargement. Laboratory values, such as the sedimentation rate and serum $\beta_2$-microglobulin levels, may rise. Untreated, acute rejection results in allograft death from vascular and tubular damage; however, rejection often responds to appropriate immunosuppressive therapy. *Accelerated* acute rejection occurs in a sensitized patient as a result of previous transplantation and blood transfusions. It is seen during the first week of transplantation.

Acute rejection is a clinical diagnosis. In the expected period with the described clinical findings, the diagnosis is fairly certain. When a clinical question still exists, allograft biopsy is often performed. Numerous scintigraphic techniques were used to aid in making this diagnosis, but most were discontinued because of nonspecificity. Renography is used to support the occasional uncertain diagnosis; to evaluate renal function, particularly when the patient requires dialysis; and most important, to evaluate blood flow and ensure viability.

The scintigraphic hallmark of acute rejection is decreased transplant perfusion and poor function. With a good bolus injection and a framing rate of 2 to 3 seconds per frame, the healthy kidney normally becomes the "hottest" structure in the field of view within one or two frames of radiotracer bolus appearance at the level of the iliac artery. Failure of the kidney to light up in the setting of adequate bolus injection suggests reduced perfusion. TACs can be helpful in confirming delayed perfusion (Fig. 13-27). A baseline study before the fifth posttransplant day is useful for comparison purposes.

With acute rejection, renal uptake and excretion are reduced. The baseline scintigrams and renograms should be used for comparison to assess the contribution of preexisting ATN. When comparing sequential TACs, the clinician should remember that ATN is most severe initially and usually resolves over 1 to 2 weeks. Thus interval changes indicating slower uptake, more prolonged retention, and less excretion typically suggest acute rejection in the appropriate interval after transplantation.

Quantitative measurements of GFR or ERPF are diminished in acute rejection. Their significance is greatest when baseline and sequential values are available to differentiate changes of acute rejection from preexisting damage due to ATN.

In addition to conventional renography, other radionuclide methods have been used for evaluation of acute transplant rejection. The colloidal particles of Tc-99m sulfur colloid (SC) become trapped within fibrin thrombi that develop in the vessels of rejecting transplants. Although this method has some utility in detecting a first episode of acute rejection, delayed return to normal makes its later use problematic. Mixed populations of indium-111 (In-111)-labeled leukocytes, In-111

lymphocytes, In-111 platelets, and gallium-67 have been tried. All accumulate in rejecting grafts, but specificity is poor.

*Chronic rejection* A delayed phenomenon, chronic rejection occurs months to years after transplantation. The course is insidious, and transplant function gradually deteriorates. In this humorally mediated process, renal perfusion, GFR, and ERPF are diminished, reflected scintigraphically as decreased perfusion, reduced and slow accumulation of tracer, and reduced urine formation (Fig. 13-28).

### Surgical complications

*Arterial stenosis* Postoperative arterial stenosis is suspected in patients who develop new hypertension after transplantation. Captopril renography can prove useful in selected cases.

*Urinary leak* Necrosis of the ureteral anastomosis in the immediate postoperative period can result in urinary leakage. When rapid, this may be easily seen on dynamic renography as increasing accumulation on sequential images (Fig. 13-29). With slower leaks a photopenic defect adjacent to the kidney may be seen initially due to the nonradiolabeled urinoma. Delayed imaging at 2 hours or later may detect increasing activity in the urinoma.

*Ureteral obstruction* Although uncommon, ureteral obstruction may be caused by kinking of the ureter, compression from an extrinsic mass (e.g., hematoma, lymphocele), intraluminal obstruction from a blood clot or calculus, and periureteral fibrosis. Some degree of collecting system dilation without significant mechanical obstruction is often seen after transplantation because of postoperative seromas and hematomas. Ureteral obstruction usually resolves spontaneously (Fig. 13-30). Fluid collections are often noted on renograms in the posttransplant period as fixed pararenal, photon-deficient areas.

*Lymphoceles* typically occur 2 to 3 months postoperatively. Because the transplanted kidney does not have lymphatic connections, disruption of lymph channels in the transplant bed can result in lymphocele formation. This may occur in up to 10% of transplants, but lymphocele is clinically important only if it displaces the kidney or impinges on the ureter or renal vascular pedicle.

## RENAL CORTICAL SCINTIGRAPHY

It is often difficult clinically to distinguish upper from lower UTI. However, the long-term complications and therapeutic implications of parenchymal infection are very different from those of lower urinary tract disease. Cortical scarring can lead to renal failure and hypertension. Cortical imaging with Tc-99m DMSA or Tc-99m GH can make this distinction.

In the past the standard method for detecting pyelo-

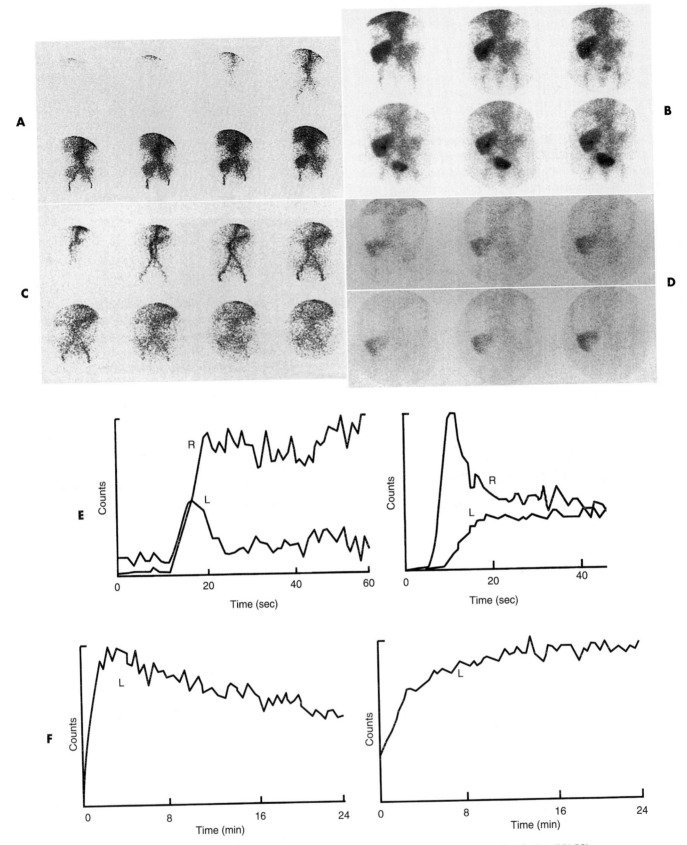

**Fig. 13-27** Acute allograft rejection. **A** and **B,** Technetium-99m mercaptylacetyltriglycine (MAG3) study at the end of the first week following transplantation. Good blood flow **(A)** and function **(B)** of the allograft in the right iliac fossa. **C** and **D,** Two days later low-grade fever, allograft tenderness, and a rising serum creatinine level developed. Follow-up flow studies show very poor blood flow **(C)** and function **(D). E,** Time-activity curves show good blood flow before rejection *(left)* but delayed flow to the transplant during rejection *(right).* **F,** Time-activity curves for 25-minute study show good function before rejection *(left)* and poor function at time of rejection *(right).*

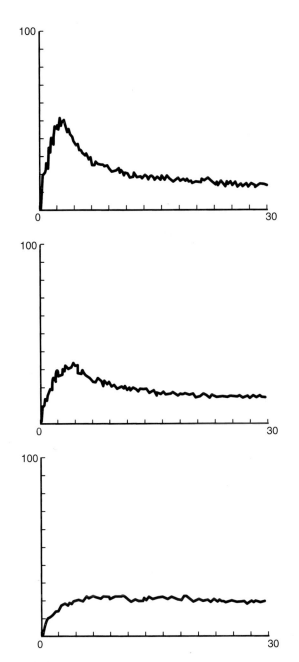

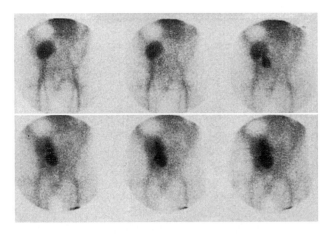

**Fig. 13-29** Postoperative urinary leak. Rapid leakage results from a disrupted surgical anastomosis. Note accumulation of radiotracer just inferior to the transplant but superior and lateral to the bladder. No bladder filling is seen.

**Fig. 13-28** Chronic allograft rejection. Time-activity curves of a patient with progressively worsening creatinine clearance over 3 sequential years (*top* to *bottom*). Each study shows poorer uptake and more delayed peak and clearance, consistent with chronic rejection.

nephritis and renal scarring was the IV urogram. Most of the epidemiological data on the incidence of acute pyelonephritis and its sequelae (scarring, hypertension, renal failure) were based on this technique. Since the mid-1980s, studies have demonstrated the superiority of radionuclide renal cortical imaging for detecting both acute pyelonephritis and renal scarring compared with IV urograms and ultrasonography.

## Pyelonephritis

Pyelonephritis usually results from vesicoureteral reflux of infected urine. Although only a portion of the cortex drained by a refluxing papilla may be involved in any one infection, the remaining cortex often becomes infected on repeated occasions until all functioning renal tissue drained by that papilla is destroyed. Repetitive infection may also occur during a single clinical episode if it is not promptly and appropriately treated. Furthermore, infection with certain strains of *Escherichia coli* has been shown to paralyze the ureter and cause a functional obstruction. For this reason pyelonephritis may be seen in the cortex of even a normally nonrefluxing papilla.

Renal infection induces rapid activation of serum complement and granulocyte aggregation at the site of infection. Vascular occlusion and renal ischemia result. In areas of acute inflammation the renal microcirculation becomes impaired because of interstitial edema, with compression of glomeruli, small peritubular capillaries, and the vasae rectae.

### Image Interpretation

Cortical scintigraphy demonstrates approximately twice as many defects as ultrasonography and four times as many defects as IV urography. Color Doppler imaging has improved the sensitivity of ultrasonography, but it remains inferior to that of scintigraphy. Preliminary studies suggest that computed tomography (CT) may be an accurate method, but no direct comparison studies have been performed. CT is more expensive, has the associated risk of contrast agent reaction, and results in a higher radiation absorbed dose to the patient.

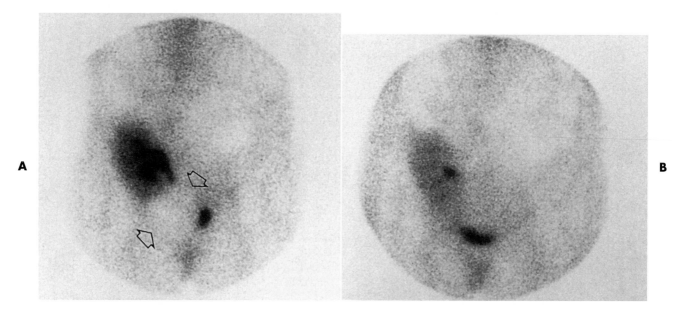

**Fig. 13-30**   Partial ureteral obstruction of renal allograft. **A,** Postoperative study showing dilated calyces and renal pelvis with an abrupt cut-off of the ureter. The adjacent, relatively photopenic area just inferior *(arrowheads)* is caused by a hematoma. **B,** Repeat study performed 3 weeks postoperatively shows complete self-resolution of the obstruction.

Ga-67 and In-111 leukocyte imaging can demonstrate infection. Delayed imaging is required (In-111 leukocytes at 24 hours and Ga-67 at 48 hours), however, and both studies are associated with a somewhat high radiation dose. Thus neither is widely used in children for this purpose.

Pyelonephritis may be seen as a solitary defect involving only a portion of one kidney, as multiple focal defects involving one or both kidneys, or as diffuse involvement of an entire kidney. A follow-up study should be performed 3 to 6 months after the acute infection to determine if the infection has resolved or if renal scarring has occurred (Fig. 13-31).

Scarring is seen as volume loss, whether focal or global. Volume loss may even occur in the absence of focal defects and present only as atrophy. More often it is seen as small or large, single or multiple, focal cortical defects or cortical thinning.

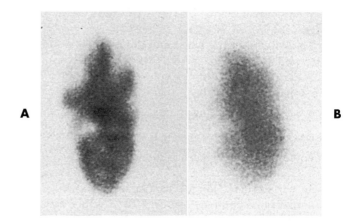

**Fig. 13-31**   Acute pyelonephritis. Technetium-99m DMSA study in 11-year-old child using a pinhole collimator. **A,** Note multiple cortical defects, particularly in the upper pole. **B,** Follow-up scan obtained 6 months later, after appropriate antibiotic therapy, shows resolution of most cortical defects.

## Mechanism of Uptake

Good agreement exists between an abnormal cortical scintigram and the histopathology of pyelonephritis in animal studies. Two mechanisms have been proposed for this tubular dysfunction: (1) the decreased uptake is caused by the decreased blood flow and ischemia associated with pyelonephritis, or (2) toxic byproducts of granulocyte lysis paralyze the active tubular transport mechanism responsible for DMSA tubular localization.

## Renal Pseudotumor

Renal cortical scintigraphy has been used for evaluating renal tumors and trauma. Intrarenal masses of any etiology do not accumulate renal radiopharmaceuticals and thus appear as "cold" or photon-deficient areas. Other imaging modalities, however, such as CT and ultrasonography, are preferable for this purpose. The one exception is the ability of scintigraphy to confirm functioning renal tissue, for example, in differentiating a renal tumor from a pseudotumor, as seen with a hypertrophied column of Bertin. The latter tissue functions normally and takes up the radiopharmaceutical.

## RADIONUCLIDE CYSTOGRAPHY

Radionuclide cystography was introduced in the late 1950s to diagnose vesicoureteral reflux and is increasingly being accepted as the technique of choice for the evaluation and follow-up of children with UTIs and reflux. The radionuclide method is more sensitive than contrast-enhanced cystography for detecting reflux and results in considerably less radiation exposure to the patient. In many centers contrast voiding urethrocystography is reserved for the initial workup of male patients to exclude an anatomical cause for reflux, such as posterior urethral valves.

### Vesicoureteral Reflux

Untreated reflux and infection are associated with subsequent renal damage, scarring, hypertension, and chronic renal failure. Vesicoureteral reflux is caused by a failure of the ureterovesical valve. The normal ureter passes obliquely through the bladder wall and submucosa to its opening at the trigone. As urine fills the bladder, the valve passively closes, preventing reflux. If the intramural ureteral length is too short in relation to its diameter or if the course is too direct, the valve will not close completely and reflux results. As a child grows, the ureter usually grows in length more than in diameter, resulting in decreased reflux and eventual resolution in 80% of patients.

Renal damage is more likely in patients with severe rather than mild or moderate grades of reflux. Reflux by itself is not pathological; that is, sterile low-pressure reflux does not cause renal injury. The intrarenal reflux of infected urine is required for damage to develop. The goal of therapy is to prevent infection of the kidney until reflux resolves spontaneously.

### Methodology

*Indirect* radionuclide cystography can be performed as part of routine dynamic renal scintigraphy with Tc-99m DTPA or Tc-99m MAG3. The child is asked not to void until the bladder is maximally filled. When the bladder is as full as can be tolerated, a previoding image is obtained. Dynamic images are then recorded continuously during voiding. After voiding is complete, a postvoiding image is obtained. The indirect method is no longer commonly used. Although its advantage is that bladder catheterization is unnecessary, upper tract stasis often poses a problem for interpretation, good renal function is necessary, and the indirect method cannot identify patients who experience reflux only during the filling phase (20%).

*Direct* radionuclide cystography is the technique performed most often. It is usually done as a three-phase procedure, with continuous imaging during filling of the bladder, micturition, and after voiding. The procedure can determine the presence or absence of reflux and measure the postvoiding residue in the bladder.

Radionuclide cystography is performed dynamically and acquired on computer (Box 13-10). The high sensitivity for detection of reflux results from the rapid acquisition of 10 seconds per frame. Tc-99m sulfur colloid or Tc-99m DTPA are the radiotracers used most often, since Tc-99m pertechnetate may be absorbed through the bladder systemically, particularly if the bladder is inflamed. A solution of 1 mCi/500 ml provides sufficient concentration.

Urinary tract catheterization of the child is an important step in the procedure, and personnel involved should use appropriate sterile technique. The catheter selected should be large enough to permit filling of the bladder within 10 minutes. The patient's cooperation is valuable to avoid premature voiding around the catheter and resultant contamination of the imaging field. As capacity is reached, voiding may occur spontaneously, especially in young children and infants.

### Radiation Dosimetry

The radiation absorbed dose is quite low. From 50 to 200 times less radiation is delivered to the gonads with the radionuclide method than with contrast cystography (Box 13-11).

### Image Interpretation

In a normal study no tracer is seen in the region of the ureters or kidneys. Any reflux is abnormal and readily detected by the presence of activity above the bladder. Reflux can be graded using criteria devised for contrast cystography (Fig. 13-32); however, anatomical resolution and the detail available with scintigraphy are significantly less than with conventional x-ray cystography. Because scintigraphy does not have adequate resolution to permit visualization of calyceal morphology, the following criteria are used to grade reflux: level reached, degree of dilation of the renal pelvis, and degree of dilation and tortuosity of the ureter. Generally, reflux is considered minimal when confined to the ureter, mild to moderate

## Box 13-10   Radionuclide Retrograde Cystography: Protocol Summary

**RADIOPHARMACEUTICAL**

Tc-99m sulfur colloid, 1 mCi

**PATIENT PREPARATION**

Insert and secure a urinary catheter.

**PATIENT POSITION**

Supine, with the bladder, ureters, and kidneys in the field of view (symphysis pubis to xiphoid).

**INSTRUMENTATION**

Camera: large-field-of-view gamma
Computer setup: $64 \times 64$ word mode
Filling: 10-sec frames for 60 sec
Prevoid: 30-sec image
Voiding: 2-sec frames for 120 sec
Postvoid: 30-sec image
Collimator: converging for newborn to 1 yr; low energy, all purpose for greater than 1 year of age

**IMAGING PROCEDURE**

Image posteriorly with camera under table.
Hang 500-ml bag of normal saline 25 cm above the table.
Inject radiotracer into the catheter.

**Filling Phase**

Fill bladder to maximum capacity with IV drip open. Bladder capacity can be estimated by the formula (age [yr] + 2) × 30 = ml.
Continue filling until the drip slows or there is backup of flow into tubing or voiding around catheter.
Observe the oscilloscope for reflux.

**Voiding Phase**

Place camera perpendicular to table.
Position patient sitting on bedpan with back to camera.
Have patient void.
Measure volume.

**Patients Too Young to Void on Request**

Change diaper and put on a preweighed dry diaper.
Deflate Foley catheter.
Record volume of saline infused at initiation of reflux and voided volume.
Weigh diaper.

**INTERPRETATION**

Total bladder volume, residual postvoid volume, and bladder volume at initiation of reflux can be determined.

Residual bladder volume (ml) =

$$\frac{\text{Voided volume (ml)} \times \text{Residual counts/min}}{\text{Initial counts/min} - \text{Residual counts/min}}$$

## Box 13-11   Radiation Dosimetry for Tc-99m Retrograde Cystography

| ORGAN | mrads/mCi |
|---|---|
| Bladder | 18-27 |
| Ovaries | 1-2 |
| Testicle | <1-2 |
| Kidneys | 0.02-0.04* |

*Mrad/ml of reflux/min of residence in collecting system.

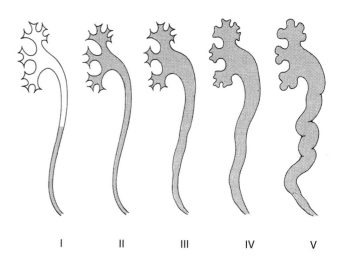

**Fig. 13-32**   Vesicoureteral grading system (International Reflux Study Committee). *I,* Ureteral reflux only. *II,* Reflux into ureter, pelvis, and calyces. No dilation; normal calyceal fornices. *III,* Mild to moderate dilation/tortuosity of ureter and mild to moderate calyceal dilation, but no blunting of fornices. *IV,* Moderate dilation and tortuosity of ureter and moderate dilation of renal pelvis. Angles of fornices obliterated, but papillary impressions maintained. *V,* Gross dilation and tortuosity of ureter and gross dilation of renal pelvis and calyces. Papillary impressions no longer visible in most calyces.

when it reaches the pelvicocalyceal system, and severe when a distended collecting system and a redundant ureter are noted (Fig. 13-33).

The volume of the bladder and the residual volume after voiding can be calculated by measuring the change in count rate before and after voiding and relating it to the urine volume (Box 13-10).

### Accuracy

Radionuclide cystography is more sensitive than the radiographic contrast technique. The radionuclide technique permits detection of reflux volumes on the order of 1 ml. In one comparison study 17% of reflux events were seen only on the radionuclide study compared with the radiographic contrast method. Repeating the filling

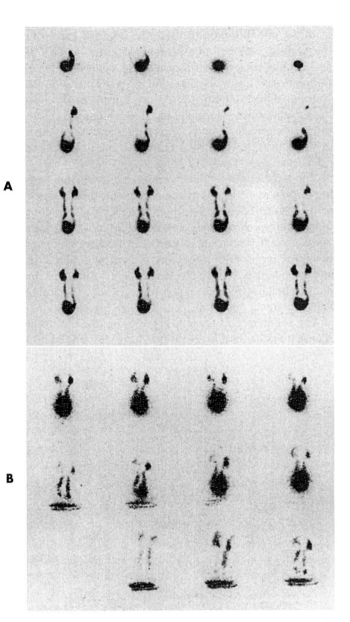

**Fig. 13-33**   Vesicoureteral reflux. **A,** During the filling phase, reflux is first seen on the right, then bilaterally. **B,** On voiding, the left side clears better than the right. Postvoiding images show bilateral pelvic reflux recurring *(bottom).* Grade II to III reflux.

and micturition phases of the radionuclide study can improve the sensitivity for detecting reflux, although this is not routinely done.

## SCROTAL SCINTIGRAPHY

Scintigraphy has been used to diagnose the cause of *acute* scrotal pain since the early 1970s. Its utility lies in the ability to differentiate acute testicular torsion from inflammation, such as epididymitis.

Testicular viability after torsion of the spermatic cord

depends on the length of time between onset of pain and surgical reduction. Atrophy may occur after as little as 4 hours of ischemia and is inevitable by 10 hours after torsion. Therefore testicular torsion is a surgical emergency. Scintigraphy can confirm the clinically suspected diagnosis of torsion and direct the patient to surgery. It can also minimize unnecessary exploration in patients with an inflammatory cause of their pain.

Color-flow Doppler imaging is increasingly used to evaluate acute scrotal pain. In addition to the technological improvements in this technique over the years, it can be done promptly in an emergency setting.

For *chronic* or painless disorders of the scrotum, ultrasonography is clearly the method of choice, and scintigraphy does not play an important role.

### Testicular Torsion

Developmental abnormalities of testicular descent and attachment predispose to spermatic cord torsion. The testicle is a retroperitoneal structure. During fetal growth the testis and its aortic blood supply descend from the midabdomen through the inguinal canal into the scrotum. The tunica vaginalis, formed as an outpouching of the retroperitoneal lining, covers the developing testis and the muscular and fascial layers of the abdominal peritoneum and descends into the developing scrotal pouch. Normally the tunica vaginalis covers the testes only anteriorly. The testis is anchored inferiorly and posteriorly through attachments to the posterior scrotal wall (Fig. 13-34).

The most common developmental abnormality leading to torsion of the spermatic cord is the *bell-clapper testis* (Fig. 13-34). This abnormality results in complete encirclement of the testis, epididymis, and spermatic cord by the tunica vaginalis, preventing normal posterior and inferior anchoring of the testis. The testis and vascular bundle are suspended freely like the clapper of a bell between the layers of the tunica. The abnormality is usually bilateral.

The incidence of torsion is tenfold higher in undescended testes than in those that have descended normally; however, the former circumstance is rare. Torsion of an incompletely descended testis above the inguinal ring is difficult to detect scintigraphically because of the large amount of background activity.

### Blood Supply

The testes and scrotum have separate blood supplies. The spermatic cord vessels supplying the *testes* include the testicular artery, which arises from the abdominal aorta just below the origin of the renal arteries, and the cremasteric and deferential arteries (Fig. 13-35). The *scrotum* receives its blood supply from the femoral and

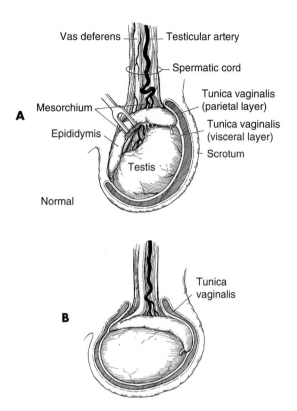

**Fig. 13-34   A,** Normal scrotal anatomy, right lateral view. The normal testis is a retroperitoneal organ with both layers of the tunica vaginalis anterior to it. The epididymis is attached to the posterolateral margin of the testis. These structures are normally anchored to the posterior scrotal wall by the testicular mesorchium. **B,** "Bell-clapper" deformity. In this congenital abnormality, which usually occurs bilaterally, the tunica vaginalis completely invests the testes. The normal posterior mesorchial anchor is absent, allowing the testis to twist on its vascular pedicle. The posterior midtesticular insertion of the testicular artery results in a horizontal lie of the testis, which is diagnostic of bell-clapper deformity.

**Fig. 13-35**   Blood supplies to the testes and scrotum. Spermatic cord vessels enter the scrotum more superiorly and vertically than scrotal vessels, which enter more horizontally and laterally. *Spermatic cord vessels* include the testicular artery, which arises from the abdominal aorta just below the origin of the renal arteries; the cremasteric artery, which arises from the inferior epigastric artery; and the deferential artery, which originates from either the internal iliac or the vesical artery. *Scrotal vessels* include the superficial external pudendal artery, arising from the femoral artery; anterior scrotal artery, arising from the deep external pudendal artery, which originates from the femoral artery below the superficial external pudendal artery; and posterior scrotal artery, which arises from branches of the internal pudendal artery, which originates from the internal iliac artery.

internal iliac arteries through the superficial, deep external, and internal pudendal arteries. These separate blood supplies can be distinguished scintigraphically. The spermatic cord has a steeper and more vertical axis than the scrotal vessels, which enter more horizontally.

## Radiopharmaceutical

Tc-99m pertechnetate is the radiopharmaceutical used for testicular scanning. It serves as a blood flow and blood pool (extracellular fluid space) radiomarker. Evidence of asymmetrical blood flow or tissue blood pool distribution is diagnostic. Inflammation and infection produce hyperemia, with increased flow-phase and tissue-phase distribution on the involved side, whereas ischemia results in decreased delivery of radiotracer.

## Methodology

Correct positioning is extremely important to compare right and left sides. A marker should be placed on the right thigh to ensure correct right/left orientation. The testicles may be supported with a scrotal sling so that the camera can be positioned as close as possible. In some patients with marked enlargement of one hemiscrotum, the scrotum may be taped to prevent the enlarged side from rotating and overlapping the noninvolved side.

Physician involvement is critical for the proper performance and interpretation of scrotal scintigraphy. The patient should be examined and testicular findings noted. Rubberized lead should be cut to size and placed immediately behind the testes to shield background thigh activity. Gentle retraction over the shield may be necessary if *testis redux* (involuntary contraction of the

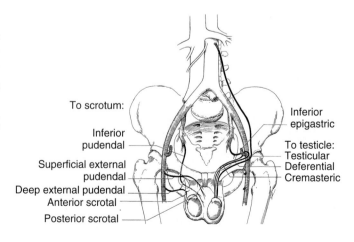

cremasteric muscle) occurs. On a late tissue phase image, a "hot" marker should be placed on the abnormal testicle to ensure correct interpretation. A lead median raphe marker placed between the testes can also aid in interpretation. The entire examination should take only 15 to 20 minutes (Box 13-12).

**Shielding**   Correct placement of an appropriate-size lead shield is critical for acquiring an interpretable study. It must be large enough to shield thigh activity behind the scrotum but not so large as to obscure iliac and

femoral vessel flow. One approach has been to use no shield during the flow phase and to place the shield before acquiring tissue-phase images. A logistically easier method is to cut and fit the shield correctly before starting the study so that no time is lost during imaging.

The study is performed with a gamma camera interfaced to a nuclear medicine computer system so that image intensity can be optimized retrospectively. Also, if necessary, selected images from the flow phase can be summed to increase count density.

In young children a converging collimator can be used for magnification and improved image resolution. A pinhole collimator has been advocated for use in very small children. However, a flow study must be done with another camera, and positioning becomes critical, since slight misalignment of the collimator orientation with the field of view can distort scrotal anatomy.

## Radiation Dosimetry

The target organ for Tc-99m pertechnetate is the stomach, followed by the unblocked thyroid (Box 13-13). The thyroid should be blocked with oral sodium or potassium perchlorate if time permits.

## Image Interpretation

A practical way of analyzing the scrotal scintigram is to divide the images into three phases: spermatic cord flow in the early dynamic flow phase, hemiscrotal flow in the late flow phase, and hemiscrotal static activity from the sequential tissue-phase images. In each phase the activity on the symptomatic side is compared with that on the opposite side.

Spermatic cord flow can be seen in the frames after tracer appearance in the iliac artery. Hemiscrotal flow appears later in the dynamic flow phase, in the region of the testicle. Blood flow is graded as increased, decreased, or equal with respect to blood flow on the asymptomatic side. Hemiscrotal tissue-phase activity is

---

### Box 13-12   Testicular Scintigraphy: Protocol Summary

**PATIENT PREPARATION**

Oral potassium or sodium perchlorate, 8 mg/kg to a maximum of 500 mg, administered 15-30 min before imaging.

**RADIOPHARMACEUTICAL**

Tc-99m pertechnetate, 10 mCi IV
Children: 250 µCi/kg (minimum, 2 mCi)

**INSTRUMENTATION**

Camera: large-field-of-view gamma
Collimator
    Adults: low energy, all purpose
    Children: converging low energy

**COMPUTER SETUP**

Magnification to limit field of view from umbilicus to junction of upper and middle thirds of the femur
Flow: 2-sec frames for 60 sec
Tissue phase: five sequential static images for 500k counts with a 10-sec delay between images to add or remove markers

**IMAGING PROCEDURE**

Position patient supine with towel roll between knees. Tape legs together at knees to prevent movement. Support scrotal contents with tape sling to allow close placement of camera.
Place individually fitted, rubberized lead shielding behind scrotum to block background. Do not obscure femoral or iliac vessels.
Tape penis up to lower abdomen so that it does not overlap scrotal contents.
Place marker on right thigh.
Start computer.
Inject radiopharmaceutical.
Acquire 60-sec flow study as described above.
Obtain five sequential images: first to third, 500k static images; fourth, hot marker on symptomatic testicle; fifth, lead marker along median raphe between testicles.

---

### Box 13-13   Radiation Dosimetry with Technetium-99m Pertechnetate Testicular Scintigraphy

| ORGAN | Rads/mCi |
|---|---|
| Stomach | 2.50 |
| Colon | 0.60 |
| Thyroid | 1.30 (unblocked) |
| Ovaries | 0.20 |
| Testicles | 0.09 |
| Whole body | 0.14 |

assessed on immediate and sequential high-count images by comparing the symptomatic and asymptomatic sides.

**Normal findings**   On flow images the iliac arteries should be seen simultaneously and should appear symmetrical in the amount of radioactivity and the time course of its passage. Because of the relatively low blood flow to the normal scrotal contents, only low-grade, diffuse, symmetrical flow is seen bilaterally. On static tissue-phase images, scrotal distribution is also low grade and symmetrical, usually somewhat less than in the thighs.

Bladder accumulation of radiotracer is increasingly seen on sequential tissue-phase images. Activity at the base of the penis may be seen in the midline and should not be misinterpreted; taping the penis to the lower abdomen minimizes this problem. Diffusion of activity into the scrotal contents on later images may decrease the contrast between structures, making image interpretation more difficult. Therefore the later images are best used for marker placement.

**Acute testicular torsion**   The scintigraphic findings in acute testicular torsion depend on the time that has elapsed since the acute event. In *early torsion,* within a few hours of onset, flow images may show no significant asymmetry during either the spermatic cord or later hemiscrotal phase. Occasionally a small projection of activity medial to the iliac artery is seen on the affected side because of activity in the proximal portion of the obstructed spermatic vessels ("nubbin" sign). On the static tissue-phase images, decreased activity may be seen in the region of the involved testicle (Fig. 13-36).

The diagnosis of early testicular torsion is often not based on the demonstration of decreased flow. With unequivocal clinical findings of an acute hemiscrotum, an apparently "negative" scrotal scintigram must be taken as evidence of acute torsion because of two factors. First, radionuclide scrotal scintigraphy often cannot distinguish "normal" from "decreased" flow. Second, compensatory changes may obscure the decreased testicular uptake that should theoretically be seen on high-count images in acute torsion. Lead shielding to reduce scatter and shine-through background activity is particularly valuable in early subtle cases.

Later in the course of torsion *(late torsion)* the image findings change significantly. Increased perfusion is actually demonstrated on the affected side as a result of scrotal flow from the pudendal arteries. The delayed dynamic flow-phase images show increased scrotal activity. The ischemic testicle is seen as an area of relatively decreased activity on static tissue-phase images. A distinct surrounding halo of increased activity develops from hyperemia of the dartos, the superficial smooth muscle in the scrotum (Fig. 13-37).

As the time since the acute torsion event elapses, the findings of hemiscrotal hyperemia, the nubbin sign, and

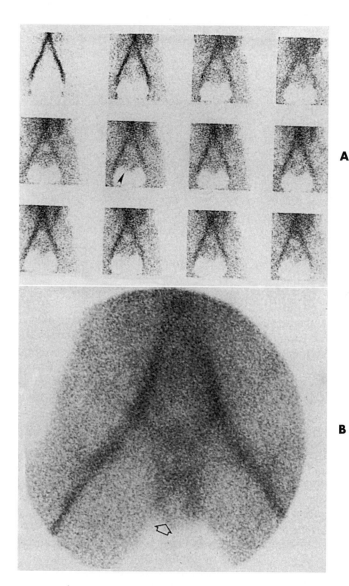

**Fig. 13-36**   Acute testicular torsion on scrotal scintigraphy. **A,** Flow phase shows minimal asymmetry, with slightly decreased flow seen on the right *(arrowhead).* **B,** Static high-count blood pool image shows decreased activity on the right *(open arrowhead),* consistent with right testicular torsion and confirmed at surgery.

the dartos halo become increasingly prominent. The term *missed torsion* is sometimes used to describe the late findings of torsion; however, *delayed torsion* is preferable and more accurate. Although the involved testis may not be salvageable, it is important to recognize a late torsion because it identifies patients who should undergo prophylactic contralateral orchiopexy, since the predisposing developmental abnormality is usually bilateral.

**Acute epididymitis**   Bacterial epididymitis and epididymoorchitis usually occur coincident with the onset of sexual activity; the peak incidence is in late adolescence

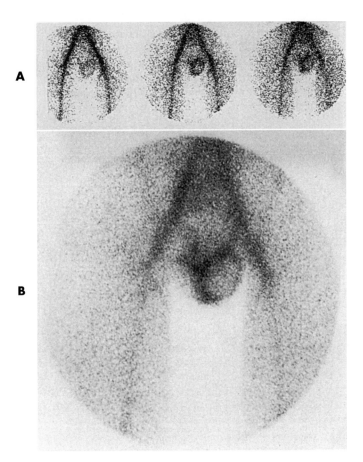

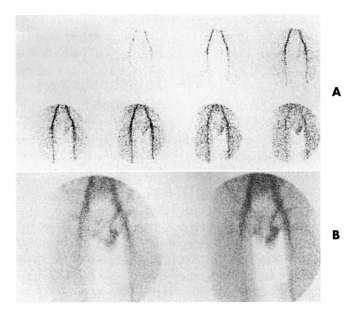

Fig. 13-37    Delayed testicular torsion on scrotal scintigraphy. Pain in the left testicle began 24 hours earlier. **A,** Two-second frames show increased flow to the left hemiscrotum. **B,** High-count blood pool image shows a halo pattern on the left, consistent with delayed torsion. At surgery this testicle was not viable and was removed. Orchiopexy was subsequently performed on the right.

Fig. 13-38    Acute epididymitis on scrotal scintigraphy. The patient complained of recent onset of pain in the left testicle. **A,** Increased flow to the left lateral scrotum. **B,** High-count blood pool images show a similar pattern of uptake, most consistent with acute epididymitis. The symptoms resolved over a week while the patient took antibiotics.

and early adulthood. Inflammatory disease in prepubertal children is more often caused by a virus.

The scintigraphic findings in acute epididymitis are dramatically different from those of acute or delayed torsion. The early dynamic-phase images demonstrate greatly increased activity in the spermatic cord vessels (Fig. 13-38). The hemiscrotal-phase dynamic images also demonstrate asymmetry with intensely increased localization on the affected side. Classically in this phase a crescent configuration of increased activity is seen laterally in the epididymis. On static images, diffusely increased uptake is seen in the region of the epididymis, but activity is normal within the testicle. With testicular involvement (epididymoorchitis) the entire hemiscrotum shows asymmetrically increased activity.

**Torsion of testicular appendage**    Torsion of one of the testicular appendages, although painful, is not serious and resolves spontaneously. Management is conservative and nonsurgical. This condition typically occurs in boys 7 to 14 years old and has a frequency

similar to that of spermatic cord torsion. Physical examination may show a palpable nodule at the upper pole of the involved testis, and a "blue dot" may be seen deep in the soft tissues with transillumination of the scrotum.

Radionuclide scrotal scintigraphy may be normal or may show evidence of low-grade inflammation. Mildly increased flow may be seen, mainly in the venous phase, as a result of inflammation of overlying dartos muscle. Tissue-phase images may show a focal area of increased activity at the upper pole.

**Other testicular disorders**    Scrotal scintigraphy is not the imaging modality of choice in most other conditions affecting the scrotal contents or testis. *Testicular abscesses* exhibit very increased flow on the dynamic-phase images. Hyperemia surrounding the abscess produces an appearance not unlike the halo seen in delayed or missed torsion. *Hydroceles* and *hematomas* appear as photon-deficient areas. Uncomplicated hydroceles are not associated with increased flow.

The appearance of *testicular tumors* is variable. They can be hyperemic with increased flow on the dynamic images and increased tracer localization corresponding to the tumor. With necrotic tumors, photon-deficient areas are seen within the lesion. The appearance can be deceptively similar to that of missed torsion, although the clinical history is usually of a longer standing process.

*Varicoceles* can have a dramatic appearance on radionuclide imaging. The later venous portions of the dynamic flow sequence demonstrate increased tracer localization in the pampiniform venous plexus. The key to the diagnosis of varicocele is late accumulation of activity in the venous structures. Tc-99m-labeled red blood cells have been used to confirm this diagnosis. Scrotal varicoceles are associated with an increased incidence of sterility.

---

## Accuracy

Testicular scintigraphy is an accurate technique for differentiating acute testicular torsion from epididymoorchitis if the examination is performed within 24 hours of the onset of symptoms. In the appropriate clinical setting, sensitivity and specificity approach 95%. The study is not as reliable if pain and swelling have been present for a longer time. The halo sign of peripheral hyperemia is nonspecific and is seen in other conditions.

## SUGGESTED READINGS

Blaufox MD, editor: *Evaluation of renal function and disease with radionuclides,* ed 2, 1989, New York, Karger.

Blaufox MD, Aurell M, Bubeck, et al: Report of the Radionuclides in Nephrourology Committee on renal clearance, *J Nucl Med* 37:1883-1890, 1996.

Blaufox MD, Fine EJ, Heller S, et al: Prospective study of simultaneous orthoiodohippurate and diethylenetriaminepentaacetic acid captopril renography, *J Nucl Med* 39:522-528, 1998.

Chen DCP, Holder LE, Melloul M: Radionuclide scrotal imaging: further experience with 210 patients. Part I and Part II, *J Nucl Med* 24:735-742, 841-853, 1983.

Eggli DF, Garcia JE: Radionuclide imaging of the acutely painful scrotum. In Van Nostrand D, Baum S, editors: *Atlas of nuclear medicine,* Philadelphia, 1988, Lippincott.

Eggli DF, Tulchinsky M: Scintigraphic evaluation of pediatric urinary tract infection, *Semin Nucl Med* 23:199-218, 1993.

Eshima D, Fritzberg AR, Taylor A Jr: Tc-99m renal tubular function agents: current status, *Semin Nucl Med* 20:28-40, 1990.

Fine EJ: Interventions in renal scintirenography, *Semin Nucl Med* 23:128-145, 1999.

Fommei E, Ghione SS, Hilson AJW, et al: Captopril radionuclide test in renovascular hypertension: a European multicentre study, *Eur J Nucl Med* 20:617-623, 1993.

O'Reilly PH: Diuresis renography 8 years later: an update, *Urology* 136:993-999, 1986.

O'Reilly P, Aurell M, Britton K, et al: Consensus report on diuresis renography for investigating the dilated upper urinary tract, *J Nucl Med* 37:1872-1876, 1996.

Tauxe WN, Dubovsky EV, editors: *Nuclear medicine in clinical urology and nephrology,* Norwalk, Conn, 1985, Appleton-Century-Crofts.

Taylor A, Nally J, Aurell M, et al: Consensus report on ACE inhibitor renography for detecting renovascular hypertension, *J Nucl Med* 37:1876-1882, 1996.

The "well-tempered" diuretic renogram: a standard method to examine the asymptomatic neonate with hydronephrosis or hydroureteronephrosis, *J Nucl Med* 33:2047-2051, 1992.

# CHAPTER 14

# Endocrine System

Studies of the endocrine system were the original procedures in nuclear medicine. When iodine-131 was made available to the medical community in the United States after World War II by the Atomic Energy Commission, thyroidologists quickly recognized that the percentage uptake of radioiodine at a fixed point in time after administration was a measure of thyroid function. This early measurement was further enhanced by suppression and stimulation interventions aimed at determining thyroid autonomy and thyroid functional reserve, respectively. By the early 1950s, gamma ray scintillation detectors had been coupled to mechanical devices to permit systematic rectilinear scanning to form functional image maps (scans) of the thyroid gland. These thyroid gland studies stimulated the early development of the nuclear medicine field.

In the ensuing decades, further advances occurred in the instrumentation and pharmaceuticals used for thyroid imaging, and scintigraphic techniques were applied to imaging other endocrine organs, with variable success. The singular strength of the radiotracer approach in the endocrine system is the ability to use a wide variety of endocrine hormone precursors and analogs to create radiopharmaceuticals that become incorporated into endocrine metabolic pathways.

## THYROID IMAGING AND FUNCTION STUDIES

Thyroid scintigraphy and radiotracer uptake studies remain an important part of the practice of nuclear medicine, although they are not used as frequently today as they were two and three decades ago. Ultrasonography and fine needle aspiration (FNA) biopsy have partially supplanted thyroid scintigraphy in the evaluation of patients with clinically palpable thyroid nodules.

Thyroid scintigraphy remains uniquely suited to determining the functional status of thyroid nodules, detecting extrathyroidal metastases from differentiated thyroid carcinoma, and establishing the thyroid as the tissue of origin of mediastinal masses. The thyroid scintigram has the advantage over cross-sectional techniques of depicting the entire gland in a single image and allowing physical findings to be correlated with abnormalities in the image.

## Radiopharmaceuticals

The principal radiopharmaceuticals employed for thyroid imaging include iodine-131, iodine-123, and technetium-99m. Iodine is a precursor in thyroid hormone synthesis. The thyroid gland traps iodine and can concentrate it in a ratio greater than 100:1 with plasma. The iodine in the gland is incorporated into thyroid hormone (organification) and subsequently bound to thyroglobulin. The pertechnetate ion ($TcO_4^-$) is trapped and concentrated by the thyroid gland but does not undergo organification or incorporation into thyroid hormone. The normally high concentration of these radiotracers in the thyroid gland affords excellent visualization of the thyroid unless thyroid uptake and function are impaired.

**Physics and dosimetry**   I-131 undergoes beta minus decay with a principal gamma photon energy of 364 keV.

The energy of the principal beta particle is 0.606 MeV, and the half-life is 8.06 days (Box 14-1). I-131 is formulated as a sodium salt for clinical use.

The presence of beta particle emissions, the relatively high energy of the principal gamma ray emissions, and the long half-life of I-131 are disadvantages to the use of this tracer. The particulate emissions and long half-life result in a higher than optimal radiation dose to the thyroid gland. This in turn restricts the size of the administered dose. The principal photon energy is higher than ideal for use with gamma scintillation cameras. Negative factors related to high energy include image degradation through septal penetration of the collimator and poor detection sensitivity in the relatively thin sodium iodide crystals of gamma cameras.

For these reasons, I-131 is not considered the agent of choice for routine diagnostic thyroid scintigraphy. However, its long half-life is well suited to delayed studies at 24, 48, and even 72 hours after injection. Delayed imaging improves tracer clearance from nontarget tissues, which is a distinct advantage in detecting thyroid cancer metastases and evaluating mediastinal masses.

In many respects, I-123 is a better agent than I-131 for thyroid imaging. The principal gamma energy is 159 keV, which is ideally suited for gamma scintillation cameras (Box 14-2). The half-life of 13.3 hours is also well suited to the time frame for most thyroid imaging and uptake studies. The mode of decay is electron capture, and there are no primary particulate emissions.

---

### Box 14-1  Iodine-131: Summary of Physical Characteristics and Dosimetry

**PHYSICAL CHARACTERISTICS**

| | |
|---|---|
| Mode of decay | Beta minus |
| Physical half-life ($t_{1/2}$) | 8.1 days |
| Photon energy | 364 keV |
| Abundance | 81% |

**DOSIMETRY***

| Organ | Rads/100 µCi (3.7 MBq) |
|---|---|
| Thyroid (15% uptake) | 78 |
| Bladder | 0.27 |
| Stomach wall | 0.15 |
| Small intestine | 0.11 |
| Liver | 0.028 |
| Testes | 0.018 |
| Ovaries | 0.012 |
| Red marrow | 0.021 |
| Total body | 0.047 |

*Sodium iodide-131 administered orally. All values assume 15% thyroid uptake. Data from product information, Mallinckrodt Medical, St Louis.

---

### Box 14-2  Iodine-123: Summary of Physical Characteristics and Dosimetry

**PHYSICAL CHARACTERISTICS**

| | |
|---|---|
| Mode of decay | Electron capture |
| Physical half-life ($t_{1/2}$) | 13.2 hr |
| Photon energy | 159 keV |
| Abundance | 83.4% |

**DOSIMETRY***

| Organ | Rads/400 µCi (15 MBq) |
|---|---|
| Thyroid (15% uptake) | 7.7 |
| Bladder | 0.16 |
| Stomach wall | 0.089 |
| Small intestine | 0.065 |
| Liver | 0.010 |
| Testes | 0.007 |
| Ovaries | 0.017 |
| Red marrow | 0.012 |
| Total body | 0.014 |

*Sodium iodide capsules administered orally. All values for thyroid uptake of 15% at time of calibration. Data from product information, Mallinckrodt Medical, St Louis.

A number of drawbacks have kept I-123 from becoming universally employed for thyroid scintigraphy. First, most methods of preparing I-123 result in longer-lived radionuclidic impurities (I-124 and I-125), with higher radiation doses to the thyroid than would be calculated from I-123 alone. Second, commercial availability has been limited, resulting in higher cost. The short physical half-life also makes it more difficult to keep I-123 reliably and routinely available.

Technetium-99m pertechnetate is a frequently used alternative to radioiodine for thyroid scintigraphy. As noted, the physical characteristics of Tc-99m are ideal for use with gamma scintillation cameras (Box 14-3). Sodium pertechnetate is readily and reliably available in nuclear medicine clinics from molybdenum-99/Tc-99m generator systems, so supply is not a problem, unlike with I-123. The lack of particulate emissions and the short half-life of Tc-99m result in the lowest radiation dose per unit of administered activity of the thyroid imaging agents.

**Pharmacokinetics** Radioiodine is rapidly absorbed from the gastrointestinal tract after oral administration. Radioactivity is detectable in the gland within minutes and, in euthyroid subjects, reaches the thyroid follicular lumen within 20 to 30 minutes. Thus the uptake and organification of iodine are quite rapid. The several-hour delay selected for imaging studies using I-123 and the 1-day delay typically chosen for studies with I-131 are dictated by the desire for background clearance and not by slow uptake in the gland. The normal range for uptake is 10% to 30% of the administered dose at 24 hours.

### Box 14-3 Technetium-99m: Summary of Physical Characteristics and Dosimetry

**PHYSICAL CHARACTERISTICS**

| | |
|---|---|
| Mode of decay | Isometric transition |
| Physical half-life ($T_{1/2}$) | 6 hr |
| Photon energy | 140 keV |
| Abundance | 89% |

**DOSIMETRY***

| Organ | Rad/mCi (37 MBq) |
|---|---|
| Thyroid | 0.130 |
| Bladder wall | 0.085 |
| Stomach | 0.05 |
| Large intestine | 0.11 |
| Red marrow | 0.02 |
| Testis | 0.01 |
| Ovary | 0.03 |
| Total body | 0.01 |

*Sodium pertechnetate administered intravenously. Data from product information, DuPont Corp, Billerica, Mass.

The pharmacokinetics for Tc-99m pertechnetate are also rapid. The tracer is typically administered intravenously for thyroid imaging studies, and the trapping process begins essentially immediately. Optimal uptake is achieved by 20 to 30 minutes, which is also selected as the time to begin imaging. At this time, approximately 0.5% to 3.75% of the radiopertechnetate is in the gland of euthyroid subjects.

The pertechnetate ion is avidly trapped but not organified by the thyroid. Concordant localization and identical scintigraphic visualization typically occur with pertechnetate and radioiodine. In a small percentage of thyroid nodules the scintigraphic pattern of radioiodine and radiopertechnetate is discordant because organification function is lost in the nodular tissue.

**Precautions** Radioiodine is excreted in human breast milk, and nursing should be stopped after diagnostic or therapeutic studies with radioiodine. With I-123, nursing can be resumed after several days if the amount used does not exceed 30 µCi. The usual imaging dosage is 100 to 400 µCi, however, and a longer interval is necessary. For I-131, nursing must be terminated for many weeks after even small doses before safe levels are achieved. With Tc-99m pertechnetate, nursing can be resumed in 24 hours.

Pregnancy is also a special precaution for studies with radioiodine. The fetal thyroid concentrates radioiodine after the tenth to twelfth week of gestation. Radioiodine crosses the placenta, and significant exposure of the fetal thyroid can occur after therapeutic doses to the mother and may even result in cretinism.

A more practical and common problem with thyroid studies is the interference of stable iodine contained in foods and medications (Box 14-4). Several non-iodine-containing drugs also affect thyroidal radioiodine uptake. The suppression of uptake may be sufficient to preclude successful imaging but is even more important in assessing the results of radioiodine percent uptake studies of thyroid function. As little as 1 mg of stable iodine can cause significant reduction of the 24-hour radioiodine uptake, and as little as 10 mg can effectively block the gland, with a 98% reduction in uptake. Radiographic contrast media are a common source of iodine in hospitalized patients that may interfere with thyroid imaging and uptake studies. A food and drug history should be obtained from all patients undergoing thyroid imaging and function studies.

### Technique

The gamma scintillation camera with pinhole collimator is the usual instrument of choice for thyroid imaging. This combination has replaced the rectilinear scanner. The combination of gamma camera and pinhole collimator offers the flexibility of obtaining multiple views of the thyroid. The magnification with the pinhole collimator allows resolution of nodules smaller than possible with parallel-hole collimators. Nodules as small as 3 to 5 mm in diameter can be detected.

**Radiopertechnetate imaging** For studies with Tc-99m pertechnetate, 1 to 10 mCi is administered intrave-

nously, with imaging begun 20 minutes after injection (Box 14-5). A standard-field-of-view gamma camera equipped with a pinhole collimator and 3- to 6-mm insert is used with a 20% window centered at 140 keV. The patient is positioned supine with the neck extended so that the plane of the thyroid gland is parallel to the crystal face of the camera. The collimator is positioned so that the thyroid gland fills approximately two thirds to three quarters of the field of view. In patients with a normal thyroid, this is achieved with a 6- to 8-cm distance from the collimator to the surface of the neck. It is useful to put a radioactive marker on the sternal notch and chin, and most laboratories use a 4- to 5-cm line marker or two point sources 4 to 5 cm apart on the neck just lateral to the thyroid lobes and parallel to their long axis (Fig. 14-1). The marker permits size estimates of observed structures, including nodules, by allowing correction for the pinhole magnification effect.

Images are obtained in the anterior and the 45° right anterior oblique (RAO) and 45° left anterior oblique (LAO) views (Fig. 14-2). Each image is obtained for

---

### Box 14-4 Nonthyroidal Causes of Increased and Decreased Thyroidal Uptake of Radioiodine

| | DURATION OF EFFECT |
|---|---|
| **DECREASED UPTAKE** | |
| **Thyroid Hormones** | |
| Thyroxine (T$_4$) | 4-6 wk |
| Triiodothyronine (T$_3$) | 2-3 wk |
| | |
| **Excess Iodine (Expanded Iodine Pool)** | |
| Lugol's solution | 2-4 wk |
| Saturated solution of potassium iodide | 2-4 wk |
| Some mineral supplements, cough medicines, and vitamin preparations | 2-4 wk |
| Iodine food supplements | |
| Iodinated drugs | |
| Iodinated skin ointments | 2-4 wk |
| Congestive heart failure | 2-4 wk |
| Renal failure | |
| | |
| **Radiographic Contrast Media** | |
| Water-soluble intravascular media | 2-4 wk |
| Oral cholecystographic agents | 4 wk-indefinite |
| Fat-soluble media (lymphography) | Months-years |
| | |
| **Non-Iodine-Containing Drugs** | Variable |
| Adrenocorticotropic hormone, adrenal steroids | |
| Monovalent anions (perchlorate) | |
| Penicillin | |
| Goitrogenic foods (e.g., cabbage, turnips) | |
| Antithyroid drugs | |
| Bromides | |
| Prior radiation to neck | |
| | |
| **INCREASED** | |
| **Iodine Deficiency** | |
| Pregnancy | |
| Rebound after therapy (thyroid hormones, antithyroid drugs) | |
| Recovery from subacute thyroiditis | |
| Choriocarcinoma, hydatidiform mole (human chorionic gonadotropin with thyroid-stimulating hormone effect) | |
| Lithium | |
| Inborn errors of thyroid hormone metabolism | |

---

### Box 14-5 Technetium-99m Pertechnetate Thyroid Imaging: Protocol Summary

**PATIENT PREPARATION**

Discontinue any medications that interfere with thyroid uptake of Tc-99m pertechnetate

**RADIOPHARMACEUTICAL**

Tc-99m pertechnetate, 1 to 10 mCi (37 to 370 MBq) intravenously

**TIME OF IMAGING**

20 min after radiopharmaceutical administration

**IMAGING PROCEDURE**

Use a gamma camera with a 3- to 6-mm aperture pinhole collimator and a 20% energy window centered at 140 keV.
Position the patient supine with the chin up and neck extended.
Position the collimator so that the thyroid fills about two thirds of the diameter of the field of view.
Obtain anterior and 45° left anterior and right anterior oblique views (move the collimator, if possible, rather than the patient).
Obtain 200k to 250k counts per view.
Mark the chin and suprasternal notch.
Note the position and mark palpable nodules and surgical scars.
Place marker sources lateral to the thyroid to calibrate size (Figs. 14-4 and 14-8).

200,000 to 250,000 counts. Marker source images may be obtained for fewer counts. It is preferable to keep the patient in one position and move the camera and collimator. This is more reproducible than moving the patient and does not distort the thyroid.

Before the patient is placed in position for imaging, a physical examination of the thyroid gland is performed to identify the location of nodules. Locations are verified in the imaging position, and during a separate acquisition a Tc-99m marker source is used to locate palpable nodules for functional correlation. If all images are obtained with a computer system, the distance calibration images as well as images obtained for nodule

localization purposes with marker sources can be readily superimposed on each other for analysis.

**Radioiodine-123** Studies with I-123 are also obtained with a standard-field-of-view gamma camera equipped with a pinhole collimator and a 3- to 6-mm insert (Box 14-6). The tracer is administered orally in

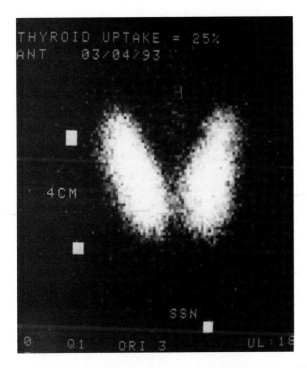

**Fig. 14-1** Normal thyroid scintigram obtained with iodine-123. The sternal notch is indicated, and electronic markers provide a 4-cm scale adjacent to the right thyroid 4-cm lobe. Radioiodine uptake is 25%.

---

**Box 14-6  Thyroid Imaging with Iodine-123 (Sodium Iodide): Protocol Summary**

**PATIENT PREPARATION**

Discontinue any medications that interfere with thyroid uptake of radioiodine.

**RADIOPHARMACEUTICAL**

I-123, 100 to 400 µCi (3.7 to 15 MBq), orally in capsule form

**TIME OF IMAGING**

At 6 and 24 hours

**IMAGING PROCEDURE**

Use a gamma camera with a 3-6-mm aperture pinhole collimator and a 20% energy window centered at 159 keV.
Position the patient supine with the chin up and the neck extended.
Position the collimator so that the thyroid fills about two thirds of the diameter of the field of view.
Obtain anterior and 45° left anterior and right anterior oblique views (move the collimator, if possible, rather than the patient).
Obtain 200k to 250k counts per view.
Mark the chin and suprasternal notch.
Note the position and mark palpable nodules and surgical scars.
Place marker sources lateral to the thyroid to calibrate size.

---

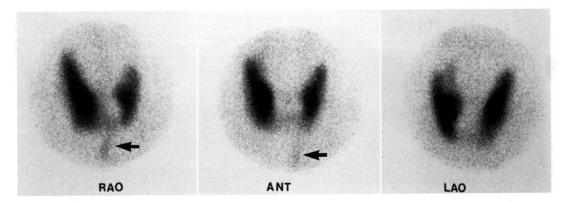

**Fig. 14-2** Anterior and right and left anterior oblique *(RAO, LAO)* views obtained with technetium-99m pertechnetate. Note the esophageal activity below the thyroid to the left midline *(arrows).*

capsule form as sodium iodide. Imaging may be accomplished at 6 and 24 hours, depending on laboratory preference. A 20% window is used and centered at 159 keV. The imaging sequence is the same as with radiopertechnetate. For each image, 200,000 to 250,000 counts are obtained. The chin and suprasternal notch are marked on the scan. All palpable nodules, masses, and scars are also noted on the physical examination and, when appropriate, by radioactive marker sources on the scan.

**Iodine-131 for thyroid carcinoma** Radioiodine is administered orally in a dose of 1 to 2 mCi (Box 14-7). A large-field-of-view gamma camera equipped with a high-energy parallel-hole collimator is used with a 20% window centered at 364 keV. For detection of thyroid carcinoma, the most important view is the anterior image of the head, neck, and chest, although obtaining views from head to pelvis is more complete. Computer acquisition is helpful to accommodate a wide range of possible count densities in the image. Many laboratories image for a fixed period, typically 10 to 20 minutes per view. The pinhole collimator may also be used to obtain higher resolution spot views of positive areas. Marker sources are used to indicate the location of the chin, suprasternal notch, and xiphoid.

Imaging is often first accomplished at 24 hours. If initial images are equivocal or negative in patients with suspected thyroid carcinoma, further delayed imaging at 48 and 72 hours is done, and longer delays may be necessary. Some laboratories acquire initial images at 48 to 72 hours.

## Normal Thyroid Scintigram

In the euthyroid adult the thyroid gland weighs approximately 15 to 20 g. It has a butterfly shape with lateral lobes extending along each side of the thyroid cartilage of the larynx (Figs. 14-1 and 14-2). The lateral lobes are connected by an isthmus that crosses the trachea anteriorly below the level of the cricoid cartilage. The detailed appearance of the gland is highly variable from patient to patient. The right lobe is often slightly larger than the left. The lateral lobes typically measure 4 to 5 cm from superior to inferior poles and 1.5 to 2 cm wide. The pyramidal lobe is a paramedian structure that arises from the isthmus, either to the right or left of the midline, and represents functioning thyroid tissue in the thyroglossal duct tract (Fig. 14-3).

The normal euthyroid subject has homogeneous and uniform distribution of radiotracer throughout the gland. Some variation in intensity may be seen in the middle or medial aspects of the lateral lobes owing to the thickness of the gland in this location. The amount of activity in the isthmus varies greatly among patients, with little or no activity in some and prominent activity in others. Likewise, in most normal adults, little or no activity is

---

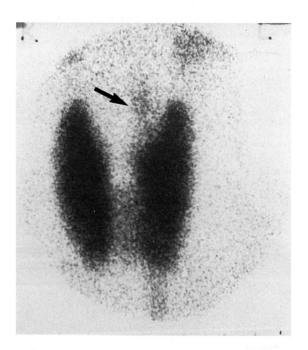

**Fig. 14-3**  Small pyramidal lobe is demonstrated arising from the medial aspect of the upper pole of the left lobe of the thyroid *(arrow)*. Small amount of activity is present below the left lobe in the esophagus. The study was obtained with technetium-99m pertechnetate, and some activity is seen in the region of the salivary glands.

seen in the pyramidal lobe. Activity is often seen in patients with Graves' disease because of hyperplasia of the tissues in the duct.

Studies using Tc-99m pertechnetate routinely visualize the salivary glands, which should not be mistaken for the thyroid or thyroid cancer metastases. Activity in the esophagus is frequently not in the midline because the esophagus is displaced by the trachea and cervical spine when the neck is hyperextended in the imaging position. The esophageal activity is more often seen just to the left of midline and can be confirmed by having the patient swallow water to cleanse the esophagus, followed by repeat imaging. Because of the later imaging time for studies with I-123 the salivary glands are not usually seen, since the tracer has been cleared.

## Clinical Applications

In current practice the major clinical applications of thyroid scintigraphy include the further evaluation of equivocal or confusing findings on physical examination and the follow-up of patients with thyroid cancers (Box 14-8).

A systematic interpretation of the thyroid scintigram requires assessment of thyroid size and configuration and the identification of focal abnormalities, including hot and cold nodules and extrathyroidal activity in the neck or mediastinum. Scintigraphic evaluation also correlates palpable abnormalities and surgical scars with scintigraphic findings (Figs. 14-4 to 14-6). This is frequently critical in assigning significance to a palpable abnormality.

**Goiter** The term *goiter* simply refers to an enlargement of the thyroid gland, but it is often qualified to indicate the cause of the enlargement. Before the addition of iodine supplements to salt and the use of periodates in food, goiter was endemic in the northern United States, scattered locations in Europe, including southern Germany, and other locations throughout the

world. These endemic goiters typically were composed of colloid nodules, and the vast majority were benign. These goiters are also referred to as *colloid nodular goiters* or *nontoxic goiters.*

The pathogenesis of nodule formation appears to be iodine deficiency–induced hyperplasia followed by the formation of functioning nodules that undergo hemorrhage and are replaced by lakes of colloid. Over time a repetition of this process leads to overall glandular

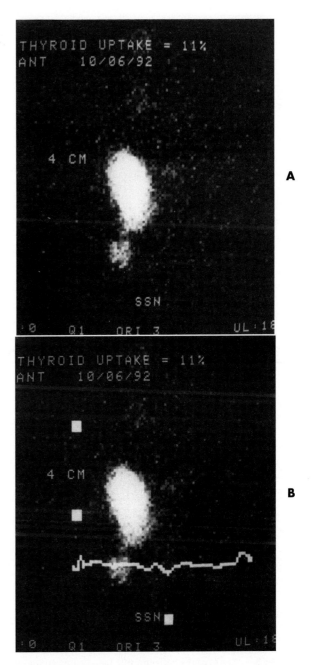

**Fig. 14-4** **A,** Thyroid scintigram in a patient who underwent thyroidectomy for thyroid carcinoma. **B,** Repeat image indicating location of surgical scar on the neck.

---

### Box 14-8 Clinical Indications for Thyroid Scintigraphy

Further evaluation of findings on physical examination
Detection of metastases in patients with thyroid carcinoma
Follow-up of radioiodine therapy for differentiated thyroid cancer
Determination of functional status of thyroid nodules
Differential diagnosis of mediastinal masses
Detection of extrathyroidal tissue (lingual thyroid)
Screening after head and neck irradiation

enlargement, with nonfunctioning colloid nodules the dominant histopathological feature.

The typical scintigraphic appearance of these benign multinodular colloid goiters is inhomogeneous uptake of tracer with cold areas of various sizes (Figs. 14-6 and 14-7). The incidence of thyroid carcinoma in endemic goiter is low (1% to 5%). If a patient has a dominant cold nodule, however, out of proportion in size to other cold areas or enlarging suddenly, it should be regarded with suspicion.

Another important cause of goiter is *Graves' disease* (toxic goiter) (Fig. 14-8 and Box 14-9). In this condition the gland is diffusely hyperplastic. The scintigraphic appearance of Graves' disease is uniform with intensely increased uptake. The pyramidal lobe is frequently seen because of hyperplasia of the thyroid tissues. In current practice Graves' disease is not generally considered an indication for obtaining a thyroid scintigram. Imaging has been used in some institutions, however, in estimating the size of the thyroid gland to calculate the dosage

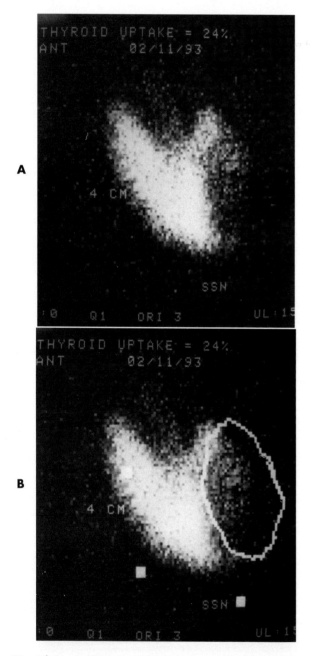

**Fig. 14-5    A,** Thyroid scintigram in a patient presenting with a large solitary nodule in the region of the left lobe. **B,** Repeat scintigram with clinically palpated outline of the nodule superimposed. The nodule is cold and measures approximately 5 × 2.5 sonometers.

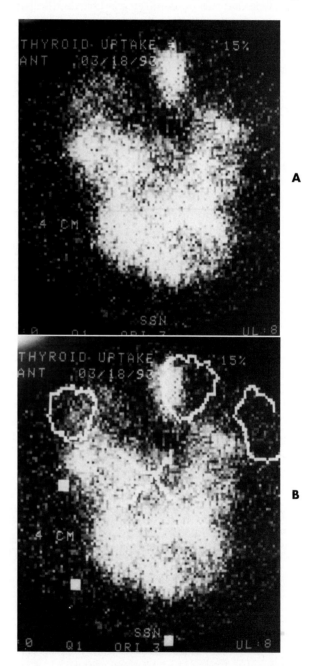

**Fig. 14-6    A,** Thyroid scintigram in a patient with a large goiter. Distribution of tracer is inhomogeneous with numerous cold areas scattered throughout the gland. **B,** Repeat scintigram with the location of three discretely palpable nodules marked on the image.

for I-131 therapy and to confirm diffuse versus nodular uptake in hyperthyroid patients.

Thyroid enlargement may be caused by thyroid carcinoma or involvement of the thyroid by other neoplasms, such as lymphoma. The thyroid may also be enlarged in active phases of thyroiditis.

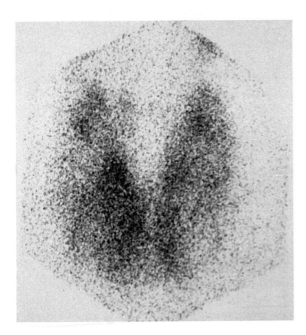

**Fig. 14-7** Typical colloid nodular goiter, with enlargement of the thyroid, inhomogeneous tracer distribution, and focal cold areas corresponding to nodules.

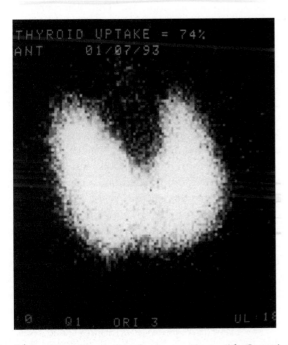

**Fig. 14-8** Thyroid scintigraphy in a patient with Graves' disease. The gland is uniformly enlarged with homogeneous tracer uptake and distribution. The radioiodine percent uptake is greatly increased at 74%.

**Thyroid nodules** Thyroid nodules are extremely common, and the incidence increases with age. Nodules are more common in women than men. The presence of multiple nodules (Figs. 14-6 and 14-7), indicating multinodular goiter, significantly reduces the likelihood of malignancy compared with the likelihood of cancer in patients with a solitary "cold" nodule (less than 5% versus 5% to 40% in surgical series). The thyroid scintigram may be used to confirm the presence of a clinically palpable nodule, to determine whether other nodules are present, and to assess the functional status of the detected nodule (Box 14-8). As noted, cold nodules as small as 3 mm in diameter may be detected using the pinhole collimator. Box 14-10 provides the differential diagnosis for thyroid nodules.

Thyroid nodules are classified scintigraphically as "cold" (nonfunctioning), "hot" (functioning), or indeterminate. The latter category may be assigned when a nodule demonstrates function equal to that of the surrounding normal thyroid. "Indeterminate" may also be assigned when a cold or nonfunctioning nodule arises from the anterior or posterior surface of the gland, with normal glandular activity superimposed over the area of the nodule on the scintigram. Although the problem is

---

**Box 14-9    Conditions Associated with Goiter**

**Graves' disease** Autoimmune disease associated with hyperthyroidism and exophthalmos. Patients typically have diffuse hyperplasia of the thyroid gland and thyroid-stimulating immunoglobulins (TSIs).

**Plummer's disease** Hyperthyroidism associated with toxic nodular goiter (one or more nodules).

**Hashimoto's disease (Hashimoto's thyroiditis)** Form of thyroiditis and autoimmune disorder often leading to hypothyroidism. Patients may experience transient hyperthyroidism ("hashitoxicosis").

**de Quervain's disease** Synonym for subacute thyroiditis, with inflammatory infiltration and destruction of thyroid cells. Often associated with transient hyperthyroidism.

**Riedel's struma (Riedel's thyroiditis)** Chronic fibrous replacement of the thyroid gland.

**Jod-Basedow phenomenon** Induction of thyrotoxicosis in a euthyroid individual after exposure to large amounts of iodine. Typically occurs in areas of endemic iodine-deficient goiter; may be seen after use of iodine contrast agents.

**Wolff-Chaikoff effect** Paradoxical blocking of iodine incorporation into thyroid hormone resulting from large amounts of iodine.

**Marine-Lenhart syndrome** Graves' disease with incidentally functioning nodules that are responsive to thyroid-stimulating hormone but are not responsive to TSIs.

## Box 14-10 Differential Diagnosis for Thyroid Nodules

**COLD NODULES**
**Benign**

Colloid nodule
Simple cyst
Hemorrhagic cyst
Adenoma
Thyroiditis (focal)
Abscess
Parathyroid cyst or adenoma

**Malignant** — ↑risk in ♂, young ♀, >40age, H₂O radiation.

Thyroid cancer
  Papillary
  Follicular
  Anaplastic
  Medullary
  Hürthle cell
Lymphoma
Metastatic carcinoma
  Lung
  Breast
  Melanoma
  Gastrointestinal
  Renal

**FUNCTIONING NODULES**

Adenomas
Hyperfunctioning adenomas

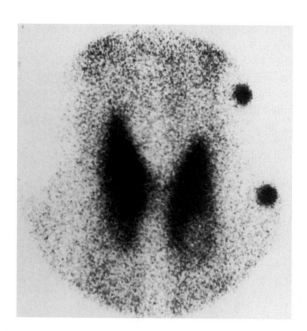

**Fig. 14-9**   Solitary cold nodule in the lower pole of the left lobe.

uncommon, the possibility of an indeterminate nodule highlights the need for close correlation between physical and scintigraphic findings. Oblique views with a pinhole collimator can be helpful in separating the nodule from adjacent thyroid tissue. For management purposes, an indeterminate nodule has the same significance as a cold nodule.

**"Cold" nodules**  The vast majority of thyroid nodules are cold or nonfunctioning (Figs. 14-5, *B,* and 14-9). In reported surgical series the incidence of thyroid carcinoma in solitary cold nodules ranges from 5% to 40%. An important factor associated with a higher likelihood of cancer is a prior history of radiation to the head and neck or mediastinum. Several decades ago external radiation therapy was commonly used to shrink the thymus gland and to treat enlarged tonsils and adenoids. Radiation up to 1000 or 1500 rads has been conclusively shown to result in an increased incidence of thyroid nodules and cancer, and concern increases when a cold nodule is detected in a patient with a history of such radiation exposure. Above 1500 rads the risk actually appears to decrease, presumably from destruction of tissue in the gland. Thyroid scintigraphy is more sensitive in detecting nodules than is physical examination and has proved useful in screening populations of irradiated patients.

Age and sex also influence the likelihood that a solitary cold nodule represents cancer. Because the incidence of benign nodules increases with age, a nodule in a young individual is a greater concern than in an older patient. Incidental nodules are also more common in women than men. Thus solitary cold nodules in young men are of particular concern. The other end of the probability spectrum is represented by a multinodular goiter in an older woman.

The thyroid scintigram cannot be used to exclude or confirm malignancy in cases of solitary cold nodules, and each physician or clinic should have a systematic approach to the workup of such patients. Some physicians advocate ultrasonography as the next step in the workup. Purely cystic lesions are rarely caused by cancer. Cancers can demonstrate cystic degeneration, however, and ultrasonography results can be misleading. Some advocate FNA biopsy without performing scintigraphy as a more direct means of establishing the histology of solitary nodules. This approach is subject to negative sampling errors and requires an experienced cytopathologist.

**"Hot" nodules**  Hyperfunctioning or "hot" nodules may be either autonomous or under hormonal feedback control (Fig. 14-10). Radiotracer uptake in autonomous nodules is not suppressed with administration of thyroid hormone (see Thyroid Function Studies). Autonomous nodules larger than 3 to 4 cm in diameter typically produce enough thyroid hormone to suppress the pituitary feedback loop. In this case the extranodular thyroid tissues are not visualized scintigraphically (Fig. 14-11). In patients with smaller hot nodules producing

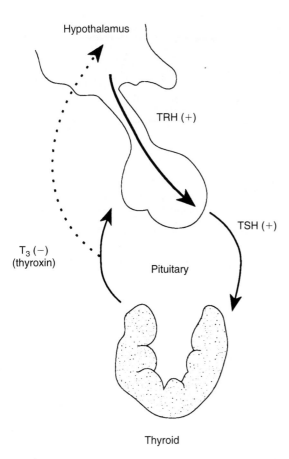

**Fig. 14-10**    Schematic of the thyroid-pituitary feedback loop. The normal thyroid is under the control of thyroid-stimulating hormone *(TSH)*. The hypothalamic production of thyroid-releasing hormone *(TRH)* and the pituitary release of TSH are decreased or suppressed as circulating levels of thyroid hormone increase.

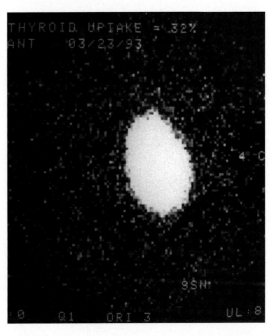

**Fig. 14-11**    Thyroid scintigram demonstrates a large, functioning nodule. No extranodular tissues are demonstrated, indicating suppression of the pituitary feedback loop. The radioiodine uptake is increased, and the patient is clinically hyperthyroid (toxic nodule).

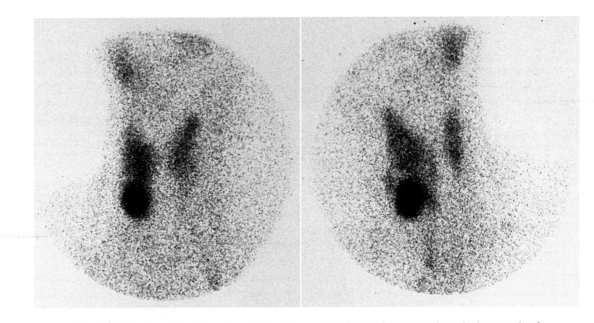

**Fig. 14-12**    Thyroid scintigraphy demonstrates a small, hot nodule arising from the lower pole of the right lobe. The extranodular thyroid tissues are clearly visualized.

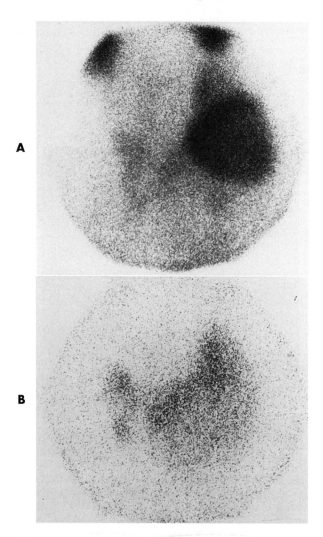

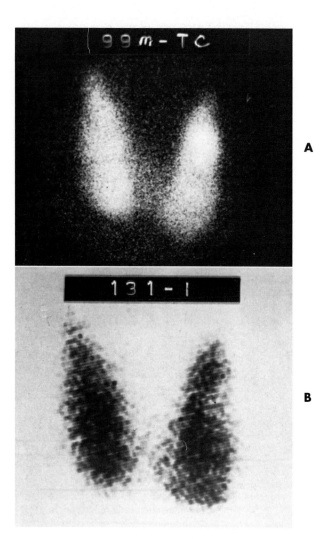

**Fig. 14-13   A,** Thyroid scintigraphy reveals a large, hot nodule in the left lobe of the thyroid. The center of the nodule appears to have less intense tracer activity than the periphery, suggesting central degeneration. **B,** Follow-up scintigraphy 1 year later reveals complete involution of the previously seen hot nodule, with residual distortion of the gland.

**Fig. 14-14   A,** Scintigraphy with technetium-99m pertechnetate reveals a functioning nodule in the left upper pole. **B,** In the corresponding iodine-131 radioiodine scintigram the nodule is cold. This is called "discordance" between radioiodine and radiopertechnetate. (Courtesy of Steven M. Pinsky, M.D., University of Illinois, Chicago.)

less hormone, significant uptake may still be visualized in the extranodular structures (Fig. 14-12). Hot nodules may undergo spontaneous involution and may have areas of cystic degeneration (Fig. 14-13).

Demonstration of radioiodine uptake in a nodule reduces the likelihood of cancer compared with solitary cold nodules. Less than 1% of hot nodules harbor malignancy, and a critical review of the literature suggests the likelihood is even lower if cancers adjacent to hot nodules are excluded.

Functioning nodules may be associated with hyperthyroidism (Fig. 14-11). This usually requires a large nodule, 3 to 4 cm or more in diameter, or multiple functioning nodules. Thyrotoxicosis associated with autonomous functioning nodules is referred to as *Plummer's disease.*

The clinical management of patients with hyperfunctioning nodules is influenced by local symptoms in the neck and the patient's euthyroid or thyrotoxic status. Locally asymptomatic hot nodules in euthyroid subjects can often be followed clinically. Some nodules continue to grow in size, with development of thyrotoxicosis. Other nodules stabilize, regress, or undergo involution.

Surgical removal, typically by lobectomy, is often recommended in thyrotoxic patients. An alternative approach is treatment with radioiodine; delivery of radiation to the hyperfunctioning tissue is selective, with sparing of the extranodular tissues. This treatment should not be used if thyroid cancer is suspected.

**"Discordant" nodules**   An important aspect of thyroid scintigraphy is the possibility of "discordance" between radioiodine and radiopertechnetate scintigrams. Because Tc-99m pertechnetate is trapped but not organified, a nodule may appear hot on pertechnetate imaging and cold on radioiodine imaging (Fig. 14-14).

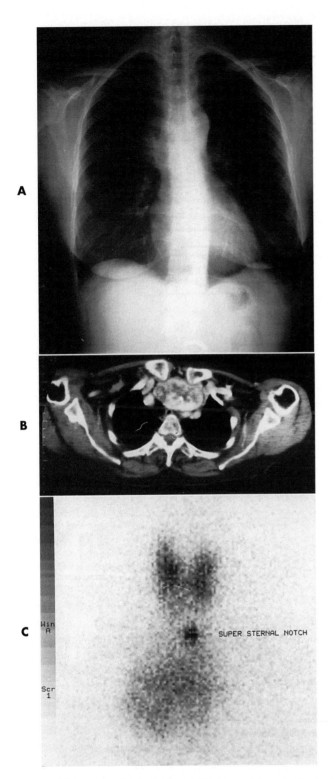

Fig. 14-15   **A,** Chest radiograph reveals a superior mediastinal mass. **B,** Computed tomography confirms the presence of the mass, which demonstrates inhomogeneous density. **C,** Subsequent radioiodine scintigraphy reveals a large substernal goiter.

This occurs in approximately 2% to 3% of radiopertechnetate hot nodules. Conservatively, a single hot nodule identified on radiopertechnetate imaging should not be considered a functioning nodule until confirmed by radioiodine studies. Case reports describe thyroid can-

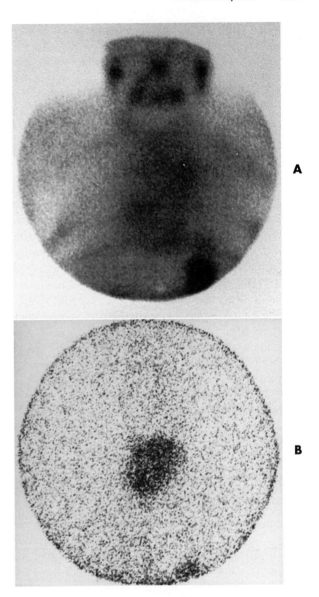

Fig. 14-16   **A,** Technetium-99m pertechnetate study in a patient with suspected substernal goiter. High background activity and activity in the large vascular structures of the mediastinum obscure the ability to visualize thyroid tissue in the mediastinum. **B,** Subsequent iodine-131 scintigraphy demonstrates uptake with good target-to-background ratio.

cers maintaining the trapping but not the organification function. The discordant nodule is a drawback to the use of Tc-99m pertechnetate for routine thyroid scintigraphy.

**Substernal thyroid** Thyroid scintigraphy is used occasionally in the differential diagnosis of mediastinal masses. Substernal thyroid tissue may result from goitrous enlargement with downward extension or from abnormal migration during development (Fig. 14-15).

The ability to perform delayed imaging after tissue and blood pool clearance of background activity is a major advantage of I-131 for this application. Tc-99m pertechnetate is not a good choice because of the high mediastinal blood pool activity at the 20- to 30-minute imaging time typically used with this tracer (Fig. 14-16).

Function and tracer uptake in substernal goiters are frequently poor, and the highest target/background ratio possible is desirable. Delayed imaging at 48 and 72 hours may be required.

The usual cervical location of the thyroid gland should always be imaged when searching for substernal goiter because the vast majority of cases demonstrate continuity with the cervical portion of the gland. Some patients have only a fibrous band connecting the substernal and cervical thyroid tissues.

**Other ectopic thyroid tissue** The thyroglossal duct runs from the foramen cecum at the base of the tongue to the thyroid. Rarely the thyroid fails to migrate from its anlage. Complete failure to migrate results in a *lingual thyroid,* which can be demonstrated scintigraphically. The typical appearance is absence of tracer uptake in the expected cervical location, with a focal or nodular accumulation at the base of the tongue. Thyroid tissue may also be found along the tract of the thyroglossal duct.

**Thyroiditis** Subacute thyroiditis (granulomatous thyroiditis, de Quervain's disease) is a nonsuppurative granulomatous inflammatory process that may affect all or part of the thyroid. The etiology is unproved but speculated to be viral. During the active phase the thyroid scintigram demonstrates decreased or absent uptake in the affected part of the gland (Fig. 14-17). Adjunctive scintigraphic methods such as gallium-67 imaging have been used to demonstrate the inflammatory nature of the process.

The clinical picture can be confusing if local symptoms are minimal. Often the patient has a history of recent upper respiratory tract infection and neck tenderness. Plasma levels of thyroid hormone are increased in the initial phase because of an outpouring of stored hormone caused by the inflammatory process in the gland. Patients may appear thyrotoxic clinically, and thyroiditis may be misdiagnosed as Graves' disease. However, the percent uptake of radioiodine is typically decreased in subacute thyroiditis. Subacute thyroiditis should always be considered before a patient is treated with radioiodine for thyrotoxicosis.

Chronic thyroiditis or *Hashimoto's thyroiditis* is characterized by a lymphocyctic infiltration of the gland. It occurs most frequently in women and may manifest with goiter or hypothyroidism. Rarely a patient presents with hyperthyroidism, and the slang term "hashitoxicosis" is used. Scintigraphic findings are highly variable and depend on the stage in the natural history during which imaging is performed. The scintigram may be normal early in the process. Later, diffuse enlargement may be demonstrated. Many patients with Hashimoto's thyroiditis eventually become hypothyroid. The scintigram often appears inhomogeneous with hot and cold areas.

Acute thyroiditis caused by suppurative bacterial infection is rare. The thyroid is typically enlarged and

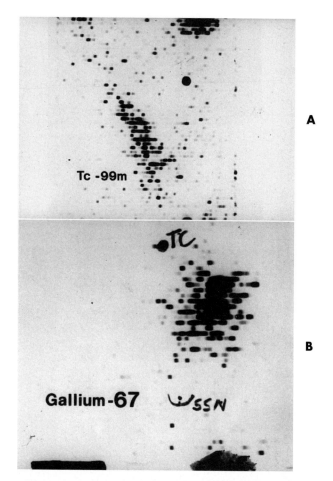

**Fig. 14-17** **A,** Technetium-99m pertechnetate scintigraphy in a patient with subacute thyroiditis affecting the left lobe. There is virtually complete lack of tracer uptake in the left lobe and decreased accumulation in the right lobe. **B,** Corresponding gallium-67 citrate scintigram obtained while the patient was still symptomatic reveals marked focal accumulation in the area of the left lobe, indicating inflammatory nature of the process.

tender. Associated focal abscess may appear as a cold nodule scintigraphically. Reidel's thyroiditis, or struma, is also uncommon; the gland is replaced by fibrous tissue.

**Thyroid cancer metastases** Extended-field-of-view images and whole body imaging are useful in detecting metastatic deposits from differentiated thyroid cancer. Follicular thyroid carcinoma can concentrate radioiodine and can be demonstrated scintigraphically. Mixed papillary-follicular carcinomas can also be demonstrated, and a high percentage of cancers classified histologically as papillary have sufficient follicular elements to be visualized. Medullary carcinomas and anaplastic carcinomas do not concentrate radioiodine and are not detected with conventional thyroid scintigraphy.

The most common sites of metastasis are locally in the lymph nodes of the neck, lung, and skeleton (Figs. 14-18 and 14-19). Nodal activity is typically focal and, if sufficiently intense, may result in a starburst pattern on

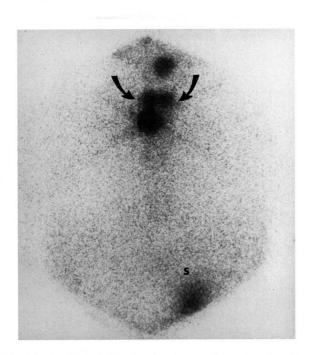

**Fig. 14-18**   Radioiodine imaging in a patient after thyroidectomy for thyroid cancer. Residual activity is seen in the thyroid bed *(arrows)*, as well as in the lymph nodes above and below the thyroid. Note the starburst artifact associated with the intense uptake in the lymph node below the thyroid bed. Uptake in lower left of the image is radioiodine in the stomach *(S)*.

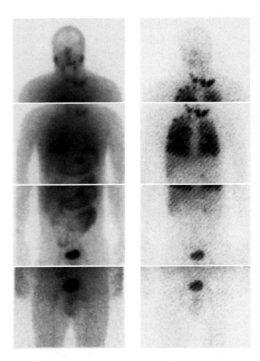

**Fig. 14-19**   Analog *(left)* and digital *(right)* composite whole body scintigrams from a patient with functioning metastatic carcinoma of the thyroid. Note the multiple foci of disease in the neck and the diffuse pulmonary uptake. Uptake in the stomach, bowel, and bladder should not be mistaken for metastatic disease. Diffuse uptake in the region of the liver is related to thyroid hormone metabolism.

parallel-hole collimators (Fig. 14-18). The intensity of uptake in residual normal tissue in the thyroid bed after thyroidectomy may preclude visualizing more subtle areas of uptake outside the thyroid. The intense activity in the thyroid bed may require shielding. Imaging is now typically performed 48 to 72 hours after radioiodine administration. More lesions are demonstrated in this time frame than at 24 hours.

The preparation of patients for follow-up imaging and the details of dose selection are controversial. In one approach, thyroid hormone replacement therapy is withdrawn for 4 to 6 weeks so that patients may achieve a maximal endogenous thyroid-stimulating hormone (TSH) response. Another approach is to switch patients to a triiodothyronine ($T_3$) preparation for a time and then discontinue the $T_3$ for 2 weeks. This protocol reduces the problem of symptomatic hypothyroidism, but its efficacy is not as well established as 6 weeks of abstinence from thyroid hormone. Some centers also have used bovine TSH before imaging. This is not considered as satisfactory for increasing I-131 uptake, and there is a significant incidence of allergic reactions to the bovine preparation. Recombinant human TSH has now been produced, however, and will probably have a better tolerance profile and renew interest in the TSH approach. Whichever approach is used, it is important

to achieve adequate uptake of tracer. Inadequate preparation can result in false negative scintigrams.

Selection of the scanning dose of I-131 is also controversial. As demonstrated more than 15 years ago, more metastatic deposits are seen with higher doses, and 5 and 10 mCi of I-131 were used for detecting metastases. Because as little as 5 mCi can "stun" thyroid cancer metastases, with less satisfactory uptake of subsequent therapeutic doses of I-131, diagnostic doses should be limited to 1 or 2 mCi.

*Thallium-201 and technetium-99m sestamibi*   Thallium-201 chloride and Tc-99m sestamibi have been used for tumor imaging, including thyroid carcinoma. The uptake is nonspecific and is seen in benign as well as malignant conditions. These tracers have not found widespread application in the initial diagnosis of thyroid cancer. Some advocate their use for thyroid cancer follow-up imaging, where differentiating uptake in normal tissue and benign lesions from tumor is not an issue. One advantage is that patients need not discontinue thyroid hormone replacement therapy before imaging. However, this approach has not found wide acceptance and should be used with caution. It may be useful for locating metastases in patients with increased thyroglobulin levels and negative radioiodine whole body scintigrams.

*Iodine-131 metaiodobenzylguanidine* I-131 MIBG localizes in neurosecretory storage vesicles of chromaffin cells. Some medullary carcinomas of the thyroid demonstrate I-131 MIBG uptake. The sensitivity is low, about 30%. Soft tissue metastases are better visualized than skeletal metastases. The low sensitivity precludes a routine role for I-131 MIBG in the workup of medullary thyroid cancer.

Indium-111 somatostatin receptor scintigraphy has also been evaluated for medullary carcinoma of the thyroid, with indifferent early results.

*Fluorodeoxyglucose positron emission tomography* The general renaissance of PET imaging has kindled interest in applying the technique for the evaluation of thyroid cancer. Early indications are that fluorodeoxyglucose (FDG) PET may offer an alternative to I-131 imaging for detection of thyroid cancer metastases. FDG PET has the advantage of being able to detect nonfunctioning as well as functioning thyroid cancers and may be important when I-131 scintigraphy is negative. FDG PET also offers the potential to distinguish thyroid nodules caused by cancer from benign causes based on the higher FDG metabolism seen in tumors.

---

### Thyroid Function Studies

**Thyroid percent uptake** The radioactive iodine uptake test was among the earliest applications of radiotracers in medicine. The degree of radioiodine uptake parallels the functional activity of the thyroid gland in producing thyroid hormone. The test is used clinically to differentiate Graves' disease from most other causes of hyperthyroidism and to guide selection of the therapeutic dose of I-131.

Thyroid uptake studies have primarily employed radioiodine-131. The test is performed with a nonimaging probe detector that has a 2 × 2-inch or larger sodium iodide crystal. Six to 10 μCi of I-131 is given orally. The sodium iodide may be either in liquid form or in solid, capsule form. From a health physics standpoint, capsules are preferable because they reduce airborne exposure of workers to radioiodine and are more convenient for handling. An early problem with commercial capsules was incomplete dissolution in the gut, resulting in falsely low 24-hour uptake values. This is no longer a problem. The radioiodine uptake test can also be performed with I-123 in conjunction with scintigraphy.

The uptake measurement is accomplished by counting uptake in the patient's neck and a standard dose of equal activity to that given to the patient in an appropriate neck phantom. The probe is typically positioned 10 inches from the anterior surface of the neck. A single-hole collimator designed to encompass the entire thyroid gland is used on the probe. Background correction may be accomplished either by using a lead thyroid shield and

**Box 14-11   Calculation of Thyroid Percent Uptake of Radioiodine**

**INPUT DATA**

Phantom count with radioiodine standard sample
Neck count
Background count

**CALCULATION**

$$\text{Thyroid percent uptake} = \frac{\text{Neck count} - \text{Background count}}{\text{Phantom count}}$$

$$\text{Radioiodine taken up in thyroid (μCi)} = \text{Percent uptake} \times \text{Patient dose (μCi)}$$

obtaining measurements with and without the shield or by counting the patient's thigh activity at the same 10-inch distance. Box 14-11 provides the formula for computing the percentage of uptake.

In the United States the normal range for uptake of radioiodine in a thyroid is 10% to 30%. Before the widespread use of periodate in bread and the iodination of table salt, the normal range was substantially higher, and each laboratory should maintain correlation records to ensure the appropriate values for normal. Box 14-4 summarizes common nonthyroidal causes of increased and decreased radioiodine uptake. A history of drug use should be obtained with the radioiodine percent uptake test.

The availability of sensitive and specific thyroid function tests, including tests for determining serum $T_4$ and $T_3$ values, has diminished the role of the radioactive iodine uptake test in determining the functional status of the thyroid. However, the test is uniquely suited to the differential diagnosis of hyperthyroidism. Uptake is classically elevated in Graves' disease and Plummer's disease and decreased in hyperthyroidism caused by subacute thyroiditis and thyrotoxicosis factitia.

The standard percent uptake test has a number of variations. If hyperthyroidism is suspected, earlier measurements (at 2, 4, or 6 hours) should be considered. In some patients with florid hyperthyroidism the uptake peaks before 24 hours and the measurement at 24 hours is misleadingly low.

**Suppression test** In the thyroid suppression test a baseline 24-hour uptake is determined. The patient then receives 25 mg of $T_3$ four times a day for 8 days. The 24-hour uptake is repeated beginning on day 7. Some residual activity may be in the thyroid, and the neck is counted before administration of the repeat uptake dose. A normal response to thyroid suppression is a fall in the percentage of uptake to less than 50% of the baseline value and less than 10% overall.

The thyroid suppression test is not often used in current practice. Its utility was in diagnosing patients with borderline Graves' disease and autonomous functioning glands. Very sensitive tests for TSH levels are now used and can accurately detect early hyperthyroidism.

**Stimulation test** The thyroid stimulation test also is infrequently used today. It was indicated to distinguish primary from secondary (pituitary) hypothyroidism. Failure to respond to exogenous TSH is indicative of primary hypothyroidism. Patients with secondary hypothyroidism have increased radioiodine uptake after TSH stimulation.

The stimulation test is performed by determining a baseline 24-hour radioiodine percent uptake. The patient then receives 10 units of TSH intramuscularly. The radioiodine uptake is repeated beginning the next day. In healthy subjects and patients with secondary hypothyroidism (hypopituitarism) the uptake should double, whereas those with primary hypothyroidism show no response.

**Perchlorate discharge test** A third interventional modification of the percent uptake test is the perchlorate discharge test. This procedure demonstrates dissociation of the trapping and organification functions in the thyroid. Dissociation occurs in rare congenital enzyme deficiencies, in certain types of chronic thyroiditis, and during therapy with propylthiouracil. The patient receives a tracer dose of radioiodine. The percent uptake is measured at 1 to 2 hours, and 1 g of potassium perchlorate is given orally. The percent uptake is measured hourly. In normal subjects or patients with hyperthyroidism on inadequate antithyroid drug therapy, less than a 10% discharge of radioiodine is demonstrated. A greater than 10% washout suggests an organification defect.

## RADIOIODINE TREATMENT OF HYPERTHYROIDISM AND THYROID CANCER

Radioiodine has been used for the treatment of hyperthyroidism for more than five decades (Box 14-12). The vast majority of patients with primary hyperthyroidism have Graves' disease (diffuse toxic goiter) and are candidates for I-131 therapy. A small percentage have one or more toxic nodules and, as discussed earlier, may also be candidates for therapy. I-131 therapy is not indicated for some causes of hyperthyroidism and could be harmful.

The selection of patients for I-131 therapy of hyperthyroidism is generally straightforward. Measurement of

**Box 14-12  Classification of Hyperthyroidism: Indications for Iodine-131 Therapy**

**POTENTIALLY INDICATED**

Graves' disease (diffuse toxic goiter)
Plummer's disease (toxic nodular goiter)
Functioning thyroid cancer (metastatic)

**NOT GENERALLY INDICATED OR CONTRAINDICATED**

Thyrotoxicosis factitia
Subacute thyroiditis
"Silent" thyroiditis (atypical, subacute, lymphocytic, transient, postpartum)
Struma ovarii
Thyroid hormone resistance (biochemical/clinical manifestations)
Secondary hyperthyroidism (pituitary tumor, ectopic thyroid-stimulating hormone, trophoblastic tumors [human chorionic gonadotropin])
Thyrotoxicosis associated with Hashimoto's disease ("hashitoxicosis")
Jod-Basedow phenomenon (iodine-induced hyperthyroidism)

serum TSH and the 4-hour and 24-hour radioactive iodine uptake essentially eliminates patients who are not candidates for therapy. Patients with Graves' disease and Plummer's disease have high uptakes and low TSH levels. I-131 therapy can be used at any age, although some physicians prefer medical or surgical therapy in children. Because maintaining a medical regimen in children is difficult, radioiodine therapy is preferred. In women, pregnancy must be ruled out before I-131 therapy. As noted, the fetal thyroid begins concentrating iodine in weeks 10 to 12 of gestation, and cretinism has occurred after therapeutic doses of I-131 during pregnancy. Women should be counseled to avoid pregnancy for 6 to 12 months after therapy in case retreatment is indicated.

The therapeutic goal in treating hyperthyroidism is to render the patient euthyroid in a reasonable length of time with a single radioiodine dose. Empirically this is achieved in Graves' disease when 80 to 120 µCi is retained in the gland per gram of tissue. Box 14-13 shows a typical calculation of an individualized treatment dose based on estimated thyroid gland weight and measurement of the 24-hour radioiodine percent uptake. Alternatively, some centers have abandoned the attempt to individualize therapy and give a standard dose in the 5- to 10-mCi range to all patients with diffuse toxic goiter. Some centers also favor higher doses for patients demonstrating rapid radioiodine turnover in the gland and for patients with Graves' ophthalmopathy.

---

**Box 14-13   Calculation of Iodine-131 Therapeutic Dose for Hyperthyroidism**

**INPUT DATA**

Gland weight: 60 g
24-hour uptake: 80%
Desired dose to be retained in thyroid (selected to deliver 8000 to 10,000 rads to thyroid): 100 μCi/g

**Calculations**

$$\text{Required dose (μCi)} = \frac{60 \text{ g} \times 100 \text{ μCi/g}}{0.80} = 7500$$

$$\text{Dose (mCi)} = \frac{7500}{1000} = 7.5 \text{ mCi}$$

---

More than 90% of patients who undergo radioiodine therapy are cured with a single dose. Therapeutic effects are not instantaneous, however, because stored hormone must be released and used. Also, most patients eventually become hypothyroid and need replacement hormone therapy. Treatment with radioactive iodine obligates the patient to lifelong follow-up.

In addition to the risk of hypothyroidism, secondary effects of radiation exposure have been a concern, including secondary cancers. It is now known that no statistically significant differences exist between patients receiving I-131 therapy and patients treated by surgery for hypothyroidism. Both groups have a higher incidence of leukemia than the general population. I-131 therapy does not reduce fertility, and congenital defects are not increased in the children of treated individuals.

Immediately after therapy, thyroid storm is a risk. Patients with florid disease and those treated with higher amounts of radioactivity are at greater risk. In older patients who have preexisting heart disease and in patients otherwise at risk, medical therapy can be carried out for several months to deplete thyroid hormone before radioiodine therapy. Beta blockers are used both before and after therapy. Some patients report local neck pain, tenderness, and swelling after I-131 therapy.

Patients with hyperthyroidism caused by toxic nodules (Plummer's disease) are generally more difficult to treat with radioiodine than patients with diffuse goiter. The tissue is relatively radioresistant, possibly because of its inhomogeneity. Radioiodine turnover may also be higher in these nodules, with a lower retained dose. For these reasons many laboratories increase the dose of radioiodine to 15 to 29 mCi. Since the extranodular tissue in the thyroid is suppressed, it is spared and may resume function after successful radioiodine therapy.

Radioactive iodine has also been used extensively in the treatment of metastases from differentiated thyroid cancers. Radioiodine is not useful for treating anaplastic and medullary tumors. Despite 50 years of experience, opinion still differs greatly on how and when to employ radioactive iodine. Much of the controversy centers on smaller, early-stage lesions, for which prognosis is already very good. Evidence is overwhelming, however, that patients with residual or recurrent differentiated thyroid cancer have improved survival with I-131 treatment. Postsurgical ablation of thyroid remnants reduces local recurrences.

Patients are prepared for therapy by discontinuing thyroid replacement hormone or suppressive therapy. A diagnostic scan is typically done to establish the presence of metastatic lesions. Thyroglobulin levels are also measured. In the past, patients had to remain hospitalized and isolated until retained activity was less than 30 mCi. The Nuclear Regulatory Commission has published a new rule (10 CFR 20 and 35) for release of patients based on the likely exposure to others. The release criterion is that an individual should receive no more than 5 millisieverts (0.5 rem) from exposure to a released patient. Patients are instructed on avoiding close contact with others, including family members.

A repeat of the whole body scintigram using the therapeutic dose is often useful. More lesions are often seen. After therapy the patient is placed back on thyroid hormone replacement or suppressive therapy. Retreatment is usually not considered for at least 6 months and preferably 12 months to avoid bone marrow suppression.

Metastatic disease is most common locally in the neck. Distant metastases are most common in the lung and skeleton. An initial dose of 150 to 200 mCi is administered after appropriate patient preparation. Repeated doses up to a total of 1 Ci may be required. Skeletal metastases are more difficult to eradicate than lung metastases. Follow-up imaging is carried out at yearly intervals until all detected metastases are eliminated. Serum thyroglobulin levels can then be followed. In patients who have had total thyroidectomies and ablation of any postsurgical remnants, elevated thyroglobulin levels indicate the presence of cancer. Imaging is then used to localize the disease.

## ADRENAL SCINTIGRAPHY

Separate classes of radiopharmaceuticals are available for scintigraphic imaging of the adrenal cortex and the adrenal medulla. Adrenocortical scintigraphy was extensively used before the development of body computed tomography (CT). Nuclear imaging studies of the adrenal cortex are not frequently performed in current practice but retain a limited utility in assessing the functional status of adrenocortical tissue when CT findings are indeterminate. In particular, incidental adrenal nodules demonstrated by CT can be assessed for functional status by adrenocortical scintigraphy.

Scintigraphic studies of the adrenal medulla and related tissues have created significant interest and have found an expanding role in contemporary practice.

## Adrenocortical Scintigraphy

**Radiopharmaceuticals**   The first successful radiopharmaceutical for adrenal visualization was I-131-19-iodocholesterol. The current agent of choice is I-131-6β-iodomethyl-19-norcholesterol (NP-59). This agent was identified as an impurity in the original formulation.

The mechanism of localization of I-131-6β-iodomethyl-19-norcholesterol by the adrenal cortex is related to the transport and receptor systems for serum cholesterol bound to low-density lipoprotein (LDL). Factors affecting cholesterol uptake into the adrenal also affect uptake of the radiopharmaceutical. An increase in the serum cholesterol reduces the percent uptake. Increases in plasma adrenocorticotropic hormone (ACTH) result in increased radiocholesterol uptake. The radiopharmaceutical is stored in adrenocortical cells and is esterified but not incorporated into adrenal hormones.

The uptake of I-131-6β-iodomethyl-19-norcholesterol is progressive over several days after tracer administration. The background clearance is also relatively slow, and for routine or baseline studies, imaging is typically performed several days after tracer injection. Background tissues demonstrating significant localization include the liver, colon, and gallbladder.

Patients should be pretreated for at least 1 day with Lugol's iodine, three drops twice daily or equivalent, to block uptake of free radioiodine in the thyroid. This is continued for 7 days.

I-131-6β-iodomethyl-19-norcholesterol is usually given in a dose of 1 mCi/1.7 m$^2$ of body surface area. The dose is administered intravenously over 1 to 2 minutes.

For routine or baseline studies, imaging is accomplished 4 to 5 days after radiopharmaceutical administration. A large-field-of-view gamma scintillation camera with a high-energy parallel-hole collimator is used, and a 20% window is centered at 364 keV. Ideally, all images are acquired with a dedicated nuclear medicine computer system. This permits a standardized time per image with intensity optimization after data acquisition. With this approach a standard imaging time of 20 minutes per view is used. The most important view is posterior and includes both adrenal glands. Anterior views may be helpful to assess adrenal asymmetry. Lateral views with a line marker source on the middle of the back are obtained to determine adrenal gland depth for percent uptake calculations and to help differentiate gallbladder uptake from activity in the right adrenal gland.

**Suppression studies**   Routine or baseline adrenocortical scintigraphy is typically employed in patients with hypercortisolism. In patients with abnormalities of the zona glomerulosa (production of aldosterone) or the zona reticularis (production of androgens), it is often desirable to suppress ACTH secretion and thus adrenal uptake of radiocholesterol in the zona fasciculata. This is accomplished by administering dexamethasone, 4 mg per day (2 mg bid) for 7 days before radiopharmaceutical administration and continuing until imaging is completed.

**Percent uptake determination**   The relative percent uptake of radiocholesterol in the adrenal is a crude marker of adrenal functional activity and may be calculated in a manner similar to the thyroid radioactive iodine uptake. A standard sample is counted on the gamma camera to determine the count rate of the injected dose. The net count rate from the individual glands is determined by background-corrected regions of interest (ROIs) defined on the posterior view. Tissue attenuation is corrected by measuring the left and right adrenal gland depths from the lateral view. The percent uptake of 6β-iodomethyl-19-norcholesterol in healthy subjects is approximately 0.16% of the administered dose per gland (range, 0.073% to 0.26%).

**Normal adrenocortical scintigram**   In normal subjects, radiotracer uptake in the adrenal cortex increases over the first 2 days after injection. Background activity is still relatively high at this time, especially in the liver, and imaging may be delayed until day 4 or 5.

The two adrenal glands are not symmetrical anatomically and most often have a different appearance scintigraphically. The right adrenal is typically applied to the superior pole of the right kidney and is slightly cephalad to the left adrenal gland. The right adrenal gland appears round and in most subjects is slightly more intense than the left. The right adrenal gland's greater intensity is caused by its more posterior location in the body with reduced soft tissue attenuation. Liver activity is also superimposed. The left adrenal gland is typically applied to the anteromedial border of the left kidney and may extend inferiorly to the renal hilum. Scintigraphically it appears more caudad and has an oval rather than a round configuration. The left adrenal gland frequently appears less intense because of its more anterior location and the lack of additive background activity from the liver.

Activity in the gallbladder may be confused with right adrenal gland activity. The gallbladder can be emptied by administering a cholecystagogue. It also may be beneficial to administer a renal agent to localize the kidneys and establish the relationship of the kidneys to the adrenal glands.

**Cushing's syndrome**   Scintigraphic patterns vary in Cushing's syndrome (Fig. 14-20). In patients with bio-

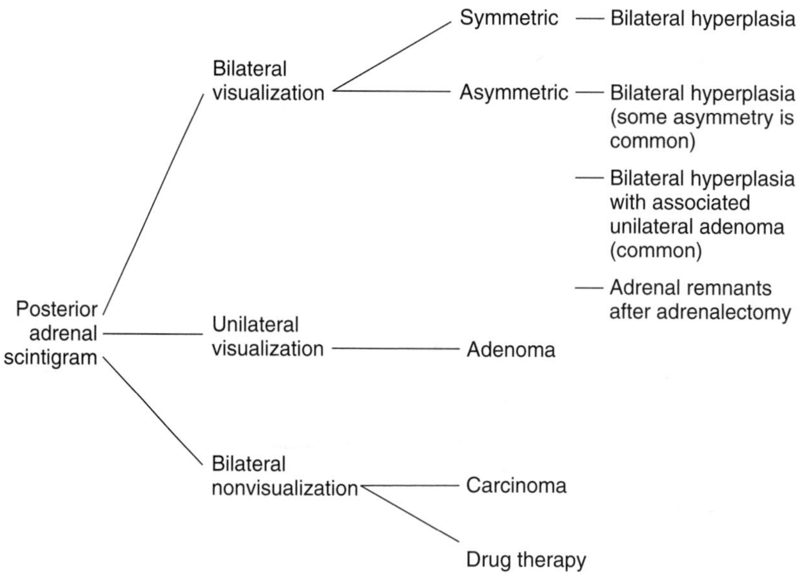

**Fig. 14-20**  Diagnostic patterns for adrenocortical scintigraphy in patients with biochemically proven Cushing's syndrome.

Posterior adrenal scintigram
- Bilateral visualization
  - Symmetric — Bilateral hyperplasia
  - Asymmetric — Bilateral hyperplasia (some asymmetry is common)
    - Bilateral hyperplasia with associated unilateral adenoma (common)
    - Adrenal remnants after adrenalectomy
- Unilateral visualization — Adenoma
- Bilateral nonvisualization
  - Carcinoma
  - Drug therapy

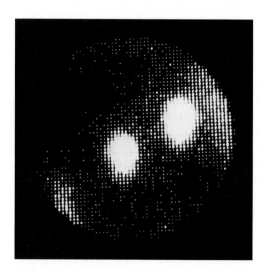

**Fig. 14-21**  Adrenocortical scintigraphy in a patient with Cushing's disease. Note the bilateral and fairly symmetrical uptake.

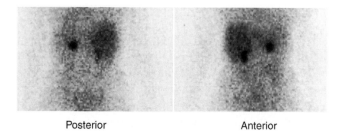

Posterior                    Anterior

**Fig. 14-22**  Adrenocortical scintigraphy in the posterior view reveals unilateral uptake in the left adrenal gland in a patient with adrenal adenoma. The anterior view shows uptake in the adenoma as well as in the gallbladder, which should not be mistaken for a lesion. This is easily accomplished by imaging on the lateral view to confirm the location of the activity.

chemically proven hypercortisolism, symmetrical visualization of the adrenals is invariably caused by adrenal hyperplasia (Fig. 14-21). The most common cause is Cushing's disease or pituitary excess of ACTH. Less often, ectopic ACTH syndromes may be the cause. The percent uptake is increased in Cushing's disease to an average of 0.5% of the injected dose per gland. The highest uptakes are seen in ectopic ACTH syndromes and adrenal macronodular hyperplasia, which result in uptakes of 1.2% ± 0.30% per gland of the injected dose. Uptakes greater than 0.26% per gland are invariably associated with Cushing's syndrome. Even in patients with Cushing's disease, however, the serum cholesterol has an inverse effect on percent uptakes.

In a small number of patients, both glands are

visualized but are asymmetrical. Mild to moderate asymmetry may be seen with hyperplasia. More striking asymmetry may result from macronodular hyperplasia, the concomitant presence of adenoma on one side, or prior surgery with asymmetrical adrenal remnants.

Unilateral visualization is classically seen in patients with glucocorticoid-producing adrenal adenomas (Fig. 14-22). The autonomous production of cortisol in the adenoma feeds back to shut off pituitary ACTH secretion and thereby shuts off uptake in the contralateral adrenal gland (Fig. 14-23).

Nonvisualization of both adrenal glands in patients with Cushing's syndrome indicates adrenal carcinoma. The tumors can be quite large and are often first manifested clinically with signs and symptoms of hormone excess. However, the function per gram of tumor tissue is typically low, and tracer uptake is insufficient to visualize the tumor. The contralateral adrenal gland is typically not visualized because the cortisol production

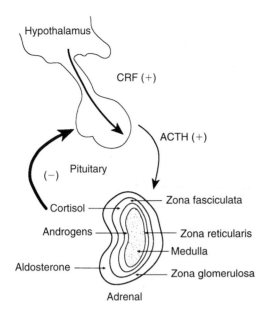

**Fig. 14-23** Pituitary-adrenal feedback loop. Function in the zona fasciculata is stimulated by adrenocorticotropic hormone *(ACTH).* Pituitary secretion of ACTH decreases as circulating levels of cortisol increase. *CRF,* Corticotropin-releasing factor.

in the cancer shuts down pituitary ACTH secretion (Fig. 14-23).

Biochemical proof of hypercortisolism and CT demonstration of a large lesion in the adrenal are considered sufficient evidence, and scintigraphy is not needed. However, if CT findings are negative or equivocal, adrenocortical scintigraphy can be helpful.

Another potential use of adrenocortical scintigraphy in patients with Cushing's syndrome, even in the era of magnetic resonance imaging (MRI) and CT, is in the detection of postsurgical adrenal remnants. These remnants may result in recurrent disease and may be difficult to localize in a surgically altered anatomy. They are readily detected by adrenocortical scintigraphy.

**Aldosteronism**  The principal clinical question in aldosteronism is the distinction of adenoma from hyperplasia. Aldosteronomas are typically small, and CT or MRI often is not diagnostic. Aldosterone is produced in the zona glomerulosa of the adrenal cortex. This hormone does not affect the pituitary-ACTH feedback loop, and the dexamethasone suppression scan is necessary in evaluating patients with aldosteronism. Normal uptake in the zona fasciculata can obscure asymmetry caused by small nodules and adenomas in the zona glomerulosa. The suppression scan is performed sequentially over a number of days. Early (less than 5 days) unilateral "breakthrough" indicates aldosteronoma. Bilateral, delayed breakthrough typically indicates hyperplasia.

**Androgen excess**  The adrenal glands may be a source of androgen excess. Scintigraphic patterns are similar to those found in aldosteronism. That is, pa-

tients with bilateral hyperplasia demonstrate bilateral breakthrough on dexamethasone suppression scans, and adenomas are characterized by marked scintigraphic asymmetry.

## Adrenomedullary Scintigraphy

Adrenomedullary scintigraphy has proved useful in the management of patients with functional adrenergic tumors. These include paragangliomas, neuroblastomas, ganglioneuroblastomas, and ganglioneuromas. Pheochromocytomas are paragangliomas that arise in the adrenal medulla. Paragangliomas are associated with a number of important familial syndromes, including multiple endocrine neoplasia (MEN) type IIA (medullary carcinoma of the thyroid, pheochromocytoma, hyperparathyroidism) and MEN type IIB (medullary carcinoma of the thyroid, pheochromocytoma, ganglioneuromas). Other associations are von Hippel-Lindau disease and neurofibromatosis.

**Radiopharmaceuticals**  Scintigraphic studies of the adrenergic nervous system became possible with MIBG, an analog of guanethidine. Localization appears to be through the type I, energy-dependent, active amine transport mechanism. The tracer is taken up and further localized in cytoplasmic storage vesicles in presynaptic adrenergic nerves. In addition to the uptake in the adrenal medulla and other adrenergic and neuroblastic tumor tissues, the tracer localizes avidly in other organs with rich adrenergic innervation, including the heart, salivary glands, and spleen. Both I-131 and I-123 have been used as radiolabels. I-123 has the advantage of a lower radiation dose to the patient, whereas I-131 facilitates delayed imaging.

**Technique**  The tracer is taken up rapidly by adrenergic tissues. To achieve sufficient target-to-background ratios, imaging is typically delayed for 1 day after tracer administration and may be repeated at 2 or 3 days.

For studies with I-131 MIBG, patients are given a blocking dose of either saturated solution of potassium iodide (SSKI) or Lugol's solution. The usual adult dose of I-131 MIBG is 0.5 mCi/1.7 m$^2$. The tracer is administered intravenously over 15 to 30 seconds. Higher doses have been used postoperatively to look for residual remnant tissues. When MIBG is radiolabeled with I-123, up to 10 mCi/m$^2$ can be administered with the same radiation dose to the patient as from 0.5 mCi/m$^2$ of I-131 MIBG.

Initial images with I-131 MIBG are usually obtained at 24 hours, with further delayed imaging at 48 and 72 hours after injection. A wide-field-of-view gamma scintillation camera equipped with a high-energy parallel-hole collimator is used for all computerized image acquisition. Computer acquisition permits a fixed time per image to be used, typically 20 minutes. The views obtained are determined by the clinical condition under evaluation.

For pheochromocytoma the posterior view of the mid-abdomen with the region of the adrenal glands is most important. Additional images from the pelvis to the base of the skull are indicated to detect extraadrenal pheochromocytoma (paraganglioma).

With I-123 MIBG, initial images may be obtained at 2 to 3 hours, with delayed imaging at 24 hours and 48 hours. Single-photon emission computed tomography (SPECT) is feasible with I-123 MIBG.

**Precautions**   A number of drugs interfere with MIBG uptake, and a drug history should be obtained before imaging. Interfering drugs include tricyclic antidepressants, reserpine, guanethidine, certain antipsychotics, cocaine, and the alpha- and beta-blocker labetalol.

**Normal metaiodobenzylguanidine scintigram**
With the usual doses employed for I-131 MIBG imaging, only faint visualization of the normal adrenal medulla is achieved in 10% to 15% of patients. Visualization increases with time, but the image remains faint. The normal adrenal medulla is visualized more frequently with I-123 MIBG and with therapeutic doses of I-131 MIBG. Early images reveal activity in the spleen, heart, salivary glands, and liver. These areas clear with time. Some bladder activity may be visualized because of free radioiodine. The colon is also seen transiently in 20% to 25% of cases.

**Clinical applications**   The greatest clinical experience with MIBG is in the evaluation of patients with suspected intraadrenal paraganglioma or pheochromocytoma. The characteristic appearance is unilateral focal uptake in the tumor (Fig. 14-24). Sensitivity for detection of pheochromocytoma is 90% or better, with a specificity greater than 95%. In approximately 10% of patients, pheochromocytoma is bilateral. In 10% to 20% the tumors are extraadrenal and are referred to as paragangliomas. As noted, pheochromocytomas are increasingly seen with other neuroectodermal disorders, including neurofibromatosis, tuberous sclerosis, Carney's syndrome, and von Hippel-Lindau disease. Paragangliomas may be found from the bladder up to the base of the skull.

Scintigraphy with MIBG is not a screening procedure for pheochromocytoma and should be applied only after biochemical tests suggest the diagnosis. Many centers first use CT to evaluate the adrenal glands. If an adrenal mass is demonstrated, the diagnosis is inferred and further workup before surgery is unnecessary. MIBG is particularly helpful in surveying the entire body for extraadrenal and metastatic lesions.

Adrenomedullary hyperplasia develops in patients with MEN IIA. This condition is difficult to diagnose with CT or MRI. MIBG scintigraphy is uniquely suited to detect medullary hyperplasia and has been used to assist decision making for timing of surgery.

MIBG imaging has been used most often for pheochromocytomas but also has been widely used in imaging neuroblastomas. Reported sensitivity is 60% to 90%, with a high degree of specificity. Other tumors demonstrating uptake of MIBG include carcinoids and medullary carcinoma of the thyroid.

The successful scintigraphic visualization of these tumors and pheochromocytoma has led investigators to attempt therapy with I-131 MIBG. Therapeutic applications are still experimental and restricted largely to patients in whom prior conventional therapies have failed.

## PARATHYROID SCINTIGRAPHY

A number of imaging techniques have been proposed for visualizing the parathyroid glands. Ultrasonography with high-resolution transducers (10 MHz) is the imaging technique of choice in most centers. Ultrasound has the additional advantage of guiding needle biopsies and even percutaneous ablation of parathyroid adenomas or hyperplastic glands. Scintigraphy has also proved useful in many institutions.

The first radiopharmaceutical used to any extent for parathyroid scintigraphy was selenium-75 selenomethionine. The rationale for this tracer is the incorporation of selenomethionine in areas of protein synthesis as an amino acid analog of methionine. Both the sensitivity and the specificity in the detection of parathyroid adenomas were poor, and this tracer has been largely abandoned.

*Technetium-99m (Tc-99m) sestamibi* and the related tracer *Tc-99m tetrofosmin* have been studied extensively as agents for parathyroid imaging. The rationale for Tc-99m sestamibi is its observed parallel uptake properties to thallium-201 and the superior image quality and better dosimetry available with the Tc-99m-labeled agents.

Early investigators observed that Tc-99m sestamibi demonstrates slower washout from parathyroid adenomas and hyperplastic parathyroid glands compared with surrounding thyroid tissue (Fig. 14-25). This permits detection of these structures by observing differential clearance over time (Box 14-14). Other centers have

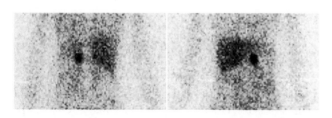

**Fig. 14-24**   Adrenomedullary scintigraphy reveals unilaterally increased uptake in the region of the left adrenal owing to pheochromocytoma.

used subtraction techniques, and more recently SPECT imaging has also provided good results (Fig. 14-26). With SPECT, early imaging can be superior to delayed imaging. Even though differential washout is slower in parathyroid lesions than in the thyroid, some adenomas demonstrate sufficiently rapid Tc-99m sestamibi clearance that they are not detectable at 2 hours.

Detection of parathyroid adenomas is more accurate than detection of parathyroid hyperplasia. Sensitivities of 90% have been reported for adenoma detection. A reasonable approach based on current information is the use of Tc-99m sestamibi and SPECT. Reprojection imaging with cinematic display is helpful in both detecting and localizing adenomas.

A more traditional scintigraphic technique uses combined Tc-99m pertechnetate and T1-201 subtraction imaging. The rationale is that thallium avidly accumulates in both parathyroid tissue and thyroid tissue, whereas Tc-99m pertechnetate accumulates only in thyroid tissue. Thus the subtraction of normalized Tc-99m pertechnetate activity from a thallium image should theoretically remove the contribution from the thyroid and leave only activity caused by T1-201 accumulation in the parathyroid glands (Fig. 14-27). If the parathyroid adenoma is adjacent to the thyroid rather than behind or in it, visualization is usually obvious without the need for subtraction.

Techniques have been described for the initial injection of either Tc-99m or T1-201, although most laboratories use T1-201 first because of its lower energy. Either

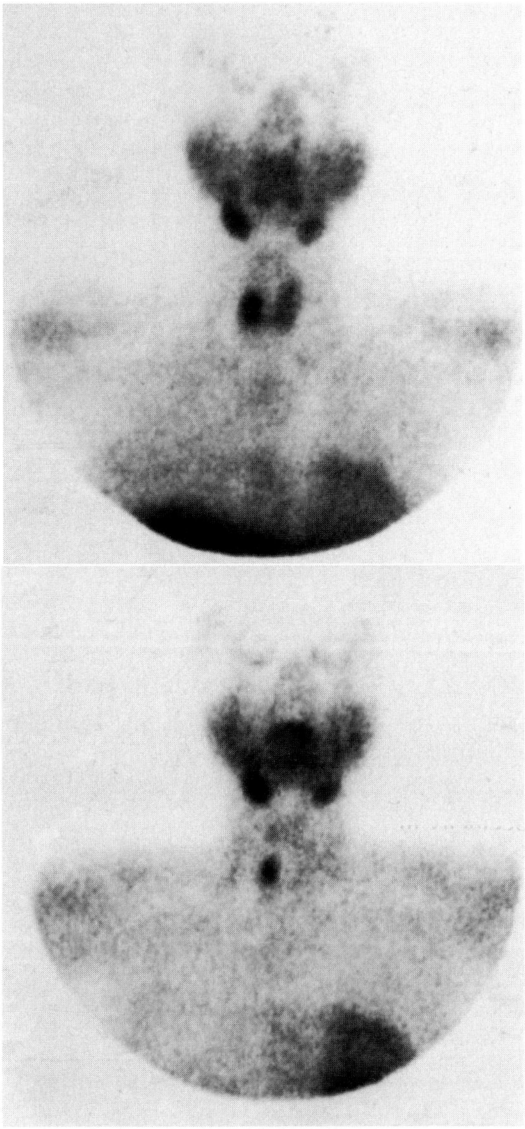

**Fig. 14-25**    **A,** Early imaging with technetium-99m sestamibi in a patient with suspected parathyroid adenoma reveals asymmetrical activity in the region of the thyroid gland. **B,** Delayed imaging at 2 hours demonstrates washout of thyroid activity and a large parathyroid adenoma.

---

### Box 14-14    Technetium-99m Sestamibi Parathyroid Imaging: Protocol Summary

**PATIENT PREPARATION**

None

**RADIOPHARMACEUTICAL**

Tc-99m sestamibi, 20mCi (740 MBq), intravenously

**TIME OF IMAGING**

Early scans at 15 minutes
Delayed scans at 2 hours

**IMAGING PROCEDURE**
**Planar**

Use a high-resolution collimator and a 20% window centered at 140 keV.
Position the patient supine with the chin up and neck extended.
Place markers on the chin and sternal notch.
Obtain anterior and 45° left and right anterior oblique views, 300k counts per view.

**SPECT Imaging**

Position patient as above.
Use a high-resolution collimater and a 20% window centered at 140 keV.
Use dual- or triple-headed SPECT camera, if available: 360° contoured acquisition arc, 3° angular sampling increment, 15 to 30 sec per view, 128 × 128 matrix with 1.5 zoom, Hanning or Butterworth filter.
Reconstruct transaxial, coronal, and sagittal planes.
Reproject images at each sampling angle.

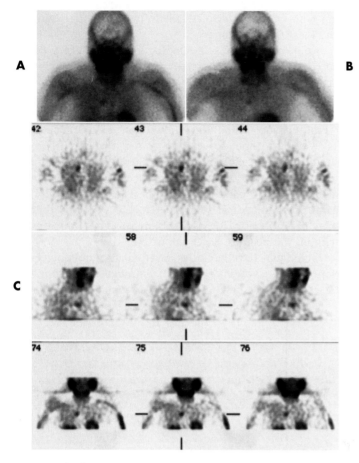

**Fig. 14-26** Immediate **(A)** and delayed **(B)** imaging with technetium-99m sestamibi (anterior views) in a patient with hyperparathyroidism reveals a suspicious area in the mediastinum that becomes less intense between images. **C,** SPECT images with reconstruction in the transaxial *(top),* sagittal *(center),* and coronal *(bottom)* planes confirms the presence of the parathyroid adenoma.

approach is probably valid. When T1-201 is administered first, images are acquired with a nuclear medicine computer system in several projections. The view thought to be most indicative of possible abnormality is selected, and the patient is repositioned in that view. A baseline T1-201 image is obtained. The patient is then given 1 to 2 mCi of Tc-99m pertechnetate, with image acquisition repeated 10 minutes after tracer administration. A normalization factor is computed by comparing the count rates on the respective thallium and pertechnetate images in areas of normal thyroid tissue. Care must be used in flagging the ROIs for normalization of the calculation to avoid abnormal areas.

The sensitivity of the technique depends on the size of the parathyroid adenoma being sought. For lesions greater than 1 g in size, sensitivity is more than 95%; it decreases for smaller lesions. The smallest lesion detectable by this technique is about 0.3 g.

The technique has a number of pitfalls. First, the relative uptake of Tc-99m pertechnetate and T1-201

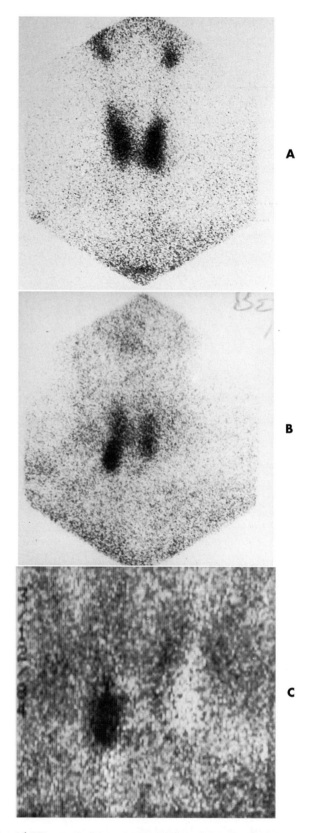

**Fig. 14-27** **A,** Technetium-99m pertechnetate scintigraphy in a patient with suspected parathyroid adenoma is essentially normal. **B,** Corresponding thallium-201 scintigraphy reveals an apparent area of increased uptake adjacent to the lower pole of the right lobe. **C,** Subtraction of the Tc-99m pertechnetate study from the T1-201 study confirms the presence of the parathyroid adenoma.

chloride throughout the thyroid gland may not be equal and constant in patients with thyroid pathology (e.g., multinodular goiter, follicular adenoma). Second, other lesions that take up T1-201, including primary metastatic cancer, can mimic parathyroid adenomas. Third, patient motion can cause misregistration of data on the two images, with inaccurate subtraction.

## SUGGESTED READINGS
### Thyroid Imaging and Function Studies
Blahd WH: Management of thyroid cancer, *Compr Ther* 19:197-202, 1993.

Chapman EM: History of the discovery and early use of radioactive iodine, *JAMA* 250:2042-2044, 1983.

Filesi M, Signore A, Ventroni G, et al: Role of initial iodine-131 whole-body scan and serum thyroglobulin in differentiated thyroid carcinoma metastases, *J Nucl Med* 39:1542-1546, 1998.

Freitas JE, Gross MD, Ripley S, Shapiro B: Radionuclide diagnosis and therapy of thyroid cancer: current status report, *Semin Nucl Med* 15:106-131, 1985.

Gross MD, Shapiro B, Freitas JE, et al: The scintigraphic imaging of the endocrine organs, *Endocr Rev* 5:221-281, 1984.

Grunwald F, Schomburg A, Bender H, et al: Fluorine-18–fluorodeoxyglucose positron emission tomography in the follow-up of differentiated thyroid cancer, *Eur J Nucl Med* 23:312-319, 1996.

Leslie WD, Peterdy AC, Dupont JO: Radioiodine treatment outcomes in thyroid glands previously irradiated for Graves' hyperthyroidism, *J Nucl Med* 39:712-716, 1998.

Park HM, Perkins OW, Edmondson JW, et al: Influence of diagnostic radioiodines on the uptake of ablative dose of iodine-131, *Thyroid* 4:49-54, 1994.

Ramanna L, Waxman A, Braunstein G: Thallium-201 scintigraphy in differentiated thyroid cancer: comparison with radioiodine scintigraphy and serum thyroglobulin determinations, *J Nucl Med* 32:441-446, 1991.

Ross DS: Current therapeutic approaches to hyperthyroidism, *Trends Endocrinol Metab* 4:281-285, 1993.

Sandler MP, Patton JA: Multimodality imaging of the thyroid and parathyroid glands, *J Nucl Med* 28:122-127, 1987.

Sandler MP, Patton JA, Gross MD, et al: *Endocrine imaging,* Norwalk, Conn, 1992, Appleton & Lange.

Singer PA, Cooper DS, Daniels GH, et al: Treatment guidelines for patients with thyroid nodules and well differentiated thyroid cancer, *Arch Intern Med* 156:2165-2172, 1996.

Uematsu H, Sadato N, Ohtsubo T, et al: Fluorine-18-fluorodeoxyglucose PET versus thallium-201 scintigraphy evaluation of thyroid tumors, *J Nucl Med* 39:453-459, 1998.

### Adrenal Scintigraphy
Dwamena BA, Kloos RT, Fendrick AM, et al: Diagnostic evaluation of the adrenal incidentaloma: decision and cost effectiveness analysis, *J Nucl Med* 39:707-712, 1998.

Gelfand MJ: Meta-iodobenzylguanidine in children, *Semin Nucl Med* 23:231-242, 1993.

Gross MD, Shapiro B, Frances IR, et al: Scintigraphic evaluation of clinically silent adrenal masses using adrenocortical scintigraphy, *J Nucl Med* 35:1145-1152, 1994.

Hay RV, Shapiro B, Gross MD: Scintigraphic imaging of the adrenals and neuroectodermal tumors. In Henkin RE, Boles MA, Dillehay GL, et al, editors: *Nuclear medicine,* St Louis, 1996, Mosby.

Sisson JC et al: Scintigraphic localization of pheochromocytomas, *N Engl J Med* 305:12-17, 1981.

### Parathyroid Scintigraphy
Apostolopoulos DJ, Houstoulaki E, Giannakenas C, et al: Technetium-99m tetrofosmin for parathyroid scintigraphy: comparison to thallium-technetium scanning, *J Nucl Med* 39:1433-1441, 1998.

Carpentier A, Jeanotte, Verreault J, et al: Preoperative localization of parathyroidism: relationship between technetium-99–MIBI uptake and oxyphil cell count, *J Nucl Med* 39:1441-1444, 1998.

Ferlin G, Borsato N, Camerani M, et al: New perspectives in localizing enlarged parathyroids by technetium-thallium subtraction scan, *J Nucl Med* 24:438-441, 1983.

Giulette TMD, Brownless SM, Taylor WH, et al: Limits to parathyroid imaging with thallium-201 confirmed by tissue uptake and phantom studies, *J Nucl Med* 27:1262-1265, 1986.

Perez-Monte JE, Brown ML, Shah AN, et al: Parathyroid adenomas: accurate detection and localization with Tc-99m sestamibi SPECT, *Radiology* 201:85-91, 1996.

# CHAPTER 15

# Pearls, Pitfalls, and Frequently Asked Questions

This chapter reinforces concepts presented in this book. Every student of medicine gathers pearls of wisdom from his or her mentors that may not fit well into a didactic treatment of a subject but that are extraordinarily valuable in day-to-day practice. Likewise, we all learn to avoid pitfalls that arise in situations but that have escaped our formal education. Also, questions posed at the viewbox or elsewhere often require assembling multiple bits of information for a correct answer, and these questions never seem to be presented in quite the same way that subject material was presented didactically.

By its nature, this chapter is neither comprehensive nor weighted to the relative importance of the topics.

## BASIC PHYSICS

**Q:** What is the difference between *isotopes, isobars,* and *isotones?*

**A:** *Isotopes* are varying forms of a given element and by definition possess the same number of protons but different numbers of neutrons. *Isobars* are atoms that have the same total number of nucleons (protons and

neutrons) but that are from different elements and thus have different numbers of protons. *Isotones* are atoms that have the same number of neutrons but that are from different elements and therefore have different numbers of protons. Remember that *isomers* are simply different energy states of nuclei of the same isotope (same atomic number, same number of neutrons, and same mass numbers).

**Q:** What is the difference between x-rays and gamma rays?

**A:** Both x-rays and gamma rays are types of ionizing radiation. By definition, x-rays originate outside the atomic nucleus, and gamma rays originate inside the atomic nucleus. The respective energy spectra for x-rays and gamma rays substantially overlap at the high-energy end of the spectrum for all forms of electromagnetic radiation.

**Q:** What is the energy equivalent of the rest mass of an electron?

**A:** 511 keV.

**Q:** What is the difference between the *rad, roentgen,* and *rem?*

**A:** These terms are frequently confused with each other but have important distinctions. *Rad* stands for radiation absorbed dose. A rad is equal to the absorption of 100 ergs per gram of absorbing material. The rad is the traditional unit of absorbed dose. The gray (Gy) is the unit of absorbed dose in the International System of Units (SI). One gray = 100 rads.

*Rem* is an acronym for *r*oentgen *e*quivalent *m*an. The rem is calculated by multiplying the absorbed dose in rads by a factor to correct for the *relative biological effectiveness* (RBE) of the type of radiation in question. The rem is the traditional unit. In the SI system the term *sievert* (Sv) is used. One sievert = 100 rem.

The *roentgen* (R) is a unit of radiation *exposure.* It is defined as the quantity of x-radiation or gamma radiation that produces one electrostatic unit of charge per cubic centimeter of air at standard temperature and pressure. In the SI system, radiation exposure is expressed in terms of coulombs per kilogram (C/kg). One roentgen is equal to $2.58 \times 10^{-4}$ C/kg air.

**Q:** Which is more penetrating in soft tissues, alpha particles or beta particles of the same kinetic energy?

**A:** Alpha particles have very low penetration in soft tissue because of their rapid loss of kinetic energy through interaction of their electrical charge with electrons in the tissues. Beta particles of the same respective kinetic energy of alpha particles have higher velocity, lower mass, and a single negative charge. They demonstrate significantly greater penetration in soft tissues, although penetration still is typically measured in millimeters.

**Q:** Define the two systems for expressing radioactive decay.

**A:** The traditional unit of radioactive decay is the *curie* (Ci). One curie is equal to $3.7 \times 10^{10}$ disintegrations per second (dps). This number was derived from the decay rate of 1 gram of radium. (Modern measurements indicate that the actual decay rate for 1 gram of radium is $3.6 \times 10^{10}$ dps.) In the SI system, decay is expressed in becquerels (Bcq). One becquerel equals one disintegration per second.

**Q:** How are the half-life and the decay constant related?

**A:** The physical *half-life* ($T_{1/2}$) of a radionuclide is defined as the time for half the atoms in a sample to decay. The half-life is expressed in units of time, typically seconds, minutes, hours, days, or years. The *decay constant* indicates the fraction of the sample decaying in a unit of time. The units of the decay constant are "per unit time" (per second, per hour). Mathematically the half-life ($T_{1/2}$) and the decay constant ($\lambda$) are related by the following equation:

$$T_{1/2} = \frac{\ln 2}{\lambda}$$

**Q:** Which is longer, the biological half-life or the effective half-life?

**A:** The effective half-life is always shorter than either the biological half-life or the physical half-life because biological clearance and physical decay take place simultaneously. In calculation of radiopharmaceutical dosimetry, the conservative assumption is sometimes made that the biological half-life is infinite. This is probably never completely correct but simplifies calculations because the effective half-life may be taken simplistically as the physical half-life.

**Q:** After a photon has undergone Compton scattering, how does the energy of the scattered photon compare to the original photon energy?

**A:** In Compton scattering the photon gives up energy to a recoil or Compton electron. The "scattered" photon has correspondingly lower energy. The amount of energy lost increases as the angle of scattering increases.

**Q:** What factors speed up or slow down radioactive decay?

**A:** Unlike chemical reactions, radioactive decay is a physical constant that cannot be sped up or slowed down by heating or cooling a specimen or by applying other physical or chemical influences.

**Q:** How many observed counts are necessary to have a percent fractional standard deviation of 5%, 2%, and 1%, respectively?

**A:** 400, 2500, and 10,000, respectively.

**Q:** What is the maximum number of electrons that can occupy the outermost shell of an atom?

**A:** Eight.

**Q:** What special term is used to designate the electrons in the outermost shell of an atom?

**A:** They are called *valence* electrons and are responsible for many of the chemical characteristics of the element.

**Q:** What is the binding energy of an electron?

**A:** *Binding energy* refers to the amount of energy required to remove that electron from the atom. Electrons in shells close to the nucleus have higher binding energy than electrons farther from the nucleus. This energy is typically expressed in terms of electron volts (eV). Remember that the binding energy for each electron shell and subshell is characteristic for the respective element; the higher the atomic number of the element, the greater the binding energy for each shell and subshell.

## RADIATION DETECTION AND INSTRUMENTATION

**Q:** What are some examples of the uses of ionization chambers in nuclear medicine?

**A:** Ionization chambers are often used in radiation survey meters and some pocket dosimeters. The radionuclide dose calibrator incorporates an ionization chamber.

**Q:** What is the purpose of the thallium impurity added to sodium iodide crystals?

**A:** The thallium is used to "activate" the sodium iodide crystal. The thallium impurity provides "easier" pathways for the return of electrons from the conduction band of the crystal to the valence bands of atoms.

**Q:** What is the relationship between photon energy and detection efficiency in a sodium iodide crystal?

**A:** For a given crystal size, detection efficiency decreases with increasing photon energy.

**Q:** Why do photopeaks appear as bell-shaped curves in pulse height spectra rather than as discrete spikes corresponding to the energy of the gamma ray?

**A:** Although gamma rays have discrete energies, the detection process is subject to statistical factors at each step of the process. The bell-shaped curve corresponding to the gamma ray photopeak reflects these statistical variations, which results in different events being measured as having slightly different energies. The better the "energy resolution" of a pulse height analyzer, the narrower the bell-shaped curve.

**Q:** In using a gamma scintillation camera, what does it mean to "set" the energy window?

**A:** Gamma cameras are equipped with pulse height analyzers that allow the operator to select a range of observed energies for accepting photons to be used in making the scintigraphic image. The "window" is usually described by giving the photopeak energy of interest and a percentage range that defines the limits of acceptance above and below the photopeak energy. A typical window for the 140-keV photon of technetium-99m is 20%, or ±14 keV.

**Q:** What are the causes of homogeneous flood field images in gamma camera quality control?

**A:** Causes include improper photomultiplier tube voltage adjustment, off-peak camera pulse height analyzer setting, crystal imperfections or damage, poor coupling of the crystal and the photomultiplier tubes, and inadequate mixing of radioactive tracer in the flood phantom.

**Pitfall:** Some nuclear medicine clinics use radioactivity in the patient to confirm the window setting. This can be a pitfall because scattered photons are included in the observed spectrum and can actually shift the apparent location of the photopeak. Ideally, a sample of the radionuclide to be imaged should be used for "peaking" in the gamma camera energy window.

**Q:** What effects do Compton-scattered photons have on scintigraphic image quality?

**A:** Compton scattered photons are the enemy! Scattered photons that fall within the acceptance limits of the energy window are included in the image. They represent false data because they are recorded in a different spatial location than the origin of the primary photon. Thus Compton scattering reduces image contrast and spatial resolution. Also, Compton-scattered photons falling outside the energy window still must be processed by the gamma camera pulse height analyzer circuitry. These rejected events contribute to dead time and reduce the count rate capability of gamma cameras.

**Q:** What photons are desired in the scintigraphic image?

**A:** Primary (unscattered) photons that arise in the organ of interest in the body and travel parallel to the axis of the gamma camera collimator field of view are the photons desired in the image. Intuitively, one may think of these as "good" photons. All other photons are "bad" photons. These include primary (unscattered) photons that arise in the object or organ of interest but travel "off axis," primary photons that arise in front of or behind the organ of interest (background photons), and all scattered photons.

**Q:** What is the purpose of the collimator?

**A:** The collimator defines the geometric field of view of the gamma camera crystal. Off-axis photons, whether they are primary photons or scattered photons, are absorbed in the septa of the collimator.

**Pearl:** Pinhole collimators allow resolution of objects below the spatial resolution of the gamma camera through geometric magnification.

**Q:** What is the theoretical advantage of an asymmetrical window?

**A:** Asymmetrical windows that encompass the gamma ray photopeak but offset to the high side contain a higher ratio of primary photons to scattered photons than do symmetrical windows. Asymmetrical windows are feasible with modern high-performance gamma cameras. In older cameras the photomultiplier tube energy response was too variable between the multiple tubes for effective use of asymmetrical windows.

**Q:** How does poor energy resolution degrade spatial resolution?

**A:** Gamma cameras with poor energy resolution have reduced ability to reject scattered photons on the basis of pulse height analysis, as well as reduced ability for accurate determination of $x$ and $y$ coordinates for spatial localization of events.

## SINGLE-PHOTON EMISSION COMPUTED TOMOGRAPHY AND POSITRON EMISSION TOMOGRAPHY

**Pearl:** Most nuclear medicine departments use 180-degree SPECT acquisition for cardiac studies and 360 degrees for imaging other organs, including the brain.

**Pearl:** For SPECT imaging the highest resolution collimator that provides sufficient count rate should be selected.

**Pitfall:** Besides equipment factors, patient motion is the most important cause of image degradation in SPECT and PET studies.

**Q:** What special importance does the biological half-life of a radiotracer have in SPECT imaging?

**A:** In SPECT imaging, data are acquired sequentially from different sampling angles. If significant biological redistribution of a radiopharmaceutical takes place between the start of data acquisition and completion, the reconstruction of tomographic images can be significantly distorted.

**Q:** What is a filter?

**A:** Filters are special mathematical functions applied to SPECT and PET data that enhance desired characteristics in the image, such as background subtraction, edge enhancement, and suppression of statistical noise. The ramp filter is designed to eliminate or reduce the star artifact.

**Q:** What is the star artifact?

**A:** The star artifact is the result of simple unfiltered backprojection of a point source.

**Q:** What are the two basic approaches to attenuation correction?

**A:** The two basic approaches are the analytical or mathematical approach and the empirical approach. In the analytical approach, attenuation correction is estimated from a model of the body part under investigation. In the empirical approach, attenuation correction is accomplished by direct measurement using transmission scanning.

**Pearl:** One of the great advantages of SPECT and PET is the ability to perform flexible reformatting of image data in multiple image planes. For cardiac imaging, short-axis, vertical long-axis, and horizontal long-axis views of the heart are typically obtained.

**Pearl:** Two quick ways of assessing patient motion during SPECT imaging are to view the projection images as a cinematic closed-loop display and to create slice sinograms. In the cinematic display, patient motion is seen as a flicker from one projection image to another. On sinograms, patient motion is seen as a discontinuity in the stacked projection profiles.

**Pitfall:** SPECT is subject to a number of artifacts. Field flood nonuniformity can result in ring artifacts. Center-of-rotation misalignment causes loss of image resolution and if severe, ring artifacts.

**Pearl:** SPECT imaging at 511 keV can be accomplished using dual-headed coincidence systems or gamma cameras equipped with special high-energy collimators.

**Pearl:** PET imaging relies on the coincidence detection of the two gamma ray photons given off simultaneously during a positron annihilation event.

**Pitfall:** The higher the overall count rate in PET imaging, the more likely the recording of "false" events owing to the presence of paired random events that appear to the detection circuitry as paired annihilation photons.

**Pearl:** The spatial resolution of PET is twice or more that of SPECT.

**Pitfall:** Spatial resolution in PET is limited by positron travel in soft tissue before decay.

**Pearl:** PET imaging with transmission attenuation correction and detector sensitivity calibration allows absolute quantitative uptake determinations.

**Pearl:** Radiopharmaceuticals for PET are extremely flexible because of the ability to incorporate carbon, nitrogen, oxygen, and fluorine radiolabels.

## NUCLEAR PHARMACY

**Q:** What relationship between the half-lives of a parent radionuclide and a daughter radionuclide is necessary for a generator system?

**A:** The parent radionuclide must have a long enough half-life to permit formulation and distribution of the generator. The daughter half-life must be reasonable for clinical application. A longer-lived parent decays to a shorter-lived daughter in all generator systems in use.

**Q:** How are parent and daughter radionuclides separated in generator systems?

**A:** Because the parent and daughter are different elements, they can be chemically separated.

**Q:** What is the major drawback of molybdenum-99 prepared by neutron activation?

**A:** When Mo-99 is prepared from Mo-98 by neutron activation, the two isotopes cannot be separated, and significant Mo-98 carrier exists in the preparation. This ultimately results in low specific concentration eluates of technetium-99m from the generator system.

**Q:** What is the difference between "transient" equilibrium generators and "secular" equilibrium generators?

**A:** In *secular equilibrium* generators the half-life of the parent is far longer than the half-life of the daughter. If the generator system is left alone, the activity of the daughter becomes equal to that of the parent. In generator systems in which the parent half-life is 10 to 100 times that of the daughter, a condition of transient equilibrium occurs if the generator is not eluted. The point of *transient equilibrium* is defined as the time at which the ratio of the daughter and parent activities becomes a constant. Because the parent half-life is longer, the daughter appears to decay with the same half-life. The Mo-99/Tc-99m generator system is an example of transient equilibrium.

**Q:** What is the practical problem with having carrier Tc-99 in the generator eluate?

**A:** Tc-99 and Tc-99m behave identically from a chemical standpoint. Therefore, if there is excessive Tc-99 in the eluate, labeling efficiency can be impaired. For example, in a kit preparation using stannous chloride as a reducing agent, there may be unreduced Tc-99 and Tc-99m left in the preparation, with the consequent presence of radiochemical impurities in the final preparation.

**Q:** When is the buildup of Tc-99 at its highest?

**A:** Because Tc-99 has a far longer half-life than Tc-99m, the longer the interval between generator elutions, the greater the buildup of Tc-99. The first elution after commercial shipment or after a long weekend will have the highest content of Tc-99.

**Q:** What is the legal limit for Mo-99 in Tc-99m-containing radiopharmaceuticals?

**A:** The Nuclear Regulatory Commission limit is 0.15 mCi of Mo-99 activity per 1 mCi of Tc-99m activity in the administered dose.

**Q:** How does the ratio of Mo-99 to Tc-99m change with time?

**A:** In any preparation in which the radionuclidic contaminants have longer half-lives than the desired radionuclide label, the relative activity of the contaminant increases with time. This is an issue for iodine-123 preparations that have longer-lived radioiodine contaminants, as well as for the Mo-99 contamination in Tc-99m preparations.

**Q:** What is the purpose of stannous ion in Tc-99m labeling procedures?

**A:** Stannous ion is used to reduce technetium from a +7 valence state in pertechnetate to lower valence states necessary for labeling a wide range of agents. The development of this approach was a major breakthrough in nuclear pharmacy.

**Q:** What constitutes a misadministration of a radiopharmaceutical?

**A:** There are four basic categories of misadministration. An agent can be given to the wrong patient, or a patient may receive the wrong radiopharmaceutical. The wrong route of administration may be used, or the administered dose may differ from the prescribed dose by greater than an allowable standard. The standard varies depending on the type of preparation.

**Q:** Describe the general response to the spill of radioactive material.

**A:** In general, the person who recognizes that a spill has occurred should notify all persons in the vicinity, and the area should be restricted. If possible, the spill should be covered. For minor spills, cleanup using appropriate disposable and protective clothing can be accomplished until background or near-background radiation levels are observed. For major spills the source of the radioactivity should be shielded. For both major and minor spills all personnel potentially exposed in the area should be surveyed, with appropriate removal of contaminated clothing and decontamination of skin. The radiation safety officer should be notified of all spills and has the primary responsibility for supervising cleanup for major spills and determining what reports must be made to regulatory agencies.

## CARDIOVASCULAR SYSTEM

**Pearl:** Think of the myocardial perfusion scintigram, whether acquired with single-photon or PET agents, as a "map" of relative blood flow to viable myocardium. That is, for activity to be recorded in the image, it must be delivered (blood flow) and taken up by a myocardial cell (viable myocardium).

**Q:** How does the extraction of thallium-201 passing through the myocardial capillary bed compare with the extraction of technetium-99m sestamibi and Tc-99m teboroxime?

**A:** Tl-201 has a myocardial extraction fraction of approximately 0.85 in normal subjects at normal flow rates. The myocardial extraction of Tc-99m teboroxime is greater, and that of Tc-99m sestamibi and Tc-99m tetrofosmin is lower.

**Pitfall:** If imaging is begun too soon after exercise in myocardial perfusion SPECT studies, the position of the heart may change during the study as the patient's respiratory rate returns to baseline. The term *cardiac creep* has been used to describe this phenomenon. Replaying the multiple projections from the SPECT data acquisition readily identifies the phenomenon. Imaging can be started in most patients by 10 to 15 minutes after exercise.

**Pearl:** The left anterior oblique (LAO) view is the single planar view in which the most lesions are seen by perfusion scintigraphy. Some departments obtain an LAO planar image before beginning a SPECT study. This also permits assessment of lung activity.

**Q:** What is the rationale for a second injection of Tl-201 versus simple delayed imaging to distinguish fixed from reversible defects?

**A:** Relying solely on delayed imaging overestimates the number of fixed myocardial defects. Internal redistribution may take longer than the usual 3- to 4-hour delay and may not even be complete by 24 hours.

**Pitfall:** Incomplete normalization does not equate with a fixed defect. Insisting on complete normalization before accepting an abnormality as not "fixed" results in underdetection of ischemic areas versus scarred areas.

**Q:** What is the relationship between the time after myocardial infarction (MI) and the sensitivity of perfusion imaging?

**A:** The sensitivity of perfusion imaging for detecting defects caused by acute MI is greatest right after the infarct and diminishes with time. This is different from "hot spot" imaging with Tc-99m pyrophosphate, in which the greatest sensitivity does not occur for a day or two after infarction.

**Pitfall:** Although myocardial perfusion scintigrams are positive immediately after infarction, it is not possible to determine whether a given defect is new or old. A given cold area may be caused by myocardial scar or acute MI.

**Pitfall:** In most laboratories the primary cause of false negative exercise studies in the diagnosis of coronary artery disease is failure to achieve adequate exercise.

**Pearl:** After exercise, significant Tl-201 localization in the liver usually indicates a poor exercise level. At peak exercise, blood flow is diverted from the splanchnic circulation.

**Pitfall:** Quantitative analysis systems that rely on databases of "normals" may not reflect the patient population in a different nuclear medicine department. Care must be taken to not rely too heavily on these databases.

**Q:** What is the mechanism of action of dipyridamole?

**A:** Dipyridamole inhibits the action of adenosine deaminase. By augmenting the effects of endogenous adenosine, dipyridamole is a powerful vasodilator.

**Q:** What effect can a cup of coffee have on a dipyridamole stress test?

**A:** Caffeine in coffee, tea, soft drinks, or foods such as chocolate can block the effect of dipyridamole pharmacological stress testing.

**Q:** What is the significance of lung uptake on Tl-201 exercise studies?

**A:** Patients with left ventricular failure during exercise have higher lung-to-heart ratios than normal subjects. Significantly increased lung uptake during exercise is a secondary sign of heart disease.

**Q:** What percentage of stenosis at rest is necessary in the coronary arteries for resting blood flow to be affected?

**A:** Coronary artery stenosis greater than 85% to 90% is required before flow is diminished at rest. Remember that not all stenoses are created equal. Long irregular stenotic segments have more effect than discrete short-segment stenoses.

**Q:** What percentage of Tl-201 localizes in the heart?

**A:** From 4% to 5% of the administered dose localizes in the heart in normal subjects.

**Q:** What factors can increase the Tl-201 washout rate from the myocardium after exercise?

**A:** Eating and the administration of glucose and insulin both can increase the washout rate.

**Q:** What is the relative biological half-time of Tl-201 in the myocardium compared with Tc-99m sestamibi and Tc-99m teboroxime?

**A:** The biological half-time for Tc-99m teboroxime is the lowest (fastest washout). Tc-99m sestamibi has the longest half-time in the myocardium, with Tl-201 having an intermediate half-time.

**Q:** Why is imaging delayed for 30 to 90 minutes after administration of Tc-99m sestamibi or Tc-99m tetrofosmin?

**A:** Although myocardial uptake is rapid with Tc-99m sestamibi and Tc-99m tetrofosmin, lung and liver uptake are also significant. These organs clear more rapidly, and thus the target-to-background ratio improves with time.

**Q:** To what part of the red blood cell (RBC) does the Tc-99m label bind?

**A:** Tc-99m binds to the beta chain of hemoglobin when the stannous pyrophosphate technique is used.

**Pitfall:** Injection of labeling materials through a heparinized intravenous line can significantly decrease the yield with in vivo RBC labeling.

**Pearl:** For multiple first-pass studies, choose an agent that is rapidly cleared from the blood, such as Tc-99m sulfur colloid or Tc-99m DTPA.

**Q:** What are the considerations for selecting the number of frames in a gated blood pool study?

**A:** Selecting the number of frames to divide the cardiac cycle is a balance between having enough frames to capture the peaks and valleys of the ventricular time-activity curve versus the need to acquire a statistically valid number of counts in each frame. In most applications, 16 to 24 frames achieves this compromise. Too

few frames will "average out" the peaks and valleys. Too many frames increases the imaging time required for a given number of counts per frame.

**Pitfall:** In calculation of the left ventricular ejection fraction, too high an estimate of the background counts per pixel will result in a falsely high ejection fraction. This can happen if the background area includes activity from the spleen.

**Pearl:** Variations in the length of the cardiac cycle can be recognized on gated blood pool studies if the time-activity curve trails off or fails to approximate the height of the initial part of the curve. Significant asymmetry (greater than 10%) of the height of the curve at the beginning and the end may indicate significant arrhythmia.

**Q:** What do amplitude and phase images portray?

**A:** Amplitude and phase images are parametric or derived images. The amplitude image portrays the maximum count difference at each pixel location during the cardiac cycle. High ejection fraction areas have high amplitude, and background areas have low amplitude. The phase image portrays the timing of cyclical activity with respect to a reference standard, usually the R wave.

**Q:** What is the hallmark of a ventricular apical aneurysm by phase analysis?

**A:** Aneurysms demonstrate paradoxical motion. Activity in the area of the aneurysm is typically 180° out of phase with the rest of the ventricle.

**Q:** What factors help to distinguish true from false aneurysms?

**A:** True aneurysms have all the layers of the heart. They typically have a wider mouth than false aneurysms and are most often located anteriorly or anteroapically. False aneurysms are caused by rupture of the myocardium, covered only by epicardium. False aneurysms classically have narrow necks and are most often located posterolaterally. Both types of aneurysm distort the ventricular contour and exhibit paradoxical wall motion.

## SKELETAL SYSTEM

**Q:** What is the difference between phosphate and phosphonate compounds?

**A:** Skeletal-seeking radiopharmaceuticals are based on both classes of compounds. The phosphate compounds are inorganic and have a basic P-O-P structure. Phosphonate compounds are organic and have a basic P-C-P structure. Both classes of compound demonstrate avid skeletal localization.

**Q:** What are the potential impurities in technetium-labeled pyrophosphate and diphosphonate compounds, based on their biodistribution?

**A:** Activity in the oropharynx, thyroid gland, and stomach suggests free pertechnetate. Activity in the liver suggests a colloidal impurity. Occasionally, activity is seen in the gut, the result of excretion of activity through the biliary system. The mechanism is not well understood. Other increased soft tissue or renal activity is usually caused by a disease process rather than tracer impurity.

**Q:** What percentage of the Tc-99m-labeled compounds is retained in the skeleton at the usual time of imaging?
**A:** In normal adult subjects, 40% to 60% of the injected dose is in the skeleton 2 to 3 hours after tracer administration.

**Q:** What is the distribution of metastatic deposits from epithelial primary malignancies in the skeleton?
**A:** A rule of thumb is that 80% of metastases are found in the axial skeleton (spine, pelvis, ribs, and sternum). The remaining are distributed equally between the skull (10%) and the long bones (10%).

**Pearl:** The majority of epithelial tumor metastases localize first in the red marrow. The skeletal tracers do not localize in the tumor tissue but rather in the reactive bone around the metastatic deposits.

**Pitfall:** A small amount of activity is frequently seen at the injection site; this should not be confused with a metastatic lesion. Likewise, variable degrees of urinary contamination on the skin may be superimposed on skeletal structures and confused with activity caused by metastatic disease.

**Q:** How can the radiation dose to the bladder, ovaries, and testes be reduced?
**A:** The radiation dose to these structures is largely caused by radioactivity in the bladder. Frequent voiding reduces the radiation dose.

**Pearl:** When using a multiple spot view technique for whole body skeletal imaging, consider obtaining pelvic views first immediately after the patient has emptied the bladder. When SPECT of the pelvic area is performed, the same consideration of emptying the bladder applies.

**Q:** What factors distinguish a superscan resulting from metastatic disease from a superscan resulting from metabolic disease?
**A:** In the usual superscan resulting from metastatic disease the increased uptake is restricted to the axial skeleton and the proximal parts of the femurs and humeri, the red marrow–bearing areas. In metabolic bone disease the entire skeleton is typically affected, with increased uptake seen in the extremities as well as in the axial skeleton. In some cases resulting from secondary hyperparathyroidism, increased activity will also be seen in the lung and stomach.

**Pearl:** Faint or absent visualization of the kidneys is one of the findings on superscans that should alert the observer. This has often been misinterpreted as indicating lack of excretion of tracer through the kidneys. In cases of superscan resulting from metastatic disease, visualization of the kidneys is faint because (1) the skeleton accumulates more tracer than usual, leaving less

available for renal excretion, and (2) owing to the increased skeletal tracer uptake, the renal activity may actually fall below the density threshold of the recording medium. For images obtained using digital computers, the presence of renal activity is readily established by adjusting the window and center on the cathode ray tube.

**Pitfall:** The greatest pitfall in interpreting skeletal scintigrams is failure to understand the inherent nonspecificity of skeletal imaging. In our zeal "not to miss the cancer," many incidental areas of abnormally increased tracer accumulation are incorrectly attributed to metastatic disease. The most common pitfalls are diagnosing areas of arthritis or prior trauma as metastases.

**Q:** Which factors favor osteoarthritis versus metastatic disease as the cause of increased activity?
**A:** Osteoarthritis has characteristic locations in the extremities. Because metastatic lesions are relatively rare below the proximal femurs or beyond the proximal humeri, osteoarthritis should be considered first in the elbows, wrists, hands, knees, and feet of older patients. Involvement of both sides of a joint is common in arthritis but unusual in metastatic disease. The lower lumbar spine is the most problematic area because both arthritis and metastases are common there.

**Q:** What is the mechanism of the "flare" phenomenon?
**A:** In some patients treated with chemotherapy for metastatic disease, regression of the tumor burden is associated with increased osteoblastic activity, presumably caused by skeletal healing. This can appear on skeletal scintigrams as a paradoxical increase or apparent "worsening" of the abnormal tracer uptake.

**Q:** What is the postmastectomy appearance of the thorax?
**A:** With radical mastectomy the majority of the soft tissue is removed from the corresponding anterior thorax. The ribs appear "hotter" than on the contralateral side. This is probably caused by a combination of less attenuation of rib activity in soft tissue and possibly some uptake associated with postsurgical healing. (Note, however, that if the patient is imaged with a prosthesis in place, the rib activity may be attenuated.)

**Q:** What factors contribute to prolonged fracture positivity on scintigrams?
**A:** Displaced and comminuted fractures and fractures involving joints tend to have prolonged positivity scintigraphically.

**Q:** What factors favor shin splints versus stress fracture scintigraphically in the tibia?
**A:** Stress fractures are classically focal or fusiform. The uptake can involve the entire width of the bone. Shin splints are classically located along the posterior tibial cortex and involve a third or more of the length of the bone. In pure shin splints a focal component should not be present.

**Pitfall:** False negative scintigrams may be seen in neonates with osteomyelitis. False negatives may also be seen in very old or debilitated patients and in patients who have received a course of antibiotic therapy before scintigraphy is performed.

## PULMONARY SYSTEM

**Q:** What is the most commonly used agent for ventilation imaging?
**A:** Xenon-133.
**Q:** What are the half-lives of Xe-133 and Xe-127?
**A:** Xe-133, 5.3 days; Xe-127, 36.4 days.
**Q:** What are the principal photon energies of Xe-133 and Xe-127?
**A:** The principal photon energy of Xe-133 used for imaging is 81 keV. The principal photon energies of Xe-127 are 172 and 203 keV.
**Q:** What is the minimum number of particles recommended for pulmonary perfusion imaging?
**A:** Pulmonary perfusion scanning assumes a statistically even distribution of particles throughout the lung. This requires at least 60,000 particles in normal adults, and many authorities recommend a minimum of 100,000 particles.
**Q:** How should the dose of technetium-99m macroaggregated albumin (MAA) be adjusted in pediatric patients?
**A:** Radiopharmaceutical doses are always adjusted with respect to radioactivity in the pediatric population. With Tc-99m MAA it is also necessary to adjust the number of particles.
**Q:** What is the size range of MAA particles?
**A:** In commercial preparations the majority of particles are 20 to 40 μm.

**Pitfall:** Withdrawing blood into a syringe with Tc-99m MAA particles may create a small radioactive embolus that shows up as a "hot spot" on subsequent images.

**Pitfall:** Failure to resuspend the Tc-99m MAA particles before administration may result in clumping of particles together and the presence of "hot spots" on subsequent imaging.
**Q:** What is the biological fate of MAA particles?
**A:** MAA particles are physically broken down in the lung. Delayed imaging performed several hours after pharmaceutical administration demonstrates activity in the reticuloendothelial system because of phagocytosis of the breakdown particles.

**Pearl:** One way to determine whether radioactivity outside of the lungs is caused by free Tc-99m or shunted Tc-99m MAA is to image the brain. Free pertechnetate should not localize in the brain, whereas Tc-99m MAA particles that gain access to the systemic circulation will

lodge in the first capillary bed that they encounter, including the capillary bed in the brain.
**Q:** What is the preferred patient position during administration of Tc-99m MAA?
**A:** Administering Tc-99m MAA with the patient supine results in a more homogeneous distribution of particles in the lung than when the patient is sitting or standing. Gravitational effects result in more basilar distribution when injection is accomplished with the patient upright.
**Q:** What is the major drawback to the use of Xe-133 for ventilation imaging?
**A:** The principal photon energy of Xe-133 is 81 keV, which is below the energy of Tc-99m. Thus imaging with Xe-133 is problematic after the perfusion portion of a V/Q study. Ideally, the perfusion study would be done first, and the patient would be positioned in the view that would best evaluate perfusion defects.

**Pitfall:** In lateral views of the lung obtained for a fixed number of counts, "shine-through" from the contralateral lung can give the false impression of activity arising from the side being imaged. This is most dramatically demonstrated in patients after pneumonectomy in whom no activity is demonstrated on anterior or posterior views but a near-normal appearance can be seen because of the shine-through phenomenon.

**Pitfall:** In analysis of perfusion scintigrams, failure to recognize the significance of *decreased* versus *absent* activity is a potential pitfall. Not every clot is 100% occlusive of the circulation. Significantly diminished activity needs to be recognized as one of the patterns caused by pulmonary emboli.

**Pitfall:** In some patients with fatty liver, retained activity in the liver on Xe-133 scans can be confused with retained activity or delayed washout at the right base. Remember that xenon is fat soluble and will show significant accumulation in patients with fatty liver.

**Pitfall:** The pulmonary hili are photon-deficient structures caused by the displacement of lung parenchyma by large vascular and bronchial structures. Failure to remember this can result in false positive interpretations, especially for defects seen on posterior oblique images.

**Pitfall:** If the patient is placed supine for V/Q imaging but the chest radiograph was obtained with the patient upright, it can be difficult to correlate findings on the examinations. For example, free fluid may collect in a subpulmonic location or obscure the lung base in the upright position. With the patient supine, the fluid may layer out posteriorly or collect in the fissures. Also, the apparent height of the lungs may be different, as may the heart size. Ideally, imaging studies should be performed with the patient in the same position for all examinations. On the other hand, if there is significant pleural fluid, it may be desirable to image the patient in more than one position to prove that a defect is caused by mobile fluid.

**Q:** What is the stripe sign?

**A:** The *stripe sign* refers to a stripe or zone of activity seen between a perfusion defect and the closest pleural surface. Because pulmonary emboli are typically pleura based, the stripe sign suggests another diagnosis, often emphysema. Rarely, in the resolution of pulmonary emboli, a stripe sign develops as circulation is restored.

**Q:** What is the physiological basis for perfusion defects in areas of poor ventilation?

**A:** The classic response to hypoxia at the alveolar level is vasoconstriction. Shunting of blood away from the hypoxic lung zone maintains oxygen saturation.

**Q:** What is the shrunken lung sign?

**A:** The lungs may appear smaller than usual in patients sustaining multiple small emboli, such as fat emboli, that distribute uniformly around the lung periphery.

**Q:** What is the classic appearance of multiple pulmonary emboli on lung perfusion scintigraphy?

**A:** Multiple pleura-based, wedge-shaped areas of significantly diminished or absent perfusion. The size of the defects may vary from subsegmental to segmental or may involve an entire lobe or lung.

**Q:** What are the most common clinical signs and symptoms in patients with confirmed pulmonary embolism?

**A:** In the PIOPED study the three most common presenting symptoms (and approximate percentage frequency) were dyspnea, 80%; pleuritic chest pain, 60%; and cough, 40%. Hemoptysis (15%) and leg pain (25% to 30%) were less common. On physical examination, lung crackles (60%) were encountered much more often than leg swelling (30%) or pleural friction rub (5%). Both the heart rate and the respiratory rate were elevated on average in the PIOPED study in patients with pulmonary embolism.

**Q:** What is the sensitivity of the high-probability scan category for detecting pulmonary embolism?

**A:** In the PIOPED study, 41% of patients with pulmonary embolism had a high-probability scintigraphic pattern.

## ONCOLOGY

**Q:** What is the mechanism of gallium-67 uptake in tumors?

**A:** Ga-67 binds to serum transferrin, which transports it to the tumor, where it enters the extracellular fluid space via the tumor's leaky capillary endothelium. It is bound to the tumor cell surface by transferrin receptors and then transported into the cell, where it binds to proteins such as ferritin and lactoferrin, which are in increased concentration in tumors.

**Q:** Ga-67 uptake is normally seen in which of the following organs?
  a. Salivary glands
  b. Lacrimal glands
  c. Thymus
  d. Spleen
  e. Breast
  f. Heart

**A:** *a-e.* Salivary gland and lacrimal gland uptake is variable. Thymus uptake may be seen in children, especially after they have received chemotherapy. The spleen has uptake, but it is low in intensity. Breast uptake is variable and is most prominent post partum. Heart visualization may be seen with myocarditis or pericarditis but is not normally seen.

**Pitfall:** Surgical wounds normally have increased uptake for 1 to 2 weeks postoperatively, and faint activity may remain for 3 to 4 weeks. Focal bone uptake may be seen after bone marrow biopsy. Contrast lymphangiography can produce prominent pulmonary uptake.

**Q:** On a scale of 1 to 3 (1 being highest), grade the likelihood of good uptake by the following tumors:
  a. Hodgkin's disease
  b. Non-Hodgkin's lymphoma
  c. Hepatocellular carcinoma
  d. Soft tissue tumors
  e. Melanoma
  f. Lung cancer
  g. Head and neck tumors
  h. Abdominal and pelvic tumors

**A:** *a*—1, *b*—1, *c*—1, *d*—1 (although T1-201 may be superior), *e*—1, *f*—2, *g*—2, *h*—3.

**Q:** Which of the following statements is associated with Hodgkin's disease and which with non-Hodgkin's lymphoma?
  a. Orderly contiguous spread of lymph node involvement in young patients.
  b. Multicentric disease with a highly variable clinical course and a high incidence of extranodal tumor involvement.
  c. Mediastinal masses are common.
  d. Abdominal involvement of mesenteric and retroperitoneal nodes is common.
  e. High cure rate.
  f. Variable clinical course that can be indolent or rapidly lethal.

**A:** Hodgkin's disease: *a, c, e;* non-Hodgkin's lymphoma: *b, d, f.*

**Pearl:** Ga-67 can be used to determine tumor viability after a course of chemotherapy or radiation therapy. It is particularly useful in determining whether posttherapy masses represent residual tumor or fibrosis, necrosis, or scarring.

**Pitfall:** A pretherapy study is important for proper evaluation of the posttherapy Ga-67 study. The pretherapy study ensures that the tumor site is gallium-avid.

**Q:** Factors affecting thallium-201 uptake in tumors cells include which of the following?

    a. Blood flow

    b. Viability

    c. Increased cell membrane permeability

    d. ATPase system

    e. Binds to intracellular proteins

**A:** All but *e.*

**Q:** T1-201 tumor imaging has been found useful in which of the following tumors?

    a. Brain tumors

    b. Primary tumors of bone

    c. Kaposi's sarcoma

    d. Breast tumors

    e. Thyroid cancer

    f. Melanoma

**A:** *a-e.*

**Q:** Technetium-99m sestamibi has been approved by the FDA for imaging and evaluation of breast masses detected with mammography or by palpation. Which of these statements is true?

    a. Its accuracy is higher for palpable than for nonpalpable masses.

    b. Its sensitivity is poor for lesions less than 1 cm in size.

    c. Fibroadenomas are always negative.

    d. It is particularly useful in patients with dense breasts or those with architectural distortion, such as previous surgery, radiation therapy, and breast implants.

**A:** *a, b, d.* Fibroadenomas are a common cause for false positives.

**Q:** Which of these statements is true regarding fluorine-18 fluorodeoxyglucose (FDG)?

    a. Uptake is normally high in the brain and heart.

    b. The mechanism of uptake is identical to that of glucose.

    c. F-18 FDG can be imaged only with a PET camera.

    d. F-18 FDG shows great promise but is not yet a clinical imaging tool.

    e. F-18 FDG PET is more accurate than CT for staging lung cancer.

**A:** *a,c,e. b.* F-18 FDG enters the cell similarly but becomes trapped within the cell because it cannot progress through the glucose enzymatic pathways. *d.* It has proven clinical utility in many tumors, including lung cancer, colorectal cancer, lymphoma, melanoma, and brain tumors.

**Q:** What are two clear indications for Tc-99m CEA-SCAN monoclonal antibody imaging of patients with colon cancer?

**A:** (1) Patients with a rising carcinoembryonic antigen level but no clinical or imaging evidence of tumor recurrence, and (2) preoperative confirmation in patients with a single known site of recurrence who are potential surgical candidates. Multiple sites would make the patient inoperable.

    **Pearl:** Tc-99m CEA-SCAN is equal in accuracy to CT in the liver and superior to CT in the extrahepatic abdomen.

**Q:** Which of the following statements are true of In-111 ProstaScint?

    a. Murine monoclonal antibody against a prostate-specific membrane antigen expressed by more than 95% of prostate adenocarcinomas.

    b. It has been approved by the FDA for localization of soft tissue metastases after prostatectomy in patients with a rising PSA and negative bone scan.

    c. Elevated human murine antibody (HAMA) titers are observed in 50% of patients.

    d. SPECT is mandatory.

**A:** *a,b,d.* HAMA elevations are seen in less than 10% of patients.

**Q:** Which of the following are true statements regarding In-111 OctreoScan?

    a. It has been approved for imaging of neuroendocrine tumors.

    b. The sensitivity for all neuroendocrine tumors is very high.

    c. It is a radiolabeled peptide and somatostatin analog.

    d. Only neuroendocrine tumors have somatostatin receptors.

**A:** *a,c. b.* Although its sensitivity for detection of most neuroendocrine tumors is very high, it has a poorer sensitivity for insulinomas and medullary carcinoma of the thyroid. *d.* Somatostatin receptors are found on a variety of nonneuroendocrine tumors, including astrocytomas, meningiomas, maligant lymphoma, and breast and lung cancer.

**Q:** How can lymphoscintigraphy yield help patients with intermediate-thickness malignant melanoma?

**A:** Lymphoscintigraphy can pinpoint the sentinel node for the surgeon, which can be localized easily at surgery with a gamma probe. The results will determine which patients require further nodal dissection and adjuvant chemotherapy.

## HEPATOBILIARY SYSTEM

**Q:** What are the two FDA-approved technetium-99m iminodiacetic acid analog (IDA) radiopharmaceuticals in use, and how are they different?

**A:** Tc-99m DISIDA and Tc-99m mebrofenin. The latter has better hepatic extraction, 98% versus 88%, and less renal excretion, 1% versus 9%. The higher extraction of mebrofenin is preferable in patients with hepatic insufficiency.

**Pearl:** Tc-99m IDA is extracted pharmacologically similar to bilirubin but is not conjugated. Tc-99m sulfur colloid is extracted by the reticuloendothelial system, including the spleen and bone marrow.

**Q:** What is the most important question to ask a patient before starting cholescintigraphy for suspected acute cholecystitis, and why?

**A:** "When did you last eat?" If the patient has eaten in the last 4 hours, the gallbladder may be contracted secondary to endogenous stimulation of cholecystokinin (CCK), and therefore radiotracer cannot gain entry into the gallbladder. If the patient has not eaten in more than 24 hours, the gallbladder may not have had the stimulus to contract and will be full of thick, concentrated bile, which may prevent tracer entry.

**Q:** What are five indications for CCK infusion?

**A:** 1. Empty gallbladder in patient fasting longer than 24 hours.
2. Differentiate common duct obstruction from normal hypertonic sphincter of Oddi.
3. Exclude acute acalculous cholecystitis if gallbladder fills.
4. Diagnose chronic acalculous cholecystitis. Confirm or exclude chronic calculous cholecystitis.
5. Assist in the diagnosis of sphincter of Oddi dysfunction.

**Q:** In what clinical settings are false positive HIDA studies likely to occur when performed to rule out acute cholecystitis?

**A:** In patients who have fasted less than 4 hours or more than 24 hours, patients receiving hyperalimentation, and those who have chronic cholecystitis, hepatic insufficiency, or concurrent serious illness.

**Pitfall:** False positive HIDA studies are most likely to occur in sick, hospitalized patients. They are much less common in outpatients. In patients who have been fasting or receiving hyperalimentation, CCK is administered in an attempt to empty the gallbladder before Tc-IDA administration.

**Q:** What is the *rim sign* sometimes seen with cholescintigraphy, and what is its significance?

**A:** The *rim sign* is increased uptake and delayed clearance of activity in the hepatic parenchyma adjacent to the gallbladder fossa. It has been associated with an increased incidence of the complications, e.g., perforation and gangrene.

**Pearl:** Increased blood flow to the region of the gallbladder as a result of severe inflammation is sometimes seen with acute cholecystitis.

**Q:** At what time after HIDA injection is nonfilling of the gallbladder diagnostic of acute cholecystitis?

**A:** One hour is defined as abnormal. However, nonfilling

of the gallbladder is diagnostic of acute cholecystitis if delayed images show no filling by 2 to 4 hours or 30 minutes after morphine administration.

**Pearl:** Delayed visualization is most often seen in chronic cholecystitis and is also seen with hepatic insufficiency.

**Q:** What is the mechanism of morphine-augmented cholescintigraphy?

**A:** Morphine increases tone at the sphincter of Oddi, resulting in increased intraductal pressure. This results in bile flow preferentially through the cystic duct, if it is patent.

**Q:** What is the most common cholescintigraphic finding in chronic cholecystitis?

**A:** A normal study. Less than 5% of patients with chronic cholecystitis have delayed filling. Other associated findings include delayed biliary-to-bowel transit time and, rarely, nonvisualization of the gallbladder or intraluminal filling defects.

**Q:** What is acute acalculous cholecystitis?

**A:** Cholecystitis without a stone occluding the cystic duct. The obstruction may be caused by debris or inflammatory changes, or the cholecystitis may be limited to the gallbladder wall because of infection, ischemia, or toxins. It occurs in hospitalized patients who have sustained trauma, burns, sepsis, or other serious illness and who frequently have an underlying chronic illness. It is associated with a high morbidity and mortality.

**Pearl:** The sensitivity of cholescintigraphy is greater than 90% for acute *acalculous* cholecystitis compared with 98% for *calculous* cholecystitis.

**Pearl:** If the clinical suspicion for acute acalculous cholecystitis is high but the gallbladder visualizes, an In-111 white blood cell study could be performed to confirm the diagnosis.

**Q:** The diagnosis of common duct obstruction is usually made by detecting a dilated common duct on sonography. In what clinical situations would cholescintigraphy be needed?

**A:** In early acute obstruction (less than 24 hours), before the duct has had time to dilate, and in patients with previous obstruction or ductal instrumentation who have baseline dilated ducts. In both these situations, cholescintigraphy can be diagnostic.

**Q:** What are the cholescintigraphic findings of high-grade common duct obstruction?

**A:** Persistent hepatogram with no clearance into biliary ducts.

**Q:** What are the cholescintigraphic findings of partial common duct obstruction?

**A:** Prominent retention of activity in the common duct, delayed biliary-to-bowel clearance, and most important, poor ductal clearance on delayed imaging or with CCK.

**Pearl:** Delayed biliary-to-bowel transit is an insensitive and nonspecific finding for common duct obstruction. Delayed bowel clearance is seen in only 50% of patients. Delayed biliary-to-bowel transit may be seen in 20% of healthy subjects. It is also seen in patients pretreated with CCK. Administration of CCK at 60 minutes will result in prompt clearance and biliary-to-bowel transit in normal subjects but not in patients with partial common duct obstruction.

**Q:** What ancillary maneuver increases sensitivity of cholescintigraphy for detection of biliary atresia?

**A:** The administration of phenobarbital for 3 to 5 days before the HIDA activates the liver enzymes. A serum phenobarbital level should be in the therapeutic range before cholescintigraphy is started.

**Q:** What are the common causes for the postcholecystectomy syndrome?

**A:** Cystic duct remnant, retained or recurrent stone, inflammatory stricture, sphincter of Oddi dysfunction.

**Pearl:** Sphincter of Oddi dysfunction is essentially a partial common duct obstruction without evidence of stone or stricture, but with elevated sphincter manometry. CCK cholescintigraphy can aid in the initial workup and the follow-up postsphincterotomy.

**Q:** What is the difference in clinical presentation and clinical course of patients with focal nodular hyperplasia (FNH) and hepatic adenoma?

**A:** FNH is asymptomatic and found incidentally, whereas hepatic adenomas often present with hemorrhage can be life threatening. Adenomas are closely associated with the use of oral contraceptives, which must be discontinued.

**Q:** What are the Tc-99m sulfur colloid scintigraphic findings in FNH and hepatic adenoma?

**A:** Hepatic adenomas do not show Tc-99m sulfur colloid uptake because they do not usually have Kupffer cells. FNH is associated with increased blood flow. Uptake may be increased, normal, or nonexistent. Two thirds of cases of FNH show some Tc-99m sulfur colloid uptake.

**Q:** What are the cholescintigraphic findings in FNH and hepatoma?

**A:** FNH shows increased flow, normal uptake, and delayed focal clearance. Hepatomas are cold on early images but often fill on delayed images (2 hours). The hepatoma is functional, but hypofunctional compared with the normal liver.

**Q:** Chronic acalculous cholescystitis is usually diagnosed on which of the following?

   a. Ultrasonography
   b. Oral cholecystography
   c. Conventional cholescintigraphy
   d. CCK cholescintigraphy

**A:** *d.* Studies a, b, and c are often normal. A low gallbladder ejection fraction (less than 35%) on CCK cholescintigraphy is diagnostic.

**Q:** The sensitivity for detecting liver hemangiomas with Tc-99m-labeled red blood cells (RBCs) depends on which of the following factors?

   a. Lesion size
   b. Instrumentation used (planar versus SPECT, single-versus multiple-headed camera)
   c. Location (e.g., superficial or deep, near large vessels)
   d. Close correlation with anatomical study (ultrasonography, CT, MRI) to ensure detection.

**A:** All true.

**Q:** Which of the following statements is true in regard to the diagnosis of hemangiomas?

   a. Ultrasonography is neither sensitive nor specific.
   b. CT is not very sensitive when strict criteria are used and not specific when liberal criteria are used.
   c. MRI is sensitive, has a distinctive pattern (light bulb sign), and is much more specific than CT or ultrasonography, but other benign and malignant tumors may have an appearance similar to hemangioma.
   d. The positive predictive value of RBC scintigraphy is very high, with few false positive studies reported.
   e. MRI is the method of choice for small lesions adjacent to large vessels.

**A:** All true.

**Q:** What are the characteristic scintigraphic findings in liver hemangioma?

**A:** Blood flow is normal. Immediate images show a cold defect, whereas delayed images acquired 1 to 2 hours after tracer administration show increased uptake within the lesion compared with the normal liver, often equal to uptake in the spleen and heart. SPECT is mandatory for smaller lesions.

**Q:** Besides FNH, what are other causes of increased focal uptake on Tc-99m sulfur colloid imaging?

**A:** Superior vena cava syndrome (with arm injection), inferior vena cava syndrome (with leg injection), Budd-Chiari syndrome, and cirrhosis with a regenerating nodule.

**Pearl:** The last two entities do not truly show an absolutely increased uptake but a relatively increased uptake compared with the surrounding liver. In Budd-Chiari syndrome the caudate has relatively more uptake because of impaired venous drainage of the remainder of the liver and subsequent decreased function. The caudate lobe retains function because of its direct venous drainage into the inferior vena cava.

**Q:** What is functional asplenia?

**A:** Nonvisualization of the spleen on a Tc-99m sulfur colloid study when the spleen is anatomically present and when functions other than reticuloendothelial extraction are intact. Functional asplenia is caused by an acquired dysfunction of the reticuloendothelial system (e.g., sickle cell anemia) or by a disruption of the blood supply (e.g., splenic artery occlusion). Functional asplenia is reversible in the case of sickle cell disease but irreversible when caused by Thorotrast irradiation, chemotherapy, or amyloid. Radiotracers with different mechanisms of splenic uptake will demonstrate the spleen, including In-111 oxine–labeled white blood cells and Tc-99m-labeled RBCs.

**Q:** In regard to regional intraarterial chemotherapy, which of the following statements is/are true?

   a. Hepatic arterial chemotherapy preferentially perfuses the tumor, with relative sparing of uninvolved liver.

   b. Systemic toxicity is directly related to the amount of chemotherapeutic agent that reaches the systemic circulation.

   c. The response to therapy can be predicted from Tc-99m macroaggregated albumin (MAA) hepatic arterial perfusion scintigraphy.

   d. Symptoms of drug toxicity can be easily differentiated clinically from the progression of liver metastases.

**A:** *a.* True. Tumor in the liver receives its blood supply primarily from the hepatic artery, whereas the normal liver receives approximately 70% of its blood supply from the portal vein.

   *b.* True. For example, arteriovenous shunting will increase the amount of chemotherapeutic agent reaching the gastrointestinal epithelium and marrow, with resulting toxicity.

   *c.* True. Evidence of proper catheter placement and perfusion of tumor nodules is associated with a good response to therapy.

   *d.* False. The symptoms are identical. Only the Tc-99m MAA study can make that differentiation by determining the adequacy of perfusion and the presence or absence of extrahepatic perfusion.

**Q:** What is the significance of the extrahepatic perfusion seen on Tc-99m MAA hepatic arterial perfusion studies in patients receiving intraarterial chemotherapy for liver metastases?

**A:** Extrahepatic perfusion of abdominal viscera, most often the stomach but also the bowel, pancreas, and spleen, is associated with a high incidence of adverse symptoms (nausea, vomiting, abdominal pain), about 45%, versus a 16% incidence of similar symptoms in patients treated identically but without evidence of extrahepatic perfusion on the Tc-99m MAA study.

## GASTROINTESTINAL SYSTEM

**Q:** What is achalasia, and how can radionuclide studies help in making the diagnosis and following the patient's course?

**A:** Achalasia is characterized by absence of peristalsis in the distal two thirds of the esophagus, increased lower esophageal sphincter (LES) pressure, and incomplete sphincter relaxation after swallowing. It is associated with symptoms of dysphagia, weight loss, nocturnal regurgitation, cough, and aspiration. The diagnosis can be confirmed by esophageal manometry. Radionuclide esophageal transit studies have a high sensitivity for making the diagnosis and can evaluate the effectiveness of esophageal dilation.

**Q:** Characterize the following statements as true or false in regard to reflux and aspiration studies:

   a. The milk study is a sensitive method for diagnosing gastroesophageal reflux.

   b. The milk study is a sensitive method for diagnosing aspiration.

   c. Frequent image acquisition improves the sensitivity of the milk study.

   d. The salivagram is a sensitive method for diagnosing aspiration.

**A:** *a.* True.

   *b.* False. Aspiration is seen only rarely on delayed imaging.

   *c.* True.

   *d.* True.

**Q:** Which anatomical portions of the stomach are responsible for solid emptying and which for liquid emptying?

**A:** Liquid emptying is largely caused by the slow contractions of the proximal fundus, whereas the distal stomach, or antrum, is responsible for the grinding and sieving of solid food.

**Q:** Which of these factors will affect the rate of gastric emptying?

   a. Meal content.

   b. Time of day.

   c. Gender.

   d. Position (standing, sitting, lying).

   e. Stress.

   f. Exercise.

   g. All the above.

**A:** *g.*

**Q:** Describe the difference in emptying patterns between solids and liquids.

**A:** Liquids empty exponentially, whereas solid emptying is biphasic, with an initial lag phase until linear emptying begins. The lag phase represents the time required for the food to be broken down into small enough pieces to allow passage through the pylorus.

**Which of the following statements are true for gastric emptying studies?**

   a. Attenuation results in an underestimation of gastric emptying when performed in the anterior view.

   b. A solid gastric emptying time-activity curve shows a rise in activity after ingestion in the anterior view.

c. The geometric mean (GM) method of attenuation correction is considered the reference standard.

d. The left anterior oblique (LAO) method of attenuation correction is superior to the geometric mean.

**A:** *a.* True.

*b.* True.

*c.* True.

*d.* False. The GM mean method is superior.

**Pearl:** Attenuation is a particular problem in obese patients. The rising activity curve is caused by food moving from the relatively posterior fundus to the more anterior antrum, closer to the camera. The LAO method of attenuation correction is an accurate and simple clinical method of correcting for attenuation, but it incompletely corrects for attenuation in some.

**Q:** When might the use of technetium-99m sulfur colloid offer advantages over Tc-99m red blood cells (RBCs) for the diagnosis of acute gastrointestinal (GI) bleeding?

**A:** With very rapid GI bleeding and vascular instability, the radiotracer can be injected and the study completed in 15 to 20 minutes. It is likely to be positive with a rapid hemorrhage when transfusions cannot keep up with the bleeding rate. The patient can then go directly to angiography; the radionuclide study will save the angiographer and patient time and contrast.

**Q:** List in increasing order the labeling efficiency of methods to label Tc-99m RBCs: in vivo, in vitro, and in vivtro.

**A:** In vivo, 75%; in vitro or modified in vivo, 85%; and in vitro, 98%. A kit in vitro method for labeling Tc-99m RBCs is now available and is the method of choice, particularly for GI bleeding studies.

**Q:** Why is the Tc-99m RBC method for detecting GI bleeding more sensitive than the Tc-99m sulfur colloid method?

**A:** Delayed imaging can be performed for up to 24 hours with RBC labeling.

**Q:** What are the criteria needed to diagnose confidently the site of bleeding on a radionuclide study?

**A:** (1) A radiotracer "hot spot" appears where there was none and conforms to bowel activity; (2) the activity increases over time; and (3) the activity moves antegrade or retrograde.

**Pitfall:** A poor label can result in bladder activity that might be misinterpreted as rectal bleeding or in gastric activity that might be construed as upper GI bleeding.

**Pearl:** Look for thyroid and salivary gland uptake when in doubt about the presence of free Tc-99m pertechnetate.

**Pearl:** A lateral view of the pelvis should be routine to confirm rectosigmoid bleeding in order to differentiate bladder, rectal, and penile activity.

**Pitfall:** Focal activity that does not move may be anatomical (e.g., kidney, accessory spleen, hemangioma, varices, aneurysm).

**Pearl:** Contrast angiography can detect bleeding rates of about 1 ml/min, versus 0.1 ml/min for the radionuclide study.

**Q:** Ectopic gastric mucosa is most often seen clinically in Meckel's diverticulum. What other gastric abnormalities may contain gastric mucosa?

**A:** Duplication of the GI tract, Barrett's esophagus, and a retained gastric antrum after gastrectomy. In addition, ectopic gastric mucosa may occur in gastrogenic cystis and has been found in the pancreas, duodenum, and colon.

**Pearl:** Studies have shown that the mucin cells in the stomach are responsible for gastric uptake of Tc-99m pertechnetate, not the parietal cells.

**Q:** What is the origin of Meckel's diverticulum?

**A:** It is the most common congenital anomaly of the GI tract and results from failure of closure of the omphalomesenteric duct of the embryo, which connects the yolk sac to the primitive foregut via the umbilical cord.

**Pearl:** This true diverticulum (Meckel's) arises on the antemesenteric side of the bowel, usually 80 to 90 cm proximal to the ileocecal valve, although it can occur elsewhere.

**Pearl:** Gastric mucosa is present in 10% to 30% of all Meckel's diverticula, in 60% of symptomatic patients, and in 98% of those with bleeding.

**Pitfall:** A number of false positive studies have been reported over the years in scans for Meckel's diverticula, including those of urinary tract origin (e.g., horseshoe kidney, ectopic kidney), those resulting from inflammation (e.g., inflammatory bowel disease, neoplasms), bowel obstruction (seen most often with intussusception and volvulus), and other areas of ectopic gastric mucosa.

## CENTRAL NERVOUS SYSTEM

**Q:** Which radiopharmaceuticals have been used for blood-brain scintigraphy?

**A:** Technetium-99m pertechnetate, Tc-99m diethylenetriamine pentaacetic acid (DTPA), and Tc-99m glucoheptonate (GH). The latter two were preferred because of their faster background clearance, lack of choroid plexus uptake, and lower radiation dose.

**Q:** What is the "flip-flop" phenomenon seen with cerebrovascular disease on conventional scintigraphy, and what is its significance?

**A:** On the flow phase, parenchymal flow is delayed on the abnormal side compared with the contralateral normal side. Thus, as the normal cortex clears, uptake in the abnormal side peaks. This may be seen with a high-grade carotid artery stenosis with or without cerebral infarction. Delayed carotid flow is seen concomitantly.

**Pearl:** A "hot nose" may be seen on the flow-phase images and delayed images as a result of shunting of blood from the internal to the external carotid system that supplies the face and nose in patients with severe carotid stenosis, brain death, psychoactive drug use, and use of other drugs that cause nasal congestion.

**Q:** What is luxury perfusion?

**A:** Increased perfusion may be seen in the region of an infarct after a recent stroke (1 to 10 days), caused by an uncoupling of blood flow from metabolism and oxygen demand.

**Q:** How is brain death diagnosed?

**A:** The diagnosis is primarily clinical. The patient must be in deep coma with total absence of brainstem reflexes and spontaneous respiration. Reversible causes (e.g., drugs, hypothermia) must be excluded; the cause of the dysfunction must be diagnosed (e.g., trauma, stroke); and the clinical findings of brain death must be present for a defined period of observation (6 to 24 hours). Confirmatory tests such as electroencephalography (EEG) and radionuclide imaging may be used to increase diagnostic certainty, but the diagnosis is primarily clinical. The radionuclide study is more specific than EEG.

**Q:** Which radiopharmaceuticals are used to evaluate brain death, and what are the advantages of each?

**A:** Tc-99m flow agents such as DTPA are inexpensive. The 60-second flow study can be interpreted at the bedside. Because Tc-99m hexamethylpropyleneamine oxime (HMPAO) or Tc-99m ethyl cysteinate dimer (ECD) fixes in the cortex, delayed static images can be obtained and interpreted for diagnosis. The clinician is not dependent on a flow study, which demands a good bolus and good timing with proper computer acquisition. However, it is more expensive.

**Q:** What is the difference in mechanism of uptake between fluorine-18 fluorodeoxyglucose (F-18 FDG) and the Tc-99m cerebral perfusion agents?

**A:** F-18 FDG is a glucose analog, and its uptake represents regional glucose metabolism. It is metabolically trapped intracellularly. Tc-99m HMPAO and Tc-99m ECD are lipid-soluble cerebral perfusion agents taken up in proportion to regional cerebral blood flow. They fix intracellularly. In most cases, cerebral blood flow follows metabolism.

**Pearl:** An example of a decoupling of metabolism and blood flow is during the acute phase of a stroke. Blood flow may be normal (luxury perfusion), but metabolism is decreased.

**Q:** How can single-photon emission computed tomography (SPECT) brain perfusion or positron emission tomography (PET) FDG imaging be useful in the differential diagnosis of dementia?

**A:** Multiinfarct dementia is characterized by multiple areas of past infarcts, recognized as areas of decreased uptake that correspond to the vascular distribuions. Alzheimer's disease exhibits a characteristic pattern of bitemporal and parietal hypoperfusion and hypometabolism. Pick's disease is associated with decreased frontal lobe uptake. AIDS-dementia complex is associated with a pattern of multifocal or patchy cortical regions of decreased uptake, seen particularly in the frontal, temporal, and parietal lobes and the basal ganglion.

**Pearl:** Although Alzheimer's disease has a characteristic bitemporal-parietal pattern on perfusion imaging, it is often *not* symmetrical. Decreased frontal lobe uptake may also be seen. This pattern cannot be differentiated from the imaging pattern of Parkinson's disease, although they typically have very different clinical presentations.

**Q:** What is the purpose of cerebral perfusion imaging in patients with seizures? What is the expected PET or SPECT pattern?

**A:** PET F-18 FDG or SPECT cerebral perfusion studies can often localize the seizure focus in patients requiring surgery (typically temporal lobectomy) for seizure control. Interictally, a seizure focus shows decreased metabolism (FDG) on PET and decreased perfusion on SPECT; increased activity is seen during a seizure (ictally). Normally, perfusion follows metabolism. In many surgical seizure centers, depth electrodes are not required preoperatively if the clinical picture, EEG, and SPECT study are all consistent as to the location of the seizure focus.

**Q:** Which radiopharmaceuticals have been found useful in imaging brain tumors, and what is their clinical utility?

**A:** F-18 FDG PET imaging demonstrates increased uptake in tumors owing to increased glycolysis. Uptake of FDG is proportional to the malignant grade of glioblastomas. PET determines tumor viability after radiation therapy. SPECT with thallium-201 and Tc-99m sestamibi can be used in a similar manner. Both Tl-201 and PET FDG can differentiate lymphoma from infection, most often toxoplasmosis, in AIDS patients. Uptake of Tl-201 or FDG is indicative of lymphoma.

**Q:** Name the radiopharmaceutical used for cisternography and the most common clinical indication for this study.

**A:** In-111 DTPA. The most common use of this radiopharmaceutical in modern practice is to confirm the diagnosis of normal-pressure hydrocephalus (NPH), an obstructive communicating form of hydrocephalus. The next most common use is to localize cerebrospinal fluid (CSF) leaks.

**Pearl:** The symptoms of NPH are incontinence, dementia, and gait disturbance.

**Q:** What is the characteristic pattern of NPH on radionuclide cisternography?

**A:** Persistent ventricular filling and evidence of a convexity block.

## GENITOURINARY SYSTEM

**Q:** What percentage of renal plasma flow is filtered through the glomerulus, and what percentage is secreted by the tubules?

**A:** Twenty percent of renal plasma flow is cleared by glomerular filtration and 80% by tubular secretion.

**Q:** Which nonradioactive drugs used to calculate glomerular filtration rate (GFR) and effective renal plasma flow (ERPF) are considered to be the reference standards?

**A:** Inulin for GFR and paraaminohippurate (PAH) for ERPF.

**Q:** Which radiopharmaceuticals are most often used clinically for measurement of GFR and ERPF?

**A:** Technetium-99m diethylenetriamine pentaacetic acid (DTPA) for GFR and iodine-131 orthoiodohippurate (OIH) for ERPF.

**Q:** What is the mechanism of renal uptake for I-131 OIH, Tc-99m mercaptylacetyltriglycine (MAG3), Tc-99m DTPA, Tc-99m dimercaptosuccinic acid (DMSA), and Tc-99m glucoheptonate (GH)?

**A:** Tc-99m DTPA, glomerular filtration; Tc-99m MAG3, tubular secretion; I-131 OIH, tubular secretion and glomerular filtration; Tc-99m GH, cortical binding and glomerular filtration; and Tc-99m DMSA, cortical binding.

**Q:** What is the percent cortical binding of Tc-99m DMSA and Tc-99m GH?

**A:** Tc-99m DMSA, 40% to 50%; Tc-99m GH, 10% to 20%.

**Pearl:** The two radiopharmaceuticals bind to the proximal convoluted tubules in the cortex.

**Q:** The radiation dose to normal kidneys from I-131 OIH is considerably higher than that of technetium-labeled agents. True or false?

**A:** *False.* The radiation dose of I-131 is high with renal insufficiency or obstruction but not in the setting of normal function. With worsening renal function, the radiation dose becomes increasingly dependent on the physical half-life of the radiopharmaceutical and less dependent on body clearance.

**Q:** Radionuclide angiography (flow study) cannot be done with I-131 OIH. Why?

**A:** The low allowable administered dose (200 to 300 mCi) results in insufficient count statistics for a diagnostic flow study.

**Q:** What is Webster's rule?

**A:** Pediatric radiopharmaceutical doses can be estimated using the formula (age + 1)/(age + 7) × adult dose.

**Q:** The time-to-peak activity of a renal time-activity curve (TAC) represents which of the following?:

    a. The end of extraction.

    b. The beginning of renal clearance.

    c. The time point at which the amount of cortical uptake of the radiopharmaceutical is equal to clearance.

**A:** *c.* Uptake and clearance are occurring simultaneously over a period because of several factors, including an imperfect bolus, the percent first-pass extraction fraction of the radiotracer, the amount of recirculating radiotracer, and the normal variability of nephron function.

**Q:** What is the proper renal region of interest (ROI) selection on the computer for the following:

    a. Diuresis renography.

    b. Captopril renography.

**A:** *a.* The ROI should include the dilated pelvis and the cortex. Because of hydronephrosis, the dilated collecting system counts predominate. *b.* A whole kidney ROI is adequate if there is no pelvic retention. Lasix is often given with the radiopharmaceutical to ensure pelvicocalyceal clearance. When there is pelvicocalyceal activity, a peripheral two-pixel cortical ROI should be selected to avoid the effect of these counts on the TAC. A drop in GFR with captopril is manifested as deterioration in the cortical TAC (delayed peak and clearance). An identical ROI should be used for the baseline comparison study.

**Q:** Differential renal function is evaluated by drawing kidney and background ROIs. The relative uptake of the two kidneys after background correction is determined. Which time interval is used to calculate differential renal function for dynamic renal scintigraphy?

    a. Entire 30-minute study.

    b. The 60-second flow study.

    c. Interval of 1 to 3 minutes.

**A:** *c.* Because cortical uptake of the renal radiopharmaceutical is of interest, the optimal interval is after the initial flow but before the collecting system has cleared, usually 1 to 3 minutes. With good function, activity may be seen before 1 minute, especially in children. Radiopharmaceuticals with higher extraction also clear faster. With Tc-99m DTPA the 1- to 3-minute interval is usually optimal, whereas with I-131 OIH the 1- to 2-minute interval is preferable because of its faster clearance. Ideally the clinician should review the dynamic frames to determine when calyceal clearance occurred and use the 60- to 90-second interval before that.

**Q:** What are the two general methods for calculating absolute GFR?

**A:** Blood sampling and camera-based methods.

**Q:** At what step in the renin-angiotensin-aldosterone cascade does captopril work? In which organ does this occur?

**A:** Captopril blocks the conversion of angiotensin I to angiotensin II in the lungs.

**Pearl:** The usual captopril dose, 25 to 50 mg, although pharmacologically effective on the renal vasculature, is usually inadequate to produce peripheral vasodilation and hypotension. However, a patient may rarely develop hypotension, requiring prompt fluid administration to maintain intravascular volume and pressure.

**Q:** In renal artery stenosis the effect of captopril is manifested by a reduction in blood flow to the kidney that can be seen on radionuclide angiography. True or false?

**A:** *False.* Blood flow is not affected by captopril. If it is poor to begin with, it will remain poor. If it is normal, no change is seen. The compensatory mechanism for maintaining GFR is renin dependent and results in decreased GFR after captopril administration.

**Q:** Which of these factors affects the accuracy of diuresis renography?
    a. State of hydration.
    b. Renal function.
    c. Dose of diuretic.
    d. Radiopharmaceutical used.
    e. Bladder capacity.
    f. All the above.

**A:** *f.* Adequate hydration is required for good urine flow and adequate response to the diuretic. A full bladder may cause a functional obstruction. Intravenous hydration and urinary catheterization are strongly suggested, especially in children. Tc-99m DTPA, Tc-99m MAG3, and I-131 OIH have all been successfully used. Because of its better extraction efficiency and good image resolution, Tc-99m MAG3 is the agent of choice in renal insufficiency. I-131 OIH can also be useful in renal insufficiency; however, poor cortical versus collecting system differentiation results from poor image resolution. Tc-99m DTPA works well in patients with good renal function. Renal insufficiency is a definite limitation to diuresis renography. The kidney must be able to respond to the diuretic challenge. Therefore the dose of diuretic must be increased in renal insufficiency, but the exact dose required is only an educated estimate.

**Q:** A good diuretic response rules out a partial obstruction. True or false?

**A:** *False.* Diuretic renography is often performed to determine the functional significance of a known partial obstruction, as in patients with cervical or bladder cancer. A poor diuretic response indicates a significant obstruction and impending deterioration in renal function if intervention is not performed. If the postdiuretic clearance is good, no immediate intervention is required.

**Q:** What is the most sensitive technique for diagnosing scarring secondary to reflux?

**A:** Tc-99m DMSA cortical imaging. Ultrasonography and intravenous urography have much lower sensitivity.

**Q:** How can radionuclide imaging differentiate upper from lower tract urinary tract infection, and why is this differentiation important?

**A:** Tc-99m DMSA shows regional dysfunction, as manifested by decreased uptake in patients with parenchymal infection. Upper tract infection has prognostic implications, since it may lead to subsequent renal scarring, hypertension, and renal failure.

**Q:** Why is radionuclide cystography preferable to the contrast method in most cases? What is the exception?

**A:** The radionuclide test is more sensitive for detection of reflux than contrast-enhanced voiding cystourethrography and results in much less radiation exposure (50- to 200-fold less) to the patient. The only exception is in the first evaluation of a male, when the better resolution of the contrast study can permit the diagnosis of an anatomical abnormality such as posterior urethral valves.

**Q:** Which is the preferred method for performing radionuclide cystography, direct or indirect?

**A:** Direct cystography, that is, cystography requiring urinary tract catheterization and infusion of radiotracer into the bladder, is a more sensitive method for detecting vesicoureteral reflux. It can be used to detect reflux during bladder filling as well as voiding, in contrast to the indirect method, which cannot be used to detect reflux during the bladder filling stage because radiotracer is flowing through the collecting system antegrade.

**Q:** What is the most common developmental abnormality leading to testicular torsion?

**A:** The bell-clapper testis.

**Pearl:** The bell-clapper testis is a congenital abnormality and usually bilateral. Prophylactic surgery is performed on the asymptomatic side.

**Q:** What is the difference in blood supply to the testes and scrotum?

**A:** The testes receive blood predominantly from the testicular artery, whereas the scrotum receives its supply from the pudendal vessels.

## ENDOCRINE SYSTEM

**Pearl:** Swallowed activity from salivary secretions on radiopertechnetate scans occasionally remains in the esophagus and can be confusing. The nature of the activity is readily established by having the patient drink water, followed by reimaging of the thyroid gland.

**Q:** What has happened to the range for normal percent thyroid uptake of radioiodine in the United States over the last 50 years?

**A:** The normal range has dropped significantly owing to iodination of salt and the use of iodine in other foods. In many laboratories the range was 20% to 45% as recently as the mid-1960s but is now 10% to 30%.

**Pearl:** Iodine-131 is preferred over technetium-99m for the detection of substernal goiter. The key factor is the ability to perform delayed imaging at 24 or even 48 hours, after vascular and background activity has cleared.

**Q:** What is the origin of lingual and sublingual thyroid tissue?

**A:** The main thyroid anlage begins as a downgrowth from the foramen cecum. Thyroid tissue may be seen anywhere along the tract of the thyroglossal duct from the foramen cecum to the usual location of the gland. However, with lingual thyroid tissue, there is usually a failure of normal development and no tissue in the normal location of the thyroid.

**Q:** What do perchlorate and thiocyanate have in common?

**A:** They are both monovalent anions that block iodine trapping competitively.

**Q:** What is the mechanism of action of propylthiouracil (PTU) and methimazole (Tapazole)?

**A:** Both PTU and methimazole are antithyroid drugs that work by preventing organification of iodine.

**Q:** What is meant by the "organification" of iodine?

**A:** In thyroid metabolism, iodide is oxidized to iodine and incorporated into tyrosine to form either mono-iodotyrosine or diiodotyrosine. A deficiency in peroxidase, which catalyzes the reaction, is a cause of congenital hypothyroidism.

**Pearl:** The recommendation is to use preparations of I-123 on the day of calibration because of the presence of longer-lived radioiodine contaminants (I-124, I-125). The longer the interval before dosage administration, the higher the relative contribution of the contaminants.

**Q:** What is the rationale underlying thyroid/parathyroid subtraction imaging?

**A:** For subtraction imaging to work best, uptake of both tracers in the organ to be "subtracted" should be identical. In the case of thyroid/parathyroid subtraction imaging with thallium-201 and Tc-99m pertechnetate, this is not always the case. Some thyroid abnormalities demonstrate T1-201 accumulation but not uptake of radiopertechnetate. When this happens, a false positive study can result.

**Q:** What medical conditions are associated with an increased incidence of paragangliomas (pheochromocytomas)?

**A:** Both forms of multiple endocrine neoplasia type II are associated with pheochromocytoma, as are von Hippel-Lindau disease and neurofibromatosis.

**Pitfall:** Autonomous nodules are not synonymous with toxic nodules. Patients with small autonomous nodules (less than 3 cm in diameter) are most often euthyroid.

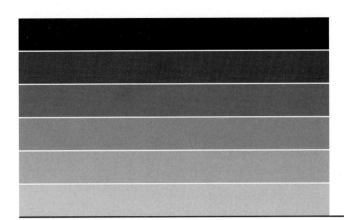

# Index

*t* indicates a table; *f* indicates a figure.